Advances in Visual Science and Eye Diseases 2

Series Editor

Ningli Wang
Beijing Tongren Hospital
Capital Medical University
Beijing, China

Advances in Visual Science and Eye Diseases presents the latest progress and achievement made in visual science and eye diseases for eye care health professionals at different links in the chain of eye care delivery including ophthalmologists, researchers, eye care service providers, health policy makers, and medical students.

The series firstly covers major blinding eye diseases, expounding on their characteristics and the latest development in pathogenesis, up-to-date researches and treatment options of the diseases in detail. Then, the series unfolds the pathogenesis, new diagnosis methods, latest surgery techniques, genetic research, animal modelling studies and translational medicine in glaucoma. Next, the series provides an overall picture on 1. the development of ophthalmology in China along with the contribution of Chinese ophthalmologists to the international community from historical perspective and sheds light on its future development directions; 2. eye epidemiological studies and achievements in blindness prevention in China; 4. holistic view on the systematic relationship between the eye and other organs as well as the relationship between eye diseases and systematic diseases. We hope readers can benefit from this series by enriching their latest knowledge in no matter visual science or clinical management of eye diseases.

Ningli Wang is a professor at Beijing Tongren Hospital affiliated to Capital Medical University, Beijing, China. He is also the director of Tongren Eye Center, Beijing, China.

More information about this series at http://www.springer.com/series/16143

Ningli Wang • Xuyang Liu • Ning Fan
Editors

Optic Disorders and Visual Field

PMPH PEOPLE'S MEDICAL PUBLISHING HOUSE Springer

Editors
Ningli Wang
Beijing Tongren Hospital
Capital Medical University
Beijing
China

Xuyang Liu
Xiamen Eye Center of Xiamen University
Xiamen
China

Ning Fan
Shenzhen Eye Hospital
Shenzhen University
Shenzhen
China

Shenzhen Eye Hospital
Shenzhen University
Shenzhen
China

ISSN 2524-566X ISSN 2524-5678 (electronic)
Advances in Visual Science and Eye Diseases
ISBN 978-981-13-2501-4 ISBN 978-981-13-2502-1 (eBook)
https://doi.org/10.1007/978-981-13-2502-1

Library of Congress Control Number: 2018967944

This Springer imprint is published by the registered company Springer Nature Singapore Pte Ltd.
The registered company address is: 152 Beach Road, #21-01/04 Gateway East, Singapore 189721, Singapore

Preface

In our clinical practice, follow-up observation is generally carried out especially on those cases with unexpected visual function loss, with a hope of finally figuring out the reasons for the impaired vision and visual field. In this way, a large number of cases have been collected. Now, we feel that it is worthy of carefully summarizing the enlightenment, experience, and lessons brought to us when we review these cases. Consequently, the book is compiled based on the analyses of more than 100 visual pathway-related cases with certain changes in the visual fields.

We have got several insights that we would like to share with the readers during the compilation of the book:

1. Typical visual field defects, such as bitemporal hemianopia caused by pituitary adenoma, usually would not be misdiagnosed. However, we have found that some "atypical" visual field changes are actually "typical" when we track carefully and such cognitive transformation process is actually the process of improvement in our understanding of these diseases.
2. We strongly feel that the multidisciplinary approach and integrated medicine contributed greatly to the analysis of the difficult and real cases.
3. There are some cases which made us feel at our wits' end, but we still obtained their final diagnoses through molecular genetics approaches that helped us find a way out.

In this book, most of the typical visual field changes have been described in the first two chapters, "Visual Field-related Anatomy of Visual Pathway" and "Interpretation of Visual Field Test." Therefore, those visual field changes that can be recognized at a first glance based on visual field impairment are not mainly discussed in this book. Although we have found the causes of visual filed defects in some cases mentioned in the book, the understanding of the primary reasons is far from enough. In another word, the pathophysiology and molecular genetics mechanisms of these diseases still need further exploration, and the further findings will be presented as one of the main contents of the book republished several years later, which means the tracking of the diseases mentioned in this book has not stopped yet. It is also worth noting that the diagnoses and analyses of these diseases still have many aspects worthy of discussing, and meanwhile, we have also consulted many experts worldwide for their opinions. Our greatest hope after the publication of the book is to hear from the experts and readers from both ophthalmology and non-ophthalmology specialties.

The book is compiled on the basis of the cases collected through years by the authors, but its compilation is completed in less than one year. Therefore, oversights and deficiencies can hardly be avoided and any correction or advice from the readers would be really appreciated.

Beijing, China Ningli Wang
Shenzhen, China Xuyang Liu
Shenzhen, China Ning Fan
July 10, 2018

Acknowledgments

The authors gratefully acknowledge the support from our colleagues including **Professors Feng Wen** and **Qingshan Chen**, etc., for their help in the analysis of retinal diseases. We also would like to express our gratitude to our postgraduates including **Xizhen Wang**, **Sheng Liao**, and **Sheng Chen** for their contribution to this book.

We wish to express our sincere thanks to doctors, as follows, for providing their valuable cases.

Junyi Chen, Eye and ENT Hospital, Fudan University, Shanghai, China

Weiwei Chen, Beijing Tongren Hospital, Capital Medical University, Beijing, China

Xuanchu Duan, The Second Xiangya Hospital, Central South University, Changsha, China

Yun Jing, Beijing Tongren Hospital, Capital Medical University, Beijing, China

Jian Wang, Beijing Tian Tan Hospital, Capital Medical University, Beijing, China

Jiawei Wang, Beijing Tongren Hospital, Capital Medical University, Beijing, China

Shihui Wei, General Hospital of the Chinese People's Liberation Army, Beijing, China

Diya Yang, Beijing Tongren Hospital, Capital Medical University, Beijing, China

Yuansheng Yuan, The First Affiliated Hospital, Kunming Medical University, Kunming, China

This work was supported by the National Natural Science Foundation of China (NSFC grants #81770924), the Science and Technology Innovation Committee of Shenzhen (No. JCYJ20160428144701106), and Sanming Project of Medicine in Shenzhen (No. SZSM201512045).

Contents

Part IV Optic Nerve Disorders

Part I

Visual Field-Related Anatomy of Visual Pathway

As the afferent pathway of vision, visual pathway refers to the overall nerve impulse conduction route, starting from the retinal photoreceptors, via optic nerve, optic chiasm, optic tract, lateral geniculate body, and optic radiation, to the visual cortical center in the occipital lobe [1]. The neuronal composition of visual pathway is as follows:

- First neurons: Visual cells in the outer layer of retina, i.e., retinal cone and rod cells
- Second neurons: Bipolar cells
- Third neurons: Retinal ganglion cells (RGCs) in the inner layer of retina
- Fourth neurons: Cells in the different layers of the lateral geniculate body

Optic nerve impulse carrying visual information forms inside the retina, which will be transmitted by three levels of neurons. First, the cone and rod cells of the photoreceptor will transmit the visual information to the bipolar cells after they receive light stimulation and then to the RGCs. After that, the axons of the RGCs will form retinal nerve fiber layers and optic nerve at the optic disc and then transmit the information to the lateral geniculate body through the optic chiasm and optic tract. Finally, the information will be projected to the visual cortex in the occipital lobe through the optic radiation sent by the lateral geniculate body.

The visual stimulation within a certain range that can be perceived by photoreceptor cells and received by a retinal ganglion cell is called the receptive field of this RGC (Fig. 1). There are about 132 million photoreceptor cells but only about one million RGCs in the human retina. Therefore, a retinal ganglion cell needs to integrate the information transmitted from multiple photoreceptor cells, i.e., one retinal ganglion cell corresponds to multiple bipolar cells, and one bipolar cell corresponds to multiple photoreceptor cells; therefore, the receptive fields of different RGCs are overlapped [2].

The macular fovea in the posterior pole of retina, where cone cells are dense, is the area with the highest visual sensitivity. In this area, there is one-to-one correspondence (1:1:1) between the three levels of neurons, and their receptive fields are not overlapped and have a minimum size, but the visual sensitivity, i.e., the resolving power, is the highest. As to the areas outside the

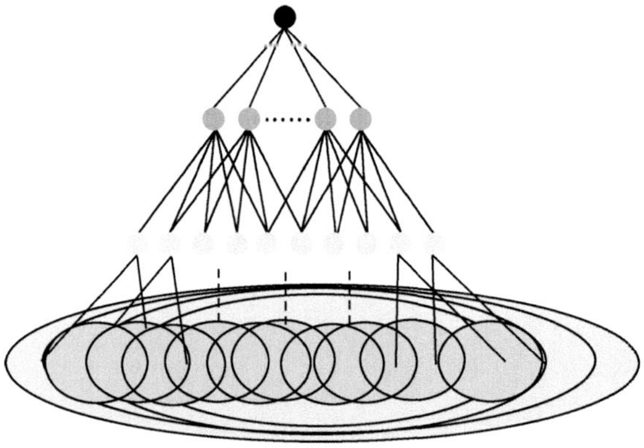

Fig. 1 Schematic drawing of the receptive field of RGCs

macular area, the cone cell density will reduce gradually with the increase of the degree of eccentricity, while the rod cells will increase in number. The connection between the three levels of cells will not be one-to-one correspondence anymore; instead, there will be a lot of crosses. The size of receptive fields and extent of their overlapping will become bigger and bigger, and the visual sensitivity will become lower and lower. The receptive fields will mutually overlap, and the sum of all receptive fields constitutes the visual field of the eye. Therefore, in a visual field figure, maybe a fairly mild defect in the central area, such as a defect smaller than 5 dB, will be considered as visual field impairment of remarkable significance. However, defects bigger than 10 dB at multiple peripheral sites may just be a relative scotoma or even a short-term or long-term fluctuation, which may not have actual clinical significance. Besides, a damage found in the first-level neurons will lead to the photoreception dysfunction of the retina in the corresponding position, which belongs to sensory disorders. Light cannot be seen when disorders are found in the second-, third-, and fourth-level neurons, not because the visual cells of the retina cannot receive light stimulation but because the nerve impulse produced by light stimulation cannot reach the visual center to form vision, which belongs to conduction disorders [2–4].

The whole course of the visual pathway from the photoreceptor of the retina to the visual cortex is arranged as per the principles of local orientation and point-to-point arrangement. Any minimal lesion in any parts of the pathway for visual perception and (or) conduction will lead to corresponding visual disorder. Therefore, like the vision, a normal visual field must rely on an intact visual pathway. The study of the anatomy of visual pathway can help us better explain the corresponding visual field changes. Or in other words, in case of real visual field defects in any form, the visual pathway is bound to have corresponding lesions after refracting media change has been excluded. This is also the main thread throughout the whole book.

Visual field-related pathway anatomy will be elaborated in this part. The specific contents of the anatomy will also be further explained in subsequent parts and chapters.

References

1. Weilong Z, Shizhen Z. Clinical anatomy series-head and neck volume. Beijing: People's Medical Publishing House; 1988.
2. Jiaqi L, Fengming L. Practice of ophthalmology. 2nd ed. Beijing: People's Medical Publishing House; 1999.
3. Haisheng L, Jiapu P. Principles and practices of visual electrophysiology. Shanghai: Shanghai Popular Science Press; 2002.
4. Honglu Y, Xiumin Y. Physiology of eye. Beijing: People's Medical Publishing House; 2001.

Retina

1

Xuyang Liu, Jia Ma, and Ningli Wang

The retina is a layer of transparent membrane lining the posterior part of the eyeball wall, whose outer surface is close to the choroid and internal surface is attached to the vitreous.

1.1 Retinal Imaging

Light is projected onto the retina through the cornea, aqueous humor, pupil, lens, and vitreous. Retinal imaging is similar to the pinhole imaging principle, which states that if you put a plate with a pinhole between a screen and an object, an inverted image of the object will be formed on the screen and the size of the image will change with the back-and-forth movement of the plate in the middle. The pupils are equivalent to the pinhole on the plate and the retina to the screen. Since light travels along a straight line, after penetrating through the pupil, the light from above will be projected onto the inferior retina. Similarly, the light from below will be projected onto the superior retina, and the light from the temporal side will be projected onto the nasal retina, while the light from the nasal side will be projected onto the temporal retina. The principle is similar to that of a camera [1, 2].

1.2 Relationship Between Anatomy and Diseases of Retina

The retina develops from the optic cup formed by neuroectoderm in the embryonic stage. The outer layer of the optic cup forms the single retinal pigment epithelium, while the inner layer of the optic cup differentiates into the retinal neurosensory layer, which is again histologically divided into nine layers from outside to inside, including photoreceptor cell layer of cone cells and rod cells, external limiting membrane, outer nuclear layer, outer plexiform layer, inner nuclear layer, inner plexiform layer, ganglion cell layer, nerve fiber layer, and internal limiting membrane. A potential gap exists between the retinal pigment epithelium and the retinal neurosensory layers. In general, retinal detachment refers to the detachment between these two layers. Modern optical coherence tomography (OCT) can now display clearly the individual layers of the retina in vivo (Fig. 1.1).

X. Liu (✉)
Xiamen Eye Center of Xiamen University, Xiamen, China

Shenzhen Eye Hospital, Shenzhen University, Shenzhen, China

J. Ma
The First Affiliated Hospital, Kunming Medical University, Kunming, China

N. Wang
Department of Ophthalmology, Beijing Tongren Hospital, Capital Medical University, Beijing, China

N. Wang et al. (eds.), *Optic Disorders and Visual Field*, Advances in Visual Science and Eye Diseases 2, https://doi.org/10.1007/978-981-13-2502-1_1

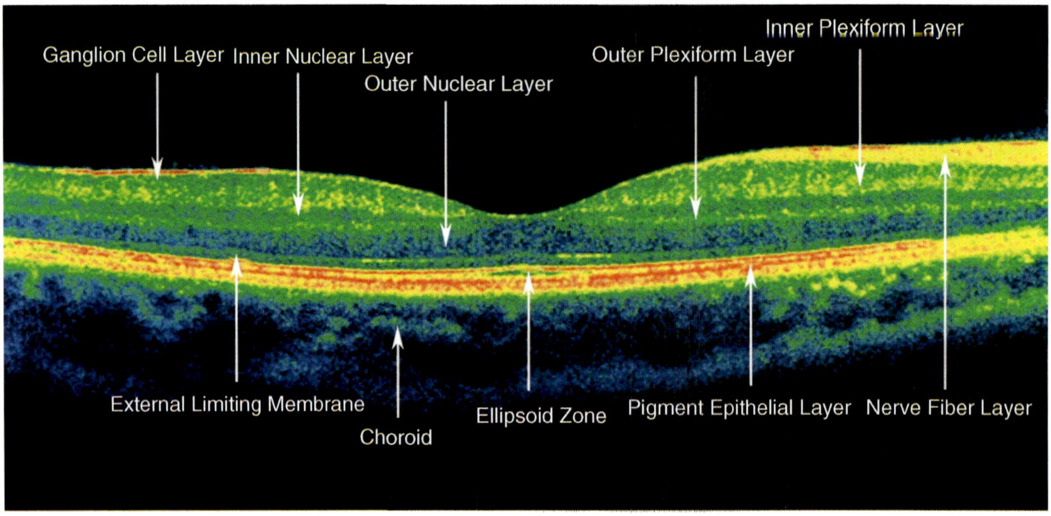

Fig. 1.1 OCT scanning image of the macula

The retina is like a cup with the rim at the ora serrata, which is located at the equator of the eyeball. There is a small shallow funnel-like sunken area about 2 mm in diameter in the posterior pole. It is called macula, which gains the name for rich lutein in this area. In its center, there is a small fovea called macular fovea, which, as the part with the most sensitive vision on the retina, mainly corresponds to the central visual field. If the macular area is impaired, mainly the central visual field will be damaged. The retina can be divided into nasal and temporal halves and superior and inferior halves by a hypothetical vertical line and horizontal line across the central fovea, respectively. The optic papilla is located at the supranasal quadrant above the horizontal line, which manifests as the physiological blind spot in visual field, because there is no photoreceptor cell here. Therefore, the physiological blind spot is situated at the inferotemporal quadrant below the horizontal line in the central visual field [3].

The diseases in different parts of the retina will result in the different visual field impairments in the reverse directions. For example, the retinal detachment in the supratemporal quadrant will lead to an inferonasal visual field defect. Age-related macular degeneration or central serous chorioretinopathy will cause central scotomas. The visual field impairments caused by retinochoroiditis, diabetic retinopathy, etc. are usually relative and multifocal, with variegated appearance of the whole visual field. The visual field defect resulting from retinal detachment is usually located in the peripheral part. In degenerative diseases, such as retinitis pigmentosa, the defect is ringlike, which is located in the mid-peripheral visual field at first and will gradually contract concentrically into tubular visual field. The degree of visual field impairment is also related to the degree of retinal tissue damage caused by a lesion. For example, as to retinal vascular occlusion, the arterial occlusion without timely treatments will produce typical absolute visual field impairment, whereas the venous occlusion will have relatively mild and variant visual field impairment.

Generally speaking, visual field defects simply caused by ocular diseases are usually fundus lesions (mainly the retina and/or optic nerve), except the impact of refracting media. Subtle changes of the central visual field sometimes can be felt by a patient with good central vision, but it is difficult to detect the corresponding fundus lesion under an ophthalmoscope. Auxiliary examinations, such as Amsler chart, OCT, fluorescein fundus angiography (FFA), electroretinogram (ERG), and visual evoked potential (VEP), will be required in such situation, and the retinopathy and/or optic neuropathy corresponding to the visual field defect can usually be found. Consequently, the retinopathy and optic neuropathy should be screened firstly when a visual field defect is observed, especially a monocular defect, and then the intracranial lesions. Conversely, a binocular visual field defect indicating an intracranial lesion also necessitates careful screening of the retinopathy or optic neuropathy in additional to visual pathway examinations, because sometimes both of them may coexist.

1.3 Retinal Nerve Fiber Layer and Glaucoma

Retinal nerve fibers, or retinal ganglion cell axons, can be divided into papillomacular bundles, temporal arcuate fibers, and nasal radial fibers (Fig. 1.2). The numbers of retinal nerve fibers sent out from the respective parts of the retina are not the same. The retinal nerve fibers sent out from the macula, which are 65% of the total retinal fibers in quantity, constitute the papillomacular bundles. They enter into the temporal side of the optic disc in a more central and straighter course and correspond to the central 5° of the visual field. A central scotoma can be observed when damage occurs in these bundles. The retinal nerve fibers sent out from the nasal half of the retina are the second most and relatively sparse. Wedge-shaped, fan-shaped, or half-side visual field defects connecting with the physiological blind spot may appear when damage occurs in these fibers. The retinal nerve fibers sent out from the temporal half of the retina are the least. These fibers, which are originated from RGCs located at the temporal superior and inferior parts of the macula, are sent from the temporal retina without mixing at the horizontal raphe, bypass the macula and the papillomacular bundles arcuately, and enter the superior and inferior poles of the optic disc temporally. The fiber course is mainly in the area between 5° and 25° around the macula, where the visual field mainly corresponds to the Bjerrum area (the paracentral area, i.e., the area between 5° and 25° of the visual field) [3].

The typical damages caused by glaucoma mainly involve thinning of the retinal nerve fiber layer and excavation of the optic disc, with focal notching of the rim. The retinal nerve fiber layer is formed by the axons of RGCs. The typical visual field defect of glaucoma is pro-chiasm damage, a nerve fiber bundle defect. The superior and inferior retinal nerve fiber layers are thicker than the nasal and temporal ones. The nerve fiber bundles run through the lamina cribrosa of the sclera. The meshes in the upper and lower poles of the lamina cribrosa are relatively big, and the arcuate fibers from the temporal retina run through this

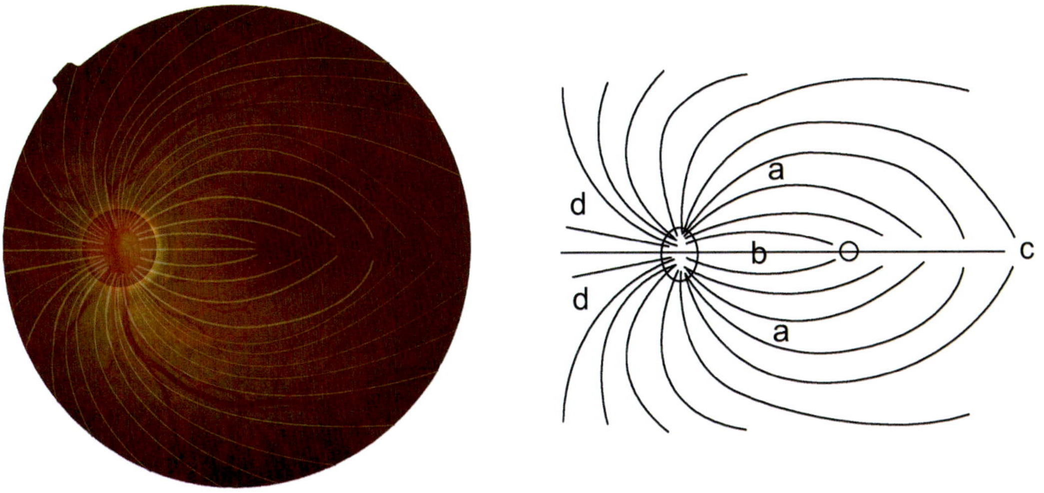

Fig. 1.2 Distribution of the central retinal nerve fibers. *a*: Superior and inferior arcuate fibers. *b*: Papillomacular bundles. *c*: Horizontal raphe. *d*: Nasal fibers

area. Furthermore, the lamellae forming these meshes are thin and fine, and the local connective tissue is relatively sparse, so these meshes are easily deformed when the intraocular pressure increases. Meanwhile, due to the absence of the support from connective tissue, the nerve fibers in these pores are susceptible to squeezing, which may lead to the disturbance or even interrupt of blood supply and axoplasmic transport, and then significant damage and corresponding visual field defect will appear. Nonetheless, the meshes at the nasal and temporal sides of the lamina cribrosa are smaller, and the lamellae are thicker and coarser with the relatively dense local connective tissue. The shear force resulting from the distortion of the lamina cribrosa and the dislocation of the meshes due to squeezed lamina cribrosa tissue under high intraocular pressure will lead to the axoplasmic flow blocking of the nerve fibers and then optic nerve damage of glaucoma.

The part of the lamina cribrosa the temporal nerve fibers run through is more susceptible to damage under high intraocular pressure due to lack of proper protection from the connective tissue. The typical visual field defects of early glaucoma are paracentral scotoma and nasal step in the Bjerrum area (the central 5° to 25° of the visual field) and correspond to the damages at the superior and inferior poles of the optic disc, enlargement of the vertical diameter of the optic cup and notch on the optic disc edge. Because the resistance to the high intraocular pressure in the meshes and the connective tissue of the part of the lamina cribrosa the radial nasal fibers and the papillomacular bundles run through is relatively strong, so the nerve fibers are not easy to be damaged at the early stage of glaucoma. This may be one of the mechanisms for the preservation of the central and temporal visual fields. It also explains why only the central tubular visual field and the temporal island of vision can be preserved in patients with advanced glaucoma.

As shown below, early glaucomatous damages can be found in the patient's right eye with a cup-disc ratio of 0.5 and the wedge-shaped defect of the inferior retinal nerve fibers (Fig. 1.3). The visual field impairments are nasal step, superior paracentral scotoma, and even small superior arcuate scotoma (Fig. 1.4). The OCT measurement reveals thinning of the inferior retinal nerve fiber layer (Fig. 1.5).

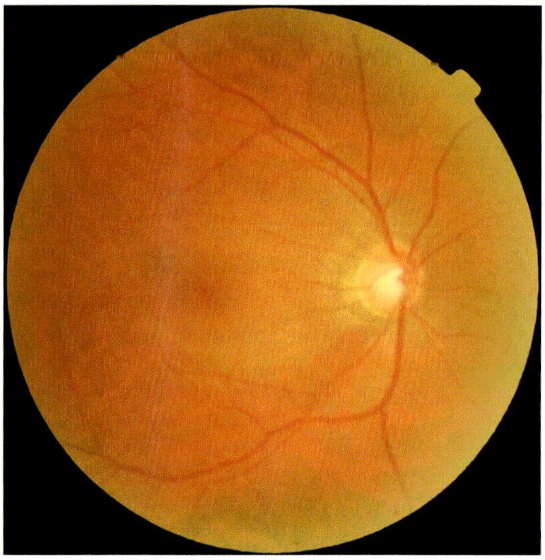

Fig. 1.3 The right fundus image of a glaucoma patient. The cup-disc ratio was 0.5. There's a wedge-shaped defect in the inferior retinal nerve fibers with narrowed cup rim

1.4 Retinal Blood Supply

The inner five retinal layers are mainly supplied by the central vascular system of the retina. The arterial and venous routes and distributions are roughly the same with no anastomotic branches. The outer five retinal layers are mainly supplied by the short posterior ciliary artery of the choroid vascular system. Both central retinal artery and short posterior ciliary artery are the branches of the ophthalmic artery which is a branch of the internal carotid artery. If there is any retinal vascular disease, it will cause corresponding tissue damage and function change (visual field impairment) [3, 4].

There is no retinal vessel in the center of the macula whose nutrition is mainly supplied by the choroidal vessels. Therefore, macula is relatively sensitive to choroidal vascular lesions. Age-related macular degeneration, commonly found in the senior population, is closely related to the changes in choroidal vessels. A series of changes

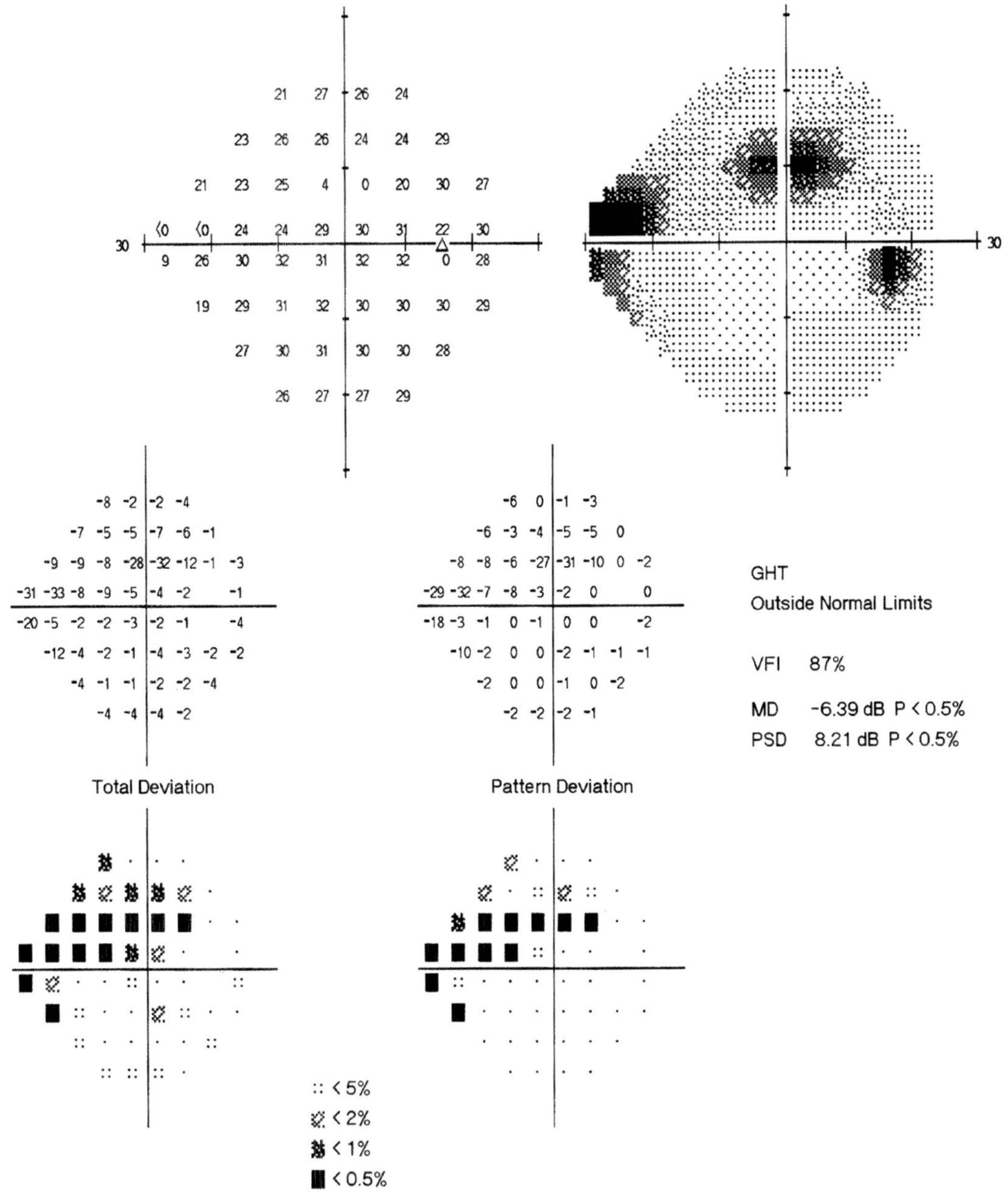

Fig. 1.4 Visual field defects of early glaucoma. Nasal step and a superior paracentral scotoma in the right eye

resulting from new vessels breaking through the retinal pigment epithelium layer into the inner retina can be found in such lesions.

The central retinal artery is one of the terminal arteries. The farthest distribution layers supplied by the capillaries of the central retinal artery are inner nuclear layer and inner plexiform layer. When the intraocular pressure becomes higher, the anatomical positions with the most serious ischemia should be the inner nuclear layer and the inner plexiform layer, and damages in these two layers can be found on an OCT scan. The area around the lamina cribrosa of the optic disc, including the lamina cribrosa and anterior area, is

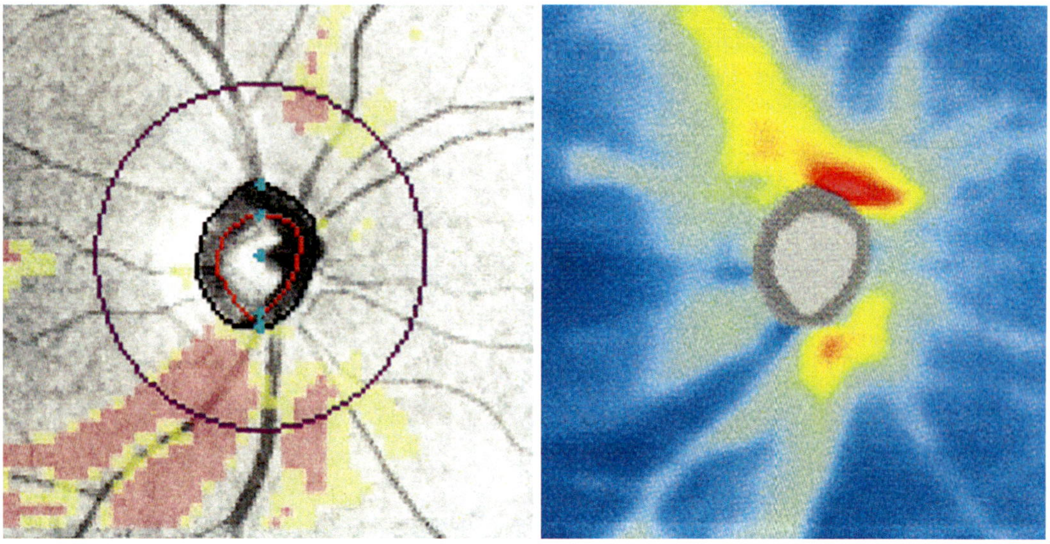

Fig. 1.5 OCT scan for the thickness of the nerve fiber layer around the optic disc in a glaucoma patient. Thinning of the inferior retinal nerve fiber layer in the right eye

supplied by 15–20 short posterior ciliary arteries. Ischemia of these arteries will cause hypoperfusion and vascular infarction of the anterior part of the optic nerve, which may lead to anterior ischemic optic neuropathy.

References

1. Haisheng L, Jiapu P. Principles and practices of visual electrophysiology. Shanghai: Shanghai Popular Science Press; 2002.
2. Honglu Y, Xiumin Y. Physiology of eye. Beijing: People's Medical Publishing House; 2001.
3. Jiaqi L, Fengming L. Practice of ophthalmology. 2nd ed. Beijing: People's Medical Publishing House; 1999.
4. Weilong Z, Shizhen Z. Clinical anatomy series-head and neck volume. Beijing: People's Medical Publishing House; 1988.

2 Optic Nerve

Xuyang Liu, Jia Ma, and Ningli Wang

The axons of RGCs gather at the level of the optic disc and then are divided into bundles, running through the lamina cribrosa of the sclera and then piercing the eyeball posteriorly to form the optic nerve.

2.1 Anatomy of the Optic Nerve

The axons sent out by RGCs, i.e., nerve fibers, gather to form the optic disc 3–4 mm nasal to the macula and then run through the lamina cribrosa to form the optic nerve. With an overall length of about 35–50 mm, the nerve is divided into four segments in anatomy, including intraocular, intraorbital, intracanal, and intracranial segments [1–3].

X. Liu (✉)
Xiamen Eye Center of Xiamen University, Xiamen, China

Shenzhen Eye Hospital, Shenzhen University, Shenzhen, China

J. Ma
The First Affiliated Hospital, Kunming Medical University, Kunming, China

N. Wang
Department of Ophthalmology, Beijing Tongren Hospital, Capital Medical University, Beijing, China

2.1.1 Intraocular Segment

This segment is the shortest segment. It starts from the optic disc and ends at the level throughout the lamina cribrosa, with a length of about 0.7–1.0 mm. It is the part easily involved by glaucoma, ischemic optic neuropathy, and increased intracranial pressure. This optic nerve segment has no medullary sheath until it runs out from the lamina cribrosa. Therefore, the diameter of the optic nerve will increase to 3–3.5 mm here. It's relatively crowded when the nerves run through the lamina cribrosa, which is one of the possible reasons for edema and congestion being more common in the optic disc. Edema can easily occur in the optic disc when the intracranial pressure is higher than the intraocular pressure.

Between the intraocular segment and choroid and sclera, there is a peripheral layer of neuroglia and connective tissue separating them from each other, which has certain protective effect on the optic nerve. For example, posterior scleritis or choroidal lesions, such as inflammation, will hardly involve the optic nerve.

2.1.2 Intraorbital Segment

This segment starts from the posterior surface of the sclera to the orbital aperture of the optic canal. With a length of about 25–30 mm, it is the

N. Wang et al. (eds.), *Optic Disorders and Visual Field*, Advances in Visual Science and Eye Diseases 2, https://doi.org/10.1007/978-981-13-2502-1_2

longest segment of all. The straight-line distance from the posterior wall of the eyeball to the optic foramen is about 18 mm. Therefore, this intraorbital segment is hidden in the orbital fat with a physiological "S" shape, which is favorable to eye movements, because it will not be stretched during eyeball moving. The visual function will not be affected within a certain period even if the optic nerve is stretched in clinical pathological exophthalmos, such as thyroid-associated orbitopathy. In addition to extraocular muscle and orbital fat, there are also other structures, such as the ophthalmic artery and its branches, oculomotor nerve, abducens nerve, trochlear nerve, and trigeminal nerve in the surrounding area of the intraorbital segment. Any lesion in the muscle cone or the orbit, including tumor, hemorrhage, traumatic foreign bodies, inflammation, edema, etc., will compress or spread to this part, thus leading to corresponding optic neuropathy and even optic atrophy.

At about 2 mm behind the eyeball, a slightly dilated area can sometimes be observed in the subarachnoid space of the optic nerve, which is usually the operating site for intraorbital optic nerve decompression. The surgeon will approach from the nasal side near the eyeball, disconnect the medial rectus, expose the medial side of the optic nerve posteriorly, and then cut open the dura mater at the dilated area of the retrobulbar optic nerve. The cerebrospinal fluid outflows, and a window 1 × 2 mm in size will be cut for continuous decompression.

2.1.3 Intracanal Segment

It's the segment of the optic nerve located inside the bony optic canal. Since it used to be considered as a foramen only, optic canal has been called optic foramen. However, it's actually a very short bony canal structure, and therefore it's also called optic canal. The lengths of respective walls, especially the length of the superior wall, are closely related to the development status of the minor ala of sphenoid. The average lengths of the superior wall and the inferior wall are 4–9 and 5–6 mm, respectively, and the average canal diameter is 4–6 mm. The longer is the optic canal, the smaller is the canal diameter, and vice versa. This segment of the optic nerve is susceptible to compression or even cross-sectional injury in the case of trauma, resulting in the corresponding visual field defects.

The running of the inferior lateral side of the optic nerve inside the optic canal is accompanied by the ophthalmic artery. The medial surface of the optic nerve is close to the bony wall of the optic canal with only optic nerve sheath between them. The bony wall here is relatively thin and medially close to the last air chamber of the sphenoid sinus and the posterior ethmoid sinus. Therefore, lesions in these sinuses can involve the optic nerve, such as retrobulbar optic neuritis. The optic nerve can also be easily damaged during superior nasal sinus operations or transsphenoidal pituitary operations. With the rapid development of the intranasal endoscopic surgery in recent years, it can show clearly the lateral wall of the optic canal after entering and gasifying the sphenoid sinus adequately (Fig. 2.1).

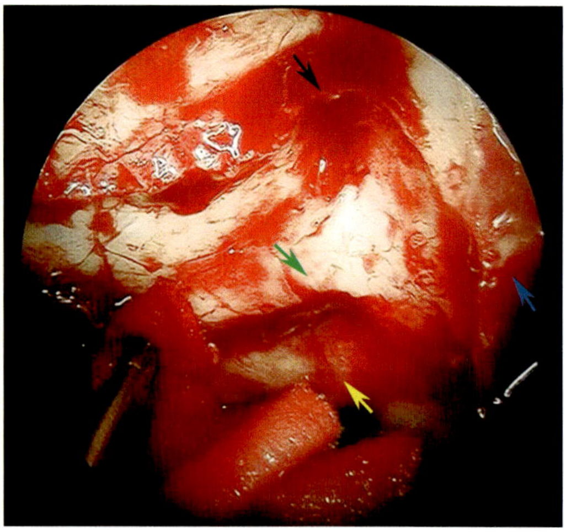

Fig. 2.1 Sphenoid sinus area under the intranasal endoscope. Under the intranasal endoscope, the blue arrow indicates the orbital apex, the black arrow indicates the superior optic recess, the green arrow indicates the optic canal, and the yellow arrow indicates the internal carotid artery

2.1.4 Intracranial Segment

Starting from the cranial access of the optic canal and ending at the optic chiasm, this segment is about 10 mm in length, and the full segment is located inside the subarachnoid space. The intraorbital and intracanal segments of the optic nerve exhibit a round-rope shape, while the intracranial segment of the optic nerve exhibits a flat-rope shape. There are many structures around it, such as internal carotid artery posterior laterally, ophthalmic artery inferiorly, and the bottom structures of the frontal lobe (which include precribrum, olfactory tract, and anterior cerebral artery) superiorly. The anterior cerebral artery and the anterior communicating artery are the common sites of hemangioma which usually involves this segment of the optic nerve, and patients usually go to see a doctor for a monocular visual field defect.

The intraorbital and intracanal segments of the optic nerve are enveloped by the optic nerve sheath. The optic nerve sheath has three layers, which are the direct continuation of the three layers of cerebral mater. The outer layer from the cerebral dura mater is called the outer sheath, which connects with the sclera anteriorly, fuses with the periosteum of the optic canal posteriorly, and links to the orbital periosteum. The inner layer from the cerebral pia mater is called the inner sheath which covers the outer surface of the optic nerve. A significant gap between the inner and outer sheaths is known as an intervaginal space, which is divided into the subdural space and the subarachnoid space by the arachnoid mater. Both the front ends of the subdural and subarachnoid spaces are blind ending in the posterior area of the sclera. They directly connect posteriorly with the intracranial subdural space and the intracranial subarachnoid space. The subarachnoid space inside the optic nerve sheath is filled with cerebrospinal fluid. The pressure inside the optic nerve sheath will also increase with the increase of the intracranial pressure.

The three layers of optic nerve sheath fuse with the periosteum at the medial superior part of the optic canal and fix the optic nerve on the bony wall of the optic canal. No fusing of the three layers of optic nerve sheath can be found in the remaining parts of the optic canal, and the intervaginal space maintains unobstructed. When intracranial mass such as meningioma of sphenoid ridge and olfactory groove compresses the optic canal or the intracranial optic nerve in an inferolateral direction, the intervaginal space of the affected side will be blocked completely, and even descending optic atrophy can be found. The increased intracranial pressure caused by the tumor will cause contralateral optic edema but no ipsilateral optic edema, which is called Foster-Kennedy syndrome.

2.2 Nerve Fiber Distribution of the Optic Nerve

At the junction between the eyeball and the foremost part of the intraorbital segment of the optic nerve, the fibers from the macula are not located in the center of the optic nerve but laterally, in which the superior macula fibers are located superolaterally and those inferior ones inferolaterally. The nasal retinal fibers lie in the medial side of macula fibers, in which the supranasal fibers are located superomedially and those inferonasal ones inferomedially. The fibers from the temporal half of the retina are divided into two parts which do not cross at the horizontal raphe, the supratemporal fibers located superolaterally and those inferotemporal ones inferolaterally. The fibers from the margin of the nasal retina, which correspond to the most temporal nonoverlapping visual field of both eyes, are located in the marginal part of the most medial part of the optic nerve here, also superior ones located superiorly and inferior ones inferiorly.

The macular fibers will move gradually toward the center of the optic nerve along with the posterior stretching of the intraorbital segment of the optic nerve until 10–15 mm behind the eyeball, where there are no central retinal vessels. Now, the temporal retinal fibers envelope the lateral side of macular fibers, with the supratemporal fibers located superolaterally and inferotemporal ones inferolaterally. The nasal retinal fibers envelope the medial side of macular fibers, with the supranasal fibers located superomedially and inferonasal ones inferomedially. The location of the nasal marginal retinal fibers remains basically unchanged.

At the end of the optic nerve close to the optic chiasm, the arrangement of optic nerve fibers is approximately the same as that at 10–15 mm behind the eyeball, but with a rotation of about 45° toward the nasal side; that is to say, all of the optic nerve fibers are rotated as a whole with the superior part rotating toward the nasal side or medially by 45°. There is a thin slice as a partition to separate the nasal retinal fibers from the temporal ones, which stretch down from the cerebral pia mater on the surface of the optic nerve. The partition formed by the cerebral pia mater is considered as the boundary sign between the optic nerve and the optic chiasm [2–10].

2.3 Blood Supply of the Optic Nerve

2.3.1 Blood Supply of the Intraocular Segment of the Optic Nerve

The optic nerve is mainly supplied by the Zinn-Haller ring. This ring is a complete or incomplete ring formed by the mutual anastomosis from 2 to 4 or more posterior ciliary arteries around the optic nerve penetrating into the sclera nasally and temporally. The arterial ring sends out many branches, forward to the choroid, inward to the optic nerve, and backward to the vascular network of the cerebral pia mater with capillary anastomosis. Meanwhile, some arterioles sent out by the short posterior ciliary arteries directly supply the anterior part of the lamina cribrosa. The central retinal artery supplies the most superficial fiber layer of the optic disc. Capillary anastomosis can also be found between the arterial ring and the central retinal artery.

2.3.2 Blood Supply of the Intraorbital Segment of the Optic Nerve

The surrounding part of the intraorbital optic nerve is supplied by the vascular network of the cerebral pia mater, which is composed of branches from the neighboring ophthalmic artery. Its branches reach into the optic nerve along the cerebral pia mater septum and further divide into anterior and posterior sub-branches after reaching the median septa. There are some small branches of the central retinal artery, about 6–12 in number, penetrating the cerebral dura mater to supply the surrounding part of the optic nerve before entering the optic nerve, and only some small branches supply the axial fibers of the optic nerve after entering the optic nerve.

2.3.3 Blood Supply of the Intracanal Segment of the Optic Nerve

It's also supplied by the branches of the vascular network of the cerebral pia mater. The vascular network here is from the regressive branches of the ophthalmic artery.

2.3.4 Blood Supply of the Intracranial Segment of the Optic Nerve

Just like the intracanal segment, this segment is also supplied by the smaller branches of the vascular network of the cerebral pia mater superiorly, which comes from the anterior cerebral artery. The inferior part is mainly supplied by the branches of the internal carotid artery with the ophthalmic artery and the anterior communicating artery playing a supplementary role [1, 11, 12].

References

1. Tianzhu Y. Clinically-oriented neurotomy. Beijing: Peking Union Medical College Press; 2002.
2. Duke-Elder S. System of ophthalmology, vol. II. London: Kimpton; 1961.
3. Wilkinson JL. Neuroanatomy for medical students. London: John Wright & Sons Ltd; 1986.
4. Arthur CG, John EH. Text book of medical physiology. 10th ed. Philadelphia: WB Saunders Company; 2000.
5. Ni C, Wang WJ, Albert DM, et al. Intravitreous silicone injection: histopathologic findings in a human eye after 12 years. Arch Ophthalmol. 1983;101(9):1399–401.
6. Shields CL, Eagle RC. Pseudo-Schnabel's cavernous degeneration of the optic nerve secondary to in traocular silicone oil. Arch Ophthalmol. 1989;107(5):714–7.
7. Budde M, Cursiefen C, Holbach LM, et al. Silicone oil associated optic nerve degeneration. Am J Ophthalmol. 2001;131(3):392–4.
8. Papp A, Toth J, Kerenyi T, et al. Silicone oil in the subarachnoidal space-a possible route to the brain? Pathol Res Pract. 2004;200(3):247–52.
9. Dong FT, Dai RP, Zheng L, et al. Migration of intraocular silicone into the cerebral ventricles. Am J Ophthalmol. 2005;140(1):156–8.
10. Yu JT, Apte RS. A case of intravitreal silicone oil migration to the central nervous system. Retina. 2005;25(6):791–3.
11. Weilong Z, Shizhen Z. Clinical anatomy series-head and neck volume. Beijing: People's Medical Publishing House; 1988.
12. Jiaqi L, Fengming L. Practice of ophthalmology. 2nd ed. Beijing: People's Medical Publishing House; 1999.

3 Optic Chiasm

Xuyang Liu, Jia Ma, and Ningli Wang

The optic nerve from each eye gathers above the sella turcica to form the optic chiasm. The anatomical region of the optic chiasm is relatively complex, with the pituitary gland located inferiorly, the third ventricle superoposteriorly, the anterior cerebral artery and the anterior communicating artery superoanteriorly, and the internal carotid arteries bilaterally. The tumor, inflammation, trauma, or vascular lesions, etc. at this site may all involve the optic chiasm [1, 2].

3.1 Relationship Between the Visual Field and the Anatomy of Nerve Fiber Distribution in the Chiasm

The left and right optic nerves gather to form the anterior angles of the optic chiasm, and the optic chiasm stretches backward to form the left and right optic tracts with joints, the posterior angles. The optic chiasm exhibits quadrilateral or oval shape cross-sectionally, and its size varies significantly. The anteroposterior diameter, transverse diameter, and superoinferior diameter are about 4–13 mm with an average of 8 mm, 10–20 mm with an average of 13 mm, and 3–5 mm, respectively. The nerve fibers here are in a half-crossing status, which ensures the formation of the binocular single vision.

Among the optic nerve fibers, only the fibers from the nasal retina cross within the optic chiasm and enter the contralateral optic tract, while the fibers from the temporal retina remain in the same side and enter the ipsilateral optic tract.

The fibers from the temporal retina run in the lateral edge of the optic chiasm, with the supratemporal fibers located dorsally and inferotemporal ones lateral-ventrally.

The routes of the fibers from the nasal retina in the optic chiasm are curved. The fibers from the inferonasal retina run along the front edge of the optic chiasm to the opposite side and form a little forward curve into the end of the contralateral optic nerve, which is called the anterior Wilbrand's knee. Then the fibers will run along the lateral edge of the optic chiasm backward to enter the ventrolateral part of the contralateral optic tract. The fibers from the supranasal retina, after entering the optic chiasm, run backward into the initial part of the ipsilateral optic tract and form a little backward curve, which is called

X. Liu (✉)
Xiamen Eye Center of Xiamen University, Xiamen, China

Shenzhen Eye Hospital, Shenzhen University, Shenzhen, China

J. Ma
The First Affiliated Hospital, Kunming Medical University, Kunming, China

N. Wang
Department of Ophthalmology, Beijing Tongren Hospital, Capital Medical University, Beijing, China

N. Wang et al. (eds.), *Optic Disorders and Visual Field*, Advances in Visual Science and Eye Diseases 2, https://doi.org/10.1007/978-981-13-2502-1_3

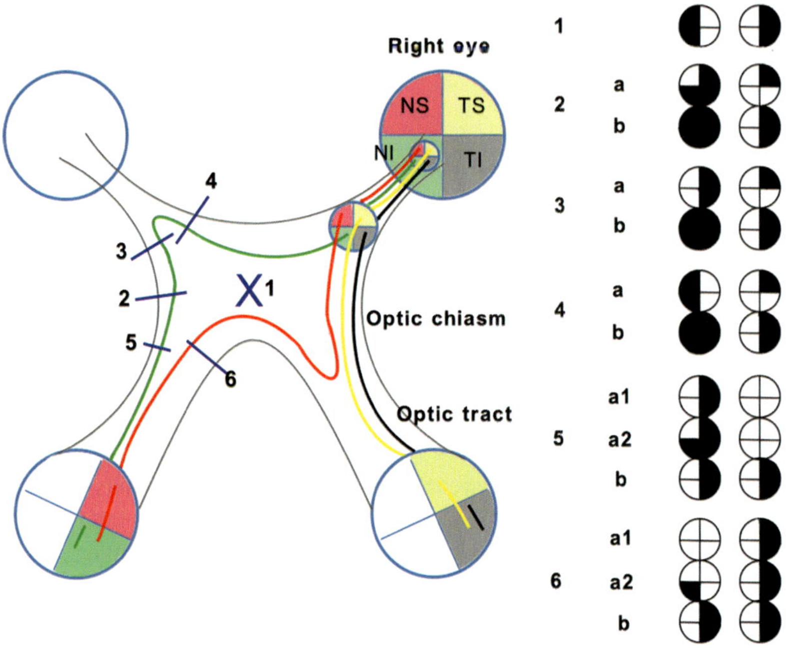

Fig. 3.1 Fiber crossing status in the optic chiasm and visual field impairment caused by damages to its different parts (the left side). The numbers 1–6 correspond, respectively, to the following different damaged parts in the optic chiasm: central part, middle-lateral part, anterolateral side, anteromedial side, posterolateral side, and posteromedial side. Panels a, a1, and a2 show the visual field manifestations at the early stage during the disease course and Panel b shows the ones at the advanced stage. NS: Supranasal quadrant; NI: Inferonasal quadrant; TS: Supratemporal quadrant; TI: Inferotemporal quadrant

the posterior Wilbrand's knee. Then the supranasal fibers will run along the posterior edge of the optic chiasm and enter the dorsomedial part of the contralateral optic tract. The posterior Wilbrand's knee is not as obvious as the anterior one, and some authors even believe it does not exist. The appearance of the anterior and posterior knees actually comes from the scattering of the fibers from the nasal retina during the process of running to the opposite side, and those fibers with the most disperse and the furthest routes will extrude into the posterior end of the contralateral optic nerve or the anterior end of the ipsilateral optic tract. The fibers from the macula can also be divided into the nasal half and the temporal half. Like the fibers from other parts of the retina, only the fibers from the nasal half cross the midline to the opposite side at the superoposterior part of the optic chiasm and then enter the contralateral optic tract. The fibers from the temporal half run backward through the lateral part of the optic chiasm and enter the ipsilateral optic tract. Some authors call the chiasm formed by the fibers from the nasal parts of the bilateral macula as the small optic chiasm in the optic chiasm.

Visual field changes in this area are very complicated and vary from part to part (Fig. 3.1). Central lesions in the optic chiasm may cause the typical bitemporal hemianopia. Nasal and inferotemporal 3/4 hemianopia in the ipsilateral side and supratemporal 1/4 hemianopia in the contralateral side will appear at the early stage of the medial lesions in the optic chiasm, and ipsilateral total blindness and contralateral temporal hemianopia will be observed at the advanced stage. Nasal hemianopia in the ipsilateral side and supratemporal 1/4 hemianopia in the contralateral side will appear at the early stage of anterolateral lesions in the optic chiasm, and ipsilateral total blindness and contralateral temporal hemianopia will also be observed at the advanced stage. Temporal hemianopia in the ipsilateral side and supratemporal 1/4 hemianopia in the contralateral side will appear at the early stage of anteromedial lesions in the optic chiasm, and ipsilateral total blindness and contralateral temporal hemianopia will be observed at the advanced stage. Nasal hemianopia, sometimes accompanied by inferotemporal 3/4 hemianopia in the contralateral side, will appear at the early stage of posterolateral lesions in the optic chiasm, and temporary contralateral temporal hemianopia, i.e., binocular contralateral homonymous hemianopia of the lesion, will be observed at the advanced stage. Temporal hemianopia in the contralateral side, sometimes accompanied by inferotemporal 1/4 hemianopia in the ipsilateral side, will appear at the early stage of posteromedial lesions in the optic chiasm, and temporary ipsilateral nasal hemianopia, i.e., binocular homonymous hemianopia at the side contralateral to the lesion, will be observed at the advanced stage [3, 4].

3.2 Relationship Between the Optic Chiasm and Surrounding Tissues and Its Impacts on Visual Field

Around the optic chiasm, there are many structures, the anterior cerebral artery and the anterior communicating artery superoanteriorly, third ventricle superoposteriorly, sellar diaphragm and pituitary gland inferiorly, cavernous sinus inferolaterally with nerves and vessels passing through it, the internal carotid artery (about 4 mm away from the lateral margin of the optic chiasm) and posterior communicating artery bilaterally, the inner root of the olfactory tract superolaterally, and corpus mammillare, tuber cinereum, and infundibulum from it (which stretches inferoanteriorly and becomes the hypophyseal stalk clinging to the posterior lobe of the pituitary gland after penetrating the posterior sellar diaphragm) posteriorly. The sella turcica is located above the body of the corpus sphenoidale in the center of the middle cranial fossa, equivalent to the midpoint of the line between the nasal root and the posterior edge of the foramen occipital magnum. As to sella turcica, there are anterior clinoid processes bilateroanteriorly and tuberculum sellae (typically has small osseous processes called middle clinoid processes on both sides) centrally. There is a sulcus prechiasmaticus between the cranial openings of bilateral optic canals in front of the tuberculum sellae. The tuberculum sellae is a transverse crest about 10 mm in width, which separates the sulcus prechiasmaticus and the pituitary fossa. In the posterior area of the tuberculum sellae lies the elevated dorsum sellae with posterior clinoid processes bilaterally. In the superior area lies sellar diaphragm composed of cerebral dura mater. The slightly sunken area at the bottom of the sella turcica is called the pituitary fossa, with carotid sulci located bilaterally.

The sellar diaphragm covers the sphenoid superiorly. It seals the pituitary fossa and forms a small cavity accommodating the pituitary gland. There is a small hole in the center of the sellar diaphragm through which the infundibular stalk runs. The optic chiasm doesn't contact with the sellar diaphragm directly. There is a basal cistern composed of the chiasmatic cistern and the interpeduncular cistern belonging to a part of the subarachnoid space, between the optic chiasm and the sellar diaphragm, and the distance is about 5–10 mm.

If the sellar diaphragm is relatively thin, the pituitary tumor will easily break through it and expand upward. When this happens, the interpeduncular cistern above the diaphragm plays a certain buffering role so that it will take some time before the tumor involves the optic chiasm. Therefore, symptoms arising from compression of optic chiasm may not appear in a pretty long time. Whether the tumor will compress the optic chiasm is closely related to the location of the optic chiasm. The tumor can compress the central part of the optic chiasm from the bottom if the optic chiasm is located completely or almost

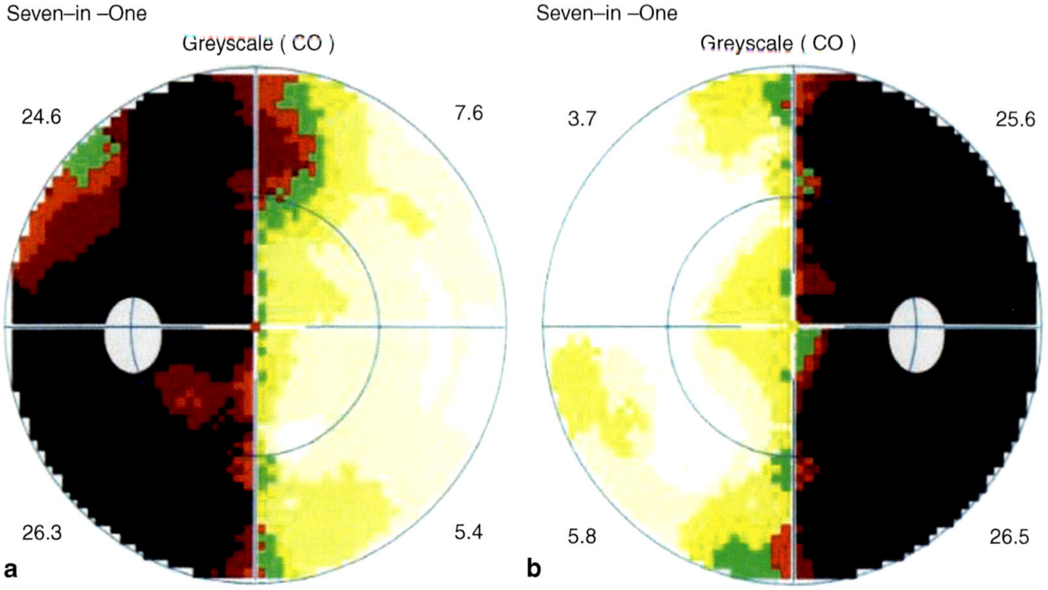

Fig. 3.2 Octopus grayscale maps of the visual field of both eyes. Vertical bitemporal hemianopia; (**a**) left eye; (**b**) right eye

completely above the sella turcica, and a typical optic chiasm-type visual field defect, i.e., bitemporal hemianopia, may be observed. The following case is the visual field change caused by the tumor compression on the central part of the optic chiasm in a patient with hypophysoma (Fig. 3.2).

The occurrence of empty sella, which is usually found in senior women, is also related to the weakness of the sellar diaphragm. In case of weak sellar diaphragm or pituitary gland atrophy, the cerebrospinal fluid will run downward into the pituitary fossa. The process is just like the orbital fat prolapse in case of weak orbital septum but from a different direction. The visual field changes in such patients can be diversified, but binasal hemianopia can usually be observed. The causes of the visual field impairment may be related to the following factors: (a) the optic chiasm is compressed downward and pushed into sella turcica; (b) the optic nerve becomes tortuous due to the herniation of the anterior part of the third ventricle into the sella turcica; and (c) incarceration of the optic chiasm into the crest of dorsum sellae.

Above the optic chiasm is the anterior end of the third ventricle, and this end forms recesses around the optic chiasm, optic recess anteriorly and infundibular recess posteriorly, respectively. When increased intracranial pressure causes ventricular enlargement, the optic chiasm will be compressed due to the enlargement of the optic recess or the infundibular recess, and typical bitemporal hemianopia will be observed, which may be misdiagnosed as pituitary tumor.

3.3 Blood Supply of Optic Chiasm and Visual Field Changes Caused by Ischemia

The blood supply of the optic chiasm can be divided into blood supply of the superior part and that of the inferior part. The superior and lateral parts are supplied by the branches of arterioles sent out from the anterior cerebral artery before the communicating branch. There are very abundant blood vessels in the inferior part, supplied by the superior hypophysial artery plexus formed by the anastomosis between the internal carotid artery, the posterior communicating artery, and the middle cerebral artery.

Bitemporal hemianopia of visual field can still be found clinically in some patients with pituitary microadenoma completely limited inside the pituitary fossa. The reason should be considered from the perspective of the blood supply of the optic chiasm and the pituitary gland. No "specialized artery" supplies the optic chiasm as revealed in anatomical studies. The optic chiasm is mainly supplied by a branch of the pituitary anterior artery from the internal carotid artery before entering the hypophyseal stalk. Lao Yuanxiu et al. have carried out a study on the blood supply of the optic chiasm in 85 cases by the method of scanning electron microscopy (SEM) following the intravascular ink infusion with tissue transparentization and vascular casting. The study has found that the capillaries entering the optic chiasm parenchyma can be divided into two parts: those in the lateral parts of the optic chiasm have more anastomoses, smaller meshes, and higher density in a back-to-forth longitudinal arrangement with penetrating branches of arterioles; and those in the middle part of the optic chiasm have less anastomoses, bigger meshes, and lower density in a left-to-right horizontal arrangement almost without any penetrating arterioles. Most importantly, the capillaries in the middle part are formed by the convergence of the ends of small vessels, and most of them come from the abrupt conversion of the lateral capillaries from longitudinal arrangement to horizontal one. Therefore, the middle part of the optic chiasm is one of the weak points of blood supply. According to the abovementioned anatomical bases, we can analyze the mechanism of bitemporal visual field defects caused by pituitary microadenoma—arterial steal syndrome (ASS). Active metabolism can usually be found in pituitary microadenoma, and the blood volume required exceeds the normal. Consequently, the pituitary microadenoma will "steal" blood from the blood vessels that simultaneously supply the optic chiasm, which interferes with the normal blood supply of the optic chiasm. Meantime, the optic chiasm is very sensitive to ischemia like other cerebral white matter of the central nerve system. Therefore, bitemporal hemianopia can be observed when there is blood supply insufficiency in the weak point of the microcirculation existing in the middle part of the optic chiasm. However, such impairment may be improved with the establishment of compensation or collateral circulation [1].

References

1. Fengming L. Chinese ophthalmology. 2nd ed. Beijing: People's Medical Publishing House; 2005.
2. Kanxing Z, Peizeng Y. Ophthalmology. 7th ed. Beijing: People's Medical Publishing House; 2008.
3. Yuansheng Y, Jia M. Essence of reading and analysis on visual field: ABC of Humphrey visual field analysis. 4th ed. Shanghai: Shanghai Popular Science Press; 2013.
4. Yuansheng Y, Hua Z. Modern clinical visual field examination. 2nd ed. Beijing: People's Medical Publishing House; 2015.

Optic Tract

4

Xuyang Liu, Jia Ma, and Ningli Wang

The optic tracts originate from the posterior part of the optic chiasm bilaterally, with a length of about 4–5 cm. The left optic tract and the right one bypass the left and right cerebral peduncles and end at the left and right lateral geniculate bodies (LGBs), respectively, where the neurons are changed accordingly. It is one part of the optic pathway fibers resulting from the rearrangement of visual fibers after the optic chiasm.

4.1 Anatomy of the Optic Tract

Starting from the posterior angles of the optic chiasm laterally, the optic tracts run between the tuber cinereum and the precribrum in a cylindrical shape and then gradually go posterolaterally in a flat bundle shape. After bypassing the cerebral peduncle, the unilateral optic tract is divided into medial and lateral roots at the tail end. The lateral root is relatively big with about 80% of its fibers are thick ones, including all of the visual fibers, and ends at the ipsilateral lateral geniculate body at the posterolateral part of the thalamus. Before that, about 20% of the visual fibers, which are the afferent fibers of the pupillary light reflex, leave the optic tract and end at the anterior pretectal nucleus in the midbrain through the brachium of superior colliculus of the quadrigeminal bodies.

The medial root is relatively small and is believed by some authors to have relationship with neither visual transduction nor visual reflex. Some authors considered that the fibers of the optic tract, which reach the superior colliculus and pretectal area through the brachium of the superior colliculus, run inside the medial root. These fibers contained are mainly the commissure fibers from the bilateral optic tracts, called Gudden's commissure, which end at the medial geniculate body and connect with the thalamic pulvinar, the pretectal area, and the superior colliculus of the midbrain. The medial root fibers are irrelevant to the vision, but they may be related to the visual reflex and the mechanism of the integrated eyeball movement.

The adjacent structures of the optic tracts include the globus pallidus, internal capsule, and lenticular nucleus superiorly, the hippocampal gyrus of the temporal lobe inferiorly, and the inferior horn of the lateral ventricle inferolaterally.

X. Liu (✉)
Xiamen Eye Center of Xiamen University, Xiamen, China

Shenzhen Eye Hospital, Shenzhen University, Shenzhen, China

J. Ma
The First Affiliated Hospital, Kunming Medical University, Kunming, China

N. Wang
Department of Ophthalmology, Beijing Tongren Hospital, Capital Medical University, Beijing, China

N. Wang et al. (eds.), *Optic Disorders and Visual Field*, Advances in Visual Science and Eye Diseases 2, https://doi.org/10.1007/978-981-13-2502-1_4

After bypassing the cerebral peduncles, which are the left and right cylinder elevations ventral to the midbrain with the interpeduncal fossa between them, the optic tracts run posteriorly along the edge of the temporal lobe and are covered by the temporal lobes, close to the pyramidal tracts and sensory fibers. Therefore, in addition to the visual dysfunction, lesions here can bring about the disorders of limb movement and sensation [1–6].

4.2 Relationship Between the Nerve Fiber Distribution of Optic Tract and the Visual Field

The fibers in the optic tracts come from the ipsilateral temporal half and the contralateral nasal half of the retina, and there are totally six types shown as follows: (a) non-crossing fibers from the temporal half of the ipsilateral macular area; (b) crossing fibers from the nasal half of the contralateral macular area; (c) non-crossing fibers from the temporal peripheral area of the ipsilateral retina; (d) crossing fibers from the nasal peripheral area of the contralateral retina; (e) crossing fibers from the supranasal quadrant of the contralateral retina; and (f) crossing fibers from the inferonasal quadrant of the contralateral retina. Among these six types of fibers, the fibers from the superior halves of the bilateral macular areas gather together, including the fibers from the supratemporal part of the ipsilateral macular area and those from the supranasal part of the contralateral macular area; the fibers from the inferior halves of the bilateral macular areas gather together, including the fibers from the inferotemporal part of the ipsilateral macular area and those from the inferonasal part of the contralateral macular area. Similarly, the fibers from the peripheral areas of the retina also gather together in terms of the superior half or superior quadrants and the inferior half or inferior quadrants, respectively. That is to say, the fibers from the supratemporal peripheral area of the ipsilateral retina and the supranasal peripheral area of the contralateral retina gather together, while the ones from the inferotemporal peripheral area of the ipsilateral retina and the inferonasal peripheral area of the contralateral retina gather together. In short, the fibers from the left parts of retina of both eyes form the left optic tract, and those from the right side form the right optic tract. The fibers from the inferior halves of both retinas, including the crossing and non-crossing ones, are located at the lateral side of the optic tract, and those from the superior halves are located medially. The fibers from the supratemporal and supranasal quadrants of the contralateral retina have no commissure with the ipsilateral ones and thereby occupy an independent position in the optic tract.

Since there are fibers from both retinas in one optic tract, visual dysfunction will frequently be found in both eyes when any optic tract is damaged. For example, as to the damage of the left optic tract, the fibers sent out from the temporal retina of the left eye is damaged, which leads to nasal hemianopia of the left eye; meanwhile, the fibers from the nasal retina of the right eye is damaged, which results in temporal hemianopia of the right eye. The lesion in the left optic tract causes the right hemianopia of both eyes, the nasal hemianopia of the left eye, and the temporal hemianopia of the right eye. Therefore, it is called contralateral hemianopia. Moreover, neither eye can catch the light from the right direction; therefore, it is also called binocular homonymous hemianopia. Any damage from the optic tract or the visual pathway after the optic tract will lead to the binocular homonymous hemianopia. However, the crossing and non-crossing fibers are not completely mixed in one optic tract, and therefore when one optic tract is damaged, the degree of involvement in the two eyes may be different, and the typical binocular homonymous hemianopia may present incomplete consistency. In general, the more anterior the lesion location is, the more inconsistent the hemianopia in the two eyes will be, while the more posterior, the more consistent.

4.3 Pupillary Light Reflex and Visual Pathway

The reflex, contraction of the pupils, or miosis in response to the light with enough intensity cast to the eyes, is called pupillary light reflex. Miosis of the illuminated eye is direct light reflex, and miosis of the other eye is indirect light reflex.

The neural pathway or the reflex arc of pupillary light reflex is still not thoroughly clear. It is commonly accepted that the cone and rod cells produce nerve impulse in response to the light illuminating the retina, which will be transmitted to the optic tract via the bipolar cells, retinal ganglion cells, optic nerve, and optic chiasm, successively. The afferent fibers therein, involved in pupillary light reflex, leave at the posterior one third of the optic tract and end at the pretectal area of the midbrain through the lateral root of the optic tract and the brachium of superior colliculus of the quadrigeminal body. These fibers do not reach the lateral geniculate body. Consequently, the visual transduction and the light reflex pathway are both blocked if there is a lesion ahead of the posterior end of the optic tract. However, only the visual transduction not the light reflex will be involved if there is a lesion at the posterior end of the optic tract. Therefore, when one optic tract is damaged, there is no miosis if the light is cast to any eye in the hemianopia direction. However, when the lesion is located in the lateral geniculate body, optic radiation, or optic cortex, miosis in both eyes will be observed if the light is cast to any eye in the hemianopia direction. This is called Wernicke's hemianopic pupillary rigidity, i.e., when the hemianopic part of the retina is exposed to the light, miosis will not be found. Damages in the anterior 2/3 of the optic tract or the posterior 1/3 and beyond can be differentiated by this method [1, 5, 7].

4.4 Blood Supply of the Optic Tract

The blood supply of the optic tract comes from the small branches of the vascular network covering the pia mater. The anterior part of the optic tract is supplied by the small branches of the anterior choroidal artery and the posterior communicating artery, while the posterior part is supplied by the thalamic anterior perforating branches of the posterior cerebral artery, anastomosing with the branches of the middle cerebral artery.

References

1. Fengming L. Chinese ophthalmology. 2nd ed. Beijing: People's Medical Publishing House; 2005.
2. Kanxing Z, Peizeng Y. Ophthalmology. 7th ed. Beijing: People's Medical Publishing House; 2008.
3. Yuansheng Y, Ma J. Essence of reading and analysis on visual field: ABC of Humphrey visual field analysis. 4th ed. Shanghai: Shanghai Popular Science Press; 2013.
4. Yuansheng Y, Hua Z. Modern clinical visual field examination. 2nd ed. Beijing: People's Medical Publishing House; 2015.
5. Hongqi W. Modern neurophthalmology. Beijing: People's Medical Publishing House; 2005.
6. Yi T, Shihui W, Siwei Y. Basis and clinical progress of visual pathway diseases. Beijing: People's Medical Publishing House; 2010.
7. Jiaqi L, Fengming L. Practice of ophthalmology. 2nd ed. Beijing: People's Medical Publishing House; 1999.

Lateral Geniculate Body

5

Xuyang Liu, Jia Ma, and Ningli Wang

The lateral geniculate body (LGB) is a part of the diencephalon.

5.1 Anatomy of the Lateral Geniculate Body

Exhibiting a saddle shape (oval shape), the LGB is a continuation of the optic tract. The LGB on one side is located lateral to the cerebral peduncle and the medial geniculate body (MGB), medial to the internal capsule, inferolateral to the thalamic pulvinar, anterior to the hippocampal gyrus, and anteromedial to the inferior horn of the lateral ventricle.

The lateral geniculate body is connected to the superior colliculus of the quadrigeminal body via the brachium of superior colliculus. There is a bundle of nerve fibers at the back entering the Wernicke area. The lateral geniculate body is composed of alternating white matter and gray matter and belongs to the low-level visual center, or subcortical center. The white matter is composed of the myelinated nerve fibers from the optic tract, and the gray matter is in fact the ganglion cell nuclei, or geniculate cell nuclei of the lateral geniculate body at the end of optic tract fibers. The gray matter is divided into two nuclei, a ventral nucleus and a dorsal one. The ventral nucleus is located medial to the dorsal one and is irrelevant to the vision. The dorsal nucleus, relatively big, which is the main part of the lateral geniculate body, is the terminal of the anterior afferent fibers of the visual pathway. The peripheral neurons of the visual pathway pass signals to the ganglion cells of the lateral geniculate body through synapse here, which send out fibers forming the optic radiation.

5.2 Relationship Between the Nerve Fiber Distribution of Lateral Geniculate Body and the Visual Field

The optic nerve fibers conducting the visual impulse in the optic tract end at the lateral geniculate body where the local positioning and arrangement of the nerve fibers are basically the same as

X. Liu (✉)
Xiamen Eye Center of Xiamen University, Xiamen, China

Shenzhen Eye Hospital, Shenzhen University, Shenzhen, China

J. Ma
The First Affiliated Hospital, Kunming Medical University, Kunming, China

N. Wang
Department of Ophthalmology, Beijing Tongren Hospital, Capital Medical University, Beijing, China

N. Wang et al. (eds.), *Optic Disorders and Visual Field*, Advances in Visual Science and Eye Diseases 2, https://doi.org/10.1007/978-981-13-2502-1_5

that in the optic tract. The human lateral geniculate body rotates inwardly by 90° to make the superior and inferior fibers located medially and laterally, respectively. The nerve fibers after neurotransmission form the posterior visual pathway, and the arrangement rotates once again and restores to the original superior-inferior organization.

The dorsal nucleus of the gray matter is composed of six curved cell layers with clear boundaries from the ventral side to the dorsal side. The contralateral nasal retinal fibers end at layers 1, 4, and 6 of the lateral geniculate body, while the non-crossing ipsilateral temporal fibers at layers 2, 3, and 5. The superior fibers outside of the macula are projected to the ventromedial area of the lateral geniculate body and the inferior ones to the ventrolateral area. The macular fibers are projected to the central part of the dorsal part and stretch from up to down to the ventral part through the respective layers. The dorsal part is bigger than the ventral one. The fibers from superior and inferior areas of the macula are projected dorsomedially and dorsolaterally, respectively. About 3/4 of the lateral geniculate body is occupied by the projection from the macula. The fibers from the most peripheral area of the contralateral nasal retina end at the foremost narrow area, with the superior and inferior fibers located medially and laterally, respectively. As the nerve fiber distribution in the optic radiation is similar to that in the optic tract, the visual field changes from lesions of the optic radiation are similar to those of the optic tract, with no specificity. The main visual field change is binocular homonymous hemianopia or quadrant hemianopia. A medial lesion of the lateral geniculate body may lead to contralateral inferior quadrant hemianopia, while a lateral lesion may result in contralateral superior quadrant hemianopia [1].

5.3 Blood Supply of the Lateral Geniculate Body

The blood supply of the lateral geniculate body comes from the small branches of the vascular network covering the pia mater, which is supplied by the thalamo-geniculate branch of the posterior cerebral artery and the branch of the middle cerebral artery. The lateral and anterior parts of the lateral geniculate body are supplied by the anterior choroid plexus artery. Homonymous hemianopia from ischemia here may focus on the superior and inferior quadrants far away from the horizontal raphe (Fig. 5.1a). On the other hand, the posterior, medial, or central parts of the lateral geniculate body are supplied by the posterior cerebral artery and the posterolateral choroid plexus artery, and homonymous hemianopia from ischemia here may focus on the area around the horizontal raphe (Fig. 5.1b). This is also one of the bases for location diagnosis.

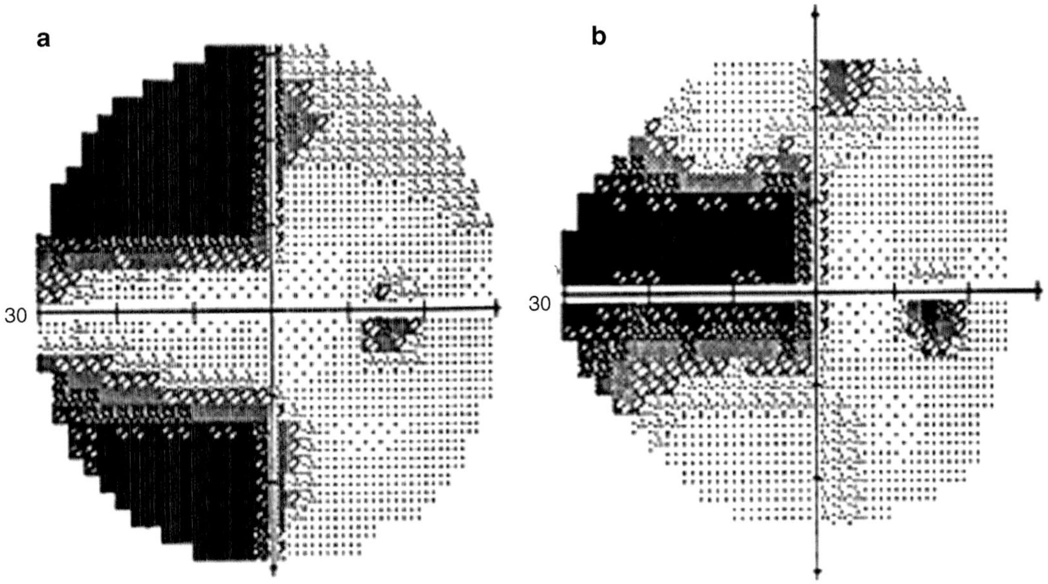

Fig. 5.1 Visual field changes of the lateral geniculate body damages caused by ischemia from different vessel sources. Panel (**a**) Visual field defects in the superior and inferior quadrants far away from the horizontal raphe caused by the ischemia in the lateral and anterior parts of the lateral geniculate body. Panel (**b**) Visual field defects around the horizontal raphe caused by the ischemia in the posterior, medial, or central parts of the lateral geniculate body

Reference

1. Yuansheng Y, Hua Z. Modern clinical visual field examination. 2nd ed. Beijing: People's Medical Publishing House; 2015.

6 Optic Radiation

Xuyang Liu, Jia Ma, and Ningli Wang

The optic radiation is also known as the geniculocalcarine tract.

6.1 Relationship Between the Nerve Fiber Distribution of Optic Radiation and the Visual Field

Starting from layers 3 to 6 of the lateral geniculate body, the optic radiation fibers run posterolaterally through the Wernicke area and form dense fiber bundles in front of the lateral ventricle called optic peduncle. It turns backward at the posterior part of lenticular nucleus of the internal capsule and runs posteriorly along with the lateral wall near the central part of the lateral ventricle, where the fibers gradually scatter and finally end at the visual center of the occipital cortex. The optic radiation fibers of one side can be divided into three bundles, dorsal or superior, external or middle, and ventral or inferior bundles. The superior and inferior bundles correspond, respectively, to the inferior and superior visual fields, while the middle bundle corresponds to the central visual field of the macula. For example, the ventral or inferior fiber damage in the right optic radiation results in binocular homonymous quadrant hemianopia that involves the supranasal quadrant of the right eye and the supratemporal quadrant of the left eye, while the dorsal or superior fiber damage in the right optic radiation leads to binocular homonymous quadrant hemianopia that involves the inferonasal quadrant of the right eye and the inferotemporal quadrant of the left eye.

Besides the afferent fibers from the lateral geniculate body, the optic radiation fibers also include the efferent fibers from the occipital cortex to the lateral geniculate body and the thalamus. The considerable parts of the efferent fibers, including dorsal and lateral parts of the optic radiation, run through the parietal lobe, in fact parietal inferior lobule. Therefore, a lesion deep in the white matter of the parietal lobe is very likely to involve this part of the optic radiation. The ventral or inferior bundles of the optic radiation run along with the lateral wall of the inferior horn of the lateral ventricle in the temporal lobe anteroinferiorly and turn backward after reaching the front end of inferior horn to form a fiber loop

X. Liu (✉)
Xiamen Eye Center of Xiamen University, Xiamen, China

Shenzhen Eye Hospital, Shenzhen University, Shenzhen, China

J. Ma
The First Affiliated Hospital, Kunming Medical University, Kunming, China

N. Wang
Department of Ophthalmology, Beijing Tongren Hospital, Capital Medical University, Beijing, China

N. Wang et al. (eds.), *Optic Disorders and Visual Field*, Advances in Visual Science and Eye Diseases 2, https://doi.org/10.1007/978-981-13-2502-1_6

called temporal loop or Meyer's loop. Then the fibers turn to the superoposterior direction and are projected to the primary visual cortex, the anterior part of the visual cortex below the calcarine sulcus. A lesion deep in the temporal lobe may involve the temporal loop and cause corresponding visual field defects, i.e., the peripheral visual field defects in the contralateral superior quadrant in both eyes.

The internal capsule is located among the thalamus, caudate nucleus, and lenticular nucleus. There are many afferent and efferent fibers of the cerebral cortex having connections with the diencephalon, brainstem, and spinal cord. These fibers become the most centralized when passing through the internal capsule and form a wide and thick white matter plate. The internal capsule connects the cerebral peduncle base of the midbrain inferiorly and scatters upward to the respective cortex layers to form the radiate corona. The internal capsule is divided into three parts, the geniculate part located intermediately at the lenticular nucleus apex with the corticobulbar tract running through it, the occipital part or posterior limb between the thalamus and the lenticular nucleus with the corticospinal tract and the fibers from the thalamus to the central gyrus running through it, and the frontal part or anterior limb between the head of the caudate nucleus and the lenticular nucleus with the frontopontine tract and fibers from the thalamus to the frontal lobe running through it. The internal capsule is the part where the sensory and motor fibers are most concentrated. There are optic radiation and auditory radiation fibers as well as the parieto-occipital-pontine tract running through the posteroinferior part of the lenticular nucleus. Symptoms of contralateral homonymous superior quadrant hemianopia, contralateral hemianesthesia, and contralateral hemiplegia (the three hemidysfunction signs) can usually be found when damage occurs in the internal capsule [1, 2].

6.2 Blood Supply of the Optic Radiation

In terms of the blood supply of the optic radiation, the anterior part is supplied by the anterior choroid branches of the internal carotid artery, the posterior part by the middle and posterior cerebral arteries, and the lateral part by the lateral striate artery from the middle cerebral artery.

References

1. Tianzhu Y. Clinically-oriented neurotomy. Beijing: Peking Union Medical College Press; 2002.
2. Fengming L. Chinese ophthalmology. 2nd ed. Beijing: People's Medical Publishing House; 2005.

Visual Cortex

7

Xuyang Liu, Jia Ma, and Ningli Wang

The occipital lobe is the advanced visual center of the human being, located at the posterior part of the cerebral hemispheres. The fibers sent out from the lateral geniculate body after neurotransmission form the optic radiation, in which the visual fibers scatter fanwise posterior to the sensory transduction tract of the posterior limb in the internal capsule. The fibers from the superior, middle, and inferior bundles are projected posteriorly, gradually gather together, and finally end at the occipital visual cortex. The pathway, from the lateral geniculate body to the occipital visual cortex, is the posterior visual pathway. The arrangements of fibers from the different parts of the retina in the visual pathway are subject to a strict order. There are different neighbor tissues around the different parts of the posterior visual pathway, with different visual field defects being possible.

7.1 Anatomy of the Visual Cortex

Primary visual cortex, also known as visual area I, or striate area, i.e., Brodmann area 17, is located at the medial side of the posterior part of the occipital lobe in the bilateral cerebral hemisphere and superior and inferior to the calcarine fissure. With a horizontal diameter of about 5 cm, the visual cortex stretches posteriorly to the occipital pole, and a small part of it with different sizes can also stretch to the lateral part of the occipital pole and even stretch anteriorly to the anterior part intersecting with the parieto-occipital fissure close to the splenium of the corpus callosum. The striate area is characterized by the clear striations in the cross section, i.e., Gennari's stria, which are white lines or striations formed in layer IV of the cortex by the medullated fibers and intracortical association fibers from the optic radiation. Calcarine fissure is an arch-shaped fissure from the occipital lobe, with a depth of about 18 mm. The anterior 1/3 segment of the fissure, relatively deep, is the main part of the calcarine fissure, while the posterior 2/3 segment, relatively shallow, is called the posterior calcarine fissure.

X. Liu (✉)
Xiamen Eye Center of Xiamen University, Xiamen, China

Shenzhen Eye Hospital, Shenzhen University, Shenzhen, China

J. Ma
The First Affiliated Hospital, Kunming Medical University, Kunming, China

N. Wang
Department of Ophthalmology, Beijing Tongren Hospital, Capital Medical University, Beijing, China

N. Wang et al. (eds.), *Optic Disorders and Visual Field*, Advances in Visual Science and Eye Diseases 2, https://doi.org/10.1007/978-981-13-2502-1_7

7.2 Relationship Between the Nerve Fiber Distribution of Visual Cortex and the Visual Field

The striate area in each hemisphere will receive the projection of the fibers from the ipsilateral temporal retina and contralateral nasal one. The retinal fibers outside of the macula are projected to the anterior part of the striate area, the fibers from the ipsilateral superior quadrant in both retinas are projected to the upper lip of the calcarine fissure corresponding to the contralateral inferior visual field, while the fibers from the ipsilateral inferior quadrant in both retinas are projected to the lower lip of the calcarine fissure corresponding to the contralateral superior visual field. The fibers from macula are projected to the upper and lower lips of the posterior part of the striate area, and sometimes the projection area can be extended for 1–2 cm transversely on the posterior surface of the occipital posterior pole. The fibers from the peripheral nasal side in one eye are projected to the most anterior part of the cortex. Macula occupies a small proportion in the total area of the retina, but the projection areas of macular and peripheral fibers in the striate area are similar in area.

Any damage in lateral geniculate body, optic radiation, or primary optic cortex in one side leads to the contralateral homonymous hemianopia. For example, in the following case, a patient with infarction of the internal capsule of the right hemisphere showed consistent left homonymous hemianopia contralateral to the lesion, which was absolute defects and without any significant change after the operation (Fig. 7.1).

However, the visual fields of both eyes are not completely overlapped. There is a nonoverlapping crescent area about 30° in size in the temporal peripheral visual field of one eye, corresponding to the contralateral nasal peripheral retinal fibers, which is projected to the most anterior part of the striate area. The lesion here can lead to a unilateral temporal crescent defect in the contralateral eye (Fig. 7.2a). Nonetheless,

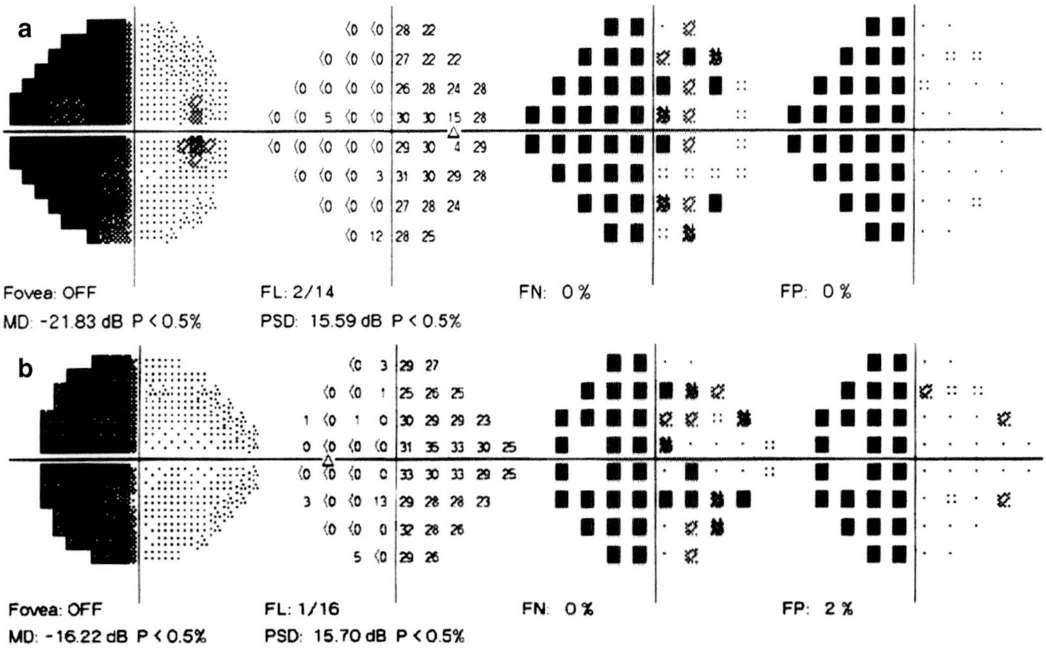

Fig. 7.1 Visual fields analysis printouts of both eyes of a patient with infarction of the internal capsule of the right hemisphere. Testing with the 24-2 strategy showed consistent left homonymous hemianopia. Panel a: right eye. Panel b: left eye

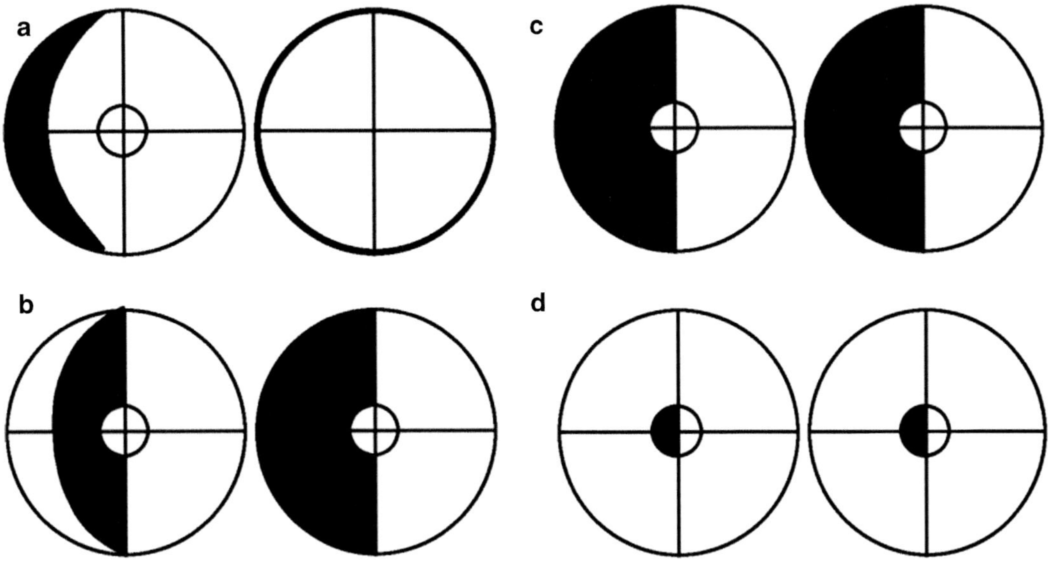

Fig. 7.2 The visual field defects caused by the damages in the visual center. Panel a: Left temporal crescent defect, caused by the damage in the most anterior part of the right visual cortex, involving the most peripheral nasal fibers of the left eye. Panel b: Left homonymous hemianopia with the macula spared and the temporal crescent spared in both eyes, caused by the damage in the central part of the right visual cortex, involving the projection area except binocular macular fibers and the most peripheral nasal fibers of the left eye. Panel c: Left homonymous hemianopia with the macula spared in both eyes, caused by the extensive damage in the right visual cortex. Panel d: Left homonymous macular splitting, caused by the damage in the right occipital pole, involving the crossing macular fibers of the left eye and the non-crossing macular fibers of the right eye

it is more common that the lesions in the postmedial part of the occipital lobe lead to binocular homonymous hemianopia with the contralateral crescent spared because of the preservation of these contralateral nasal peripheral retinal fibers (Fig. 7.2b).

Moreover, the contralateral homonymous hemianopia, caused by the damages to the optic radiation or primary visual cortex on one side, is always demarcated from the healthy halves of the visual fields via non-straight boundary lines which detour the central area; that is to say, the whole macular vision or central vision in both eyes is retained, a phenomenon clinically called macular sparing (Fig. 7.2c). It's a specific manifestation of the optic radiation and visual cortex damage, but its mechanism is still unclear. The phenomenon corresponding to it is binocular contralateral homonymous macular splitting or homonymous hemianopic central scotoma, caused by the lesion of the occipital pole on one side, in which the macular central visual field is divided into two parts by the vertical boundary line (Fig. 7.2d).

Concerning the mechanism of macular sparing, neuroanatomists, ophthalmologists and neuro-ophthalmologists once tried to give various explanations, but still no anatomical evidences are available. In one of the explanations, the primary visual cortex is supplied by the calcarine arteries from the posterior cerebral artery, while the lateral surface of the cerebral hemisphere is mainly supplied by the branches of the middle cerebral artery except the superior edge from the frontal pole to the occipital pole. There are anastomotic branches between the ends of middle cerebral artery branches and the calcarine arteries in the pia mater before entering the brain parenchyma. When embolism occurs in the calcarine artery, collateral circulation can be set up via this route to a certain degree; thus, the function of the rearmost end of the primary visual cortex or the macular visual area can be retained. Besides, the extensive scattered projection of the macular fibers in the occipital lobe is another possible reason [1, 2].

7.3 Blood Supply of the Visual Cortex

The blood supply of visual cortex mainly comes from the three branches of the posterior cerebral artery, including the posterior temporal artery, calcarine artery, and parieto-occipital artery. The striate area is mainly supplied by the calcarine artery, with supplementation from the small branches of the posterior temporal and parieto-occipital arteries. The posterior part of the occipital pole is also supplied by the terminal branches of the middle cerebral artery.

Therefore, the infarction of any branch of the anterior choroidal artery or the middle and posterior cerebral arteries will lead to the contralateral homonymous hemianopia. When the optic radiation or the visual cortex is involved, macular sparing will appear, but macular splitting may be observed if the lesion is located posteriorly. In case that the posterior occipital pole is supplied simultaneously by the calcarine artery, posterior temporal artery and middle cerebral artery, macular sparing may sometimes manifest although the calcarine artery infarction is observed.

References

1. Fengming L. Chinese ophthalmology. 2nd ed. Beijing: People's Medical Publishing House; 2005.
2. Meiyu L. Glaucoma. Beijing: People's Medical Publishing House; 2004.

Part II

Interpretation of Visual Field Test

Visual field, as the name suggests, is the area in which objects can be seen in our vision. As far back as about 400 B.C., Hippocrates, the father of medicine, firstly proposed the concepts of "visual field" and "visual field defect" according to the "hemianopia" state in which patients are able to see only in half of their normal visual fields. Two thousand years later, scientists, including Albrecht von Graefe, Groenouw, Traquair, etc., gradually introduced visual field testing into clinical ophthalmology. They have found that different visual field impairments can be produced by ocular or central nervous system diseases, and the conditions of visual field can be used for staging and locating diagnosis of diseases. Moreover, they also have illustrated the concepts of "island of vision" and "isopter," making visual field develop from a 2-D concept to the 3-D one with the added dimension of visual sensitivity. With regard to visual field testing, starting from the simplest face-to-face examination, to the initial simple visual field screen, to arc perimeter and Bjerrum screen, and then to Goldmann hemispheric projection perimeter, etc., ophthalmologists have researched and developed various perimeters. With the inception, development, and application of automated perimeters, the sensitivity of visual field testing has been improved significantly, and clinical visual field testing has entered a new epoch.

Visual field testing plays a quite important role in the clinical diagnosis and follow-up observation of ocular and nervous system diseases. As far as ocular diseases are concerned, including visual pathway diseases, some present very typical visual field changes, such as bitemporal hemianopia arising from compression by pituitary tumor of the optic chiasm and contralateral homonymous hemianopia resulting from posterior visual pathway diseases. There are still some atypical visual field changes which usually don't point to certain diseases but can frequently be definitively diagnosed through analysis and other examinations, which, from the perspective of visual field, can explain the mechanism of such visual field changes. Among them, there are also some typical visual field changes that do not tell at first glance, which, therefore, are also "atypical." This book focuses on the discussion of atypical visual field changes. This part introduces the basic knowledge of visual field.

Physical and Physiological Bases of the Visual Field

8

Jia Ma, Ning Fan, and Ningli Wang

When an eye fixates on any object in the space, it can not only see clearly the object but also can see objects in a certain space around the fixation point. The summation of the space one eye can see is called the visual field (VF) of this eye. It needs to be noted here that only the space perceived or seen by the tested eye, when it stares at or fixates on the object without any movement, can be called as visual field. Such scale is determined by the distance between the fixating eye and fixation object and the size of the object in the space. Meanwhile, the real visual field, as mentioned above, is a three-dimensional concept, which contains not only the spatial extent that can be perceived around the fixation point but also the visual sensitivities at different positions in the space.

J. Ma
The First Affiliated Hospital, Kunming Medical University, Kunming, China

N. Fan
Shenzhen Eye Hospital, Shenzhen University, Shenzhen, China

N. Wang (✉)
Department of Ophthalmology, Beijing Tongren Hospital, Capital Medical University, Beijing, China

8.1 Units and Standardization

Like vision testing, visual field testing is actually used to test the perception of human eyes to light, belonging to a psychophysical examination. Compared with the central visual acuity tested by visual chart, it is peripheral vision. Essentially, light is a kind of electromagnetic wave. The wavelength range of electromagnetic waves which can be detected by human eyes is between 390 and 770 nm, called visible light. Different wavelengths correspond to different light colors. Normal human eyes are most sensitive to green light with a wavelength of 555 nm but cannot perceive infrared ray over 770 nm or ultraviolet ray less than 390 nm.

The perception of human eyes to light is actually the results of the interaction between the physics of light energy and the physiology of vision. Although Watts, the unit of electromagnetic radiation energy, has been adopted in physics as the unit of luminance, the relevant efficiency of human eyes in perceiving light with different wavelengths should also be taken into consideration in visual field testing. That is luminance flux. Therefore, an ancient unit of luminance flux, viz., apostilb (asb), can be found in actual visual field tests and literature which has been used as the unit of luminance. The background luminance of a perimeter can vary between 0 and 1000 asb [1, 2].

N. Wang et al. (eds.), *Optic Disorders and Visual Field*, Advances in Visual Science and Eye Diseases 2, https://doi.org/10.1007/978-981-13-2502-1_8

Meanwhile, a perimeter measures the visual function by the sensitivity of the tested eye to light. Light sensitivity is the minimum visible luminance which can be represented by the intensity of the light stimulus shown. The light stimuli of Goldmann perimeter have been adopted as the standard currently, and a tenth of their logarithmic units are used as the unit of light sensitivity, i.e., decibel (dB). For example, 10,000 asb is equivalent to the stimulus intensity of Goldmann optical filter 4e, and the logarithmic unit is 0.0. It represents the strongest stimulation that the perimeter can produce. But the tested eye cannot perceive that luminance; therefore, the light sensitivity is 0 dB. Hundred apostilb is equivalent to the stimulus intensity of optical filter 2e, and the logarithmic unit is 1.0, i.e., 10 dB. The weakest stimulation that an automated perimeter can produce is 0.08 asb which corresponds to the light sensitivity of 51 dB, an ideal value beyond the reach of human eyes [1].

Therefore, for a current automated perimeter, in addition to the standardizations of operation and statistical software, the most important is the standardizations in color and luminance of the background light and the stimuli. Only in this way can comparability be realized during the analysis. Of course, even if standard luminance has been adopted for the background light and the light stimuli, the image luminance projected on the retina will still be influenced by the pupil size, the direction and eccentricity of the entering light beam, as well as the opacity of the refractive media.

8.2 Differential Light Threshold

How to understand that the retinal light sensitivity in the visual field test is the minimal visible luminance? It can be understood through the differential light threshold. Under a constant background illumination, the visibility of the light stimuli is 50%. When light stimuli with different intensities are presented repeatedly at one point of the visual field, the dark light stimuli are always invisible with a visibility rate of 0, and the bright ones are always visible with a visibility rate of 100%. If the probability of detecting a light stimulus with certain intensity is 50%, this stimulation intensity can be considered as the differential light threshold of the test point. There is a concept of threshold here just like doorsill actually. The eyes will detect the existence of light when their capability is strong enough to pass the doorsill or threshold. Therefore, differential light threshold is opposite to light sensitivity. The higher the threshold, the higher light stimuli intensity required and the lower the perception to light, i.e., the light sensitivity is relatively low, and vice versa. When the detection is conducted using a size-III white light stimulus following the standard strategy, the weakest stimulation that can be seen by a normal young person at the central fixation point is the maximum sensitivity which is slightly lower than 40 dB. The normal sensitivity within the 30° of the central visual field is between 20 and 40 dB. The sensitivity will reduce significantly if there is any visual field defect. The absolute defect produced in the visual field where the brightest light stimulus cannot be identified is called a blind area [1].

8.3 Light Threshold Fluctuation

As we have known, a visual field test is a psychophysical test, and there are many factors that may lead to variations in the visual field test results of the same patient or even variations in the results at specific sites. Whether the variations are the true visual field impairment or improvement or the interference from other factors needs to be determined.

The dispersion of light threshold results at the same test point in one visual field test usually within 20 min is called short-term fluctuation (SF). Generally, SF of normal people is 1–2 dB. In some diseases such as glaucoma, increase of light threshold dispersion or SF may be manifested firstly at the point before the appearance of confirmed scotoma. The main factors influencing SF include the test method for light threshold, retinal light sensitivity, the cooperation of the patient, false-positive rate and false-negative rate, etc. SF is the foundation for evaluating local visual field defects, i.e., the decrease of local light sensitivity becomes significant only when it exceeds SF.

The light thresholds measured at different times may be different, due to the difference in the physiological response of the visual system and due to the impacts of learning effect, the mental state of the patient, ocular pressure fluctuation, etc. The inconsistency of light thresholds between two tests at different times is called long-term fluctuation (LF). Generally, homogeneous LF of a normal person is 1–1.2 dB and nonhomogeneous LF 0.8–1.3 dB. LF is the premise for quantitative reexamination and comparison of visual field. Only when the LF fluctuates within the normal range can the follow-up evaluation of visual field be carried out [2].

References

1. Xiaoming C, Yuansheng Y. Modern clinical visual field test. Beijing: People's Medical Publishing House; 2000.
2. Yuansheng Y, Jia M, Hui Z. Principle for humphrey visual field test and analysis. Beijing: People's Medical Publishing House; 2005.

9 Normal Visual Field

Jia Ma, Ning Fan, and Ningli Wang

9.1 Normal Visual Field

9.1.1 Definition

Sufficient understanding of what is a normal visual field is the premise to identify abnormal visual fields, especially a mildly abnormal one. A normal visual field includes two key points, spatial extent and light sensitivity, as mentioned above, which is a three-dimensional concept:

(a) The absolute boundary of the visual field should reach a certain target.

A normal visual field extends more than 90° temporally, 60° nasally and superiorly, and 70° inferiorly. The visual fields of both eyes can overlap at the nasal side to form a binocular visual field of 210° horizontally and 130° vertically, with a nonoverlapping 30° area temporally in each eye. The most effective visual field of a single eye is within 30° of fixation, where the clear visual image and color information can be provided, which is also a key area for modern visual field evaluation.

(b) The light sensitivities of each point in the whole visual field should be normal.

There should be no area with light sensitivity reduction or scotoma in a normal visual field except the physiological blind spot. The light sensitivity at the central fixation point is the highest in a normal visual field and will decrease gradually with the increase of eccentricity.

9.1.2 Island of Vision

A 3D island with not only floor area but also different altitudes in different parts has been described above. This is the island of vision described by Traguair. The area of the island of vision represents the extent of the visual field, and the altitude represents light sensitivity (Fig. 9.1). Each point on the retina corresponds to a position on the island of vision. The light sensitivity of the central fixation point, corresponding to the macular fovea, is the highest, i.e., the peak of the island of vision. The light sensitivities of the peripheral visual field corresponding to the peripheral parts of the retina are relatively low, which constitute the peripheral parts of the island of vision with

J. Ma
The First Affiliated Hospital, Kunming Medical University, Kunming, China

N. Fan
Shenzhen Eye Hospital, Shenzhen University, Shenzhen, China

N. Wang (✉)
Department of Ophthalmology, Beijing Tongren Hospital, Capital Medical University, Beijing, China

N. Wang et al. (eds.), *Optic Disorders and Visual Field*, Advances in Visual Science and Eye Diseases 2, https://doi.org/10.1007/978-981-13-2502-1_9

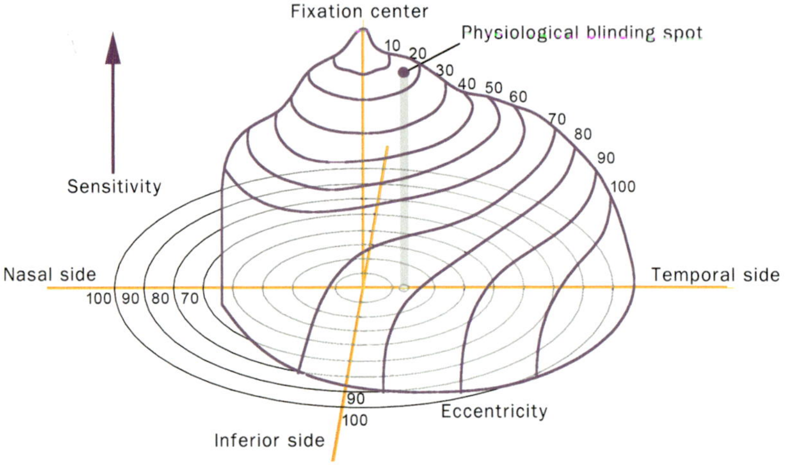

Fig. 9.1 Correspondence between retinal nerve fibers and visual field. A: Optic papillae (Fundus) / Physiological blinding spot (Visual field) B: Macula (Fundus) / Central fixation spot (Visual field) NS: Supranasal quadrant; NI: Inferonasal quadrant; TS: Supratemporal quadrant; TI: Inferotemporal quadrant

relatively low altitudes. Since the nerve fibers of temporal retina are relatively concentrated, the gradual altitude reduction of the corresponding nasal island of vision with the increase of eccentricity is relatively precipitous, while that of the temporal island is relatively gentle. The physiological blind spot is a vertical deep cave formed temporal to the peak. Cutting the island vertically through any longitude, we can obtain a 2D section drawing. The vertical axis of the section represents the altitude or the light sensitivity of each point, while the horizontal axis represents the degree of eccentricity on this longitude [1–5].

9.1.3 Isopter

The vertical altitude of any point on the island of vision is the light sensitivity of this point. The connecting line of the points at the same vertical latitude, or the connecting line of the points with the same light sensitivity, is called the isoheight of the island of vision, or isopter in the visual field. Multiple isopter loops with different sizes can be mapped from the different light sensitivities on the island of vision. As mentioned above, the distances between isopter loops in different parts with different degrees of eccentricity are varied. The slope in the center of the normal island of vision is relatively gentle and the isopter distance is relatively wide. However, the slope in the peripheral part of the island, especially the nasal one, is relatively precipitous, and the isopter distance is relatively narrow. Kinetic perimetry shows the isopters for different light stimuli, while static perimetry shows the outline of the island of vision (Fig. 9.2).

9.1.4 Physiological Blind Spot

The optic disc itself has no visual cells and is thus with no photoreceptive function. Therefore, there is an absolute scotoma in the paracentral area of visual field temporally, called the physiological blind spot, or the blind spot. With a relatively constant position and range, it is 15.5° temporal to the central fixation point and 1.5° inferior to the horizontal raphe, with an area of about 6–8°. The blind spot corresponding to the optic disc is an absolute scotoma, i.e., the stimulus cannot be perceived no matter what kind of stimulation intensity, while the scotoma around the absolute scotoma corresponding to the retina peripheral to the optic disc is a relative scotoma. The light sensitivity of this part is relatively low and the stimulus can be perceived with increased intensity. Some diseases may be manifested as enlargement of the physiological blind spot.

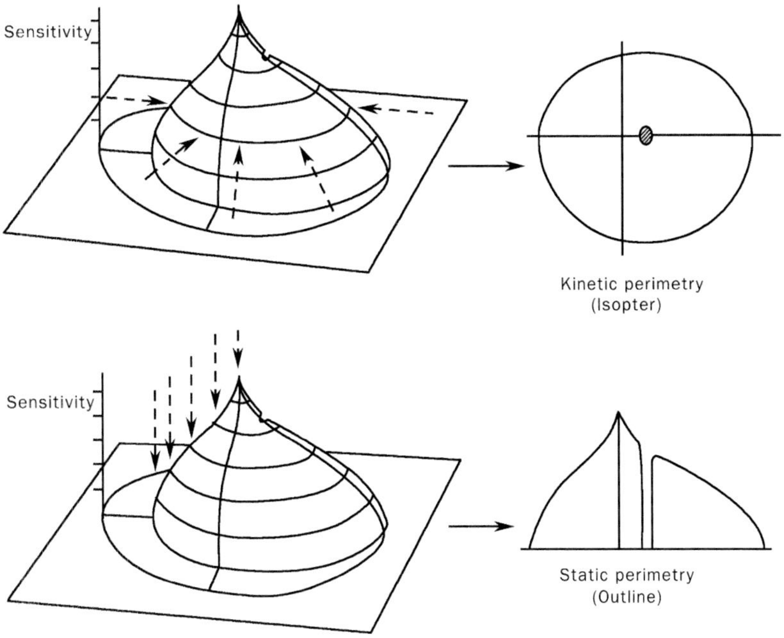

Fig. 9.2 Horizontal and vertical section drawings for island of vision

9.1.5 Symmetry of Normal Visual Fields

The sizes of isopter loops of both eyes of a normal person are generally equivalent, their shapes are basically identical, and the average light sensitivities of the central visual field are also almost the same. With the central fixation point as the center, the horizontal and vertical midlines divide the visual field into four quadrants. The temporal, nasal, superior, and inferior quadrants of the visual field correspond to the nasal, temporal, inferior, and superior quadrants of the retina, respectively, with the macular fovea as the center (Fig. 9.3). Clinically, the visual field within 30° radius of fixation is called the central visual field. Since most RGCs are distributed here, the central visual field is the most commonly concerned area in the visual field test. The area between 5° and 25° is customarily called the paracentral area or the Bjerrum area, which is the most important part in the visual field test for glaucoma. The area out of 30° is called the peripheral visual field [6].

9.2 Physiological and Psychological Factors Affecting Visual Field

9.2.1 Age

Age is one of the principal factors affecting nearly all psychophysical examinations. The RGCs and their nerve fibers will degenerate with the increase of age, the development of cataract will also decrease the actual intensity of the stimuli, and the response time will be prolonged, and therefore, the average sensitivity of the retina will decrease, and the isopter will constrict concentrically. In an automated perimeter, the total deviation probability can correct for every full year for the same point to remove the impact of age, and meanwhile, the pattern deviation probability can remove the impact produced by refractive media opacity resulting from factors such as age once again, thus making the test results closer to the real damages.

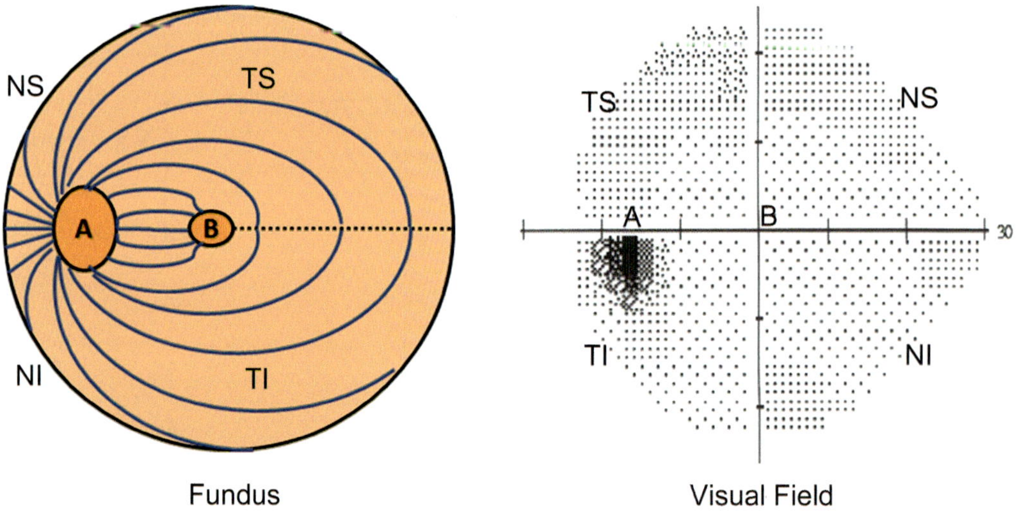

Fig. 9.3 Correspondence between retinal nerve fibers and visual field

9.2.2 Fixation Condition

Good fixation is essential to complete the visual field test. Those with poor fixation for whom even the physiological blind spot cannot be located will have a poor precision of the visual field test. Since the physiological eye movements exist, including random eye movements and inherent nystagmus, absolute fixation in human eyes is almost impossible in a general visual field test. Random eye movements can be overcome through training and voluntary cooperation, but inherent nystagmus cannot be controlled manually. In an automated perimeter, there is an excellent fixation tracing system and fixation loss evaluation that can conveniently screen out the unreliable tests.

9.2.3 Light or Darkness Adaptation of the Tested Eye

Under the darkness adaptation, the light sensitivity of the retina except the macular fovea will increase, and the peak of the island of vision will become relatively flat. Conversely, the function of the macula becomes the best under the light adaptation. Therefore, constant background illumination is required for a perimeter, not only to form a certain comparison with the light stimuli but also to maintain the adaptation state of the retina. The standard background illumination for most perimeters is 31.5 asb, close to the darkest intensity of photopic vision that can be perceived under the common office illumination. The tested eyes should adapt adequately the consistent background illumination of perimeter in each test, otherwise, different visual field results may be obtained due to the different stress states of the retina.

9.2.4 Pupil Size

The retinal illumination is about proportional to the square of the pupil diameter. The pupil being too big or too small will affect the visual field test results, and the impact of the latter is more significant. The former will affect the retinal imaging quality because of the increasing optic aberration effect of crystalline lens and the decreasing depth of focus. The latter will reduce the amount of light entering the eyes and the actual retinal illumination, and then the decreasing average light sensitivity or the concentric constriction of isopter may appear. The diameter of the pupil is usually required to be bigger than 2.5 mm in a visual field test.

9.2.5 Refractive Error

Uncorrected refractive errors do not allow the light stimulus to form a single focus on the retinal plane, and the blurred object image has a slightly bigger area and lower luminance compared with the actual one. The peripheral retina has better space accumulation effects, where the increased stimulation intensity resulting from the increase of image area can compensate the decrease of stimulation intensity caused by the luminance reduction. Therefore, the impact on the peripheral visual field test is relatively small. The central retina with relatively poor space accumulation effects will produce false diffuse decrease of light sensitivity or isopter concentric constriction. Therefore, the various refractive errors of a patient should be corrected routinely in the visual field test of the central 30°, especially when small light stimuli are used. It should also be noted that additional correction for accommodation should be given to a patient in light of the test distance of current automated perimeters to avoid the decrease of light sensitivity caused by refractive blurred vision.

9.2.6 Learning Effect and Degree of Cooperation

The isopter in a second test is slightly bigger than that obtained in the initial visual field test. Such effect of visual field enlargement resulting from the familiarity with the test procedure is called learning effect. The learning effect is more significant in the test of peripheral visual field. The impact of the learning effect will become smaller with the increase of the number of retests. Whether a patient cooperates or focuses on the test will greatly affect the visual field test results, and educational level is the key factor. The higher the educational level, the bigger the tested area of visual field may be obtained.

9.2.7 Upper Eyelid Location and Optical Frame Edge

The extent of the superior visual field is the narrowest 60° due to the existence of the upper eyelid, and the superior visual field may be further blocked in many patients with ptosis or blepharoptosis. False images of concentrically constricted visual fields will also be observed when a patient wears glasses with relatively thick optical frame edges during the test. Therefore, these influencing factors should be avoided as far as possible in the test.

9.2.8 Examination Duration

Excessively long duration of the visual field test can make a patient tired and lead to the increase of false-negative errors, and the results will be unstable and unreliable. The duration of a common visual field test should not exceed 15–20 min for each eye. The test duration may vary from method to method. Current automated perimeters have shortened considerably the test duration without affecting the reliability of the test results through advanced algorithm.

It needs to be pointed out that a correct visual field test result may often require repeated tests due to the presence of multiple influencing factors. This is extremely important for the discussion of "atypical" visual field changes in this book because it should be determined firstly whether such visual field change has reflected the real condition of a patient's visual field. In comparison, it is rare for a typical visual field change to show a relatively big distortion. All of the visual field printouts included in this book were the actual reflection of patients' visual field conditions, and those extremely rare results with relatively poor reliability had been indicated in the text [1, 7].

References

1. Xiaoming C, Yuansheng Y. Modern clinical visual field test. Beijing: People's Medical Publishing House; 2000.
2. Yuansheng Y, Jia M, Hui Z. Principle for humphrey visual field test and analysis. Beijing: People's Medical Publishing House; 2005.
3. Neil TC, Russell PE. Visual field testing with the humphrey field analyzer: a text and clinical atlas. New Jersey: SLACK Incorporated; 1999.
4. Ulrich S. Visual field defects: essentials for neurologists. J Neurol. 2003;250(4):407–11.
5. Heijl A. Essence of reading and analysis on visual field (translated by Yuan Yuansheng, Zhong Hua, Ma Jia). Shanghai: Shanghai Popular Science Press; 2013.
6. Yi T, Shihui W, Siwei Y. Basis and clinical progress of visual pathway diseases. Beijing: People's Medical Publishing House; 2010.
7. Yuansheng Y, Hua Z. Modern clinical visual field test. Beijing: People's Medical Publishing House; 2015.

Visual Field Test

10

Jia Ma, Ning Fan, and Ningli Wang

10.1 Basic Principle of Visual Field Test

Clinically, we usually carry out the monocular visual field test on the two eyes separately so that a comparison between them can be conducted. Sometimes, a binocular visual field test may be performed in situations such as tests for drivers. The fixation status of the tested eye should be emphasized repeatedly, whatever the test type. Light stimuli with certain intensity are presented dynamically or statically on the background with uniform illumination under the fixation status to determine the differential light threshold or the area where it is visible [1–4].

10.1.1 Kinetic Perimetry

The weakest intensity of stimuli just perceivable at a point in the visual field is the light sensitivity of this point, or light threshold for short. The connecting line of neighboring points with the same threshold or light sensitivity is called the isopter of this stimulus with such intensity. This stimulus cannot be seen at points out of the isopter (subthreshold stimulation), can just be seen on the isopter (threshold stimulation), and can always be seen at any point within the isopter (suprathreshold stimulation). Therefore, an isopter is the boundary line between areas where the stimulus with certain intensity is visible and invisible. In a kinetic perimetry or kinetic test, the light stimulus with certain intensity is presented from the peripheral area (where it is invisible) to the central area (where it is visible) and then presented reversely to detect the position where the stimulus can just be seen, which is crossed twice to map the isopter of this intensity. In the visual field analysis printouts, there are different isopters of the light stimuli with different intensities (Fig. 10.1). A kinetic test can conveniently and quickly find the obvious visual field constriction or depression but easily neglect the local small and deep defects inside the visual field. It's usually used in the screening for visual pathway diseases.

In clinical practice, it's difficult for bedridden patients, children, or patients with mental retardation to complete the relatively complicated perimeter testing. In this case, the confrontation method, which is more straightforward, can be adopted to rapidly test the general condition of

J. Ma
The First Affiliated Hospital, Kunming Medical University, Kunming, China

N. Fan
Shenzhen Eye Hospital, Shenzhen University, Shenzhen, China

N. Wang (✉)
Department of Ophthalmology, Beijing Tongren Hospital, Capital Medical University, Beijing, China

N. Wang et al. (eds.), *Optic Disorders and Visual Field*, Advances in Visual Science and Eye Diseases 2, https://doi.org/10.1007/978-981-13-2502-1_10

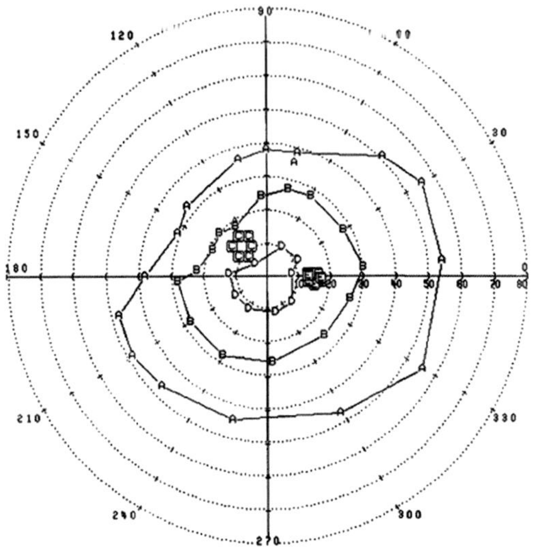

Fig. 10.1 Different isopters obtained from a kinetic visual field test

those patients' visual fields. There are many ways to carry out this method, but the basic principle is the same as that of a kinetic test. The patient covers the non-tested eye with one hand and stares at the contralateral eye of the examiner with the tested eye or stares at the examiner's nasal tip with a distance of around 1 m or 50 cm. Then, the examiner presents or moves a target, such as cotton swab, finger, pointolite, etc., between them from the peripheral area to the central area under the condition that the fixation of the tested eye is ensured. The visual field of the patient is determined through the comparison of the perception between the patient and the examiner. If double targets are used in the test, two identical targets are placed respectively on the two sides of the middle line, and a relative visual field defect may exist if the target is perceived to be darkened, and an absolute defect may be considered if only one target is seen. It's also a relatively quick and effective method to detect whether there is hemianopia.

Regardless of manual or instrument-assisted testing, generally, the extent of a normal monocular visual field, due to the impacts of the orbit, eyelid, and nose, is 60° superiorly, 75° inferiorly, 60° nasally, and 100° temporally, with the outer boundary contouring an irregular oval. The center of the physiological blind spot is 15.5° temporal to the fixation point and 1.5° inferior to the horizontal raphe. Its vertical diameter is 8° and horizontal diameter 6°. Corresponding to the outline of the island of vision, the isopter loop is a slightly horizontal oval, and the distance between different isopters is relatively sparse temporally and relatively crowded nasally.

10.1.2 Static Perimetry

A series of light stimuli with different intensities are presented at one point in a static perimetry or a static test of visual field. The intensity of the stimulus with 50% visibility is defined as the threshold (value in dB) or the light sensitivity of this point. In the static test, a suprathreshold stimulus potentially visible is presented at the tested point firstly. If the stimulus is seen, the intensity of the stimulus is decreased progressively by a step size of 4 dB till the stimulus becomes invisible to the tested eye, and then the intensity is increased progressively by a step size of 2 dB till the stimulus becomes visible. This intensity is determined as the light sensitivity or light threshold of that point. It may suggest a visual field defect if the light threshold at the point in the visual field increases, i.e., the light sensitivity decreases. The static test can easily find local defects in the visual field, but the test duration is relatively long and the procedure is complicated. An automated perimeter has made it possible for the automation and standardization of the threshold calculation of all points and the tracing of patients' responses during the test, thus significantly improving the comparability among the results obtained from different tests.

After the threshold test, a computerized automated perimeter will automatically perform the comparison between the tested value and the normal value for the same age group at each corresponding point and will present the visual field test results in ways including numeric printouts, grayscale maps and probability plots, etc. (Fig. 10.2).

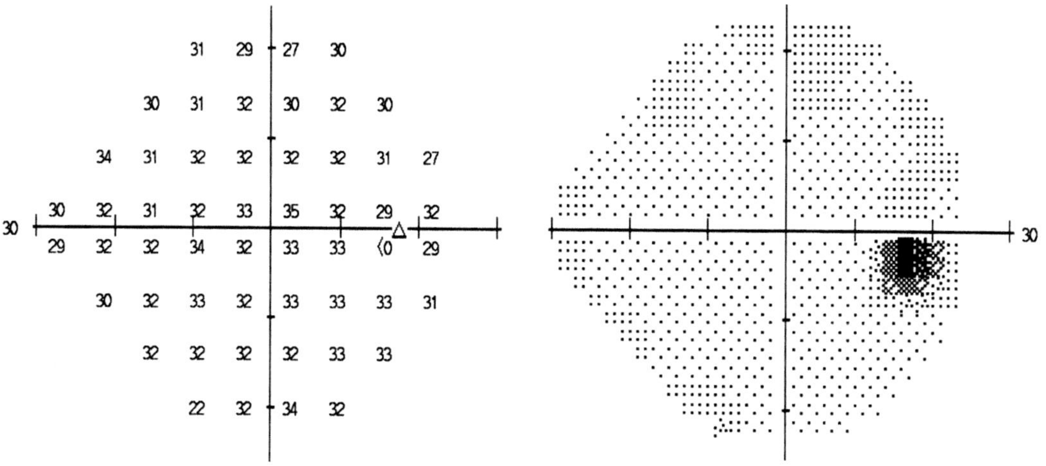

Fig. 10.2 A threshold value printout and a grayscale map produced in a static perimetry

10.1.3 Suprathreshold Test

The light stimulus belongs to the suprathreshold stimulation if its intensity is within the range of the isopter. Abnormality of visual field may exist, such as isopter depression and a local scotoma, if the suprathreshold light stimuli visible theoretically cannot be seen in the range of an isopter. A suprathreshold test, or screening test, is usually used for the screening for glaucoma or nervous system diseases. It can quickly reveal some significant visual field impairments, after which additional kinetic or static tests may be performed for further diagnoses.

10.2 Visual Field Tests in Clinical Practice

With the development of the science and technology, the types of perimeters have changed rapidly since the nineteenth century. It has developed from the tangent visual field screen, arc perimeter, Amsler's grid at the early stage, to Goldmann perimeter, which is the golden standard for the kinetic test, and finally to the computerized automated perimeters with Humphrey perimeter and Octopus perimeter as their representatives. Visual field testing has entered a historic new chapter. Of course, either the instrument-assisted tests or the confrontation methods, usually adopted in the first-line clinical practice, are nothing else but the kinetic, static, or suprathreshold tests mentioned above in terms of their basic principles. The advantages of automated perimeters include the visualized test results and advanced follow-up analysis software. Here, we would like to take the basic Goldmann perimeter and Humphrey/Octopus automated perimeter as the representatives to introduce briefly how to understand and apply the visual field test results.

10.2.1 Goldmann Perimeter and Its Light Stimuli

The Goldmann perimeter is a hemispheric projecting perimeter which was once the most widely used manual perimeter in the world. Its projection screen for light stimuli is a hemispheric-like bowl in shape, with the inner surface being uniform white background. The light stimuli are the light spots projected on the background with uniform illumination. The background illumination, the size and brightness of light stimuli, and testing distance can all be standardized. As the test standard, Goldmann light stimulus series have continued to be used in current computerized automated perimeters. There are three adjusting slots, respectively, separating the brightness of light stimuli into 5 gears of a, b, c, d, and e, increasing progressively by 0.1 logarithmic unit; 4 gears of 1, 2, 3, and 4, increasing progressively by 0.5 logarithmic unit; and 6 gears of 0, I, II, III, IV, and V, with the areas of the light spots being 1/16, 1/4, 1, 4, 16, and 64 mm^2, respectively. A series of standard light stimuli with different intensities can be obtained through different combinations of the gears in the three adjusting slots. All the Goldmann standard stimuli are far smaller than the physiological blind spot in size. The Goldmann perimeter can be used flexibly in the tests of the central or peripheral visual field and is mainly used in kinetic isopters mapping and suprathreshold screening [1].

10.2.2 Computerized Automated Perimeter

Standardized automated perimeter (SAP) is mainly used for static tests to analyze quantitatively visual field defect depth through testing the light sensitivity of a patient, thus describing the severity of the visual field defects.

10.2.2.1 Instrument Settings of Automated Perimeters

Humphrey perimeter is a fully automatic projection perimeter. In particular, the projection screen for the HFA II perimeter has been changed from the original hemispheric shape into a bullet shape, which has minimized the difference in vision clarity caused by the spherical surface. The standard background illumination of the perimeter is 31.5 asb, close to the minimal brightness of photopic vision, i.e., daily brightness of natural light, which has been internationally recognized as the standard of background illumination. Moreover, the visibility of an object under the photopic vision depends more on the contrast light luminance rather than absolute luminance, and the changes in pupil size and the color and transparency of the crystalline lens have relatively small impacts on the test results. The light stimulus intensity of the perimeter varies from 0.08 to 10,000 asb, i.e., varies from 0 to 51 dB. The stimuli sizes are identical with the Goldmann stimuli of levels I–V. The commonly used stimulus is a 0.43° Goldmann Size III stimulus with a presentation duration of 200 ms. Sometimes, a Goldmann Size V stimulus can be used for the tests on patients with serious visual field defects. The commonly used test is the white-on-white test, i.e., a test carried out with a white Size III stimulus on a white screen. The Octopus perimeter is a hemispheric projection computerized perimeter with a background illumination of 4 asb. The presentation duration is just 100 ms, and the intensity of the stimulus can be only 1000 asb, thus avoiding the possibility of the disperse effect caused by strong stimulation and reducing the false-positive rate.

10.2.2.2 Test Patterns for Automated Perimetry

It's impossible for us to test all the points in the visual field in actual operations. Therefore, different test patterns have been designed in automated perimeters according to the island of vision of normal human eyes and the characteristics of different visual field impairments. The points that are vulnerable to injury are screened by sample survey to constitute the different grids for different tests. An expert visual field examiner can select effective tests according to different diseases and focus on some vulnerable areas so that the sensitivity and specificity of the test can be improved. Humphrey and Octopus perimeters have different test patterns to carry out the threshold test, screening test, and automatic screening through the combination of the aforementioned two tests, etc., but their analysis softwares are almost the same. Different patterns can be used to carry out quantitative, semiquantitative, or qualitative analyses for abnormal visual fields, follow-up monitoring of disease changes, and observation of therapeutic effects and outcome via comparison with the baseline visual field [1, 4, 5].

Threshold Test Patterns

Although the extent of a normal visual field is relatively large, most of the diagnostic visual field tests focus on the area within 30° of the fixation, i.e., the central visual field, because most of the RGCs are distributed in this area. Humphrey threshold test patterns commonly used are standard testing grids (Figs. 10.3 and 10.4), including central 30-2, 24-2, 10-2, macular threshold, peripheral 30/60-2 patterns or tests, etc. Besides, there are also tests for neurological diseases, such as temporal crescent. Among these test patterns, the 30-2 pattern can detect 76 points within 30° of the fixation, and the 24-2 pattern can detect 54 points that not only cover the central 52 points within the central 24° of the 30-2 pattern but also highlight the 2 points at nasal 30°. The point intervals of both patterns are 6°. The latter shortens the test duration significantly without loss of diagnostic information; meanwhile, it can better avoid the artifact effects produced by trial lens and eyelids. There are similar test patterns in Octopus perimeter, such as 32 and G1, which have become the most frequently used patterns. The 10-2 pattern can be adopted to carry out the elaborate test on the 68 points in 10° of the center with a point interval of 2°, for the observation of the residual visual function in those patients with serious visual field impairments with only the central island of vision left. The test for glaucoma mainly focuses on the central visual field rather than the peripheral one due to the great peripheral sensitivity variation. For diseases of the central nervous system, most of the diagnostic information also appears in the central visual field. Therefore, 30-2 and 24-2 patterns have become the most commonly used.

Screening Test Patterns

The grids for the screening test patterns are similar to those for the threshold test patterns, which are mainly used in general surveys, the physical examinations for special occupational workers, or tests for special diseases. For example, it can be used to detect whether the patients in ophthalmic or special clinics have certain special types of visual field defects. For patients with suspected optic neuritis, the screening test should focus on the macular area for central scotoma. For patients with suspected glaucoma, the glaucoma screening pattern should be selected to test whether there is a paracentral scotoma or a nasal step. For patients with suspected pituitary tumor, the hemianopia test pattern should be selected to mainly determine whether there is vertical hemianopia. The screening patterns have also adopted in some cases mentioned in this book.

Other Patterns

Some types of Humphrey perimeters are equipped with the kinetic test pattern which can be used to

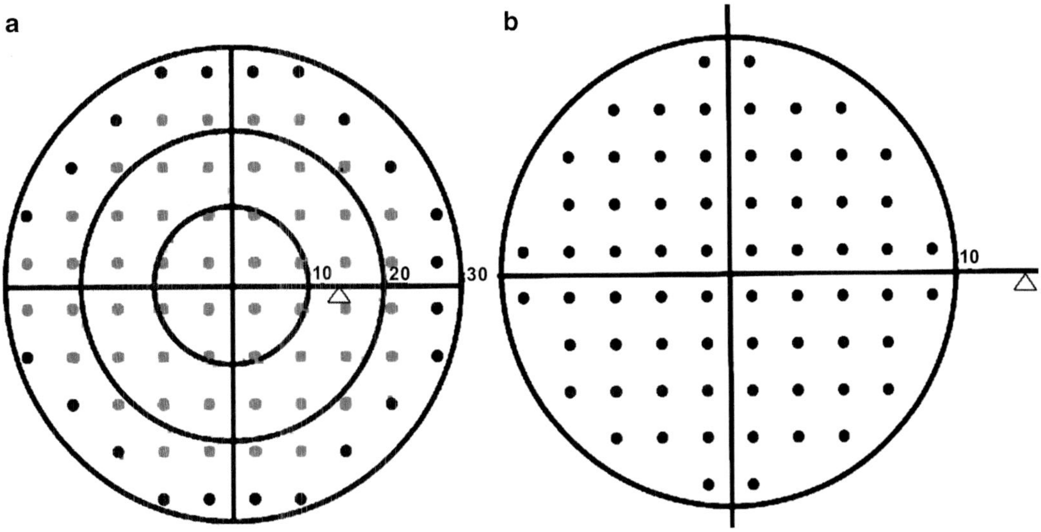

Fig. 10.3 The grids of 30-2, 24-2, and 10-2 patterns. Panel a, 30-2 pattern with gray and black points and 24-2 pattern with gray points; Panel b, 10-2 pattern

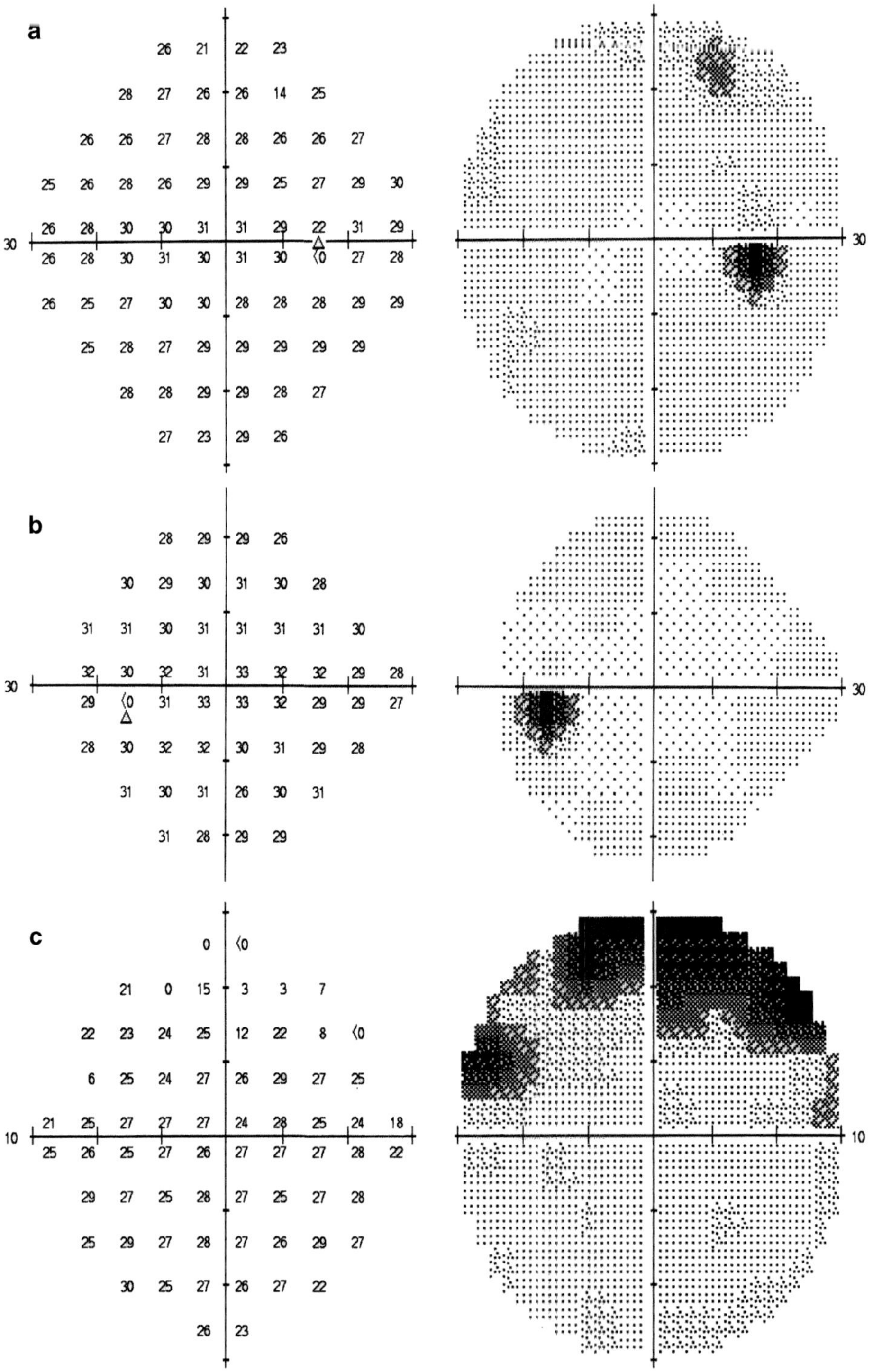

Fig. 10.4 Numeric printouts and grayscale maps of the above three patterns. Panel a, 30-2 pattern; Panel b, 24-2 pattern; Panel c, 10-2 pattern

map the isopters of the peripheral visual field. In the automated diagnosis pattern, suprathreshold stimuli can be used firstly, and then a quantitative threshold test can be used to detect the defect depth, if any visual field defect is observed. Besides, as a pattern specific to the Humphrey perimeter, custom pattern can be used to carry out testing with the diagnosis grids designed by the examiner himself/herself, which is quite practical.

10.2.2.3 Strategy Selections for Automated Perimeters

Besides all the test patterns, the reasons why automated perimeters are advanced also lie in the advanced algorithms which can provide different light stimuli presentation protocols based on the different strategies selected. Taking Humphrey perimeter as an example, the strategies have developed from the earlier full threshold and FastPAC to the later Swedish interactive thresholding algorithm standard (SITA standard) and then to SITA Fast. SITA Fast can shorten the test duration by 3/4 without efficiency decrease, which significantly reduces the false results from the lower patient compliance due to the long-time operation. Generally, for patients having difficulties with the testing, SITA Standard is preferred, while for patients with testing experience or young patients, SITA Fast is preferred. Of course, it is advised that each doctor select one preferred strategy as the standard for each patient, because standardization will make it possible to compare between the results obtained from different tests.

Although perimeters look very complicated, the test principle remains unchanged. A visual field examiner should not only be familiar with the test patterns, strategies, and skills of perimeters but also master the different characteristics of visual field changes in various diseases. For instance, whether there is paracentral scotomas or a nasal step should be paid attention to for glaucoma, central scotoma for optic neuritis, and vertical hemianopia for pituitary tumor. An expert examiner can select an effective test pattern, even combine several test strategies according to different diseases, and focus on some vulnerable areas, so that the sensitivity and specificity of the visual field test can be improved significantly.

10.3 Analysis on Results of Automated Perimeters

10.3.1 Printouts

Regardless of the STATPAC analysis of Humphrey or the CO analysis of Octopus, the printouts for the test results of computerized automated perimeters are different because different diseases are tested with different tests, but they always contain general patient data, test pattern, strategy, reliability indices, gaze tracking record, and a series of analysis maps [1, 4–6] (Figs. 10.5 and 10.6).

10.3.1.1 General Patient Data and Test Parameters

Printouts of visual field analysis always include the general data of the patient and examination parameters, such as name, age, test time, size and color of the light stimulus, background luminance, test duration, and the degree of correcting lens. All these records not only support the specific analysis of the visual field but also are beneficial to follow-up tests under the same conditions as far as possible for a comparative analysis.

10.3.1.2 Numeric Printouts

The actual sensitivities of each testing point obtained from two examinations during the threshold test and expressed in dB values are printed in a plot, and this plot is called a numeric printout. Furthermore, the defect depths expressed in dB values resulting from comparison between the detected sensitivity and the normal sensitivity at the same point of the corresponding age group are printed in a plot, and this plot is called the total deviation numerical plot. Meanwhile, the difference between the actual threshold value detected from each point and the expected value without considering the refractive media opacity are printed in another plot, and this plot is called the pattern deviation

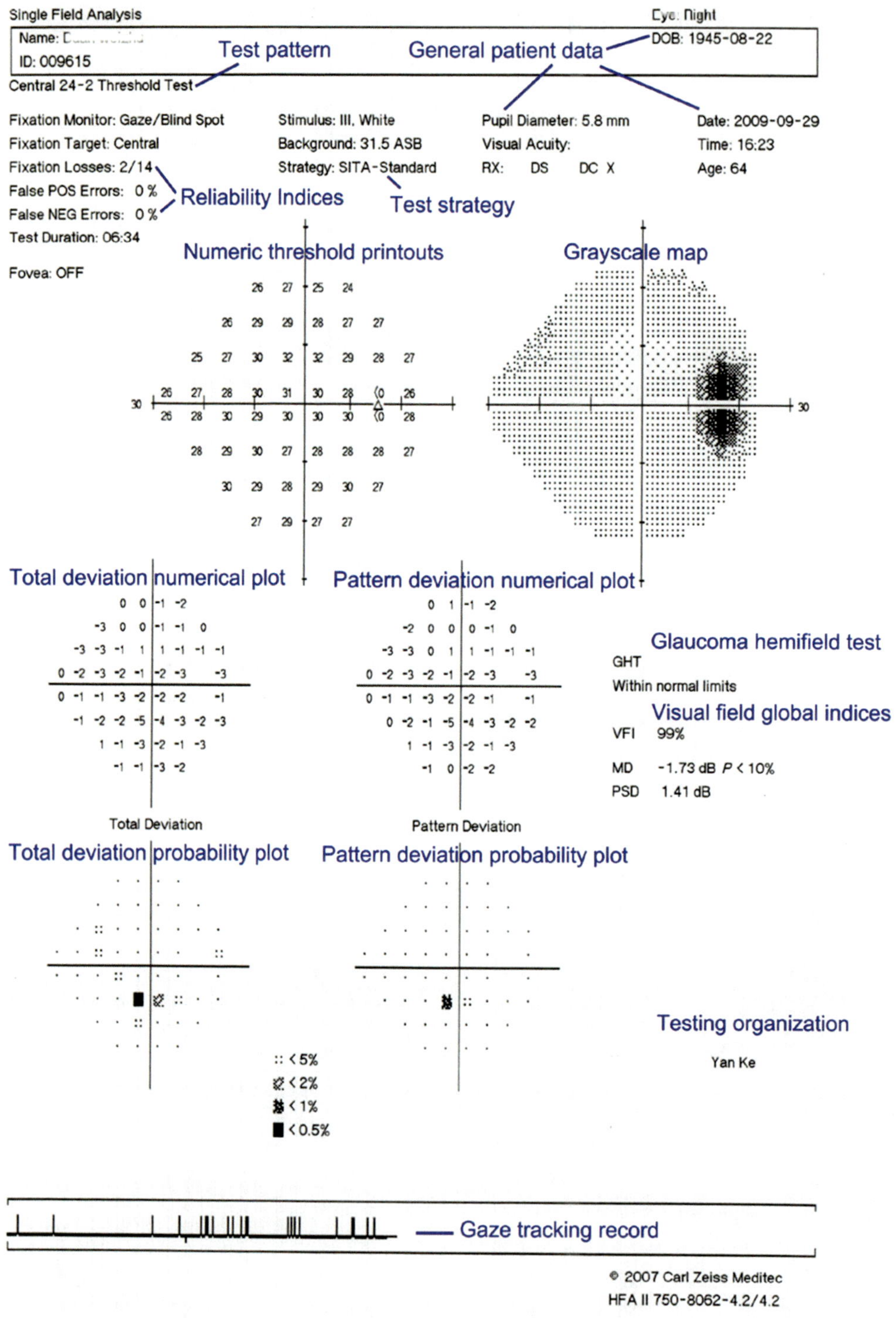

Fig. 10.5 Single field analysis (SFA) printouts of STATPAC analysis in Humphrey perimeter

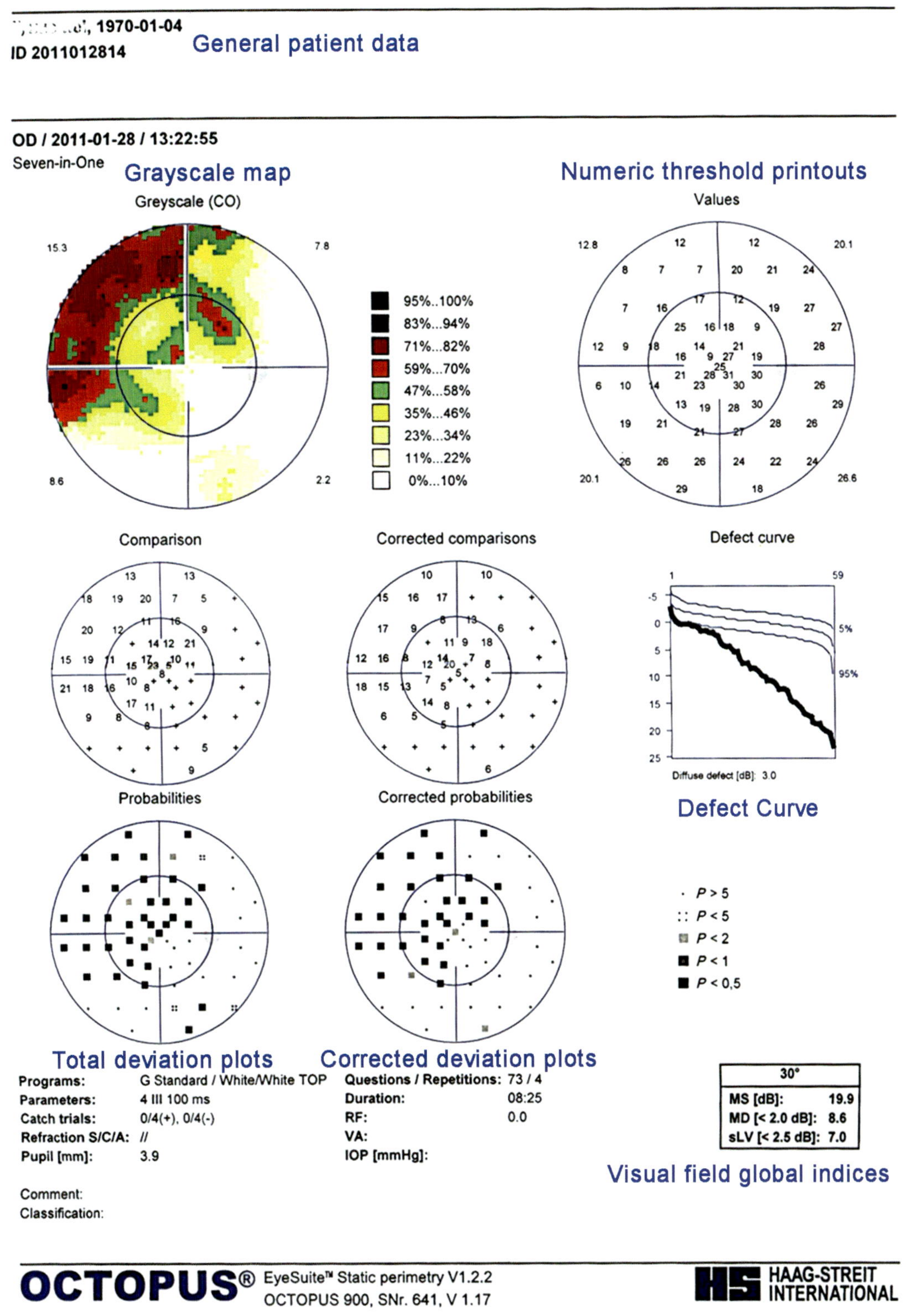

Fig. 10.6 SFA printouts of CO analysis in Octopus perimeter

numerical plot. All these numerical printouts can exhibit the defect severity to doctors and patients in a visualized and straightforward fashion. However, due to the interference of eccentricity on the dB value, the occurrence or progression of visual field impairment cannot be judged correctly through these printouts without abundant experience.

10.3.1.3 Grayscale Map

The different unprocessed dB values of sensitivity at each point are expressed by different grayscales, and the conversion ratio between grayscale and dB value are printed at the bottom of printout. The bigger the dB value, the lighter the grayscale; the smaller the dB value, the darker the grayscale. A darker grayscale indicates a lower light sensitivity in this area. In this way, an apparent picture on the island of vision and local defect can be shown to the doctor. In the normal visual field, the grayscale is the lightest at the central fixation point and the darkest at the physiological blind spot and darker and darker toward the peripheral areas. No darker areas should be found in the same grayscale range in the normal visual field. But since comparison between these grayscales and the normal range has not been carried out, we cannot identify the visual field loss with statistical significance from the printouts. Sometimes mild lesion may be easily neglected due to the general high or low sensitivity at the early stage of disease. Therefore, grayscale maps are usually used to analyze false visual field loss or serious visual field defects.

10.3.1.4 Probability Statistics Analysis Plots

As mentioned above, total deviation numerical plot and pattern deviation numerical plot are obtained by calculating the deviation between the detected value and the estimated normal value based on large-sample-size normal value database. Variance analysis or empirical pattern is adopted further to estimate whether the deviation is a defect or normal variation. Appropriate symbols at points are used to indicate the points with sensitivities lower than those in the normal population in the same age group by 5%, 2%, 1% or 0.5%. The darker the symbol, the higher the possibility of a defect. The total deviation probability plot and pattern deviation probability plot in Humphrey (corrected probability plot in Octopus) are thus obtained. For example, when a 2% symbol appears, it indicates that 98% of the normal population in the same age group are expected to have higher sensitivity values than the detected one at this point, so the change at this point is significant. The result is obtained after comparison with the empirical probability values in the visual fields of the normal population and correction for the physiological attenuation of sensitivities from the central to the peripheral visual field. Therefore, the visual field change reflected by the result is relatively objective. Especially for early local defects, pattern deviation probability plot can further correct the visual field change resulting from the refractive media opacity and distinguish them from other diseases, so it is the most meaningful analysis focusing on the mild but statistically significant variation in the single field analysis. Clinically, the impact of cataract is suggested if general sensitivity reduction appears in total deviation probability plot but no change in normal pattern deviation probability plot. On the contrary, trigger-happy mentioned below is usually indicated in a patient if the patient has a worse result in pattern deviation probability plot than the one in total deviation probability plot.

10.3.1.5 Glaucoma Hemifield Test

On the basis of the probability analysis, Asman et al., according to the anatomy characteristics of the running of retinal nerve fibers and the different patterns of glaucoma damages in superior and inferior hemifields, divided the superior and inferior hemifields of the central 30° of 30-2 or 24-2 test into five pairs of mirror-image zones respectively, with the horizontal raphe as the boundary. In the comparison between the superior and inferior hemifields, the following brief warning words can be used to classify the visual fields, "within normal limits," "borderline," "general reduction of sensitivity," or "outside normal limits." This is the glaucoma hemifield

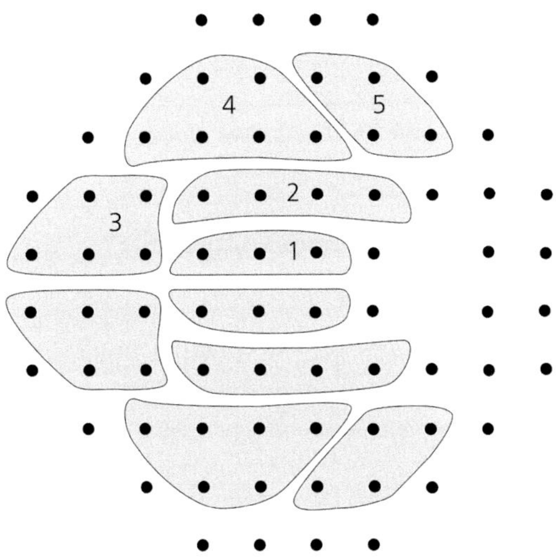

Fig. 10.7 Mirror-image areas of superior and inferior hemifields in GHT

test (GHT), which is very useful in distinguishing the early change of visual field in glaucoma (Fig. 10.7), especially for beginners. However, the test is not sensitive for determining the visual field loss caused by nervous system or retinal diseases [4–6].

10.3.1.6 Symbol Printouts

Symbol printouts are used for the suprathreshold test as a part of the screening test, with several symbols representing whether the stimulus can be seen or not and whether a defect is a relative one or an absolute one. The printouts can give doctors an initial impression on the visual field condition, but they are just an initial reference, because they cannot determine the depth of visual field defects.

10.3.1.7 Defect Depth Maps

Sometimes the perimeter will give a 3-in-1 printout including grayscale, defect depth, and threshold values, when the visual field impairment is too serious to obtain the specific numerical or probability analysis. It's an original expression without age correction or probability symbols. The map is a straightforward presentation of results but still has no standardized data and cannot be analyzed in statistics.

10.3.2 Reliability Analyses

As visual field testing is a psychophysical test, the testing process of a computerized automated perimeter relies completely on the patient's response. In order to monitor whether a patient's fixation is available or whether excessive false-positive or false-negative responses exist, the automated perimeter is equipped with the "capture experiment" program to quantify the false-positive rate, false-negative rate, and fixation loss rate, through which the authenticity of the test results can be determined. Besides the value of fraction or percentage, the printouts will also use "XX" to indicate the unreliable indices. It's a priority to determine the reliability of the results during the visual field analysis. Any unreliable results should be removed or tested repeatedly.

The reliability of all the visual field reports mentioned in this book meets the requirements, and a few tests with relatively poor reliability have been indicated in the text. The information about reliability indices is not shown in the visual field reports due to limited space [1, 4–6].

10.3.2.1 False-Positive Response Errors

The false-positive response error score (FP) measures a patient's response even without seeing any stimulus. The reason may be a kind of habitual implication resulting from the mechanical sounds or the rhythm produced by the projection of light stimuli. Any response to the mechanical sounds proportionally presented by the automated perimeter without actual stimuli will be recorded as false-positive response. Some anxious patients, who are eager to see the most or even all of stimuli during the test, will try their best to press frequently the response button even without seeing any stimulus, which results in many false-positive responses. Consequently, the threshold values at some test points may reach such a level as nobody can see, representing a typical "trigger-happy" visual field featuring an abnormally bright or even completely white image with disappearance of the physiological blind spot in the grayscale map. In this case, the patient should complete the test again under guidance. FP should be lower than 15%, or a retest will be required. And the further guided progression analysis (GPA) will also remove automatically the results with FP higher than 15%.

10.3.2.2 False-Negative Response Errors

False-negative response error score (FN) is used to assess the self-control and attention of the patient. The perimeter will present a brightest stimulus in an area for which the threshold value has been obtained, and it will record a false-negative response if the patient fails to respond, which means distraction. High FN indicates that retinal light sensitivities are relatively low in the results. FN should be lower than 33% in a Humphrey perimeter.

10.3.2.3 Fixation Loss

An automated perimeter projects the stimuli proportionally and randomly onto the physiological blind spot area to assess patient's gaze stability. If the patient responds to these stimuli, the perimeter will record it into fixation loss (FL). FL must be lower than 20%, otherwise the test result will be considered unreliable.

In a Humphrey perimeter, there's a gaze tracking system, which can measure the changes of fixation direction with an accuracy of 1° and automatically record fixation directions every time the stimulus is presented. A chart with different up-and-down fluctuation lines is used to reflect different fixation conditions. The lines above the baseline denote the fixation loss during the whole test, and a maximum fixation error of 10° or more can be indicated. The lines below the baseline show the failure of the machine to detect a certain fixation direction, such as due to a blink during a stimulus presentation. In addition to being printed out as a part of the result, the line chart is also displayed on the screen during the whole test process, which helps the examiner monitor the test.

10.3.3 Visual Field Global Indices

Since the threshold values of different points have been quantified in a computerized automated perimeter, whether the visual field is normal or whether a defect is diffuse or localized, etc. can be analyzed further through quantitative indicators such as visual field global indices [4]. The common indices include:

10.3.3.1 Mean Sensitivity (MS)

MS refers to the arithmetic mean of the light sensitivities at each point in the visual field, which reflects the mean light sensitivity of the retina. This index is still displayed by an Octopus perimeter but not by a Humphrey perimeter.

10.3.3.2 Mean Deviation (MD)

MD refers to the difference of light sensitivities between the tested eye and those of normal people from the same age group. It is the weighted mean of the values at each point in total deviation numerical plot, and it reflects the extent of decrease of the whole retinal light sensitivity. In normal people, MD fluctuates around 0 dB. The bigger the negative value, the more serious the visual field loss. However, it cannot reflect whether there is any local damage. The Octopus perimeters also provide an accumulative defect curve, which can provide a status of the whole deviation from the normal visual field. It shows whether the mean deviation is within the normal range of confidence interval. Extensive depression of the visual field is indicated if it is far lower than the normal limit, but it cannot reflect the local damage condition, either.

10.3.3.3 Visual Field Index (VFI)

VFI is the enhanced version of MD. It's less influenced by cataract and more sensitive to central visual field changes, which can correspond better to the ganglion cell loss. The VFI value of a normal visual field approximates 100%, while the VFI of a blind eye approximates 0%.

10.3.3.4 Pattern Standard Deviation (PSD)

PSD is an index in the Humphrey perimeter to determine whether there is localized damage. The PSD of a normal visual field is 0. It will increase when there is any localized damage and then decrease when the localized damage reaches certain severity and turns into more serious diffuse damage. Therefore, PSD values are all positive but nonlinear and exhibit a parabolic change pattern. They cannot be used for staging or progression analysis.

10.3.3.5 Corrected Loss Variance (CLV)

CLV is an index in the Octopus perimeter to determine whether there is localized damage. The CLV of a normal visual field or in case of diffuse depression fluctuates around 0. CLV will increase if there are localized visual field defects, such as scotomas and localized depression. It will not be influenced by measuring errors.

10.3.4 Visual Field Baseline and Follow-Up

10.3.4.1 Testing Conditions for Baseline and Follow-Up of Visual Field

Some patients, especially those with glaucoma and nervous system diseases, need regular follow-up tests on visual field to monitor progressions or therapeutic effects, which makes it necessary to develop a certain baseline for their visual fields. The first visual field test is not necessarily the best candidate for baseline. Due to learning effect, there's a big difference in the results between the first test and the second one. It can be adopted as the baseline if these two test results are equivalent. However, a third test should be carried out if the difference is relatively big. The results of the latter two tests can be adopted as the baseline if they are consistent, or the mean value of the multiple results can be used as the baseline for the future follow-up.

As mentioned above, in order to make the results more comparable, the same test method should be used in the follow-up, such as the same perimeter, the same pattern, the same pupil size, and the same correcting lens. Testing shall be carried out again in short time to verify the change if it is found in the comparison between the retest result and the baseline. Only repeatable results can lead to a correct conclusion. The follow-up interval depends on the progression speed of the disease. The patient must carry out the visual field follow-ups regularly with an interval of 3–12 months once the visual field defect is confirmed, while for primary open angle glaucoma with slow progression, the visual field retest can be conducted at intervals from 6 months to 1 year. The baseline should be reset if there're significant changes in the treatment regimen or the disease condition.

10.3.4.2 Impact of Physiological Fluctuations

As mentioned above, visual field test results can be used to determine disease progression or improvement only after exclusion of physiological fluctuation effects and test deviations. Short-term fluctuation (SF) is a detection deviation, while long-term fluctuation (LF), which can be observed in both normal and abnormal visual fields, is the most important basis for follow-ups and comparisons of visual fields. Visual field progression or improvement can be determined only when the quantitative change of visual field surpasses the physiological fluctuation. Visual field progression is mainly manifested as darkening or enlargement of the scotoma or emergence of new scotoma in the former normal area of the visual field. Therefore, follow-up tests should focus specially on the quantitative evaluation of the original scotoma and the detection of any new scotoma.

10.3.4.3 Follow-Up Methods

During the follow-up, multiple test results can be directly compared point to point, or the comparative analysis software in the computerized perimeter can be used to carry out the point-to-point comparison between the current results and the baseline automatically. For the points with normal baseline sensitivities, a decrease of 5 dB can be deemed as significance, while for those already with abnormal baseline sensitivities, a decrease of 8–10 dB may be just physiological fluctuation.

With the development of automated perimeters up to today, there have been so many follow-up softwares that can be used for analysis. Overview printouts (Fig. 10.8) can be used to

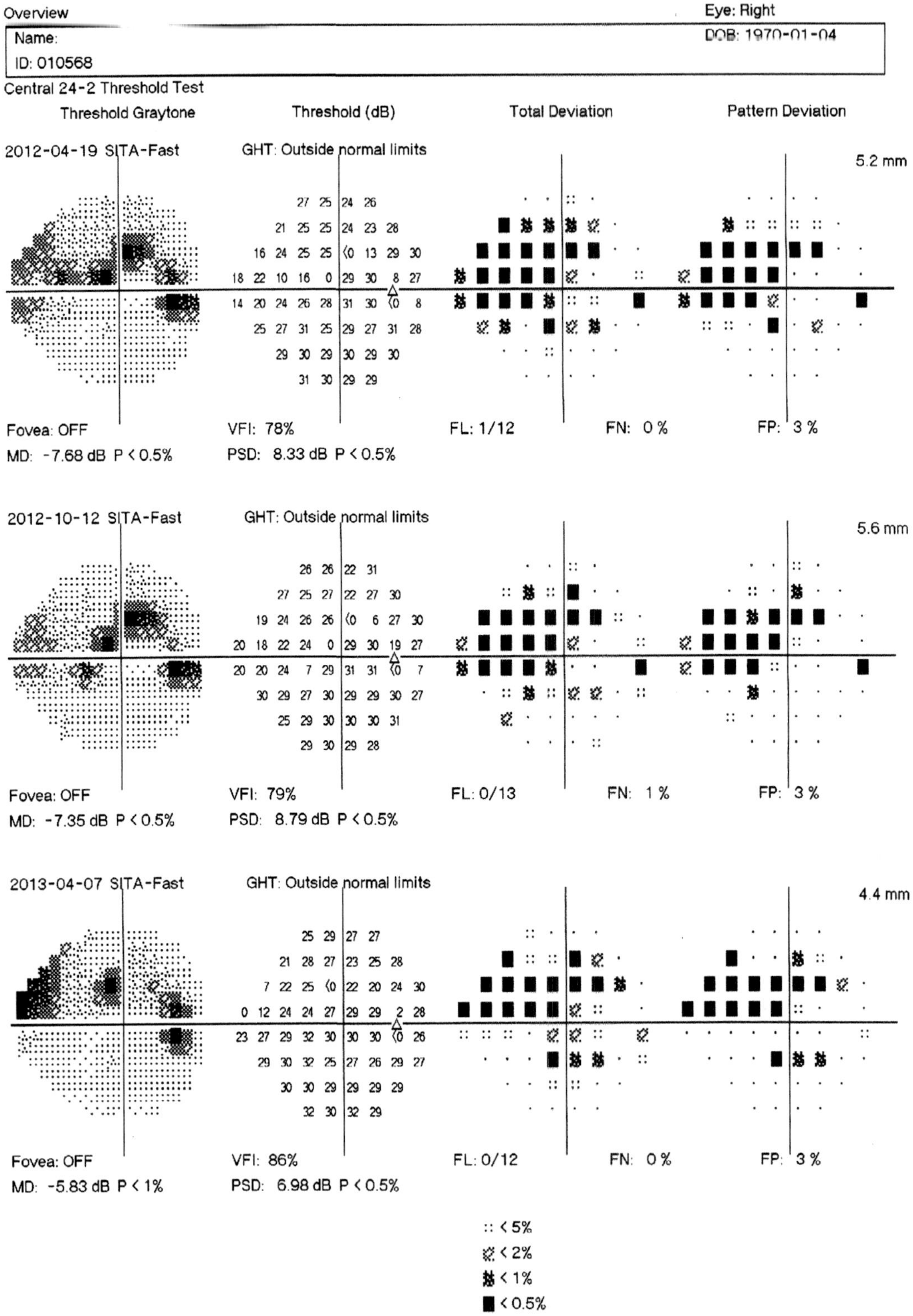

Fig. 10.8 An overview printout of a visual field follow-up test

conduct straightforward comparisons by arranging the numeric printouts, grayscale maps, and deviation plots from multiple test results through the same pattern. The box plots, MD regression analysis, glaucoma change probability (GCP), etc., which have been installed in the system, can also be used to carry out the MD comparison. The current mainstream is guided progression analysis (GPA) in Humphrey perimeter. It contains two kinds of analyses, event analysis—glaucoma change probability maps (GCPMs)—and VFI trend analysis (Fig. 10.9).

GCPMs are used to identify the progression of glaucoma, which use brief warning words, including "possible progression" or "likely progression" to show the area with a visual field change that exceeds the variation range obtained from most glaucoma patients, and a repeatable change with statistical significance is possibly related to glaucoma progression.

Regression analysis on the summative indices, such as VFI or MD, is a tendency analysis that uses the linear regression analysis on VFI change versus the time to evaluate the rate of progression (ROP), expressed as "annual loss percentage." The linear regression line can also be projected or extrapolated to the future 5 years to predict the trend of the visual function under the current unchanged interference conditions. It's used to distinguish whether the visual field is progressing rapidly at a very dangerous speed which will threaten the useful vision in the expected life, or the visual field is progressing very slowly with no need for more active interventions. Besides the presence of visual field progression, more and more ophthalmologists now pay attention to the progression rate during the management of glaucoma patients. If the progression speed is far slower than the elapse of a patient's remaining life, or the progression does not stop after various treatments, or additional treatment will bring more side effects or even influence the patient's quality of life seriously, what is our selection for treatment, alteration, or toleration?

Certainly, ophthalmic examinations have entered the age of big data, requiring the storage and allocation of a large quantity of databases. All the original data and analysis results of Humphrey perimeters can be stored into the FORUM system, which, combined with other examinations including structural damage examinations, etc., may allow more comprehensive and straightforward analysis and evaluation on patients [1, 4–6].

10.3.5 Impact of Examiner on the Visual Field Test

A test with manual perimeter relies completely on the operation of the examiner. An automated perimeter works according to the computer programs. But the skills of the examiner are also quite important in the automated perimetry. The placement of patient's seat and position height, refractive status and selection of additional accommodation lens, explanation and education about the test for the patient, determination of central isopter threshold and physiological blind spot, control of fixation loss and test duration, etc. are all factors that will influence the reliability of the visual field results. Admittedly, as for a modern automatic perimeter, except the arrangement and guidance for patients which require the examiner's work, the whole visual field test processes, even fixation monitoring and results recording and printing, are accomplished automatically by a computer, which can maximally reduce the subjective impacts from the examiner or the analyzer.

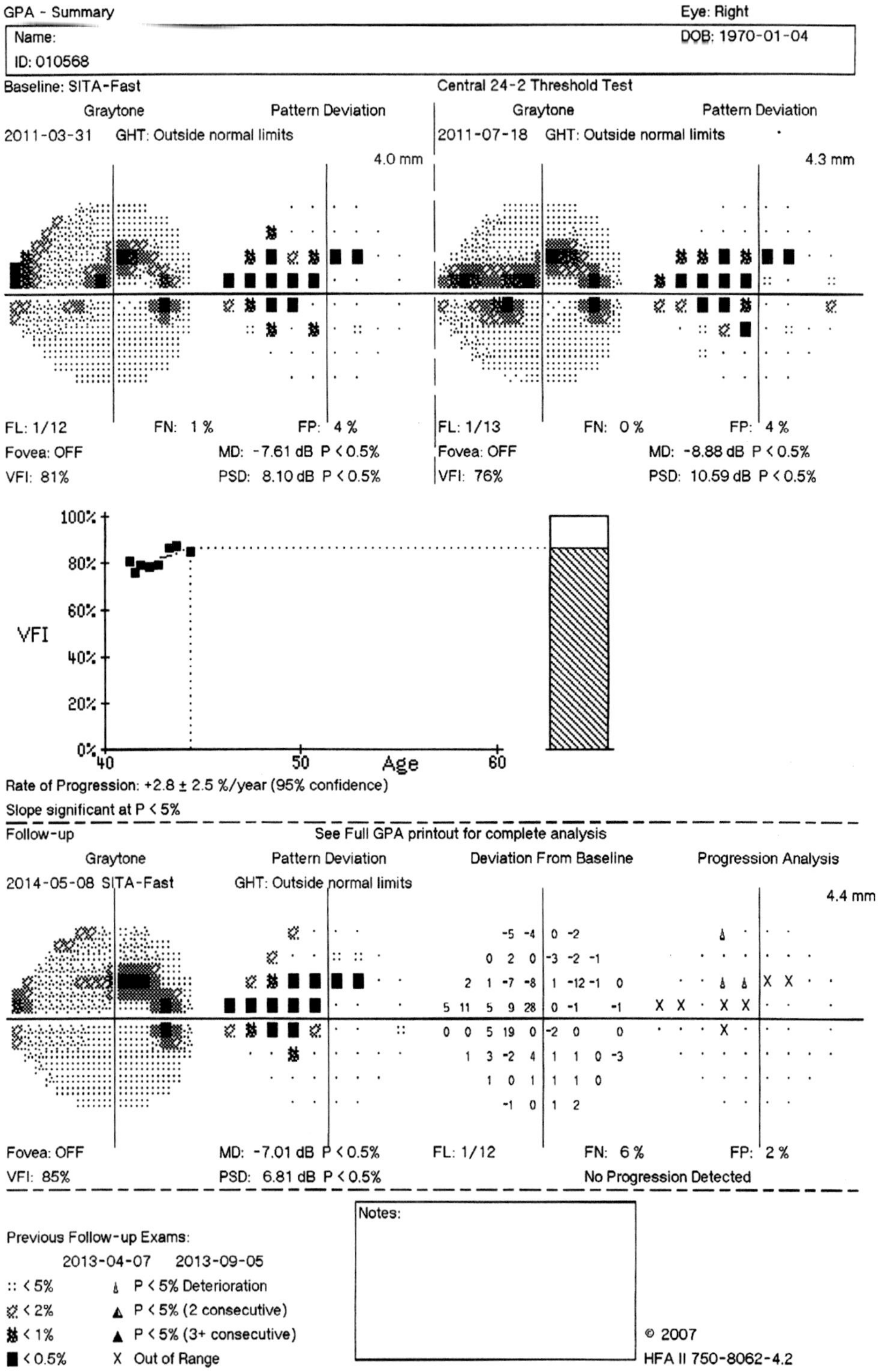

Fig. 10.9 A GPA printout of a visual field follow-up test

References

1. Xiaoming C, Yuansheng Y. Modern clinical visual field test. Beijing: People's Medical Publishing House; 2000.
2. Neil TC, Russell PE. Visual field testing with the humphrey field analyzer: a text and clinical atlas. New Jersey: SLACK Incorporated; 1999.
3. Yi T, Shihui W, Siwei Y. Basis and clinical progress of visual pathway diseases. Beijing: People's Medical Publishing House; 2010.
4. Yuansheng Y, Hua Z. Modern clinical visual field test. Beijing: People's Medical Publishing House; 2015.
5. Yuansheng Y, Jia M, Hui Z. Principle for humphrey visual field test and analysis. Beijing: People's Medical Publishing House; 2005.
6. Heijl A. Essence of reading and analysis on visual field (translated by Yuan Yuansheng, Zhong Hua, Ma Jia). Shanghai: Shanghai Popular Science Press; 2013.

11 Abnormal Visual Fields

Jia Ma, Ning Fan, and Ningli Wang

An abnormal visual field refers to the condition of clinically and statistically significant light sensitivity deviation at various points in the visual field from the normal island of vision. It can be manifested as localized or general sensitivity change (Figs. 11.1, 11.2, and 11.3). Defect area and severity (in dB value of sensitivity) are usually adopted to describe such changes. A visual field defect has many manifestations and is closely related to the pathways of the whole nerve fibers and the lesion location. The manifestations of visual field will be different according to the damage location and pathology. Therefore, the patterns of visual field defects have important clinical significance in localization diagnosis, and they will be described in detail later in this chapter.

Since there is overlapping in the visual fields of both eyes, many diseases cannot be perceived by patients even when significant visual field defects occur. Meanwhile, these manifestations cannot arouse the attention of patients and non-ophthalmologists at the early stage of diseases because they will not affect the central vision, and patients will not see an ophthalmologist until the defects reach the advanced or late stage and affect their lives. However, in these cases, the opportunities for early diagnosis and treatment have already been missed [1–7].

The cases in this book are analyzed by adopting visual field as the main thread. The authors have felt deeply the importance of early visual field testing during their clinical practice. It is visual field testing that first indicated the abnormality in a patient and helped us determine what examinations should be performed next in many cases mentioned in the book.

J. Ma
The First Affiliated Hospital, Kunming Medical University, Kunming, China

N. Fan
Shenzhen Eye Hospital, Shenzhen University, Shenzhen, China

N. Wang (✉)
Department of Ophthalmology, Beijing Tongren Hospital, Capital Medical University, Beijing, China

11.1 Scotoma

Every suprathreshold light stimulus within the isopter should be able to be perceived and responded to at each point. If such stimulus at a certain point cannot be perceived, the light sensitivity will weaken and the threshold increase, and then a scotoma will be formed. It's a relative

N. Wang et al. (eds.), *Optic Disorders and Visual Field*, Advances in Visual Science and Eye Diseases 2, https://doi.org/10.1007/978-981-13-2502-1_11

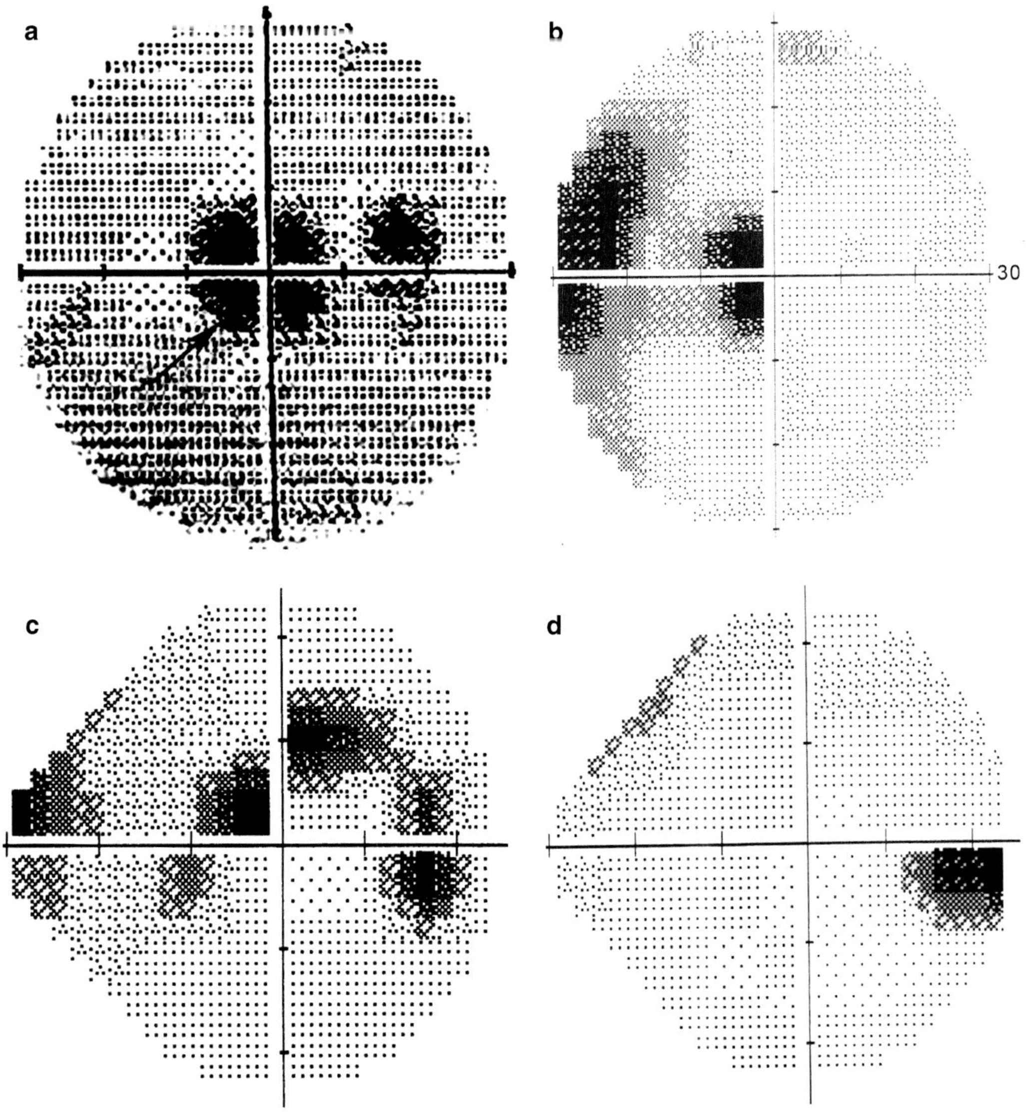

Fig. 11.1 Scotomas. Panel a, central scotoma; Panel b, cecocentral scotoma; Panel c, paracentral scotoma; Panel d, enlargement of the physiological blind spot

scotoma if the stimulus can be perceived after its intensity is increased or its color changed, and it's an absolute scotoma if the stimulus still cannot be perceived even when the brightest stimulus is given. The physiological blind spot is a typical absolute scotoma. Scotomas are described in terms of its location, area or shape, and defect depth.

11.1.1 Central Scotoma

A central scotoma refers to a scotoma located at the central fixation point accompanied by central vision decrease. The central scotoma is mostly caused by damages in the macula or papillomacular bundle, such as macular disease, optic neuritis, and hereditary optic neuropathy, etc.

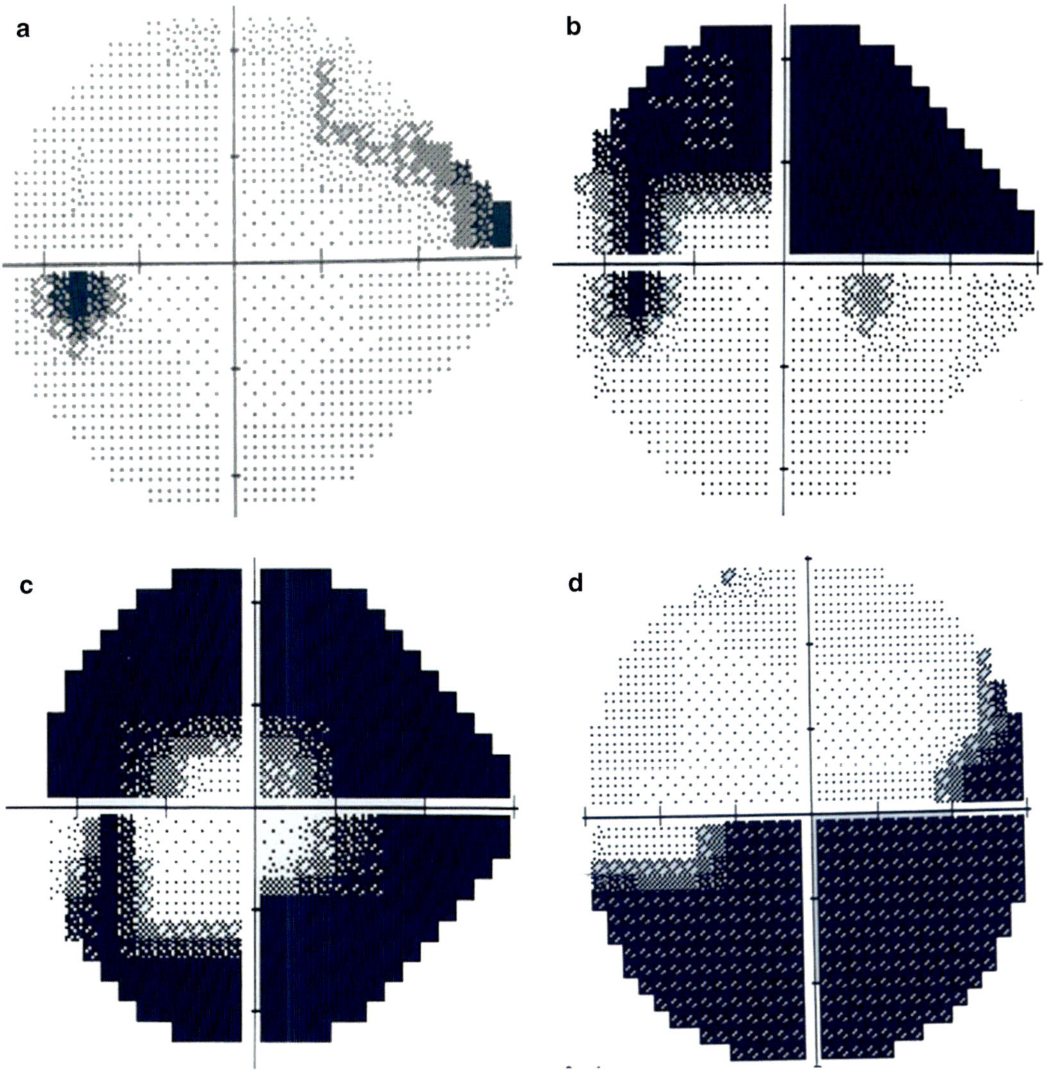

Fig. 11.2 Scotomas. Panel a, nasal step; Panel b, arcuate scotoma; Panel c, annular scotoma; Panel d, sectoral defect connected with the physiological blind spot

11.1.2 Cecocentral Scotoma

A cecocentral scotoma refers to a dumbbell-shaped scotoma composed of a central scotoma connected with the physiological blind spot, possibly resulting from damages to the papillomacular bundle. It is more commonly observed in patients with optic neuritis, glaucoma, and toxic or nutritional deficiency optic neuropathies from tobacco and alcohol abuse.

11.1.3 Nasal Step

A nasal step is a special manifestation of damage to the retinal nerve fiber bundle temporal to the

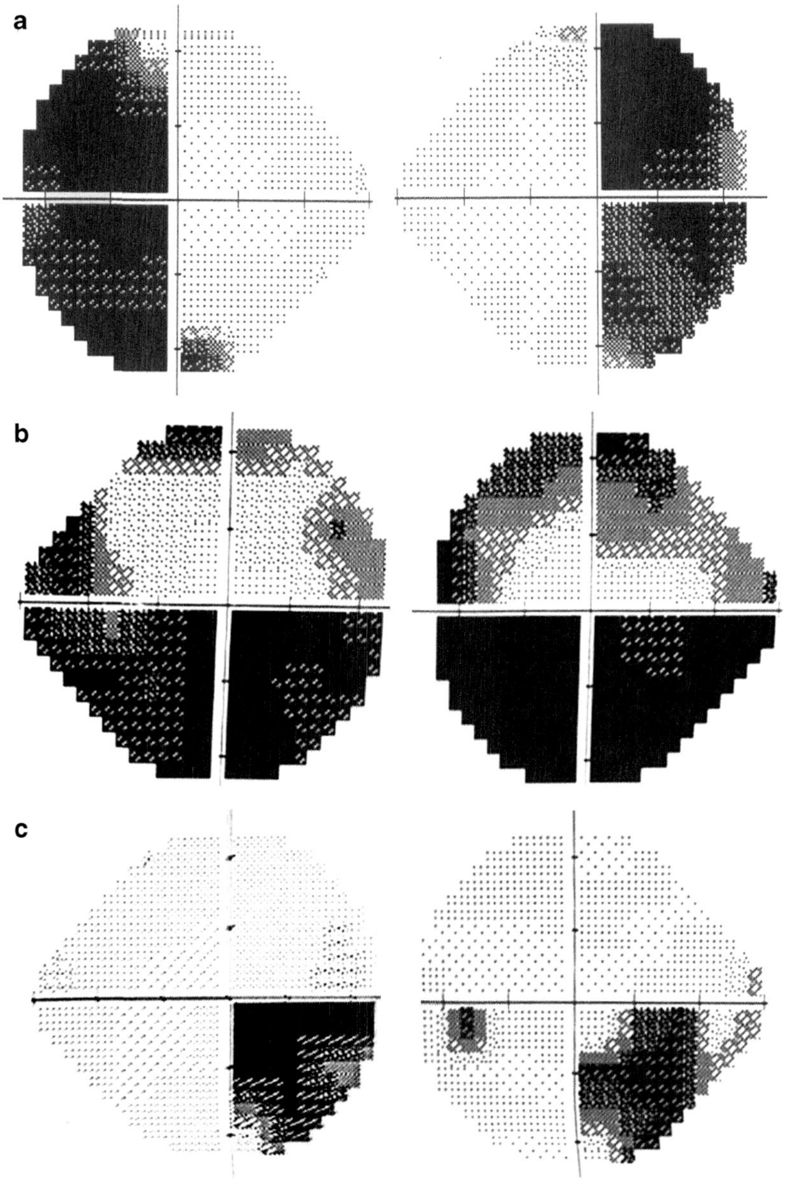

Fig. 11.3 Hemianopia. Panel a: Bitemporal hemianopia. Panel b: Bilateral inferior altitudinal defect. Panel c: Homonymous right inferior quadrantanopia

macula, where the visual field impairments below and above the nasal horizontal raphe are inconsistent and a step-like change is formed due to nonmatching or inconsistent defect depths. As the typical manifestation of visual field change in early glaucoma, it is of important significance for the early diagnosis of and public health screening for the disease.

11.1.4 Paracentral Scotoma

A paracentral scotoma is a scotoma in the superior or inferior area stretching from the physiological blind spot within the Bjerrum area of central 5–25°. With a diameter of more than 5° and a depth of more than 5 dB, it's manifested as defects at multiple neighboring points in automatic perimeter. Several paracentral scotomas will then connect with each other and develop gradually into an arcuate scotoma, which is caused by damage to the arcuate nerve fibers around the papillomacular bundle. It is commonly observed at the early stage of glaucoma.

11.1.5 Arcuate Scotoma

An arcuate scotoma is located above or below the fixation point and connected with the physiological blind spot. It stretches in an arch shape with a wide nasal part and a narrow temporal part, usually in the Bjerrum area. It is a typical visual field defect in glaucoma, and sometimes it can be caused by lesions of the optic chiasm or the ischemia of the optic disc.

11.1.6 Annular Scotoma

The superior and inferior arcuate scotomas surround the central fixation area, connect at the nasal horizontal raphe without crossing, and form a annular scotoma. It's usually observed in glaucoma. The inferior part below the nasal horizontal raphe is usually slightly wider than the superior one, which gives a step-like shape, due to the difference in sensitivities to the damage between the superior and inferior parts.

11.2 Localized Defects

11.2.1 Temporal Sectoral Defect

A temporal sectoral defect is manifested as fan-shaped or wedge-shaped with the apex pointing to the physiological blind spot in the temporal visual field. It can be an early visual field change of glaucoma or a typical change of ischemic optic neuropathy.

11.2.2 Quadrantanopia

It's also called quadrant hemianopia, i.e., the visual field defect occupies one quadrant. The defect is usually seen in visual pathway damage behind the optic chiasm and usually manifested as homonymous impairments of the visual fields.

11.2.3 Hemianoptic Visual Field Change

The defect that occupies one half of the visual field is called hemianopia, bounded usually by the vertical midline, sometimes by the horizontal midline. Hemianopia can be divided into homonymous (right or left) or heteronymous (bitemporal or binasal) and symmetrical or asymmetrical ones. The edges of the defect can pass through the fixation point. It is commonly seen in lesions of or behind the optic chiasm. Hemianopia can also avoid the central fixation area, and a small part of the visual field can be retained within the central 3°, which is called as macular sparing. It is possibly because the posterior part of the visual cortex in the occipital lobe is the macular fiber projection area, which is dual-supplied by the middle cerebral artery from the carotid artery system and the posterior cerebral artery from the vertebral artery system, difficult to be entirely damaged. However, if the damage only involves the posterior pole of the occipital lobe, hemianopia can also be observed in the central 3° area, which is called as macular splitting. A transverse half-field defect is also called an altitudinal defect, usually observed in damages to the superior or inferior retina. Detailed discussion about hemianopia will be presented in the chapter about posterior visual pathways.

11.3 Concentric Constriction of Visual Field and Tubular Visual Field

A concentrically constricted visual field has relative or absolute defects in the peripheral area of the whole visual field with the tendency of developing concentrically. Concentric constriction can be functional or organic. The former is found in hysteria while the latter in retinitis pigmentosa, retrobulbar optic neuritis, optic nerve atrophy, advanced glaucoma, etc. Only a tubular visual field will be left at the advanced stage of concentric constriction.

It needs to be pointed out here that a common visual field test usually focuses on the central 30°, but if damages including localized visual field depression or concentric constriction, etc. are involved, the test area should extend to 60°, or even 90°, namely, the full visual field, as with the kinetic test, to be able to truly reflect the visual field change. Only when the visible range is smaller than 30° at the advanced stage can the defect be found in the central visual field test.

11.4 General Reduction of Sensitivity

General reduction of sensitivity refers to the relatively low sensitivity in the whole visual field. It is usually determined by comparison with the threshold values in normal visual field and frequently analyzed with MD. The depression is diffuse. It is usually observed in diffuse damages to the retina, optic nerve, or visual pathway. It can also be caused by preretinal factors, such as senility, refractive media opacity, too small a pupil, and uncorrected refractive error.

11.5 Enlargement of the Physiological Blind Spot

Enlargement of the physiological blind spot should be considered when its vertical and transverse diameters are bigger than 9.5° and 7.5°, respectively. The enlargement can generally be found in all directions and is usually seen in optic disc edema, myelinated nerve fiber, peripapillary chorioretinal atrophy of high myopia, neuroretinitis, and glaucoma, etc. Artifact may be produced due to the egress and ingress of the great retinal vessels at the superior and inferior poles of the optic disc. Therefore, the transverse enlargement of the physiological blind spot is sometimes more relevant.

What needs to be made clear is that a white-on-white visual field is used for all routine tests. However, due to the different sensitivities of cone cells to different colors, the visual field areas of normal people tested with different color stimuli are different. From outside to inside, the isopters are white, blue, red, and green in sequence, with the intervals being about 10°. Some diseases selectively produce damages on the visual field of a certain color. For instance, the constriction of the blue visual field is the most significant in diseases of the outer layer of the retina or choroid diseases, so the visual field is tested with the most sensitive blue stimuli. As for optic neuropathies, it is constriction of the red visual field that is the most significant.

In conclusion, visual field test is one of the most widely used diagnostic methods in the ophthalmic clinical practice and scientific research, which can provide a great amount of visual function information. Visual field test can be a key to revealing diseases and plays the role of localization diagnosis and qualitative diagnosis. However, visual field test belongs to subjective examination and is closely related to the cooperation of the patient and his/her understanding of the procedures. The most in-depth studies of the visual field still focus on glaucoma and neuro-ophthalmology. Moreover, visual field manifestations may be varied and unpredictable due to the diversity and complexity of the lesions. Therefore, it can also be a mist interfering with the diagnosis. For example, what is the origin of the lesion? Is it caused by one disease or multiple diseases? Does certain damage to the visual pathway conform to the visual field defect? All these questions need to be answered by us one by one. Meanwhile, the process of answering these questions is also the process for us to form clinical thinking and understand the nature of diseases. To throw a sprat to catch a whale, this chapter has just introduced the basic theory and method of visual field test. How to effectively use the structure and function damages for early diagnosis, how to focus on the visual field changes to analyze diseases, and how to make the atypical visual field changes and their corresponding lesions reveal themselves through progressive analysis as if reeling silk from cocoons are the key points of this book.

References

1. Xiaoming C, Yuansheng Y. Modern clinical visual field test. Beijing: People's Medical Publishing House; 2000.
2. Yuansheng Y, Jia M, Hui Z. Principle for humphrey visual field test and analysis. Beijing: People's Medical Publishing House; 2005.
3. Heijl A. Essence of reading and analysis on visual field (translated by Yuan Yuansheng, Zhong Hua, Ma Jia). Shanghai: Shanghai Popular Science Press; 2013.
4. Yuansheng Y, Hua Z. Modern clinical visual field test. Beijing: People's Medical Publishing House; 2015.
5. Shihui W, Jingxiang Z. Neuro-ophthalmology review manual. Beijing: People's Medical Publishing House; 2015.
6. Sevim K, Molly G, et al. Peripheral field loss: something old, something new. Surv Ophthalmol. 2008;53(4):397–402.
7. Miller N, Subramanian P, Patel V. Walsh & hoyt's clinical neuro-ophthalmology: the essentials. 3rd ed. Philadelphia: Wolters Kluwer; 2016.

Part III

Retinal Diseases

12 Why Is AZOOR "Occult"?

Ning Fan, Xuyang Liu, and Jiantao Wang

Acute zonal occult outer retinopathy (AZOOR) is a group of diseases observed in one or both eyes with damages to broad zones of the outer retina. Initial symptoms include photopsia, visual field defects, and sometimes an enlarged blind spot. On initial presentation, the central visual acuity may not be affected, and the fundus may appear normal, easily leading to the misdiagnosis of AZOOR. The visual field examination plays an irreplaceable role in the diagnosis and follow-up observation of the disease. Two typical cases have been selected to elucidate AZOOR in this section.

12.1 Case 1

12.1.1 Case Presentation

A 27-year-old female presented with photopsia in the right eye for 1 week. No accompanying symptoms including distorted vision, red eyes, and eye pain were present. In addition, histories of trauma, systemic diseases, and familial diseases were also denied.

The uncorrected visual acuity (UCVA) was 20/25 OU, and the best corrected visual acuity (BCVA) was 20/20 with refractive correction (−1.00DS) OU. The intraocular pressure was normal in both eyes. On examination, the anterior segments and the fundus were unremarkable in both eyes.

12.1.2 Case Analysis

The patient's chief complaint was photopsia in the right eye. However, the BCVA was normal, and the slit-lamp examination, ophthalmoscopic examination, and fundus examination with the three-mirror lens revealed no positive signs. Photopsia is a nonspecific symptom, and the patient denied any discomfort including distorted vision, shadow in the vision, etc. The most likely causes include organic diseases or functional disorders of the vitreous, retina, or optic nerve. Other examinations such as visual field and electrophysiologic examinations are required to evaluate the visual function. The visual field examination is the simplest and easiest to carry out and can also help with the qualitative analysis and localization of the lesion.

The visual field examination revealed a scotoma extending from the physiological blind spot in the temporal side of the right eye (Fig. 12.1), and the visual field in the left eye was normal.

N. Fan · J. Wang (✉)
Shenzhen Eye Hospital, Shenzhen University, Shenzhen, China

X. Liu
Xiamen Eye Center of Xiamen University, Xiamen, China

Shenzhen Eye Hospital, Shenzhen University, Shenzhen, China

N. Wang et al. (eds.), *Optic Disorders and Visual Field*, Advances in Visual Science and Eye Diseases 2, https://doi.org/10.1007/978-981-13-2502-1_12

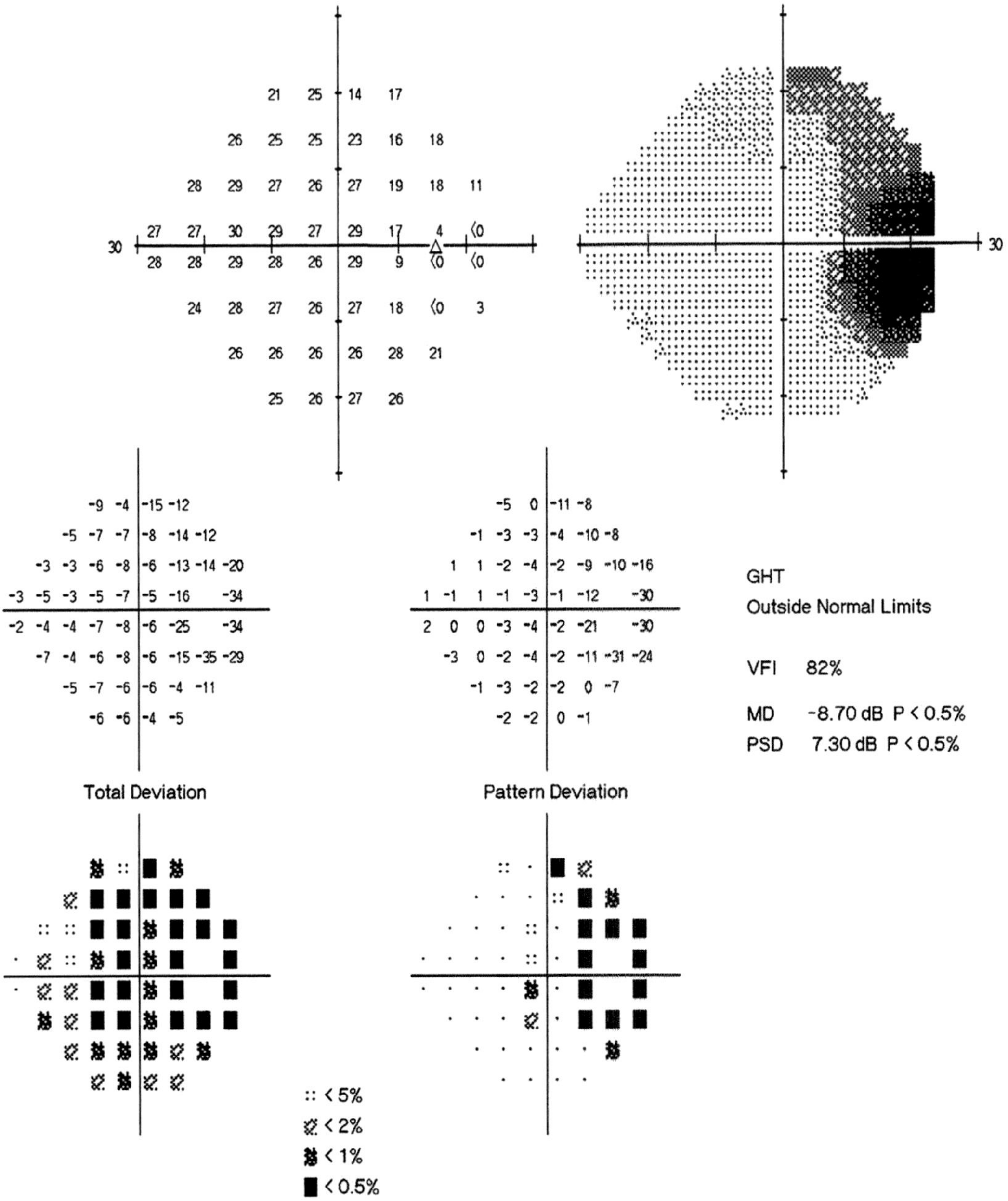

Fig. 12.1 Humphrey visual field analysis printout for the right eye. A scotoma extending from the physiological blind spot in the temporal visual field of the right eye was obtained with the 24-2 test

The visual field impairment suggested that the patient might have organic lesions. The lesions were localized in the optic disc, the peripapillary retina, and the optic nerve according to the visual field impairment features. The patient was a young female, and the common optic nerve disease seen in young females is optic neuritis. The relative afferent pupillary defect (RAPD) was negative although only unilateral optic function damage was observed, and the medical history showed no pain upon eye movements. These findings did not support the diagnosis of optic neuritis. The fundus examination by the three-minor lens showed no abnormality. Therefore, the next examination was optical coherence tomography (OCT) on the retina to find out whether there was any abnormality.

The OCT demonstrated absence or irregularity of the IS–OS photoreceptor line and the retinal pigment epithelium (RPE) in the area between the optic disc and the macular in the right eye (Fig. 12.2).

Structure change, whose lesion extent reflected the visual field impairment, was observed by OCT in the outer layer of the retina between the optic disc and the macula. In order to further unravel the focal characteristic and confirm whether the lesion was a primary disease or a secondary disease caused by changes such as ischemia or inflammation, etc., fundus fluorescein angiography (FFA) was then performed.

FFA showed transmitted fluorescence at the RPE level around the optic disc of the right eye, and retinal vessel staining and leakage could be found (Fig. 12.3).

The condition was preliminarily diagnosed to be acute zonal occult outer retinopathy (AZOOR) in the right eye. It needs to be differentiated from retrobulbar neuritis. The pattern visual evoked potential (P-VEP) examination was also completed.

The P-VEP examination showed that the amplitude and latency of the P100 wave were within the normal range in both eyes. Slight reduction of the amplitude in the right eye was revealed when compared with that in the left eye (Fig. 12.4). The amplitude reduction of the P100 wave was not in accordance with the visual field damage in the right eye. It may be caused by macular involvement, and therefore optic neuritis was excluded.

12.1.3 Final Diagnosis

The final diagnosis was acute zonal occult outer retinopathy (AZOOR) in the right eye.

12.1.4 Case Review

The patient was a young female complaining of photopsia in one eye. The central visual acuity, slit-lamp examination, and fundus examination showed no abnormality. The onset of the disease is occult. Is it a functional abnormality or an organic disease? The patient had no high myopia and the refractive media was transparent. The vitreous body and the retina showed no abnormality. Besides, the central vision was normal and the pupil was sensitive to the light. No pain upon eye movement was present. The diagnosis of optic neuritis was not supported. However, the central 24-2 visual field showed temporal visual field impairment, and the lesion was localized in the posterior polar region of the retina (nasal area of

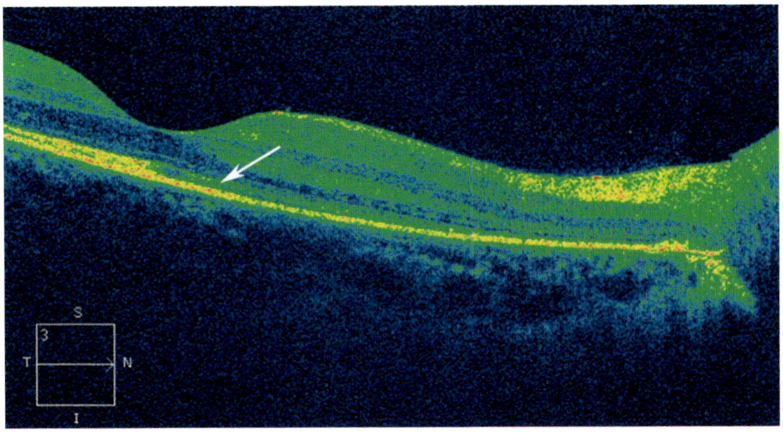

Fig. 12.2 Macular OCT image of the right eye. OCT with 9 mm linear scanning showed the absence or irregularity of the IS–OS photoreceptor line and the RPE (white arrow) in the area between the optic disc and the macular in the right eye

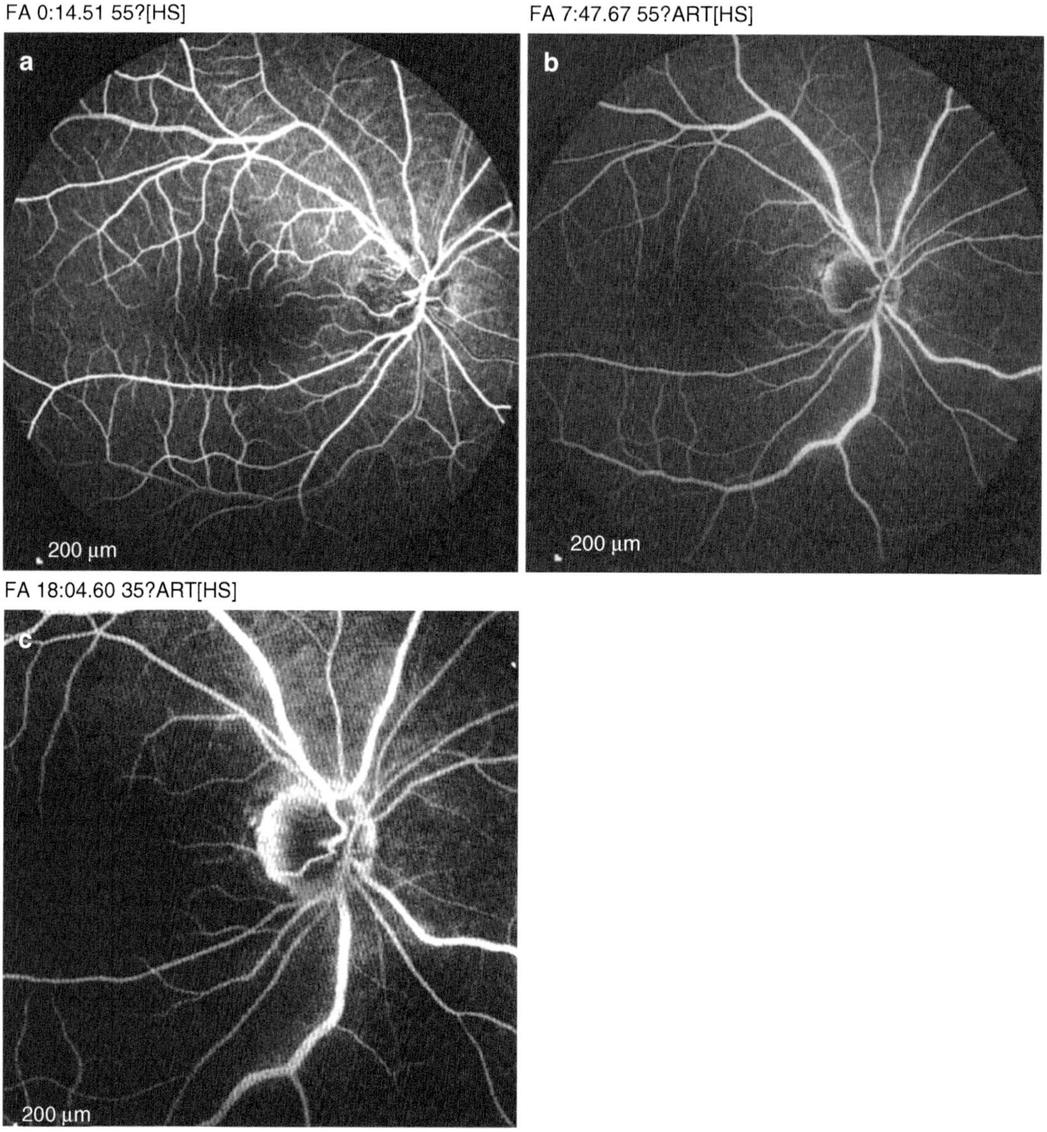

Fig. 12.3 FFA images of the right eye. Panel a and b: FFA showed transmitted fluorescence at the RPE level around the optic disc. Panel c: Retinal vessel staining and leakage could be found

the macula) or the optic nerve (including the optic disc). High-resolution OCT on the area revealed the pathologic basis for the visual field change. The further examination of FFA excluded vascular or inflammatory retinal diseases. The VEP excluded the optic neuropathy. The patient was finally diagnosed with acute zonal occult outer retinopathy.

12.2 Case 2

12.2.1 Case Presentation

A 28-year-old female complained of visual field loss and central visual acuity decrease for 1 month. The patient had high myopia of nearly 700 diopters in both eyes. Histories of other eye

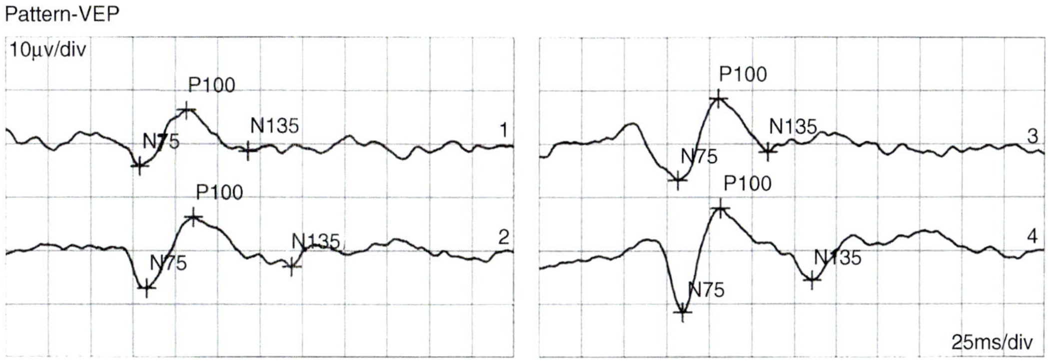

Channel	N75 [ms]	P100 [ms]	N135 [ms]	N75-P100	P100-N135
1 R-1 1,0	79	107	143	10.5µv	7.64µv
3 L-1 1,0	82	106	134	15.4µv	10µv
2 R-1 0,15	83	111	169	13.4µv	9.34µv
4 L-1 0,15	85	107	161	19.5µv	13.5µv
Normals	-	90-116-90-116	-	-	-

Channel	Stimulus	Ampl., Range, Filter
1 R-1 1,0	MON Patt. Rev. CB, 1?Full Field, Ctr:97% 1.5Hz, Avg:68	1, +/-100µv 1-50Hz
2 R-1 0,15	MON Patt. Rev. CB, 0?5' Full Field, Ctr:97% 1.5Hz, Avg:52	1, +/-100µv 1-50Hz
3 L-1 1,0	MON Patt. Rev. CB, 1?Full Field, Ctr:97% 1.5Hz, Avg:51	1, +/-100µv 1-50Hz
4 L-1 0,15	MON Patt. Rev. CB, 0?5' Full Field, Ctr:97% 1.5Hz, Avg:55	1, +/-100µv 1-50Hz

Fig. 12.4 P-VEP examination printouts of the both eyes. The P100 wave was normal in both eyes, while light reduction of the amplitude in the right eye was revealed when compared with that in the left eye

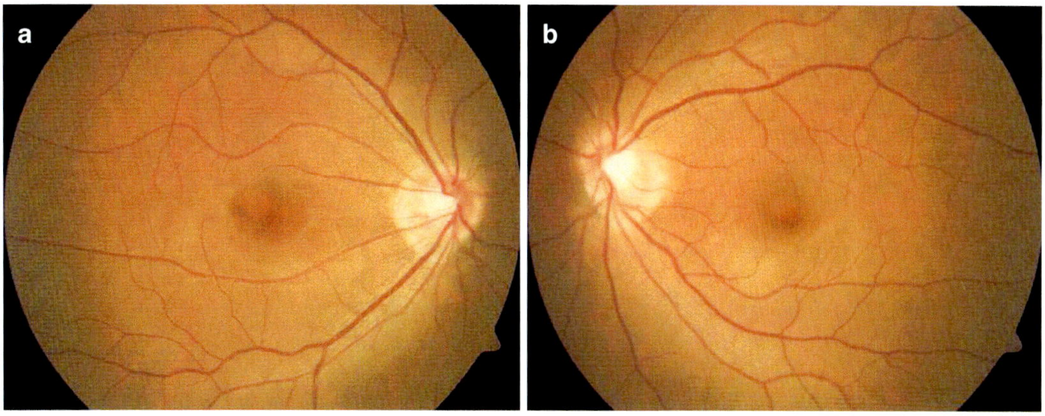

Fig. 12.5 Fundus photographs. The optic disc was pink in color with a clear boundary in each eye. Mild lacquer cracks were revealed. Panel a: Right eye. Panel b: Left eye

diseases and systemic diseases, trauma, and familial diseases were denied.

The BCVA was 20/50 with myopic correction (−6.50DS) OD and 20/20 with myopic correction (−7.00DS) OS. The intraocular pressure was normal in both eyes. Slit-lamp examination of her anterior segments was unremarkable in both eyes except that the relative afferent pupillary defect (RAPD) was weak positive in the right eye. The fundus examination was also unremarkable in both eyes except that mild lacquer cracks were found (Fig. 12.5). Standardized automated perimetry revealed temporal visual field defect in the right eye with a vertical boundary (Fig. 12.6) and normal visual field in the left eye.

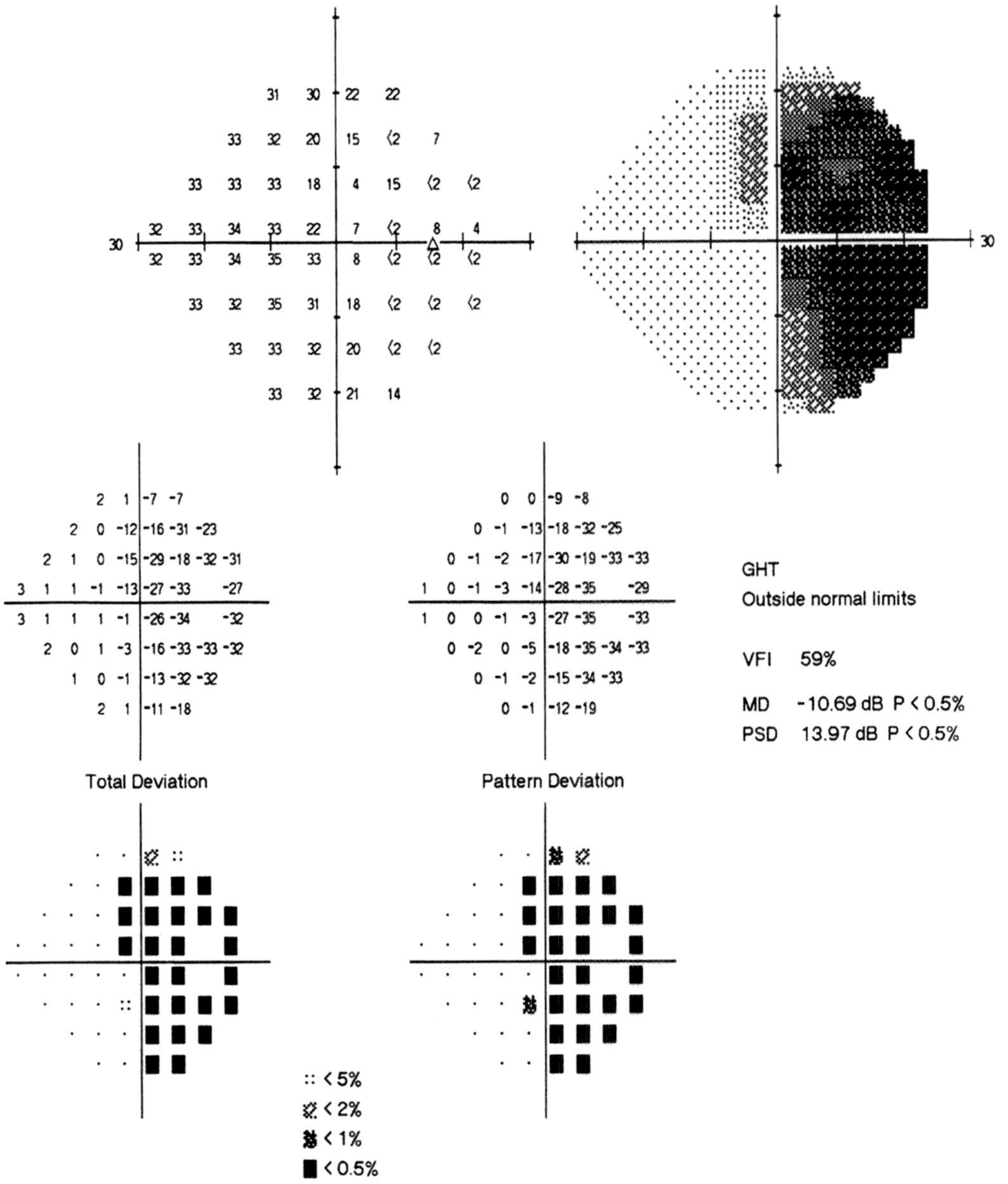

Fig. 12.6 Humphrey visual field analysis printout for the right eye. A temporal visual field defect was seen in the right eye

12.2.2 Case Analysis

The patient was a young female with high myopia and experienced central vision decrease accompanied by weak positive RAPD in the right eye. The preliminary diagnosis was retrobulbar optic neuritis based on the symptoms and negative signs obtained from the fundus examination, and retinal diseases still could not be excluded. Visual field examination showed unilateral temporal hemianopsia, but where was the lesion located? Was its anatomic site in the sellar area, the optic nerve, or the retina?

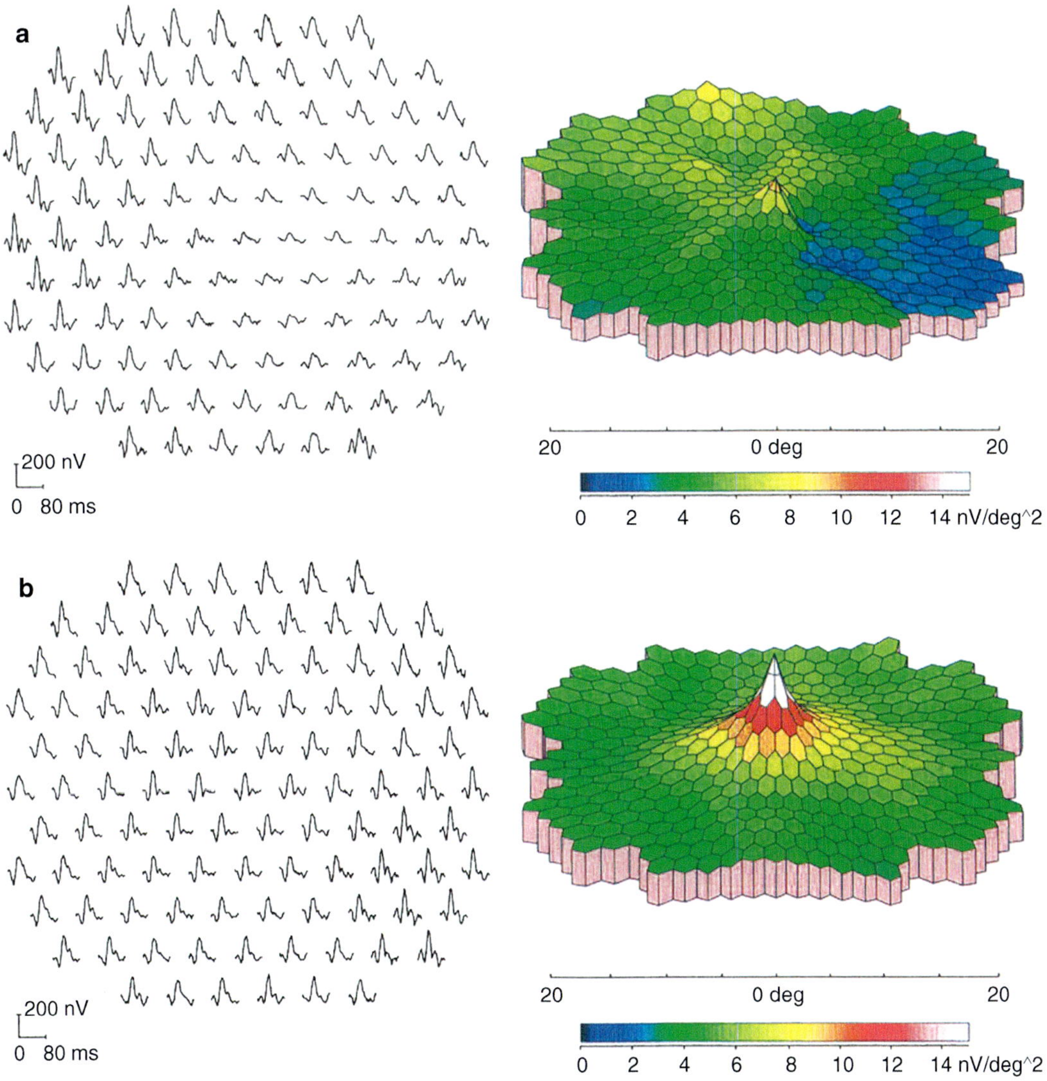

Fig. 12.7 mf-ERG images. Panel a: The low response area in the macula that adjoined the optic disc in the right eye. Panel b: Normal response in the posterior pole of the retina in the left eye

Magnetic resonance imaging (MRI) of the pituitary gland revealed no abnormality. Multifocal electroretinogram (mf-ERG) showed a low response area between the macula and the optic disc in the right eye and normal response in the posterior pole of the retina in the left eye (Fig. 12.7).

The P-VEP examination demonstrated normal waveform, a moderate delay in the latency, and a mild reduction in the amplitude at low spatial frequencies and normal waveform, a moderate delay in the latency, and normal amplitude at high spatial frequencies in the right eye. The P-VEP examination of the left eye was normal (Fig. 12.8).

A sellar lesion was excluded based on pituitary gland MRI. The abnormality found in the P-VEP examination of the right eye suggested that the lesion was very likely to be in the macula or the optic nerve. The abnormal mf-ERG wave was in accordance with the visual field impairment,

Pattern-VEP

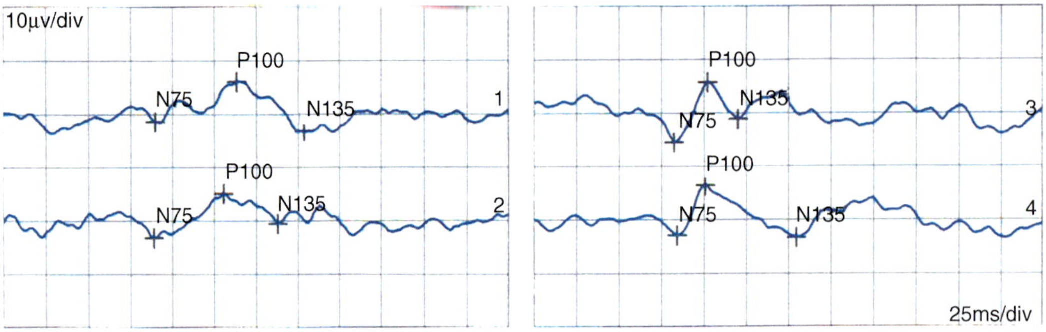

Channel	N75 [ms]	P100 [ms]	N135 [ms]	N75-P100	P100-N135
1 R-1 1,0	90	139 (!)	179	7.49µv	9.28µv
3 L-1 1,0	83	102	120	11.2µv	6.84µv
2 R-1 0,15	89	131 (!)	163	8.25µv	5.59µv
4 L-1 0,15	85	101	155	9.3µv	9.68µv
Normals	-	90-116-90-116	-	-	-

Channel	Stimulus	Ampl., Range, Filter
1 R-1 1,0	MON Patt. Rev. CB, 1?Full Field, Ctr:97% 1.5Hz, Avg:77	1, +/-100µv 1-50Hz
2 R-1 0,15	MON Patt. Rev. CB, 0?5' Full Field, Ctr:97% 1.5Hz, Avg:100	1, +/-100µv 1-50Hz
3 L-1 1,0	MON Patt. Rev. CB, 1?Full Field, Ctr:97% 1.5Hz, Avg:62	1, +/-100µv 1-50Hz
4 L-1 0,15	MON Patt. Rev. CB, 0?5' Full Field, Ctr:97% 1.5Hz, Avg:99	1, +/-100µv 1-50Hz

Fig. 12.8 P-VEP examination printouts. Normal waveform, a moderate delay in the latency, and a mild reduction in the amplitude at low spatial frequencies and a normal waveform and a moderate delay in the latency and normal amplitude at high spatial frequencies were seen for the P100 wave in the right eye. The P100 waveform, latency, and amplitude were normal in the left eye

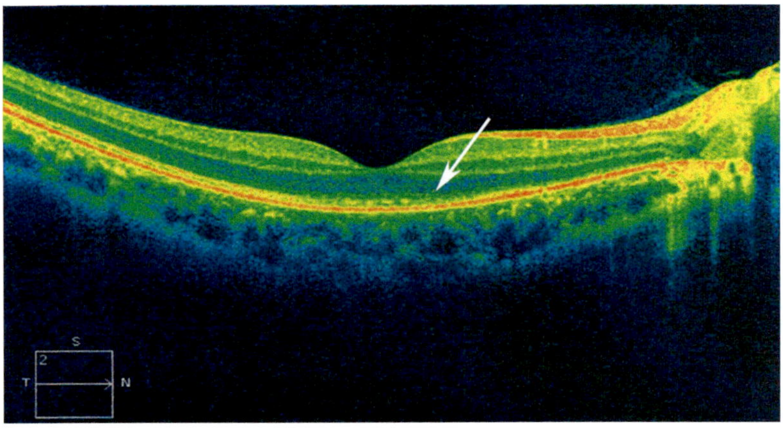

Fig. 12.9 Macular OCT image of the right eye. The OCT showed irregular shape and even partial loss of the ellipsoid zone and the RPE between the optic disc and the macula, and the lesion had expanded beyond the fovea

which indicated that it was most likely for the retinopathy located in the macular and optic disc area. Therefore, high-resolution OCT with linear scanning was performed on this area, and the FFA examination was also performed.

The OCT showed absence or irregularity of the ellipsoid zone and the RPE between the optic disc and the macula, and the lesion had expanded beyond the fovea (Fig. 12.9).

The FFA examination showed no abnormality (Fig. 12.10).

The diagnosis of acute zonal occult outer retinopathy was supported by the following: the OCT indicated that the focus location conformed to the site with abnormal mf-ERG and visual field impairment; the patient was a young female with high myopia and acute visual field defect; and FFA examination showed no abnormality.

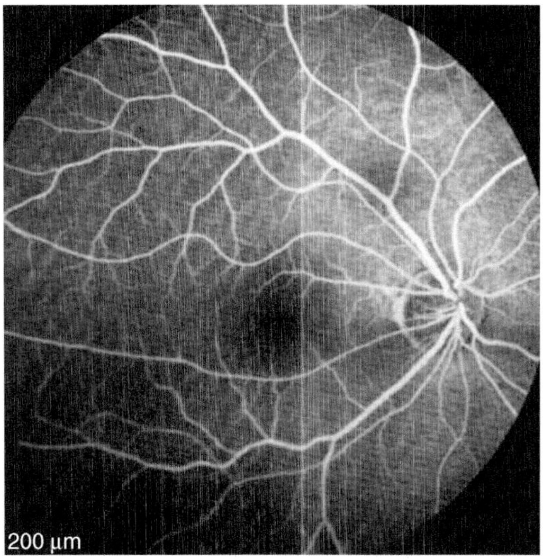

Fig. 12.10 FFA image of the right eye. No abnormality was found in the FFA image of the right eye

12.2.3 Final Diagnosis

The final diagnosis was acute zonal occult outer retinopathy in thc right eye.

Symptomatic treatments, including hormone treatment, coenzyme Q treatment, mecobalamin treatment, circulation improving, etc., were given to the patient. Follow-up has continued for 7 months so far, and the patient's visual field has improved significantly. The following figures present the visual fields of the patient obtained at 6 weeks, 4 months, and 7 months after disease onset (Fig. 12.11).

12.2.4 Case Review

This AZOOR case was extremely easy to be misdiagnosed as retrobulbar optic neuritis. The patient had decreased central vision accompanied by weak positive RAPD, negative fundus examination, abnormal VEP examination, and normal FFA in the right eye. The change in the outer layer of the retina observed by OCT was easy to be neglected or even be attributed mistakenly to low image resolution.

Unilateral temporal hemianopia is a special visual field change and should be paid attention to. On one hand, the lesion localization shall be expanded to the sellar area. On the other hand, the attention should be focused on the retina between the optic disc and macula lutea during diagnosis. The disease was definitively diagnosed based on the consistent damages (OCT, visual field, mf-ERG) found in the structure and function of the retina in this area. The retrobulbar optic neuritis is to be excluded because a macular lesion can also lead to abnormal P-VEP. The AZOOR diagnosis was further supported by the observations during several months' treatment and follow-up.

12.3 Discussion

AZOOR was systemically described by Gass for the first time [1]. "Acute" refers to acute loss of regional function accompanied by photopsia in unilateral/bilateral visual field(s); "zonal" refers to function loss in one/multiple retinal zone(s); "occult" refers to the fact that the fundus lesion is occult and not easy to be observed; "outer" refers to the fact that the lesion was mainly in the photoreceptor layer, and the RPE can also be involved, and more serious involvement can be observed in the cone cells than in rod cells by ERG; and "retinopathy" classifies it into a lesion of the retina. It's a rare fundus disease and the disease cause is still unclear. Gass reported that 28% of AZOOR patients also suffer from other systemic diseases, such as multiple sclerosis, graft versus host disease, etc. AZOOR is characterized by retinal photoreceptor damage and can be observed in one eye or in both eyes. It's more frequently found in young females. Its initial manifestations in most patients include sudden photopsia, temporal visual field loss, and absence of significant abnormality in the fundus upon examination. Missed diagnosis or misdiagnosis as retrobulbar optic neuritis has been reported due to its nonspecific symptoms and occult signs. The retinal abnormalities found by OCT examination include irregular interface between the inner and (or) outer segment of the photoreceptor, damaged outer nuclear layer, irregular RPE, and (or) retina

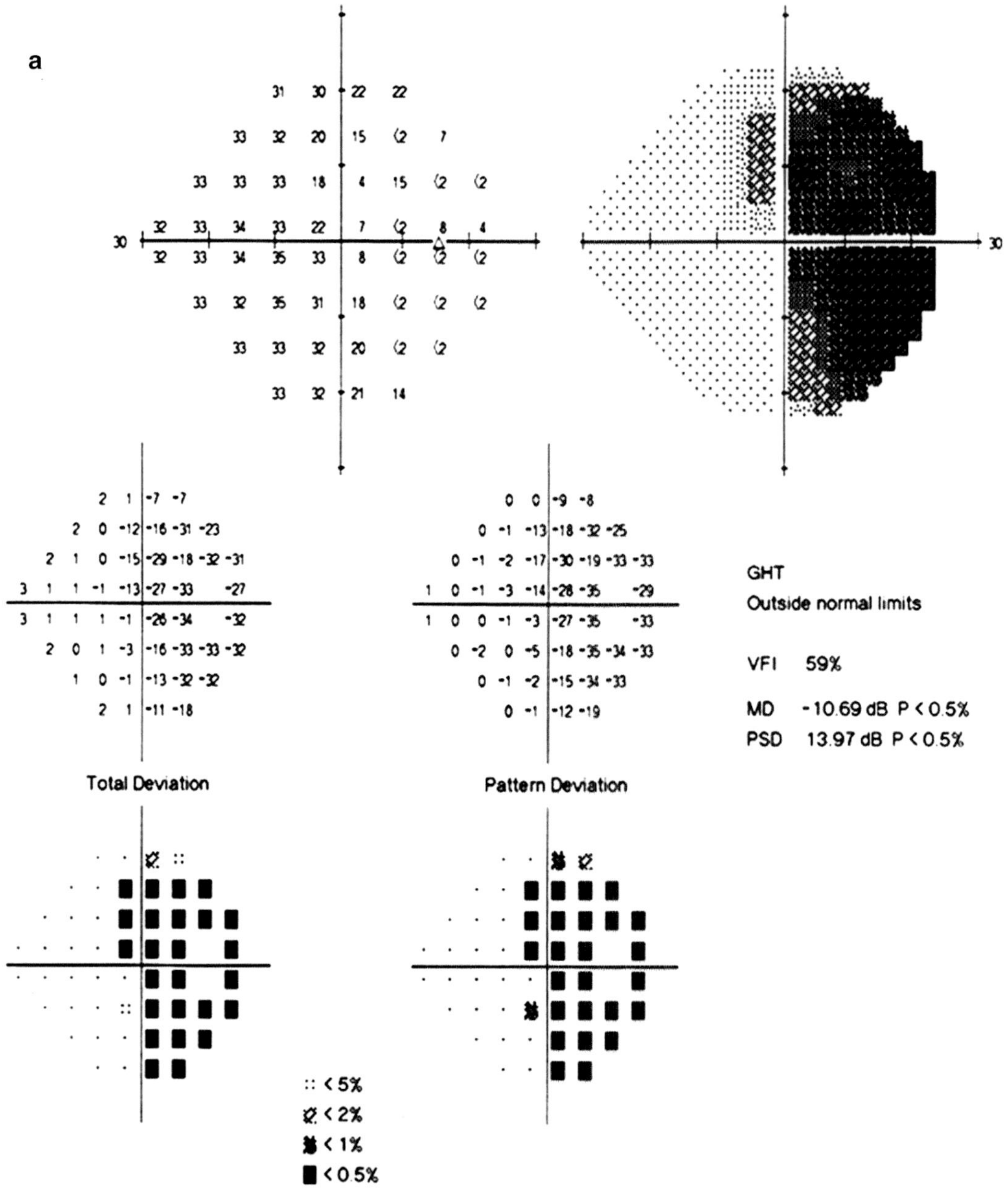

Fig. 12.11 Humphrey visual field analysis printouts for the right eye at follow-up visits. Reexamination of central visual field (24-2) at the follow-up visits revealed gradual shrink of the temporal defect in the right eye. Panel a: 6 weeks after disease onset. Panel b: 4 months after disease onset. Panel c: 7 months after disease onset

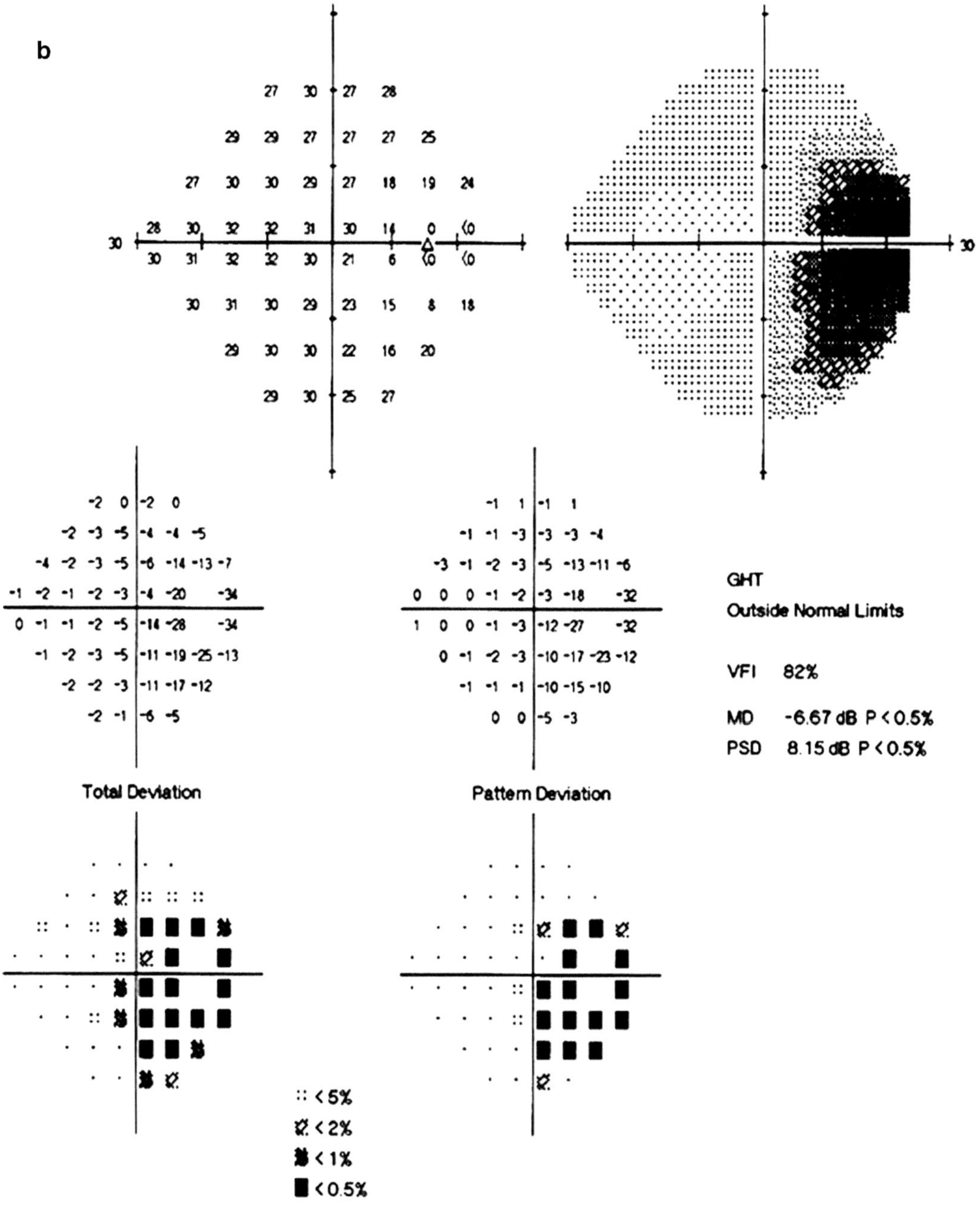

Fig. 12.11 (continued)

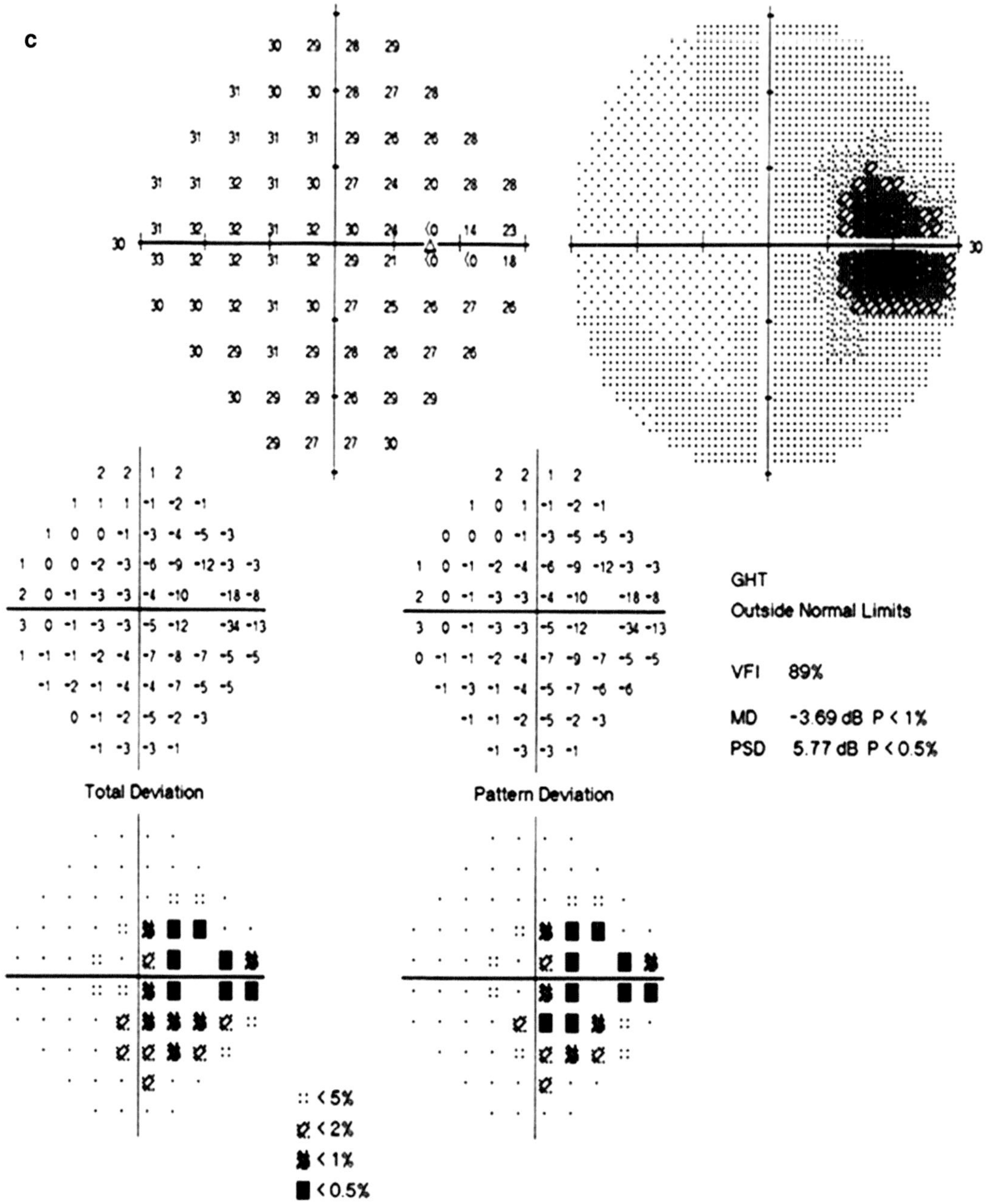

Fig. 12.11 (continued)

thinning. All these changes will lead to corresponding abnormalities in the visual field and mf-ERG.

Some authors believe that AZOOR includes a group of relevant acute and idiopathic diseases, such as multiple evanescent white dot syndrome (MEWDS), acute idiopathic blind spot enlargement syndrome (AIBSES), presumed ocular histoplasmosis (P-PHP), multifocal choroiditis and panuveitis (MCP), punctate inner choroiditis and panuveitis (PICR), acute macular neuroretinopathy (AMNR), etc.

It's often the routine visual field examinations that give us the early cues for an AZOOR diagnosis. As one of the optic function examination methods, visual field examination is convenient and easy to perform. It can be used to exclude this disease. Visual field change is also one of the characteristic manifestations of AZOOR. Enlargement of the physiological blind spot can be found in 75% of the diseased eyes with or without other visual field defects. The common visual field defects include peripheral field constriction accompanied by enlargement of the physiological blind spot and annular defect accompanied by enlargement of the physiological blind spot. Besides, some other studies have shown that island-like visual field defects are a characteristic of AZOOR. The symptoms of visual field defect are usually stable in the first 6 months after disease onset, but gradual aggravation can be found in some patients.

The above two cases suggest that the AZOOR needs to be excluded when the visual field defect is of unknown cause and especially when extensive areas of the temporal side are involved. Other assistant examinations, such as OCT, FFA, electrophysiologic examination, etc., can also be adopted to analyze the causes of the visual field impairment.

The cause and pathogenesis of AZOOR are still unclear. The hypothesis of "primary infection of photoreceptor cells in the retina" has been proposed by Gass. He believes that microorganism such as virus will infect the photoreceptor cells near the optic disc and the ora serrata where the photoreceptor cells are exposed due to defects of the neuroepithelium and thus easily invaded by the pathogenic microorganisms. The infection may not lead to disease immediately, but relevant symptoms of the disease will be observed when the immune response to the infected cells starts in the host. The initial infection site proposed in the abovementioned hypothesis can explain why the visual field defect is more usually found in the physiological blind spot and peripheral visual field. Besides, Gass also believes that this basic mechanism can explain such complicated syndromes as AZOOR [1, 2].

The hypothesis of "autoimmunity" proposed by Jampol and Becker [3] states that the disease is associated with a predisposition to autoimmune diseases and that the MEWDS, MFC, PIC, and AZOOR are autoimmune or inflammatory diseases with similar genetic basis. Some scholars believe that the abovementioned eye diseases are more common in healthy young females, which is just similar with other systemic autoimmune diseases. Specific major histocompatibility complex (MHC) genes and non-MHC genes determine the susceptibility of different individuals to diseases. These genes, together with other genes, as well as environmental factors, jointly influence the phenotype of the disease. Multiple autoimmune diseases can coexist in a susceptible individual, and multiple body parts including the eyes will be influenced. The patient may suffer from AZOOR, multiple evanescent white dot syndrome, and other systemic autoimmune diseases [4].

Besides, some other factors are also considered to be possibly related to the occurrence and progression of AZOOR. Choroidal circulation damage is also speculated by some scholars to be involved in the disease's onset [5]. The study of Ara-Iwata et al. has proposed that a phosducin gene mutation may be related to the occurrence of AZOOR. However, there is no reported inherited case of AZOOR up to now.

AZOOR is a self-limiting disease in most cases. The treatment methods mainly include systemic application of corticosteroid hormones, immunosuppressive agents, and different antimicrobial agents (for patient with viral or fungal infections), but their therapeutic effects are still to be confirmed. The follow-up study carried out by Gass et al. on the patients found that stable visual field defects were present in 77% of the patients, and different degrees of improvement in vision and/or visual field were shown in 26% of the patients at 6 months. A 3-year follow-up study revealed recurrence in 31% of the patients [2]. It is currently believed that the visual prognosis of most AZOOR patients is good, and even complete recovery can be expected. But there are also cases in which the condition gradually aggravates. For instance, a patient who was followed for 13 years in a study still developed chorioretinal atrophy and progressive visual field damage despite hormone and immune regulation therapies [6].

References

1. Gass JD. Acute zonal occult outer retinopathy. Donders Lecture: the Netherlands Ophthalmological Society, Maastricht, Holland, June 19, 1992. Retina. 1993;23(23):79–97.
2. Gass JD, Agarwal A, Scott IU. Acute zonal occult outer retinopathy: a long-term follow-up study. Am J Ophthalmol. 2002;134(3):329–39.
3. Jampol LM, Becker KG. White spot syndromes of the retina: a hypothesis based on the common genetic hypothesis of autoimmune/inflammatory disease. Am J Ophthalmol. 2003;135(3):376–9.
4. Gass JD. Are acute zonal occult outer retinopathy and the white spot syndromes (AZOOR complex) specific autoimmune diseases? Am J Ophthalmol. 2003;135(3):380–1.
5. Saito M, Saito W, Hashimoto Y, et al. Correlation between decreased choroidal blood flow velocity and the pathogenesis of acute zonal occult outer retinopathy. Clin Exp Ophthalmol. 2014;42(2):139–50.
6. Hoang QV, Gallego-Pinazo R, Yannuzzi LA. Long-term follow-up of acute zonal occult outer retinopathy. Retina. 2013;33(7):1325–7.

13 Bitemporal Visual Field Defects Mimicking Chiasmal Compression in Eyes with Retinal Disorders

Ning Fan, Xuyang Liu, and Jiantao Wang

A problem in the sellar area is the first impression that comes into the mind of an ophthalmologist when he/she sees a patient with bitemporal hemianopia, and thanks to that, many intracranial lesions have been found. As the typical and characteristic visual field changes resulting from a damage in the middle part of the optic chiasm where the major nerve fibers come from the nasal sides of binocular retina, bitemporal hemianopia is commonly caused by space-occupying lesions, such as pituitary adenoma, meningioma, craniopharyngioma, and other multiple pathogenic factors, such as inflammation, infection, trauma, and vascular disorders. Therefore, is symmetrical bitemporal visual field impairment always caused by lesions of the chiasm? If not, how to avoid making a diagnosis only by experience? The following cases may bring us some enlightenment.

N. Fan · J. Wang (✉)
Shenzhen Eye Hospital, Shenzhen University, Shenzhen, China

X. Liu
Xiamen Eye Center of Xiamen University, Xiamen, China

Shenzhen Eye Hospital, Shenzhen University, Shenzhen, China

13.1 Case 1

13.1.1 Case Presentation

An 18-year-old female with a history of gradually narrowing of peripheral visual field of the right eye presented with decreased vision in this eye for several months. No accompanying symptoms including headache, red eyes, eye pain, distorted vision, pain upon eye movement, etc. were present. In addition, histories of night blindness (nyctalopia), trauma, and systemic and familial diseases were also denied.

The best corrected visual acuity (BCVA) was 20/125 OD and 20/20 OS. Intraocular pressure was normal in both eyes. Slit-lamp examination of her anterior segments was unremarkable in both eyes except that the relative afferent pupillary defect (RAPD) was negative in the right eye. Fundus examination revealed that the vitreous was clear and the optic disc was pink in color with a clear boundary; extensive map-like atrophy foci could be observed in the posterior polar area, and great choroidal vessels accompanied by hyperpigmentation were seen inside the atrophy foci (Fig. 13.1). Standardized automated perimetry showed a bitemporal visual field defect roughly delimited by the center line in the central 30° visual field (Fig. 13.2).

N. Wang et al. (eds.), *Optic Disorders and Visual Field*, Advances in Visual Science and Eye Diseases 2, https://doi.org/10.1007/978-981-13-2502-1_13

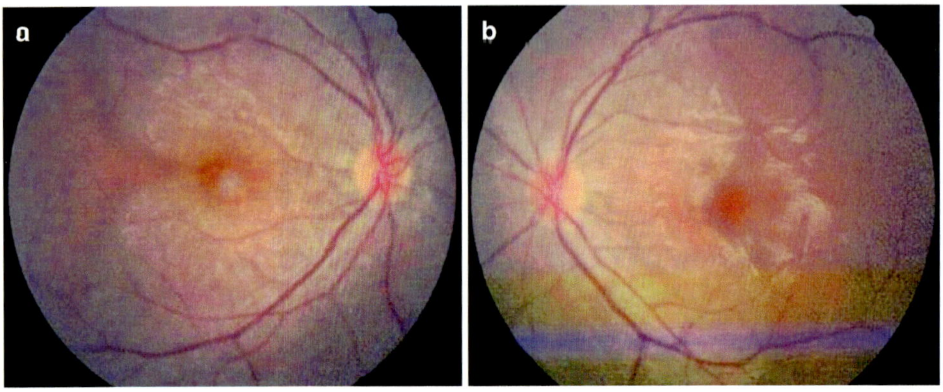

Fig. 13.1 Fundus photographs. The optic disc was pink in color with a clear boundary in both eyes. A large scale of map-like atrophy foci could be observed in the posterior polar area, and great choroidal vessels accompanied by hyperpigmentation were seen inside the atrophy foci. Panel a: Right eye. Panel b: Left eye

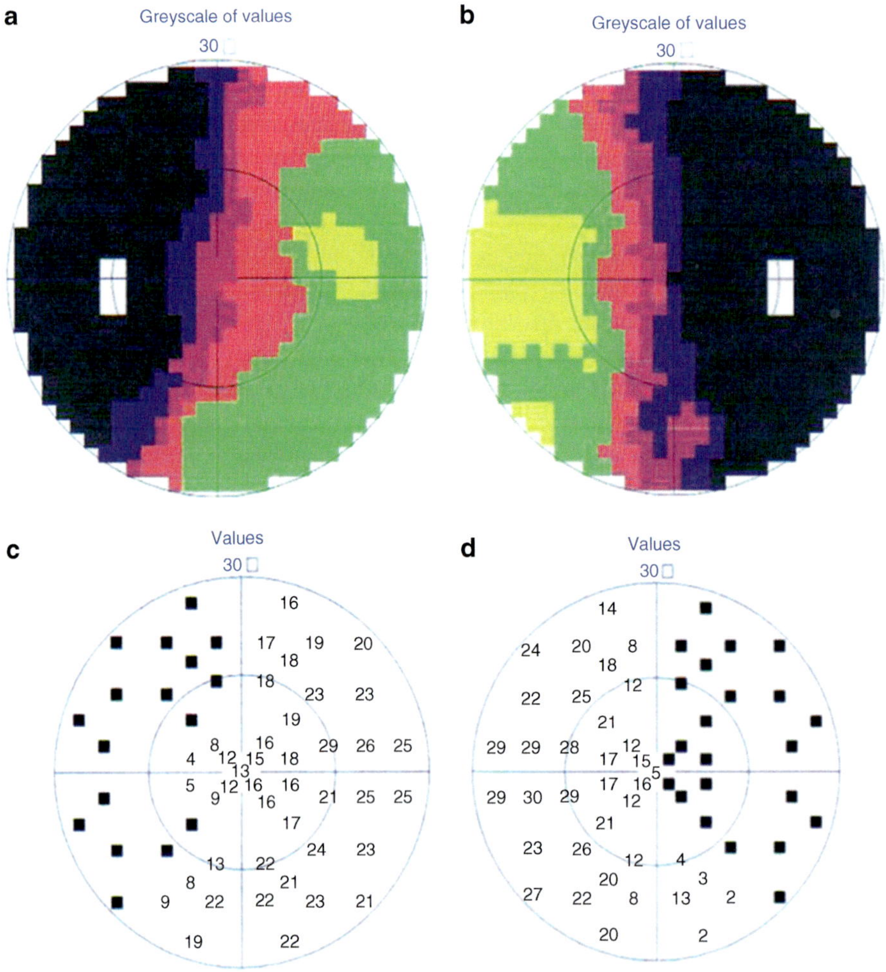

Fig. 13.2 Octopus grayscale and numeric printouts. A bitemporal visual field defect roughly delimited by the center line could be seen. Panel a: Grayscale printout for the left eye. Panel b: Grayscale printout for the right eye. Panel c: Numeric printout for the left eye. Panel d: Numeric printout for the right eye

13.1.2 Case Analysis

The patient had been initially diagnosed at the ophthalmology department of another hospital, and sellar lesions were suspected. She was then transferred to the neurology department, but no suspicious focus was observed after a series of examinations, and she was finally transferred to our hospital for diagnosis and treatment. The most conspicuous characteristic of the disease found in the patient was the symmetrical bitemporal visual field impairments. Vertical boundaries could be observed, and the lesions found in the two eyes were roughly symmetrical. The findings conformed to the typical visual field characteristics of middle optic chiasm damage caused by space-occupying lesion in the sellar area. We observed carefully the patient's ocular fundi after the sellar lesion was excluded. Significant color difference could be seen between the two sides of the macula lutea, and the macula was roughly the boundary of the lesion in both eyes. The fovea was involved in the right eye, which could explain why the central vision showed significant decrease. Therefore, the possibility of bilateral retinopathy was relatively high.

The patient was a young female, and the possibility of optic neuropathy could not be excluded according to the visual field change. However, the vision of the right eye was significantly poorer than that of the left eye. But the RAPD was negative, and no pain upon eye movements was observed in the right eye. These findings didn't conform to the typical manifestation of optic neuritis. Therefore, we chose to examine the retina and macula with OCT and VEP. Meanwhile, screening for optic neuropathy was also carried out. OCT revealed that the thickness of the retinal nerve fiber layer (RNFL) was normal in both eyes (Fig. 13.3). Structure distortion and even disappearance in the photoreceptor layer and the retinal pigment epithelium (RPE) layer could be observed in the nasal side of the fovea in the left eye, and the thickness of the fovea was 180 μm. Meanwhile, disappearance of the structures of the photoreceptor layer and the RPE layer with the thinning of the fovea (thickness, 51 μm) was also observed in the right eye (Fig. 13.4).

P-VEP test showed no typical P-VEP waveform in the right eye and a delay in the latency of the P100 wave under large check stimulation and normal latency and amplitude of the P100 wave under small check stimulation in the left eye (Fig. 13.5).

The OCT results suggested outer retinal layer lesions in both eyes: significant lesions could be observed in the photoreceptor layer and RPE layer, the fovea in the right eye was involved, and the lesion in the left eye was close to the fovea, which was consistent with the damage to the visual field and vision. The OCT measurements of the peripapillary RNFL thickness were normal in both eyes. The P-VEP results obtained from both eyes didn't conform to the visual field findings but were in accordance with central visual acuity results. Based on the OCT findings and the medical history, the optic neuropathy can be excluded. The severe abnormality found in the P-VEP of the right eye suggested serious ganglion cell lesion in the macula. The mild abnormality found in the P-VEP of the left eye suggested relatively mild ganglion cell lesion in the macula.

Therefore, the possible diagnoses included the following: (a) sellar lesion (excluded); (b) bilateral retinopathy; (c) bilateral chorioretinopathy; and (d) retrobulbar optic neuritis (excluded). FFA and indocyanine green angiography (ICGA) were required to confirm the diagnoses of retinopathy and choroidopathy.

FFA showed extensive map-like weakly fluorescent choroidal atrophy foci surrounding the optic discs in both eyes at the early phase, and great choroidal vessels could be seen inside the foci. Extensive and patchy fluorescent coloring mixed up with hypofluorescence from blocking by RPE lesion was found inside the atrophy foci at the late phase of the angiography. The macula of the right eye was observed with damaged foveal avascular zone. A mildly damaged foveal avascular zone was revealed in the macula of the left eye. The optic disc fluorescence was normal in both eyes (Fig. 13.6).

ICGA revealed an area of sparse and reduced number of choroidal capillary vessels with the optic disc as the center in both eyes,

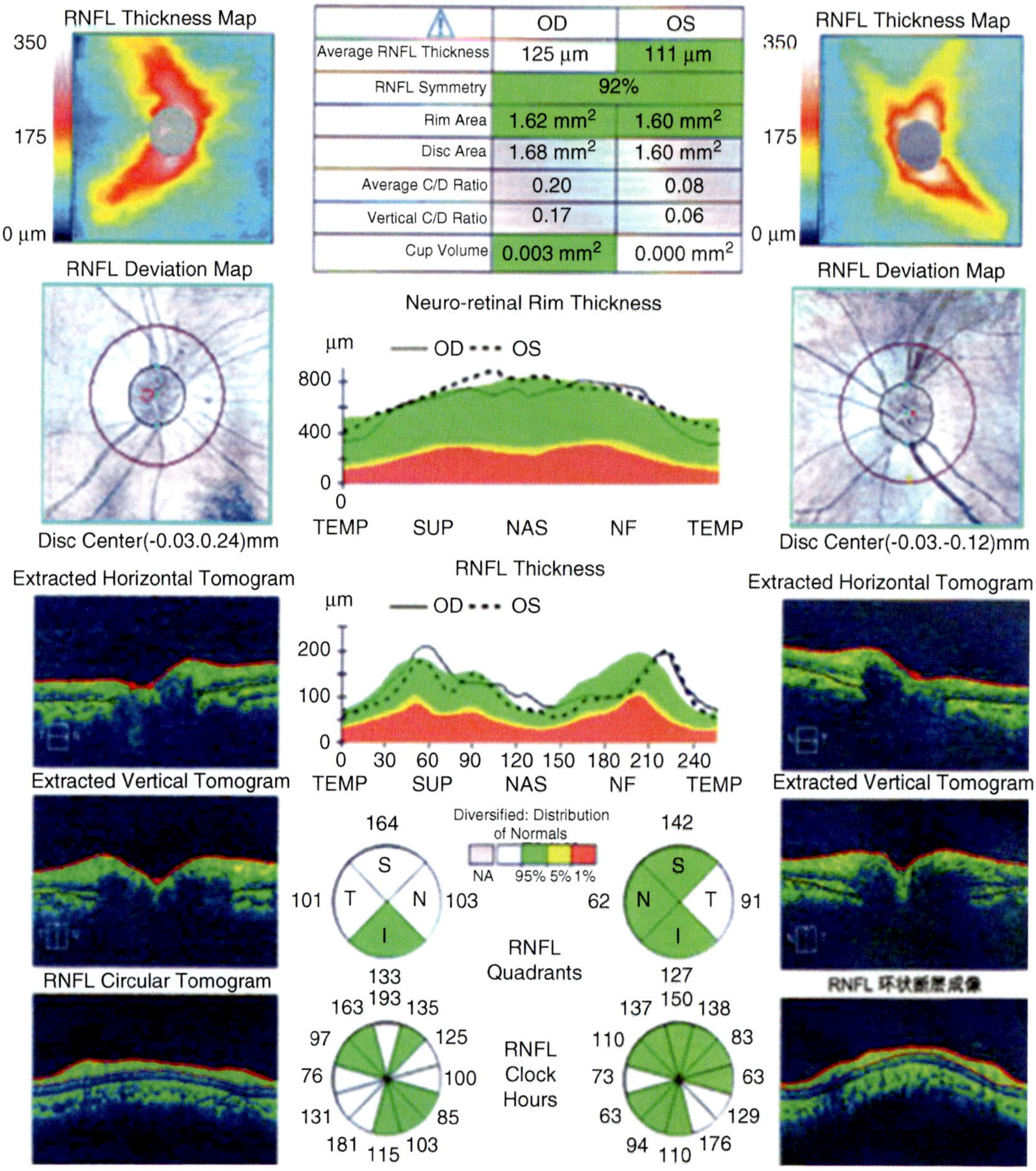

Fig. 13.3 OCT measurement printouts for the RNFL thickness. The peripapillary RNFL thickness was within the normal range in both eyes

and the areas in the two eyes were roughly symmetrical (Fig. 13.7).

The fundus showed extensive map-like depigmented peripapillary atrophy foci and exposed choroidal vessels, which made the fundus appear to be with lacquer cracks, in both eyes. The OCT results suggested significant lesion in the photoreceptor cell layer and the RPE layer. The FFA and ICGA both revealed that the lesion originated from the outer layers of the retina and the choroid. The foci were relatively static and no fluorescence leakage in the vascular wall was observed. No coexistence of active and old foci was shown. Therefore, serpiginous choroiditis, active inflammation, and vascular lesions could be excluded. An inquiry on the medical history of

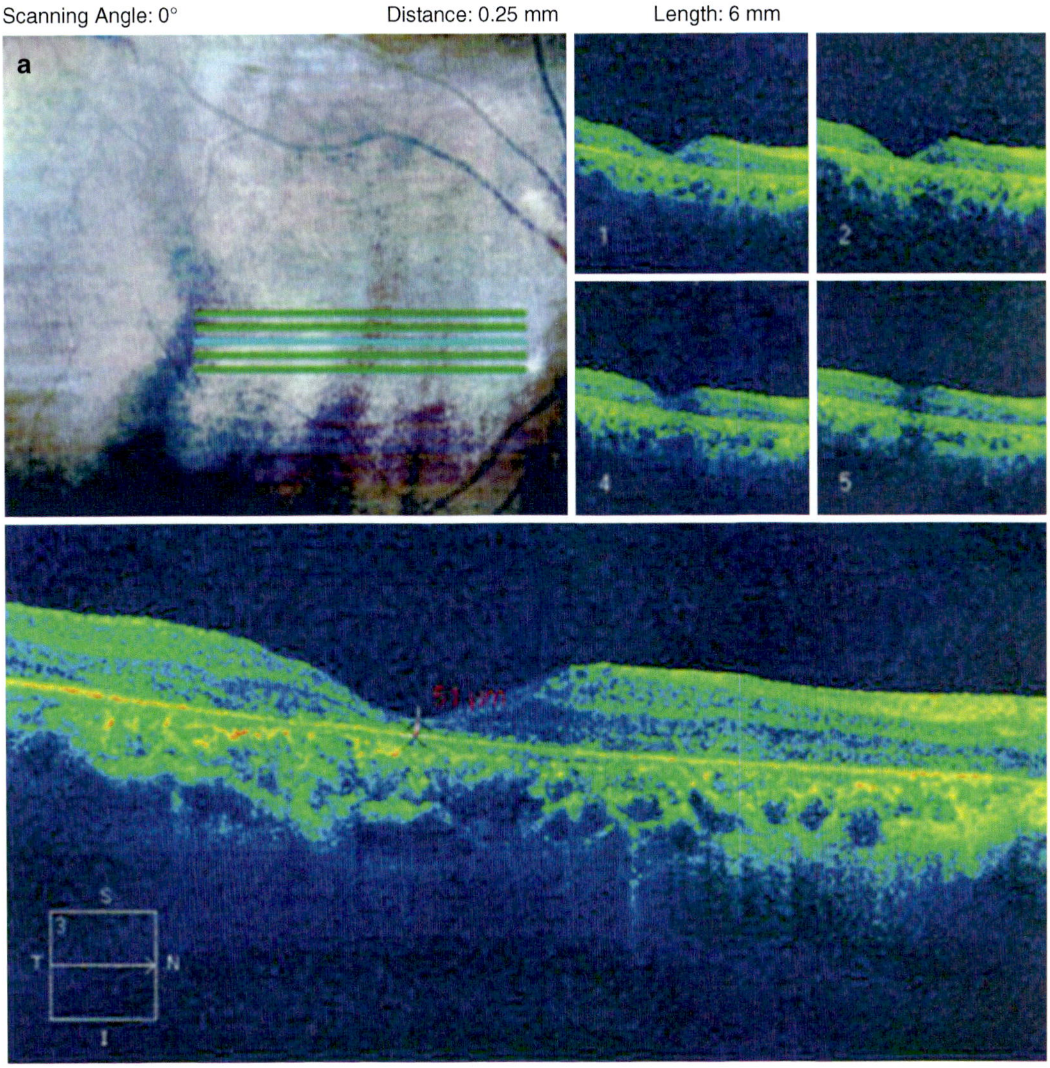

Fig. 13.4 OCT printouts of the macula. Panel a: Disappearance of the photoreceptor and RPE layers were shown in the macula, and the fovea thickness was only 51 μm in the right eye. Panel b: Structure distortion and even disappearance in the photoreceptor and RPE layers could be observed in the nasal side of the fovea, and the fovea thickness was 180 μm in the left eye

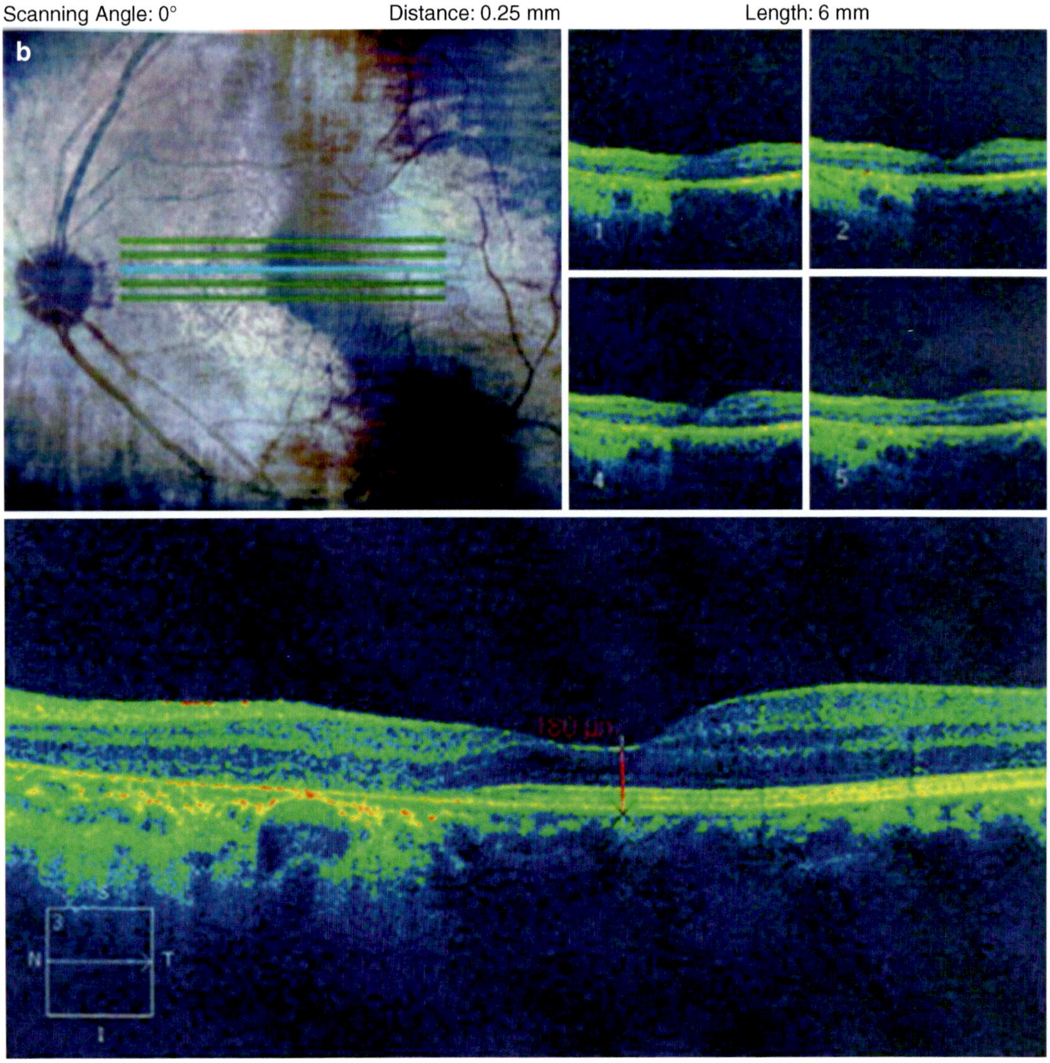

Fig. 13.4 (continued)

the patient was carried out. The patient told us that symptoms similar to those of cold, such as high fever and dizziness, were shown before disease onset. Based on this and the fact that the visual field impairment and central vision involvement were consistent with the fundus foci in addition to the medical history, the condition was considered to be bilateral old chorioretinitis.

Since the retinal foci were restricted to the peripapillary area, there should be residual normal peripheral visual field in the temporal side. We asked the patient to undergo a 60° visual field examination (Fig. 13.8), and the results showed that the real situation of the visual fields of both eyes was that there was a giant scotoma in the temporal side, which was in accordance with the manifestation of the fundus foci.

The patient has been followed for 7 years so far, and vitamins have been given for supportive treatment. The disease condition of the patient has been stable, and no progression was observed in the visual field and fundus foci, which supports the diagnosis of bilateral old chorioretinitis. The foci found in the patient were static and no wax pallor change was revealed in the optic disc. No accompanying manifestations, such as retinal

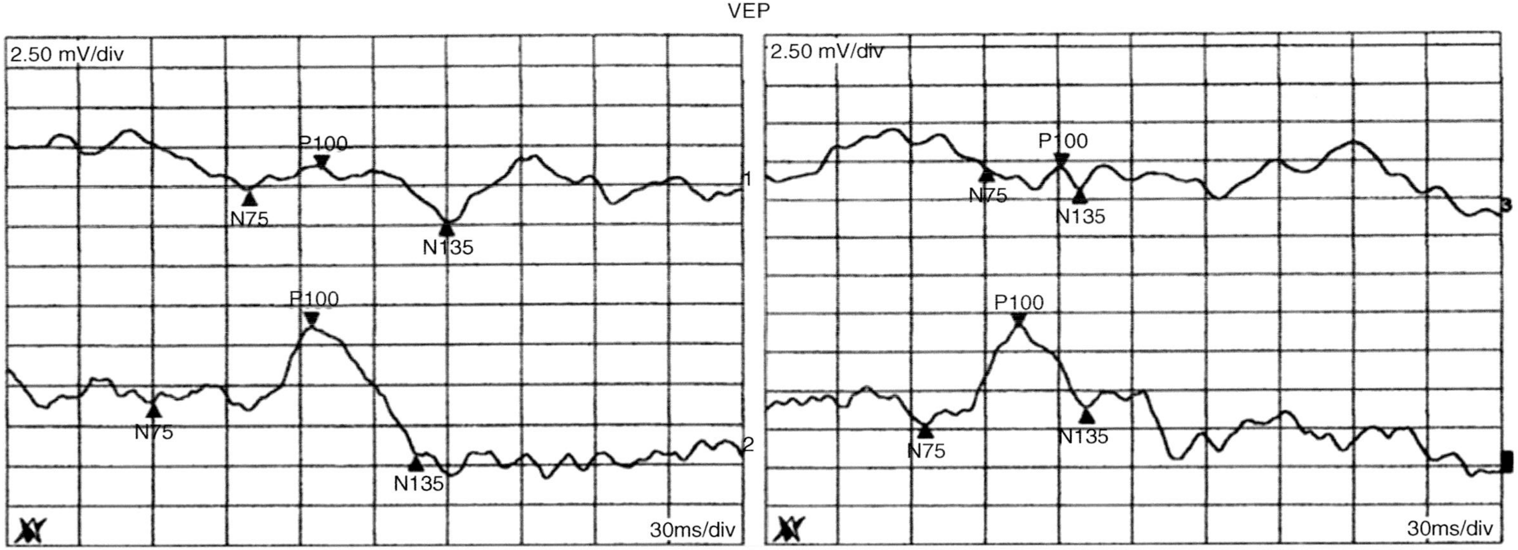

No	Description	Settings	N75	P100	N135	N75-P100	P100-N135
1	right	Pattern Rev., 1°5' Full Field, Ctr:97% 0.9Hz	99ms	128ms	179ms	1.5µV	3.6µV
	Comment:						
2	left	Pattern Rev., 1°5' Full Field, Ctr:97% 0.9Hz	60ms	124ms	166ms	4.6µV	7.9µV
	Comment:						
3	right	Pattern Rev., 0°42' Full Field, Ctr:97% 0.9Hz	90ms	121ms	128ms	35nV	1.4µV
	Comment:						
4	left	Pattern Rev., 0°42' Full Field, Ctr:97% 0.9Hz	65ms	103ms	131ms	6.4µV	5.3µV
	Comment:						

Fig. 13.5 P-VEP analysis printouts. No typical P-VEP waveform was observed in the right eye. A delay in the latency of the P100 wave under large check stimulation and normal latency and amplitude of the P100 wave under small check stimulation were observed in the left eye

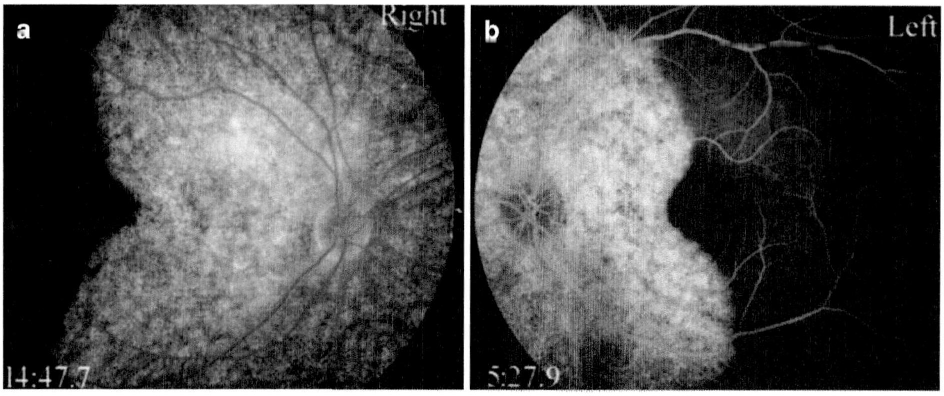

Fig. 13.6 FFA images. Extensive and patchy fluorescent coloring mixed up with hypofluorescence from blocking by RPE lesion was found inside the atrophy foci at the late phase of the angiography. Panel a: The macula lutea of the right eye was observed with damaged foveal avascular zone. Panel b: A mildly damaged foveal avascular zone was revealed in the macula lutea of the left eye

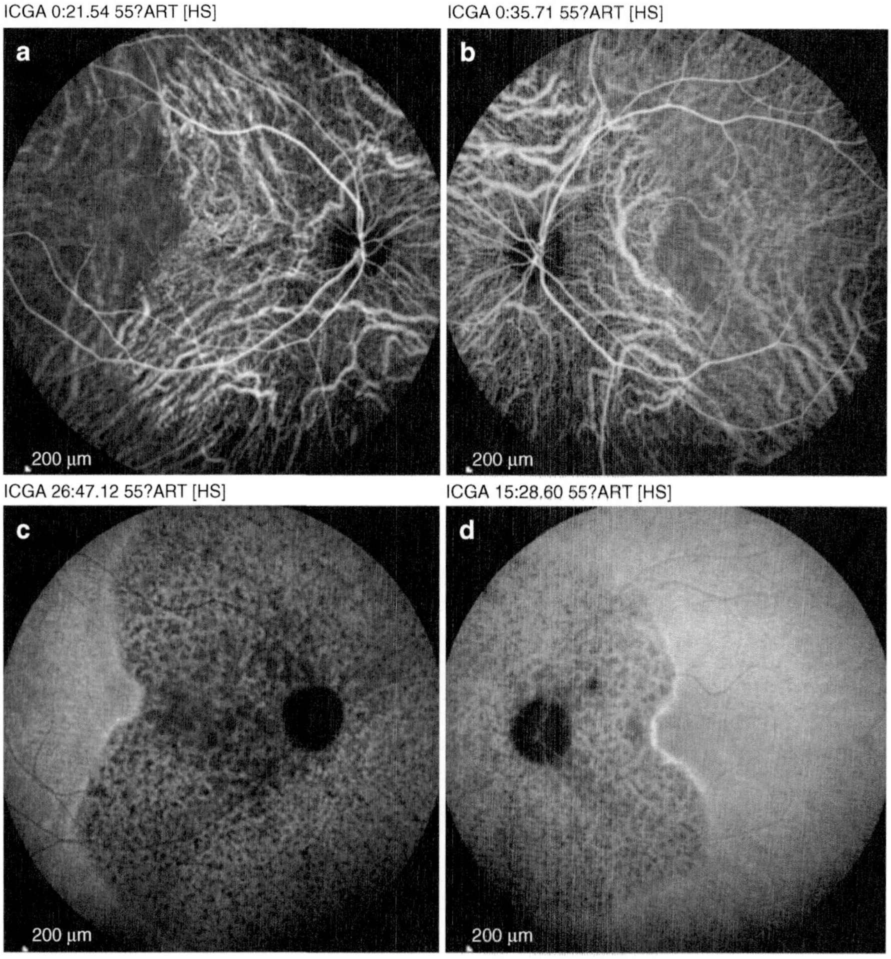

Fig. 13.7 ICGA images. ICGA revealed an area of sparse and reduced number of choroidal capillary vessels with the optic disc as the center in both eyes, and the areas in the two eyes were roughly symmetrical. Panel a: Early phase of angiography for the right eye. Panel b: Early phase of angiography for the left eye; Panel c: Late phase of angiography for the right eye. Panel d: Late phase of angiography for the left eye

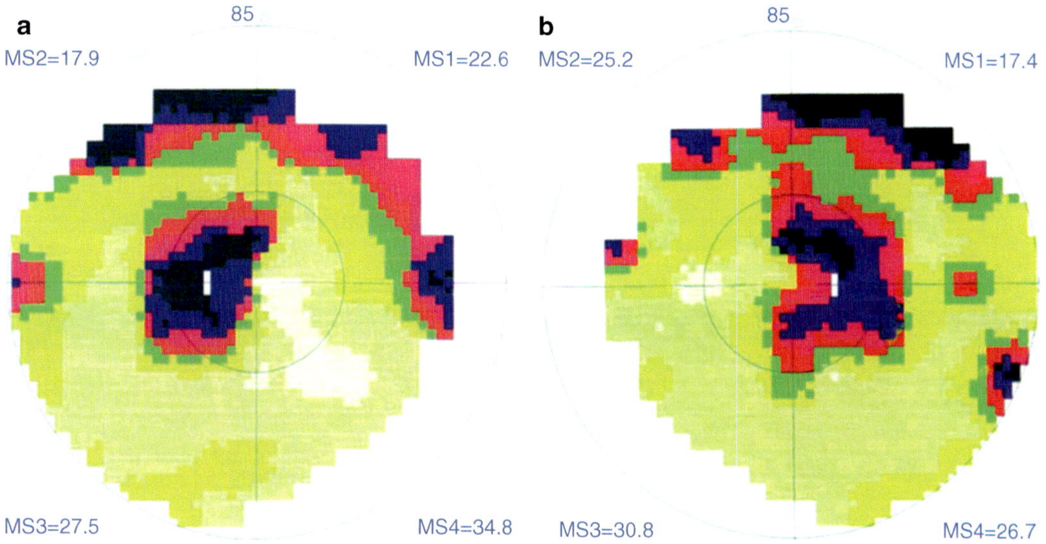

Fig. 13.8 Octopus grayscale printouts of the visual fields. The 60° visual field examination showed a giant scotoma in the temporal side in both eyes. Panel a: Left eye. Panel b: Right eye

vessel thinning and bone spicule intraretinal pigmentation, were seen. Based on these findings, peripapillary pigmentary retinal degeneration could be excluded.

13.1.3 Final Diagnosis

The final diagnosis was bilateral old chorioretinitis.

13.1.4 Case Review

The visual field manifestations were special, and the lesion mainly involved the outer layers of the retina in both eyes. Fever was observed before the disease onset, and the disease condition was static in the 7-year follow-up. Therefore, the diagnosis of bilateral old chorioretinitis was supported by the above findings, and the disease cause might be related to systemic viral infection [1, 2]. Visual field examination with the 60-2 strategy suggested a giant scotoma in both eyes, which was consistent with the fundus lesions' extent. It helped us to have a comprehensive understanding on the patient's disease. It's also worth pointing out that routine imageological examination of the head is still essential in such cases to identify whether there is a concomitant sellar lesion even when the visual field change can be explained by a confirmed retinal choroidal lesion. On the other hand, the retinopathy may not be observed in the initial diagnosis if pupil dilation is not performed. Therefore, the patient is usually required to receive imageological examination of the head and then visit the neurology department. The doctor shall order the patient to return to the ophthalmology department for reexamination regardless of the imageological examination results, so that missed diagnosis of bitemporal hemianopia caused by retinopathy can be avoided. A similar situation is found in the following case.

13.2 Case 2

Hu Yuzhang

13.2.1 Case Presentation

A 45-year-old female patient complained that something blocked her visions of both eyes. No accompanying symptoms, including bilateral visual acuity decrease, distorted vision, red eyes, eye pain, headache, etc., were present. Histories of night blindness, trauma, other eye diseases, systemic diseases, and familial diseases were denied.

The BCVA was 20/20 OD and 20/25 OS. Slit-lamp examination of her anterior segments was unremarkable in both eyes. Fundus examination also revealed nothing remarkable at the posterior poles (Fig. 13.9).

Standardized automated perimetry showed a symmetrical bitemporal visual field defect with partial involvement of the nasal side in the central 30° visual field (Fig. 13.10).

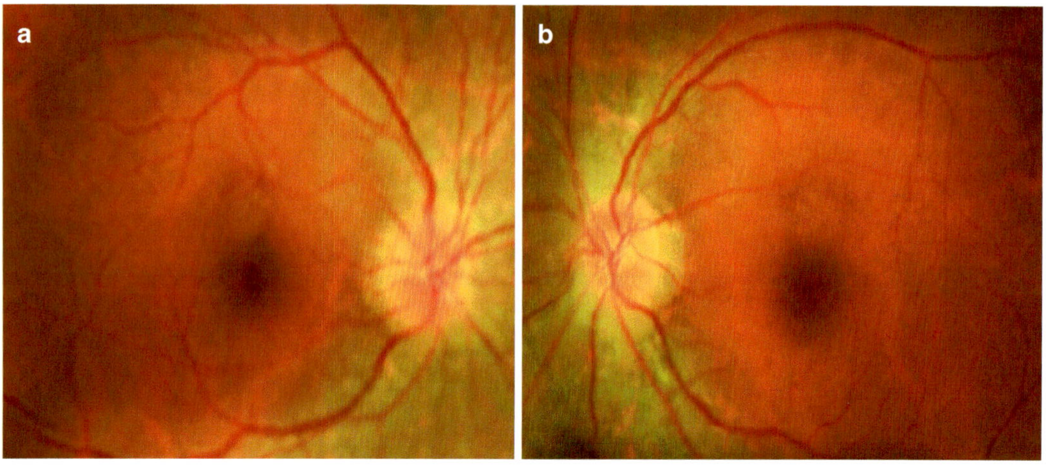

Fig. 13.9 Fundus photographs. Fundus examination showed nothing remarkable at the posterior poles of both eyes. Panel a: Right eye. Panel b: Left eye

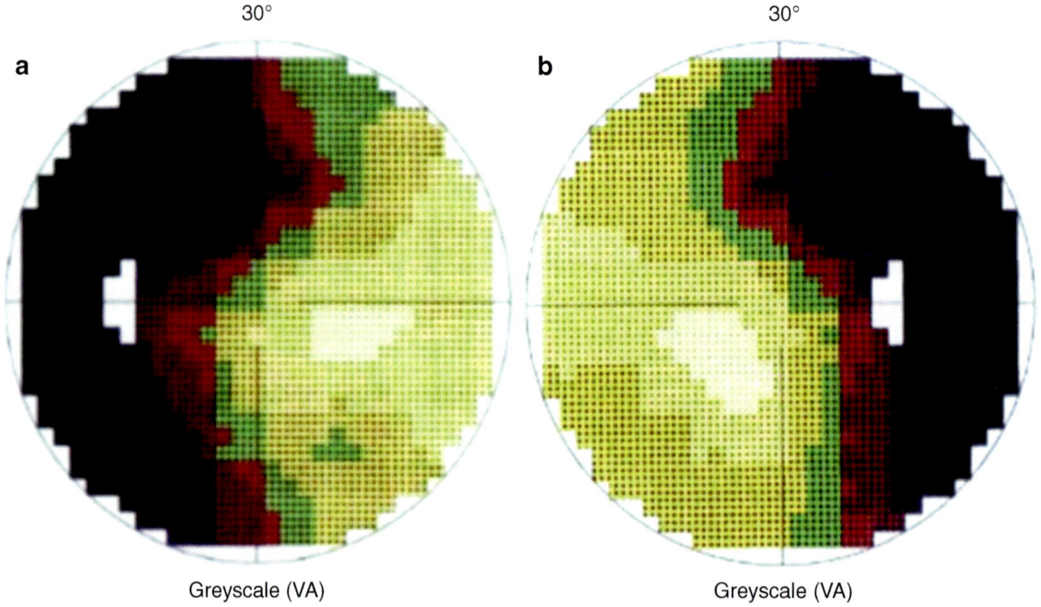

Fig. 13.10 Octopus grayscale printouts for the visual fields. A symmetrical bitemporal visual field defect with partial involvement of the nasal side could be observed in the central 30° visual field. Panel a: Left eye. Panel b: Right eye

13.2.2 Case Analysis

The chief complaint of the patient was blocked vision in both eyes. Visual field examination showed roughly symmetrical bitemporal visual field defects, and the defects had expanded beyond the vertical boundary. The examinations of the anterior and posterior segments of the eyes showed no abnormality. Therefore, middle optic chiasm damage caused by sellar lesion was considered, and pituitary gland MRI was performed. The result was negative. The result was still negative after enhanced scanning was carried out. The patient had visited multiple domestic major hospitals for treatment, and no abnormality had been revealed in multiple head MRI examinations. Then the patient visited the Department of Ophthalmology of West China Hospital. The possible diagnoses include bilateral optic neuritis, bilateral retinopathy, bilateral acute zonal occult outer retinopathy (AZOOR), and Leber's hereditary optic neuropathy (LHON).

Fundus examination after pupil dilation revealed bone spicule-like intraretinal pigmentation and vascular attenuation in the nasal and inferonasal retina in both eyes. The foci in the two eyes were symmetric in pattern (Figs. 13.11 and 13.12). OCT showed disappearance of the ellipsoid zone, atrophy and thinning in the involved retina, and choroid in the right eye (Fig. 13.13).

Fundus autofluorescence (FAF) demonstrated hypofluorescence in the nasal foci in both eyes. Fundus fluorescein angiography (FFA) showed hyperfluorescence in the nasal side (corresponding to the site in the FAF), and no significant leakage was observed at the late phase (Fig. 13.14).

In the electrophysiological examination, dark-adapted 0.1ERG suggested severe lowering of the amplitude of the b-wave in both eyes; dark-adapted

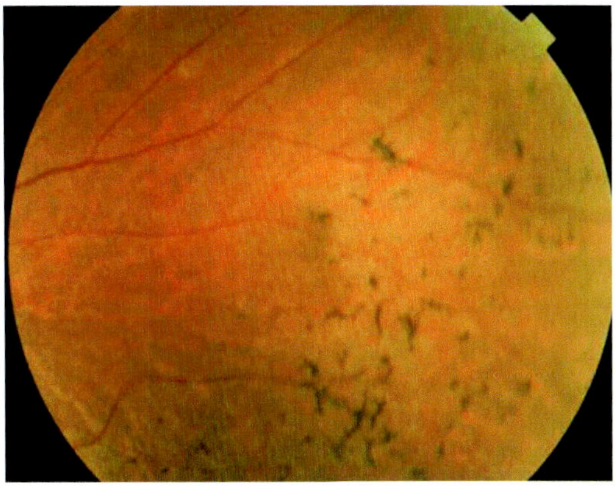

Fig. 13.12 Photograph of the nasal peripheral fundus. Bone spicule-like pigment changes were shown in the nasal peripheral retina of the right eye

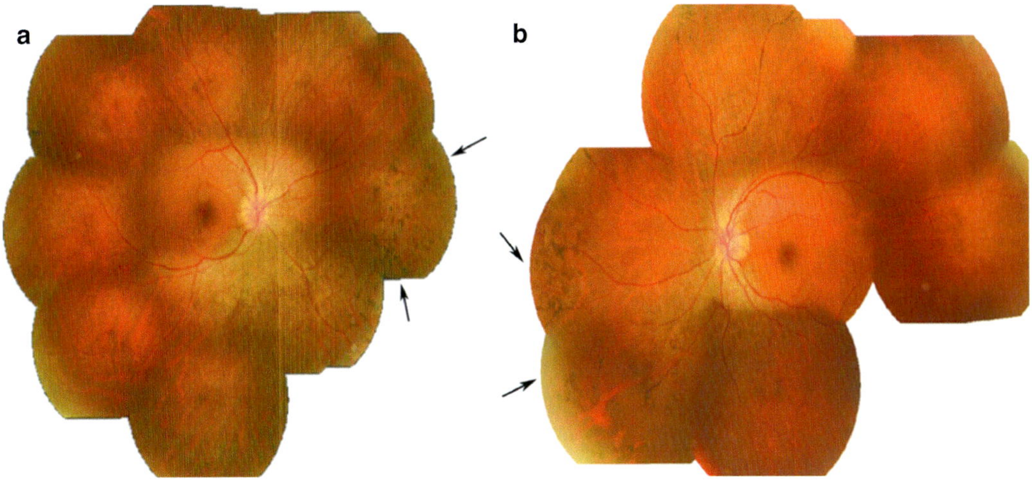

Fig. 13.11 Montage images of fundus photographs. Bone spicule-like intraretinal pigmentation and vascular attenuation in the nasal and inferonasal retina were seen in both eyes (black arrow). The retinal disease of the both eyes was symmetric. Panel a: Right eye. Panel b: Left eye

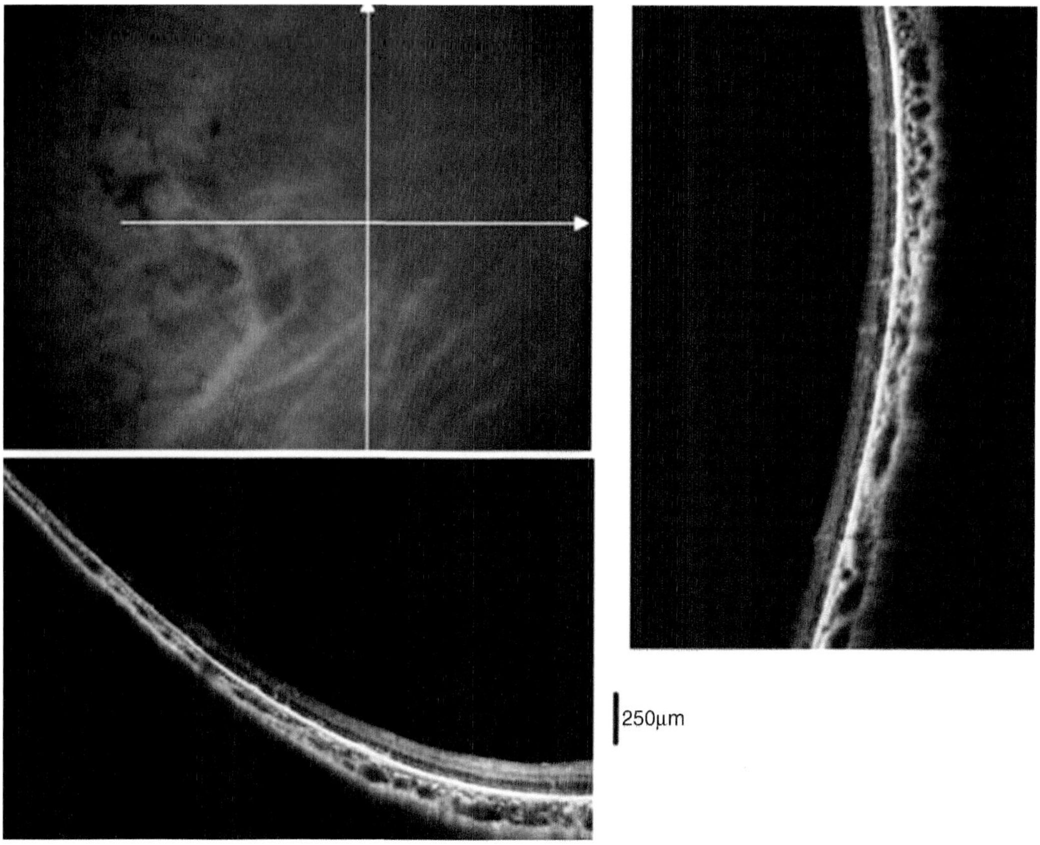

Fig. 13.13 OCT scanning images for the nasal peripheral retina. OCT showed disappearance of the ellipsoid zone, atrophy and thinning in the involved retina, and choroid in the right eye

3.0ERG suggested severe lowering of the amplitudes of the a- and b-waves in both eyes; dark-adapted 3.0 oscillatory potentials suggested severe lowering of the amplitudes of multiple wavelets in both eyes; light-adapted ERG showed mild and moderate abnormality; and the P-VEP results were normal.

Sector retinitis pigmentosa was suspected based on the foci found in the nasal peripheral retina in fundus examination after pupil dilation. The findings from further OCT, FFA, and ERG examination all supported this diagnosis.

The autofluorescence of the foci was hypofluorescence, but hyperfluorescence was shown in FFA in both eyes. This is because the fundus autofluorescence mainly originated from the lipofuscin contained in the RPE cells in vivo. Because atrophy and apoptosis of the nasal RPE cells in this patient, the nasal autofluorescence was weak. The background fluorescence of the choroid was not blocked by the RPE during the FFA, and that's why hyperfluorescence was exhibited. The amplitudes of a- and b-waves in both eyes showed severe reduction in dark-adapted 0.1ERG and 3.0ERG during the flash electroretinogram (FERG) examination. The results suggested that the retinitis pigmentosa of the patient mainly involved the rod cells. Since there was no significant abnormality in other parts of the retina, the changes revealed by P-VEP and light-adapted ERG examinations were relatively mild.

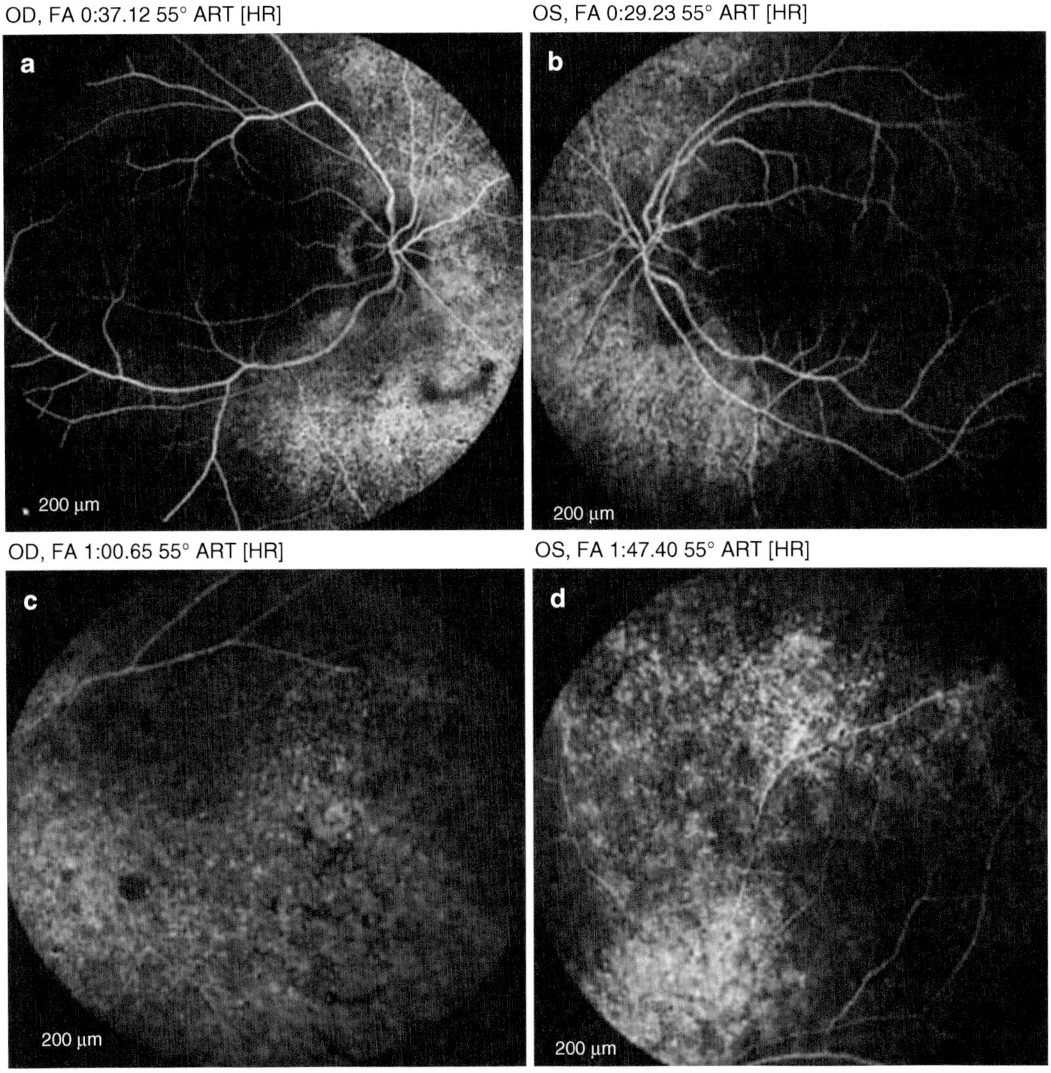

Fig. 13.14 FFA images. FFA showed hyperfluorescence in the nasal retina, and no significant leakage was observed at the late phase in either eye. Panels a, c: Right eye. Panels b, d: Left eye

13.2.3 Final Diagnosis

The final diagnosis was bilateral sector retinitis pigmentosa.

13.2.4 Case Review

The patient initially resorted to the department of ophthalmology. Since typical bitemporal hemianopia was shown and no abnormality was found in undilated fundus examination, she was then transferred to the department of neurosurgery and received head imaging. The possibility of retinopathy should also be taken into consideration, and the cause of bitemporal hemianopia should also be explored from the perspective of ophthalmology in addition to visual pathway (especially the sella turcica) lesion screening when no abnormality is found in the head to avoid unnecessary intracranial lesion screenings. Meanwhile, it's very important for a neurologist to keep alert for the bitemporal hemianopia resulting from retinopathy.

13.3 Case 3

13.3.1 Case Presentation

A 69-year-old female patient complained that something blocked her bilateral temporal-side visual field for half a year. The bilateral visual acuity of the patient showed mild decrease. No accompanying symptoms, including red eyes, eye pain, headache, distorted vision, etc., were present. Histories of night blindness and systemic discomfort, trauma, eye disease, systemic disease, and familial diseases were denied.

The BCVA was 20/32 OD and 20/40 OS. Slit-lamp examination of her anterior segments was unremarkable in both eyes except that the lens was mildly to moderately opaque in both eyes. The fundus examination was also unremarkable in the posterior poles (Fig. 13.15).

Standardized automated perimetry showed a bitemporal visual field defect (Fig. 13.16).

Careful fundus examination was carried out after the pupils were dilated and peripheral retinas were observed. Bilateral symmetric bone spicule-like pigment changes could be found in the nasal and inferonasal quadrants of the retinas, accompanied by the vascular narrowing (Fig. 13.17). The findings from further FFA, ERG, etc. supported this diagnosis.

13.3.2 Final Diagnosis

The final diagnosis was bilateral sector retinitis pigmentosa.

13.3.3 Case Review

In sector retinitis pigmentosa, the lesions are limited to one or two quadrants of the fundus and in fan-shaped distribution or occupy half of the fundus. The lesions are usually located in the two inferior quadrants. The inferonasal quadrant is more frequently affected if only one quadrant is involved. Complaint of night blindness is not common. The diseased areas in the two eyes are usually symmetric, and the disease progression is slow. The retinal vessels that supply the lesion area become thinner, and the visual field defect often corresponds to the lesion area. Dark-adapted ERGs show more serious changes in electrophysiological examinations. The disease is usually inherited in an autosomal dominant manner [3, 4].

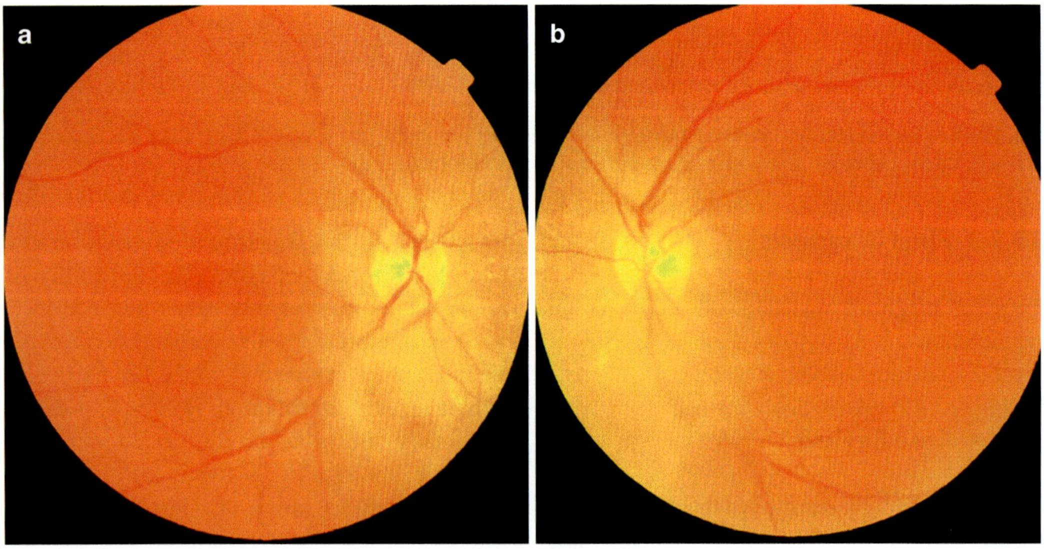

Fig. 13.15 Fundus photographs. Fundus examination showed nothing remarkable in the posterior poles. Panel a: Right eye. Panel b: Left eye (imaging quality was affected by the cataract)

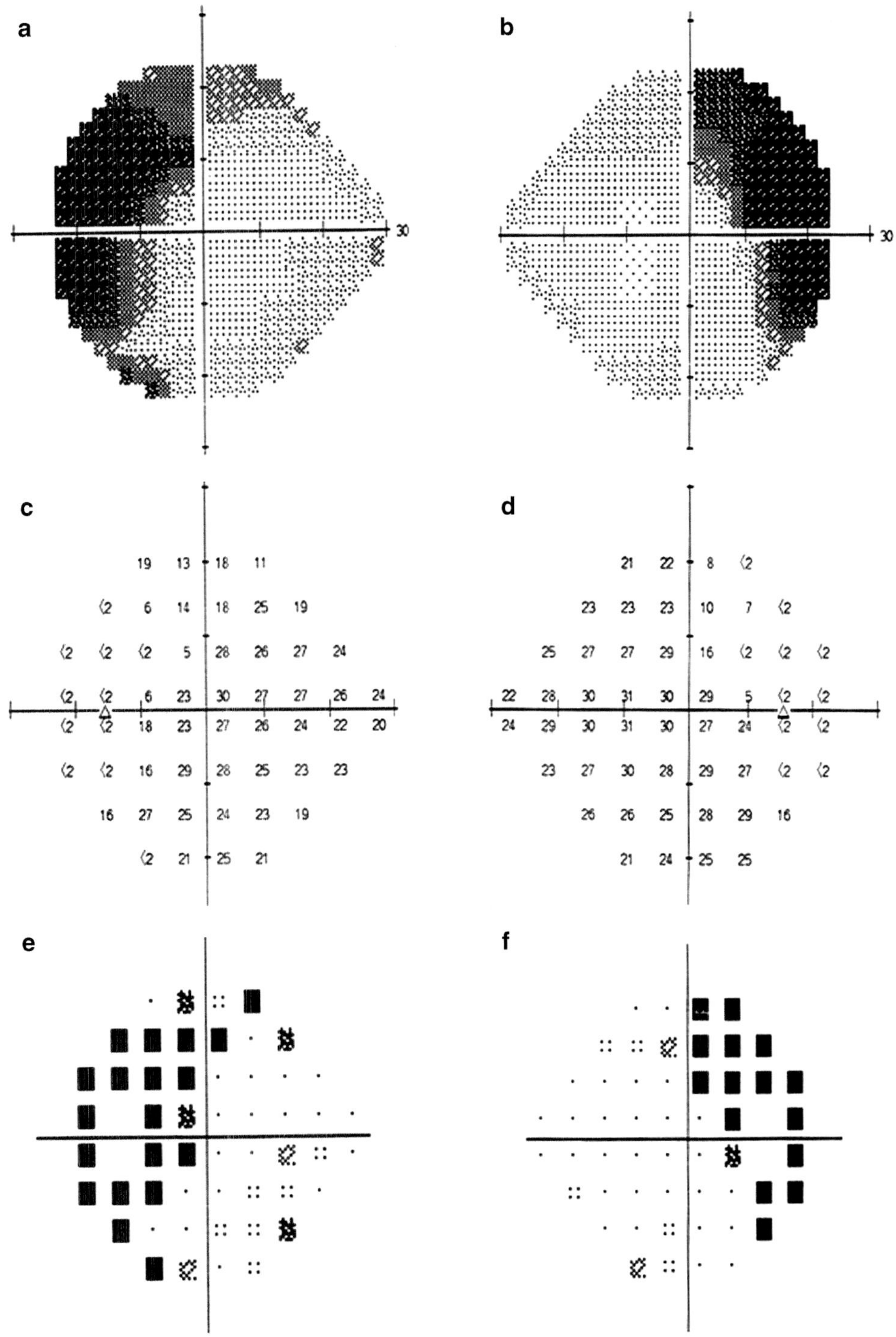

Fig. 13.16 Humphrey threshold numerical values and grayscale plot printouts for both eyes. The 24-2 test showed bitemporal visual field defects. Panel a: Grayscale plot printout for the left eye. Panel b: Grayscale plot printout for the right eye. Panel c: Threshold numerical value printout for the left eye. Panel d: Threshold numerical values printout for the right eye. Figure e: Pattern deviation plot for the left eye. Figure f: Pattern deviation plot for the right eye

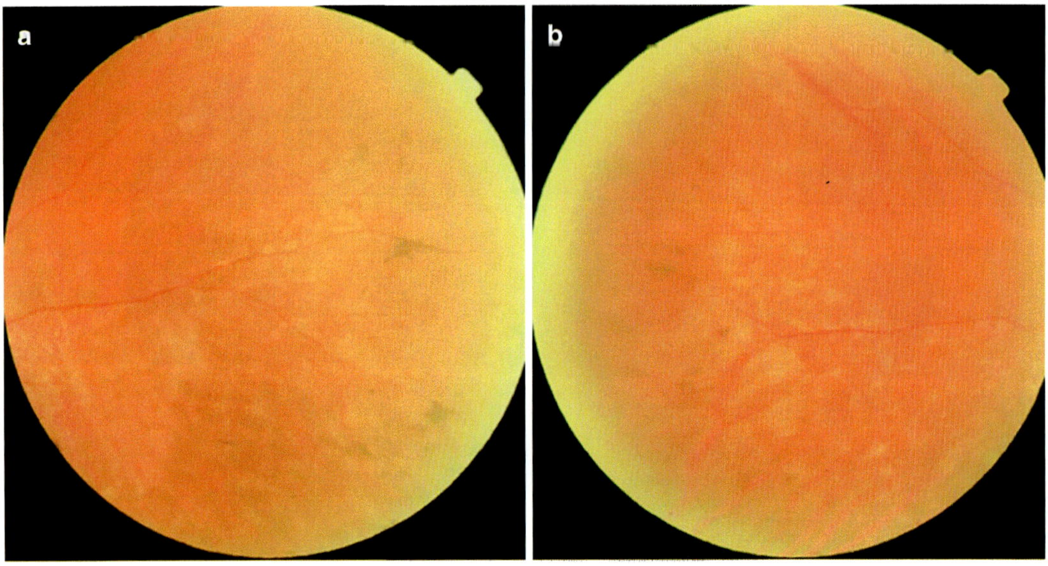

Fig. 13.17 Fundus photographs of the nasal peripheries in both eyes. Bilateral symmetric bone spicule-like pigment changes could be found in the nasal and inferonasal quadrants of the retinas, accompanied by the vascular narrowing. Panel a: Right eye. Panel b: Left eye (imaging quality was affected by the cataract)

The keys to the diagnoses in Cases 2 and 3 are the discovery of the foci and bone spicule intraretinal pigmentation in the nasal peripheral retina through careful examination after the pupil was dilated. It's not difficult to obtain the diagnosis. However, the lesion is very easy to be mistakenly localized in the sellar area according to the special visual field manifestations before adequate eye examinations are performed. It can be mistaken for optic chiasm damage, and consequently unnecessary psychological and financial burdens may be brought to the patient.

13.4 Discussion

The visual fields in the above three cases all exhibited symmetrical bitemporal damages, while the final diagnoses were old retinal choroiditis and sector retinitis pigmentosa. Missed diagnosis or misdiagnosis can easily happen due to special visual field manifestations (very misleading in diagnosis), occult fundus foci, and slow disease progression.

Besides, routine imageological examinations are still essential in such cases to identify whether there is a concomitant sellar lesion even when the special visual field change observed can be explained by the confirmed retinopathy.

Unilateral or bilateral sector retinitis pigmentosa is rare clinically when compared with the primary retinitis pigmentosa which is a group of progressive malnutritional degenerative diseases. Bietti firstly described the clinical characteristics of this disease in 1937. In sector retinitis pigmentosa, only isolated areas in the fundus can be observed with bone spicule-like changes, vascular attenuation, and peripheral atrophy with slow or no progression. The disease is usually found in the lower quadrants or nasal quadrant of the retina and may be accompanied by ERG abnormalities and visual field defects consistent with the lesion extent. Most of the patients have no night blindness complaint. The clinical manifestations and optic function damages are different from those of the primary retinitis pigmentosa [3, 4].

The following questions come to our minds regarding the above cases: (a) Why are the bilateral lesions symmetrical? (b) Why is the retinochoroiditis located around the optic disc? (c) Why does retinitis pigmentosa start from the peripheral retina? (d) Why is the macula consistently uninvolved?

There are no clear answers to the above questions yet and only some speculations can be given. The bilateral symmetrical lesions suggest that it may be associated with systemic factors and anatomic and developmental abnormalities of the retinas. The similarity between the peripheral retina and the optic disc is that they are both in the margin of the retina and are the common starting and ending points of the choroid and the RPE. But what's the role of such anatomic characteristics in the susceptibility to the disease? The fovea has no retinal vessels and it's not easy to be involved. It's speculated that the disease is closely related to the retinal vessels (not choroidal vessels), and it may have connection with such diseases as retinal vasculitis. The progression of sector retinitis pigmentosa is slow or even static, suggesting that some self-protection mechanisms may hinder the disease progression. Further studies are still needed, among which studies at the molecular level are of even higher value.

It's also worth pointing out that the diagnoses in the above three cases are subject to further discussion and follow-up studies. But the focus of this section is to emphasize that attention should be paid to the bitemporal visual field defects caused by retinal diseases.

References

1. Zhang H. Atlas of ocular fundus diseases. Beijing: People's Medical Publishing House; 2007.
2. Noble KG. Peripapillary (pericentral) pigmentary retinal degeneration. Am J Ophthalmol. 1989;108(6):686–90.
3. Van Woerkom C, Ferrucci S. Sector retinitis pigmentosa. Optometry. 2002;76(5):309–17.
4. Saperstein DA. Sector retinitis pigmentosa with bitemporal visual field defects and macular hole. Retina. 2001;21(1):73–4.

14 Acute Monocular Quadrantanopia and Retinal Diseases

Ning Fan, Xuyang Liu, and Jiantao Wang

Sudden unilateral quadrantanopia caused by retinal diseases often has characteristic presentations, such as acute onset and severe visual acuity defect. It usually affects a quadrant of the visual field, suggesting connection with retinal vascular disorders. Two typical cases are given below.

14.1 Case 1

14.1.1 Case Presentation

A 60-year-old male patient presented with sudden loss of his inferior visual field of the right eye for 3 days. No accompanying symptoms, including red eyes, eye pain, distorted vision, etc., were present. Histories of trauma, eye diseases, systemic diseases, and familial diseases were denied.

The best corrected visual acuity (BCVA) was 20/63 OD and 20/25 OS. In both eyes, the intraocular pressure was normal, and slit-lamp examination of the anterior segments was unremarkable except that mild opacity of the lens was revealed bilaterally. Fundus examination showed edematous opacification of the supratemporal retina in the distribution of the occluded vessel, and a white embolus could be observed in the supratemporal arteriole in the right eye. The C/D ratio was 0.7 with normal rim in both eyes (Fig. 14.1).

Visual field examination revealed an inferotemporal visual field defect in the right eye (Fig. 14.2), and the visual field of the left eye was normal.

Red-free fundus photography of the right eye revealed a white embolus clearly in the supratemporal arcade arteriole. Fundus fluorescein angiography (FFA) of the right eye showed that there was fluorescence leakage of the arteriole blocked by the embolus; the macula was involved by the local nonperfusion area in the supratemporal region (Fig. 14.3).

14.1.2 Final Diagnosis

The final diagnosis was branch retinal artery obstruction in the right eye.

14.1.3 Case Review

This case is a typical case of branch retinal artery occlusion. The patient was a senior male, and edematous opacification of the supratemporal retina in the distribution of the occluded vessel could be observed at 3 days after onset. The superior macula

N. Fan · J. Wang (✉)
Shenzhen Eye Hospital, Shenzhen University, Shenzhen, China

X. Liu
Xiamen Eye Center of Xiamen University, Xiamen, China

Shenzhen Eye Hospital, Shenzhen University, Shenzhen, China

N. Wang et al. (eds.), *Optic Disorders and Visual Field*, Advances in Visual Science and Eye Diseases 2, https://doi.org/10.1007/978-981-13-2502-1_14

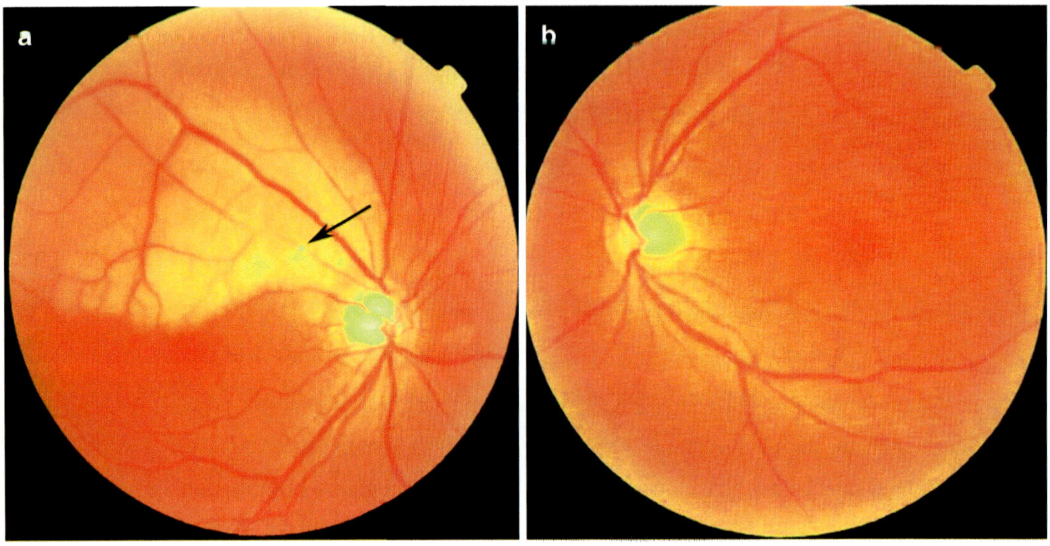

Fig. 14.1 Fundus photographs. Panel a: Edematous opacification of the supratemporal retina in the distribution of the occluded vessel was shown, and a white embolus (black arrow) could be observed in the supratemporal arcade arteriole. Panel b: The C/D ratio of the left optic disc was 0.7 and the normal retina was shown

was also involved. Red-free fundus photography and FFA showed clearly an embolus in the supratemporal arcade arteriole. The visual field manifestation was a sudden and dense visual field defect in the inferior quadrants extending from the blind spot.

14.2 Case 2

14.2.1 Case Presentation

A 25-year-old male patient presented with acute vision decrease in the left eye for 10 days. The patient had suddenly experienced vision loss in the left eye without any obvious trigger 10 days before. No accompanying symptoms, such as red eyes, eye pain, headache, etc., were present. The patient had received hormone therapy at another hospital based on the diagnosis of neuroretinitis, and the vision had shown slight improvement. Histories of trauma, other eye diseases, and familial diseases were denied. He had a systemic disease history of congenital ventricular septal defect, which was without discomfort symptoms and needed no treatment.

The BCVA was 20/800 OD and 20/20 OS. The intraocular pressure was normal in both eyes. Slit-lamp examination of his anterior segments was unremarkable except that the relative afferent pupillary defect (RAPD) was positive in the left eye. Fundus examination revealed mild opacity in the vitreous of both eyes, mild edema in the optic disc and macula, and edematous opacification in the tongue-shaped retinal area between the optic disc and the macula, without hemorrhagic or exudative foci in the left eye. A cilioretinal artery could be observed in the temporal side of the optic disc in the right eye (Fig. 14.4).

Visual field examination revealed diffuse depression but worse loss superiorly in the visual field of the left eye, and the light sensitivity decrease was especially serious in the area ranging about 20° around the central region extending from the blind spot (Fig. 14.5).

14.2.2 Case Analysis

The patient was a young male with one eye diseased and had a history of ventricular septal

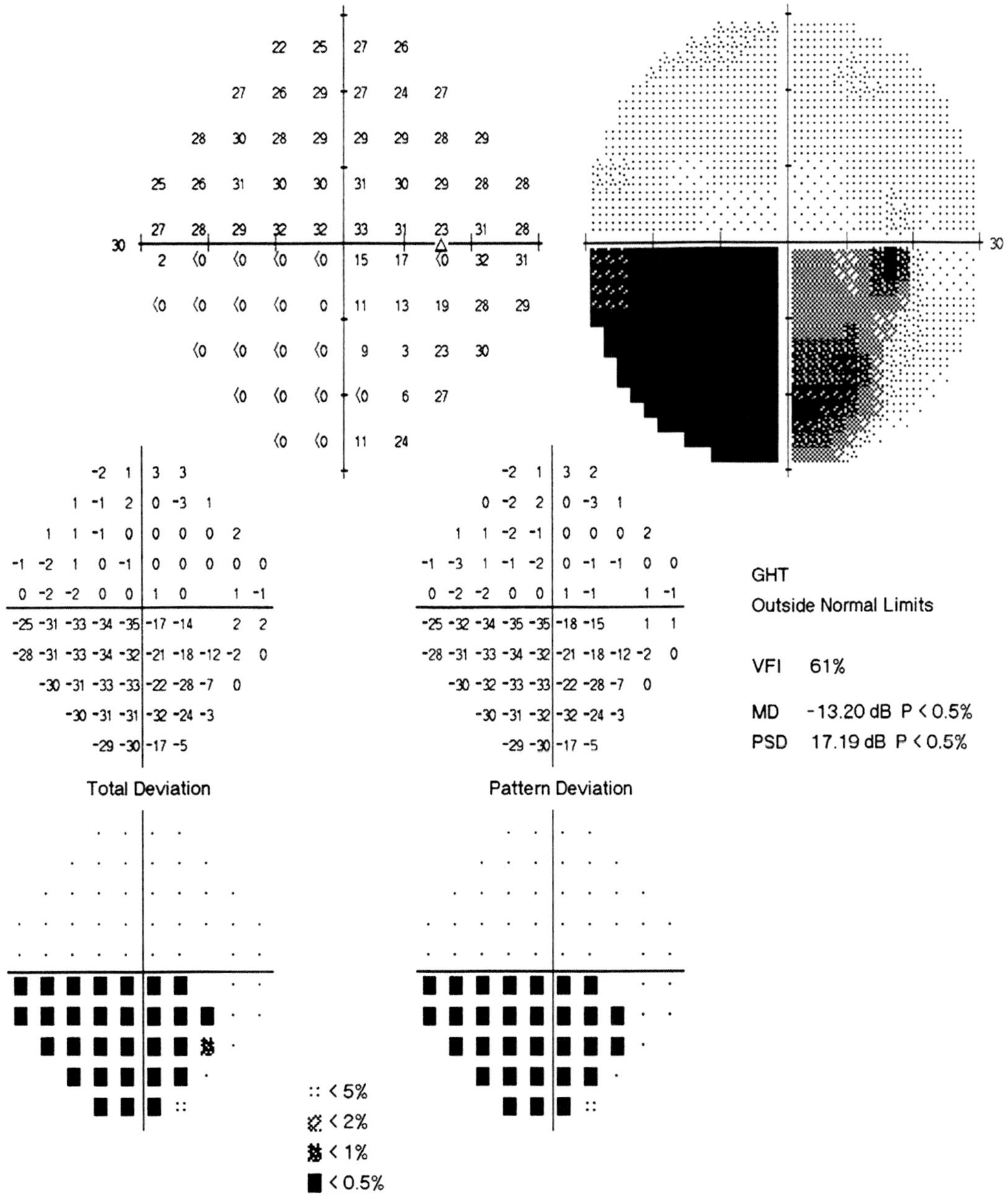

Fig. 14.2 Humphrey visual field analysis printout for the right eye. Standardized automated perimetry with the 24-2 test showed inferior temporal visual field impairment in the right eye

defect. Acute serious vision decrease was observed in the left eye and had lasted for 10 days. Drugs, including hormones, etc., had been used and vision improved a little. Fundus examination revealed optic disc and macula edema and edematous opacification in the tongue-shaped retinal area between the optic disc and the macula. Hemorrhage or exudation was not found. Cilioretinal artery could be observed in the right eye. Visual field examination with the 24-2 test revealed diffuse depression but worse loss superiorly in the visual field, and the light sensitivity

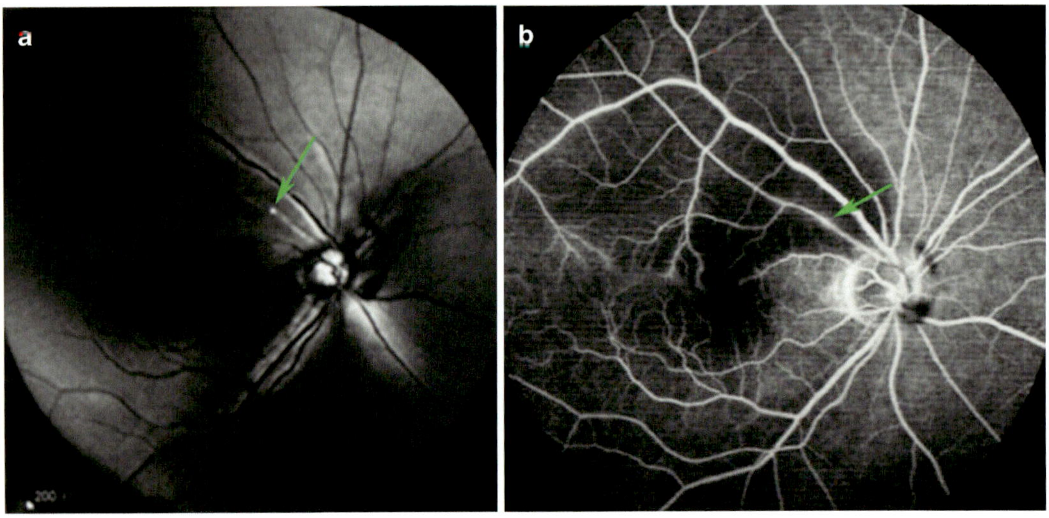

Fig. 14.3 Red-free fundus photograph and FFA image of the right eye. Panel a: Red-free fundus photography revealed an embolus (green arrow) inside the artery. Panel b: FFA indicated fluorescence leakage of the arteriole blocked by the embolus, and the macula was involved by the local nonperfusion area in the superior region

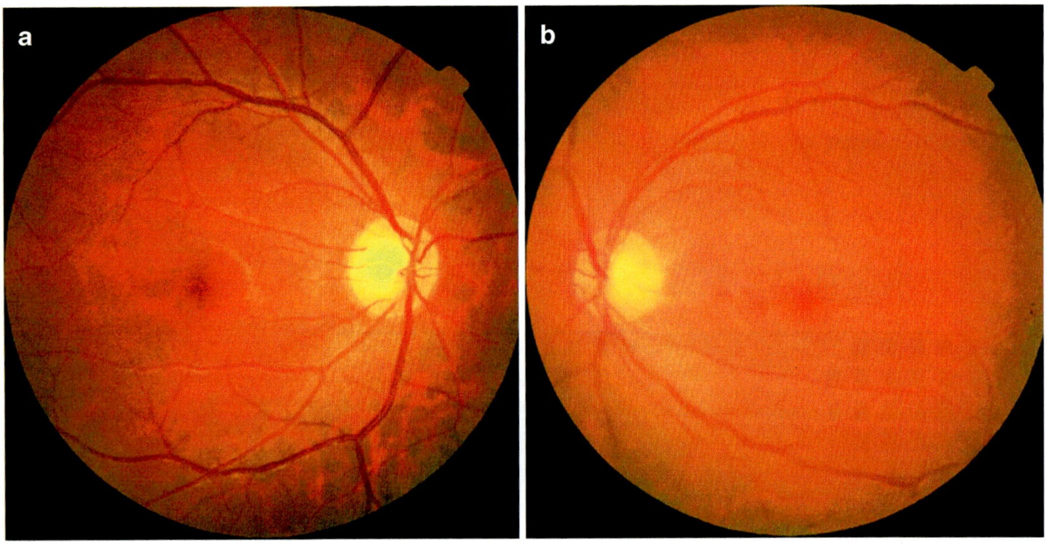

Fig. 14.4 Fundus photographs. Panel a: A cilioretinal artery could be observed in the temporal side of the optic disc in the right eye. Panel b: In the left eye, there was mild edema in the optic disc and the macula and edematous opacification in the tongue-shaped retinal area between the optic disc and the macula, without hemorrhagic or exudative foci

decrease was especially serious in the area ranging about 20° around the central region extending from the blind spot. The diffuse light sensitivity reduction was possibly related to poor central visual acuity. According to the abovementioned case characteristics, the disease onset of the young patient was acute and serious. The extent of the local edema focus in the retina corresponded to the area with the most serious visual field impairment. The visual field had a dense defect that involved a quadrant and extended from the blind spot. Therefore, our first thought

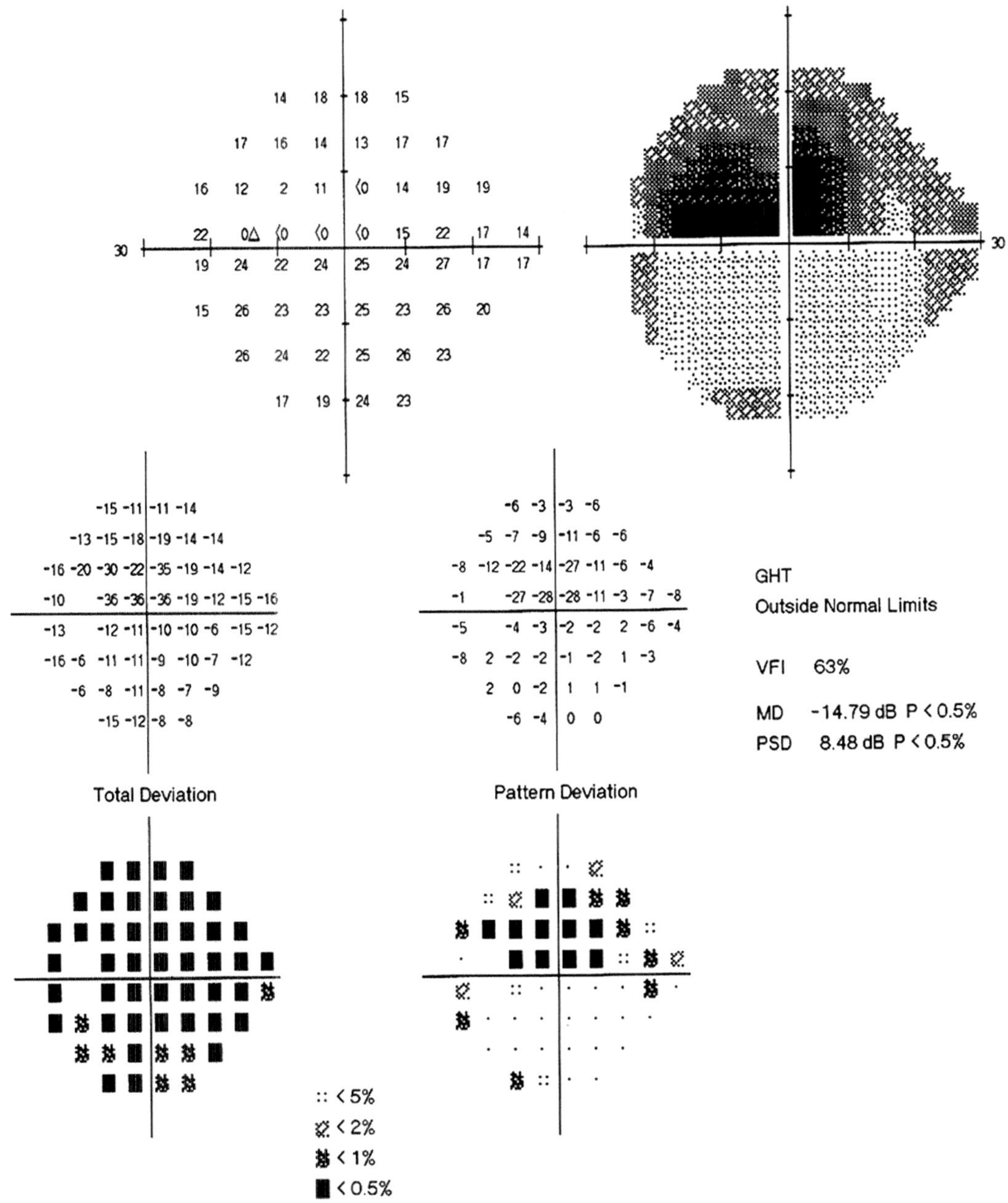

Fig. 14.5 Humphrey visual field analysis printout for the left eye. Visual field examination with the 24-2 test showed diffuse depression but worse loss superiorly in the visual field of the left eye, and the light sensitivity decrease was especially serious in the area ranging about 20° around the central region extending from the blind spot

was vascular occlusion disease of the retina, such as branch retinal artery (cilioretinal artery) occlusion of the retina. But what's the origin of the embolus? The patient was a young male, so was the embolus a result of the ventricular septal defect combined with valvular heart disease? Cardiac color ultrasound needed to be completed, and consultation with the department of cardiology was also needed. The patient's disease had lasted for 10 days, and oral drugs including hormones had been used. The symptoms showed subjective improvement, and perhaps the signs of early retinal hemorrhage, effusion, and vasculitis had disappeared. However, the possibility of optic neuritis or occlusion caused by local arteriolitis could not be excluded. Besides, the possibility of concomitant ischemic optic neuropathy could not be excluded as well. FFA was then carried out to confirm the diagnosis.

Fundus fluorescein angiography (FFA) demonstrated that the filling of the cilioretinal artery in the left eye was significantly delayed and was later than that of the central retinal artery. Mild leakage of the cilioretinal artery could be observed in the late phase (Fig. 14.6). The diagnosis of cilioretinal artery occlusion in the left eye was supported by the FFA findings. In normal situations, the filling of the cilioretinal artery should be earlier than that of the retinal artery. The patient's cilioretinal artery filling was significantly later than that of the central retinal artery. Mild leakage of the cilioretinal artery could be observed in the late phase of the angiography. Optic neuritis was excluded by FFA. Cardiac color ultrasound and consultation with the department of cardiology were completed. The ventricular septal defect was not accompanied by valve abnormality. The thrombus' origin could not be explained.

An inquiry on the patient's medical history was carried out, and the patient found the medical record made by another hospital where he visited

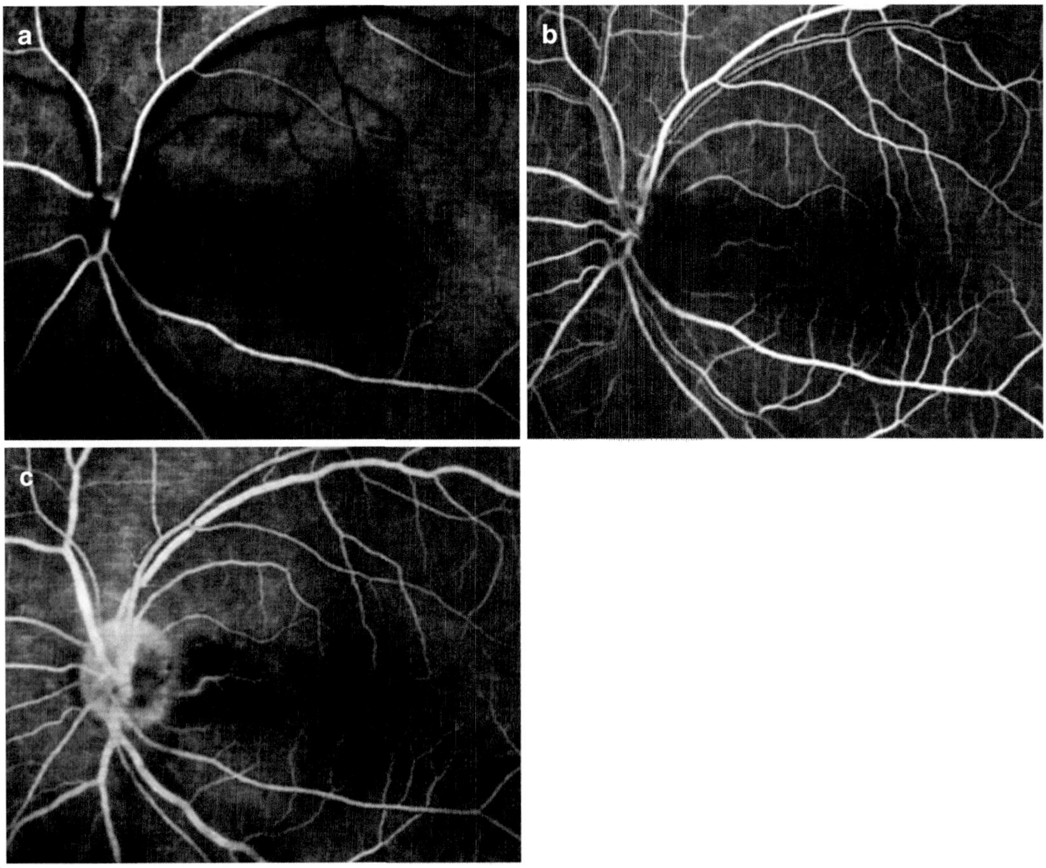

Fig. 14.6 FFA images. Fundus fluorescein angiography (FFA) demonstrated that the filling of the cilioretinal artery in the left eye was significantly delayed and was later than that of the central retinal artery. Mild leakage of the cilioretinal artery could be observed in the late phase. Panel a, b, and c were captured at 13 s, 18 s, and 12 min after injection, respectively

4 days after onset. According to the medical record of the left eye, the BCVA was hand motion; mild mixed congestion and pigmented keratic precipitates (KPs) were observed, anterior chamber flare was positive, pupil was round with a diameter of 3 mm, RAPD was positive, mild inflammatory opacity was revealed in the vitreous body, optic disc edema, peripapillary retinal hemorrhage and exudation were shown (Fig. 14.7). The diagnosis was neuroretinitis. Oral prednisone (50 mg) and the tobramycin-dexamethasone eye drops were given. The patient felt that the vision was improved slightly. He visited our hospital 6 days later.

The hemorrhage, edema, and exudation found in the retina of the patient at the early stage of the disease do not conform to the signs of cilioretinal artery occlusion caused by a thrombus. Vascular occlusion caused by cilioretinal arteritis was considered to be the cause after the uveitis observed in the anterior and posterior segments of the eye was also taken into consideration. Anti-inflammation treatment with hormone was effective. The inflammation in the anterior segment of the eye had resolved, and edema in the optic disc and the macula was observed at the residual focus when the patient visited our hospital for treatment. Oral drug treatments for vasodilation and circulation improvement were given, and the dose of oral hormone was reduced gradually. The patient's condition had been stable all the time.

The reexamination was carried out 1 month after disease onset, and the patient felt that no significant change was shown in the vision. Eye examination showed that, in the left eye, the BCVA was 0.04, the anterior segment was unremarkable, mild opacity was shown in the vitreous body, the boundary of the optic disc was clear, edema absorption was observed, slightly pallor was exhibited in the temporal rim, the macula was free from edema, and thinning with white sheathing of the cilioretinal artery was seen (Fig. 14.8).

Optical coherence tomography (OCT) of the macula of the left eye revealed that the thickness of the fovea was 163 μm and structure was normal 1 month after disease onset (Fig. 14.9).

The observations from the 1-month follow-up after disease onset supported the diagnosis of cilioretinal artery occlusion. The optic disc and retina edema resolved 1 month after disease onset, and thinned and white-sheathed cilioretinal artery

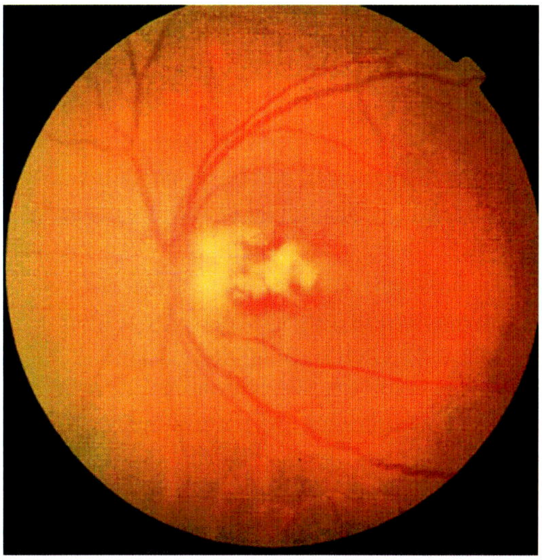

Fig. 14.7 Fundus photograph of the left eye 4 days after disease onset. Optic disc edema with peripapillary retinal hemorrhage and exudation in the area between the optic disc and the macula was seen

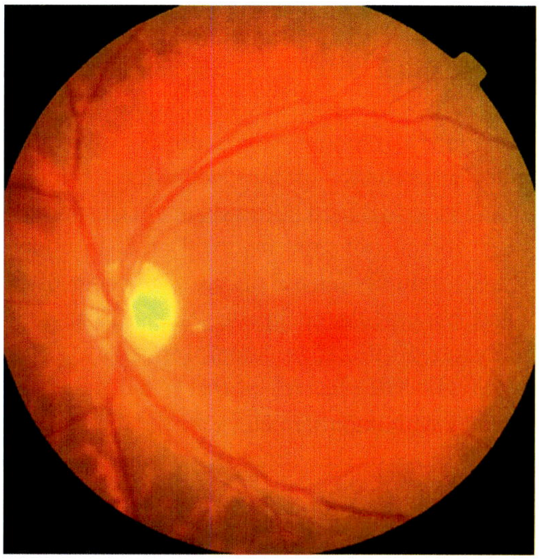

Fig. 14.8 Fundus photograph of the left eye 1 month after disease onset. The boundary of the optic disc was clear and edema absorption could be observed. Slightly pallor was exhibited in the temporal rim. The macula was free from edema. White sheath formation could be seen in the cilioretinal artery

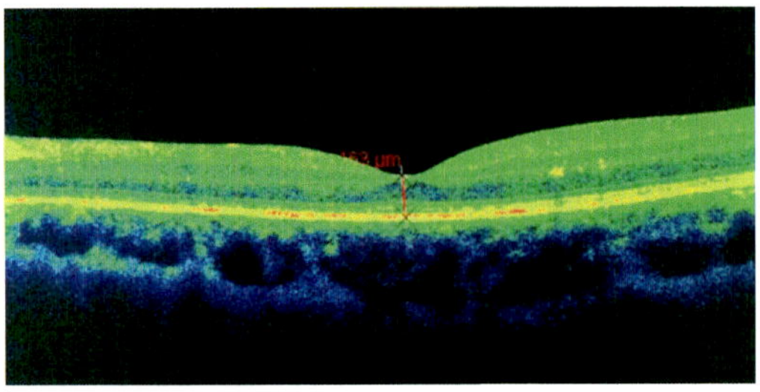

Fig. 14.9 Macular OCT image 1 month after disease onset. The thickness of the fovea in the left eye was 163 μm and the shape was normal

was observed. However, the patient's visual function was not improved significantly because it's difficult to reverse the retinal damage resulting from the arterial occlusion.

14.2.3 Final Diagnosis

The final diagnosis was cilioretinal artery occlusion in the left eye.

14.2.4 Case Review

The key to the diagnosis in this case was the visual field defect that involved only a quadrant and extended from the blind spot. Vascular obstruction disease of retina was considered after we also took the fundus manifestations into consideration, and finally the patient was diagnosed with cilioretinal artery occlusion through FFA. The visual field defect extent corresponded to the retinal ischemia involved area. In young patients, retinitis-related diseases are more often found, but vascular occlusion was rare. The morbidity rate of cilioretinal artery occlusion is about 5.46% [1]. The changes in the visual field provided us with important clues for the diagnosis.

The cause of the cilioretinal artery occlusion found in this case was considered to be related to the local arteritis. The uveitis in the anterior and posterior segments of the eye and local hemorrhage and exudation found at the early stage of the disease do not conform to the clinical characteristics of the retinal artery occlusion caused by an embolus, but arteritis could explain such findings. Thinning and white sheath formation could be observed in the cilioretinal artery in the 1 month after disease onset. The edema absorption in the macula and the optic disc was shown, but the patient's visual function exhibited no significant improvement. These FFA findings and the manifestations supported the diagnosis of cilioretinal artery occlusion. The patient had a history of congenital ventricular septal defect, but the possibility that the embolism may be caused by heart and valve diseases was excluded after the cardiac color ultrasound screening and consultation with the department of cardiology.

14.3 Discussion

Two retinal artery occlusion cases with different origins have been discussed in this section. The diseased sites in both cases are the terminal arteries. Acute ischemia and hypoxia of retina tissues will result, which will cause retinal edema and tissue necrosis, once such arteries are blocked. And the consequent visual field manifestations are visual field defect and serious reduction of light sensitivity in the corresponding distribution areas of the blocked artery.

The damages to visual acuity, visual field, and fundus manifestations depend on the site and severity of the retinal vascular occlusion. Branch retinal artery occlusion is usually located in the great vessels or the bifurcations of the great vessels around the optic disc, and white or light yellow particles (emboli) can be observed inside the blocked vessel. Quadrantal or sectoral edema can be found in the retina supplied by the blocked artery at the early stage of the disease. The edema in the junction of the ischemic zone is more significant, and cherry-red spots will appear if the macula is involved. FFA shows that the filling of the blocked arterioles and corresponding venules is delayed when compared with the unblocked ones. And sometimes fluorescent leakage can be observed in the vessel blocked by the embolus. The retinal edema resolves after 2–3 weeks, and then thinning accompanied by white sheath formation can be found in the blocked arterioles. Sometimes, the change in the vascular shape is not significant, the macula is not involved, and the central visual acuity is still fine. But the damage of the blocked arterioles to the retina is usually irreversible. In such situations, the changes in the visual field can provide us with important clues for the diagnosis of the disease.

Cilioretinal artery occlusion is even rarer with a detection rate of 7–29.6% by ophthalmoscopy and 32–40.2% by FFA [2, 3]. They are usually located in the temporal side of the optic disc. Twenty-three cases of cilioretinal artery occlusion reported by Brown et al. [2] have shown the following three types of clinical manifestations: (a) simple cilioretinal artery occlusion; (b) cilioretinal artery occlusion combined with central retinal vein occlusion (CRVO); and (c) cilioretinal artery occlusion combined with ischemic optic neuropathy (ION). The severity of vision decrease depends on whether the macula is involved. The prognosis for patients with concomitant CRVO and ION is poorer.

The second patient in this section is considered to have cilioretinal artery occlusion caused by local arteritis, and the supporting evidences are as follows: (a) symptoms of arteritis, such as uveitis of the anterior and posterior segments and local hemorrhage, exudation, and edema of the retina, could be found at the early stage of the disease; (b) the filling of the cilioretinal artery found upon FFA showed significant delay and was later than that of the central retinal artery. Mild leakage could be observed in the cilioretinal artery at the late phase of the angiography; (c) thinning and white sheath formation in the cilioretinal artery, absorption of the edema in the macula and optic disc, and absence of significant improvement in the patient's visual acuity and visual field could be observed at the advanced stage of the disease.

Studies have found that the occurrence of retinal artery occlusion is related to the encoding gene of methylenetetrahydrofolate reductase (MTHFR). MTHFR is a key enzyme for the metabolism of folic acid and methionine. MTHFR catalyzes the conversion of 5,10-methylenetetrahydrofolate to 5-methyltetrahydrofolic acid and is thus involved in the in vivo synthesis of purines and pyrimidines and the methylation of DNAs, RNAs, and proteins as an indirect methyl donor. Meanwhile, it also serves to maintain the normal in vivo level of homocysteine [4].

The C677T genotype of the MTHFR gene is more important, and the occurrence rate of this polymorphism in white Americans, Europeans, and Latin Americans is about 40–50% but lower in Asian Americans and African Americans. MTHFR activity in individuals carrying C677T is lower, and consequently an increase of the cysteine level occurs. Cytotoxicity and endothelial injury can be caused, and hyperplasia of the vascular smooth muscle cells will be stimulated. Meanwhile, the coagulation and fibrinolysis systems of the body will be damaged, and finally atherosclerosis will result. In this way, C677T increases the risks of cardiovascular diseases, such as coronary heart disease, cerebral infarction, etc., and it's also a critical risk factor for retinal vascular occlusion. Folic acid metabolism abnormality, which may aggravate the retinal ischemia through oxidative stress damage, is more common in individuals carrying MTHFR C677T versus MTHFR wild-type patients [4, 5].

Among the current treatment options for retinal artery occlusion, drugs such as Ocufolin are helpful, in addition to the conventional treatments. The main ingredients of Ocufolin are methylfolate salt and *N*-acetylcysteine, so it can alleviate the folic acid metabolism defect [5].

The above studies suggest that it's necessary to detect the molecular genetic background, such as the MTHFR gene, for patients with retinal artery occlusion.

References

1. Huirong Z. Atlas of ocular fundus diseases. Beijing: People's Medical Publishing House; 2007.
2. Brown GC, Moffat K, Cruess A, et al. Cilioretinal artery obstruction. Retina. 1983;3(3):182–7.
3. Brown CJ. Preservation of retinal structure and function after cilioretinal artery occlusion: a case report. Int Med Case Rep J. 2016;9:29–34.
4. Heifetz M, Birk RZ. MTHRF C677T polymorphism affects normotensive diastolic blood pressure independently of blood lipids. Am J Hypertens. 2015;28(3):387–92.
5. Qi Z, Hoffman G, Kurtycz D, Yu J. Prevalence of the C677T substitution of the methylenetetrahydrofolate reductase (MTHFR) gene in Wisconsin. Genet Med. 2003;5(6):458–9.

15 BRVO vs BRAO: What Are the Differences in Visual Field Changes?

Ning Fan, Xuyang Liu, and Jiantao Wang

Visual field defects will occur if branch retinal vessels are occluded. The extent and severity of the visual field defects can roughly reflect the vessel distribution area and severity of the retinal damage. The extents of involvement of branch retinal vein occlusion (BRVO) and branch retinal artery occlusion (BRAO) are similar, but the natures of the two diseases are different. BRVO mainly involves the venules and will correspondingly cause chronic ischemia and hypoxia of the retina, whereas BRAO mainly involves the arterioles with the characteristics of acute ischemia, hypoxia, and even severe edema and necrosis of the retina [1–3]. The similarities and differences of the two diseases in terms of visual field defects will be discussed in this section through two cases and literature review.

N. Fan · J. Wang (✉)
Shenzhen Eye Hospital, Shenzhen University, Shenzhen, China

X. Liu
Xiamen Eye Center of Xiamen University, Xiamen, China

Shenzhen Eye Hospital, Shenzhen University, Shenzhen, China

15.1 Case 1

15.1.1 Case Presentation

A 62-year-old male patient presented with vision decrease in the left eye for over a month. No accompanying symptoms, including red eyes, eye pain, headache, shadow in the vision, etc., were present. The patient has been suffering from hypertension for years, and the medication was irregular. Histories of other eye diseases, trauma, and familial diseases were denied.

The uncorrected visual acuity (UCVA) was 20/32 OD and 20/100 OS, and the best corrected visual acuity (BCVA) was 20/20 with myopic correction (−0.50DS) OD and 20/50 with myopic correction (−1.75DS) OS. The intraocular pressure was normal in both eyes. Slit-lamp examination of his anterior segments was unremarkable except that the lens in both eyes showed mild opacity.

Fundus examination revealed that the optic discs of both eyes were red with a clear boundary and the C/D was 0.3. In the left eye, a dilated and tortuous occluded vein could be observed in the supratemporal arcade, while intraretinal hemorrhages in a wedge-shaped pattern delineated the area drained by the occluded vein; cotton-wool spots were also seen, and hemorrhage and edema were shown in the macula (Fig. 15.1).

Standardized automated perimetry showed an inferior visual field defect extending from the blind spot delimited by the horizontal line which

N. Wang et al. (eds.), *Optic Disorders and Visual Field*, Advances in Visual Science and Eye Diseases 2, https://doi.org/10.1007/978-981-13-2502-1_15

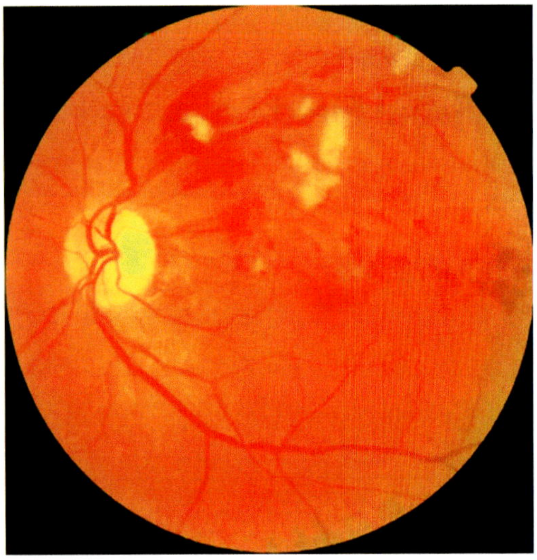

Fig. 15.1 Fundus photograph. A dilated and tortuous occluded vein could be observed in the supratemporal arcade, while intraretinal hemorrhages in a wedge-shaped pattern delineated the area drained by the occluded vein; cotton-wool spots were also seen, and macular hemorrhage and edema were shown in the left eye

could be found in the left eye, and the central region was also involved (Fig. 15.2).

Optical coherence tomography (OCT) revealed cystoid macular edema, intraretinal fluid, inner-segment-outer-segment abnormalities, and a large cyst, with the fovea thickness being 517 μm (Fig. 15.3). Fundus fluorescein angiography (FFA) showed tortuous and dilated branch retinal veins, staining, and leakage in the occluded vessels, a large nonperfusion area, and involvement of the macula by the foci in the left eye (Fig. 15.4).

15.1.2 Final Diagnosis

The final diagnosis was branch retinal vein occlusion in the supratemporal arcade of the left eye.

15.1.3 Case Review

The patient's chief complaint was vision decrease in the left eye. Intraretinal hemorrhages in a wedge-shaped pattern and tortuous and dilated venules were shown in the supratemporal arcade of the retina. The FFA examination revealed tortuous and dilated branch retinal veins, staining, and leakage in the occluded vessels and a large nonperfusion area. Visual field examination showed defects (relative scotomas) in the corresponding visual field of the drainage area of the blocked venules. The OCT demonstrated cystic edema and hemorrhage of the macula in the left eye, which were the cause of decreased central vision.

15.2 Case 2

15.2.1 Case Presentation

A 60-year-old male patient presented with sudden loss of his inferior visual field of the right eye for 3 days. No accompanying symptoms, including red eyes, eye pain, distorted vision, etc., were present. Histories of trauma, eye disease, systemic disease, and familial diseases were denied.

The BCVA was 20/63 OD and 20/25 OS. In both eyes, the intraocular pressure was normal, and slit-lamp examination of the anterior segments was unremarkable except that mild opacity of the lens was revealed bilaterally. Fundus examination showed edematous opacification of the supratemporal retina in the distribution of the occluded vessel, and a white embolus could be observed in the supratemporal arteriole in the right eye (Fig. 15.5). The C/D ratio was 0.7 with normal neuroretinal rim in both eyes.

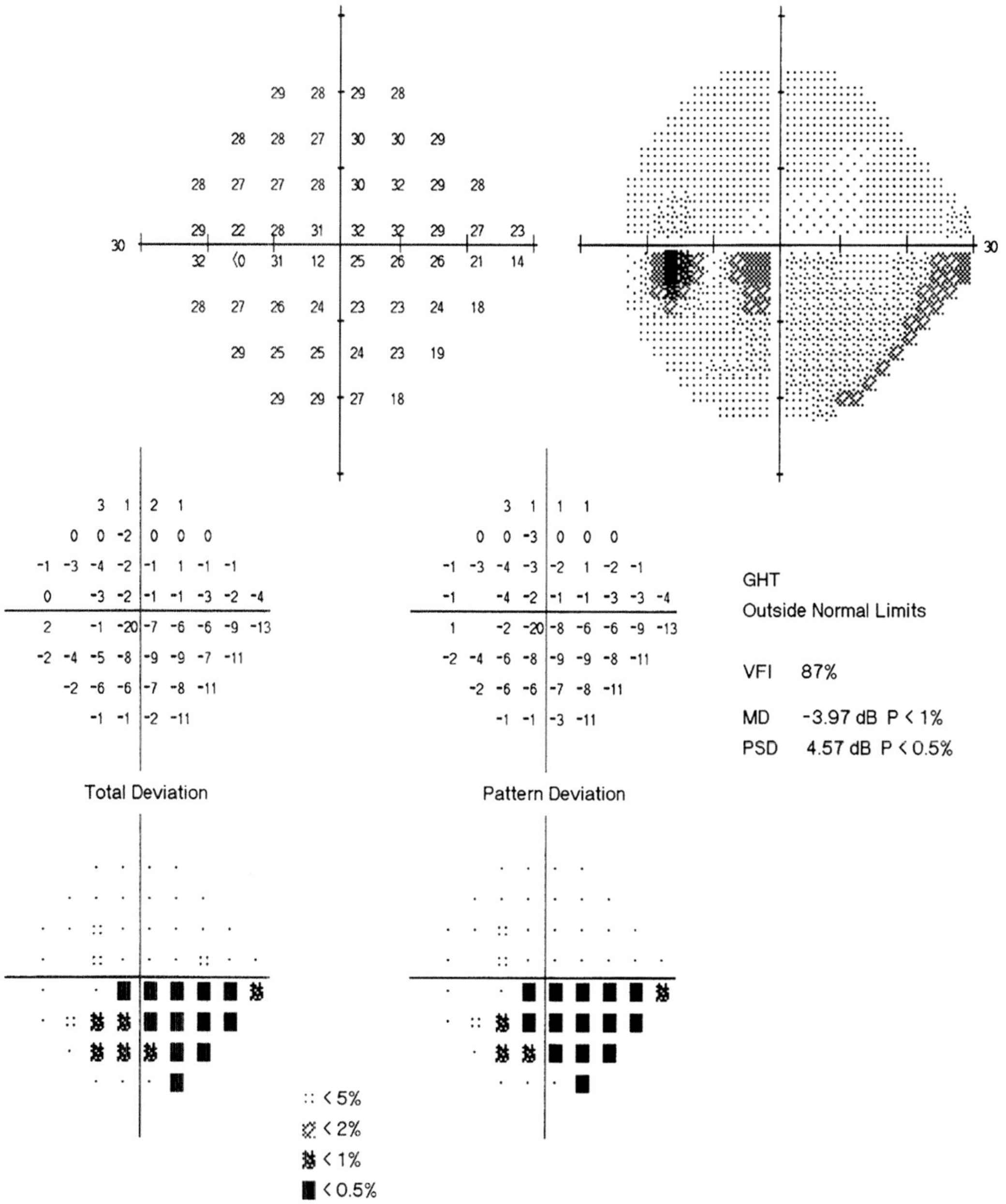

Fig. 15.2 Humphrey visual field analysis printout. Visual field examination with the 24-2 test showed an inferior visual field defect extending from the blind spot delimited by the horizontal line which could be found in the left eye, and the central region was also involved

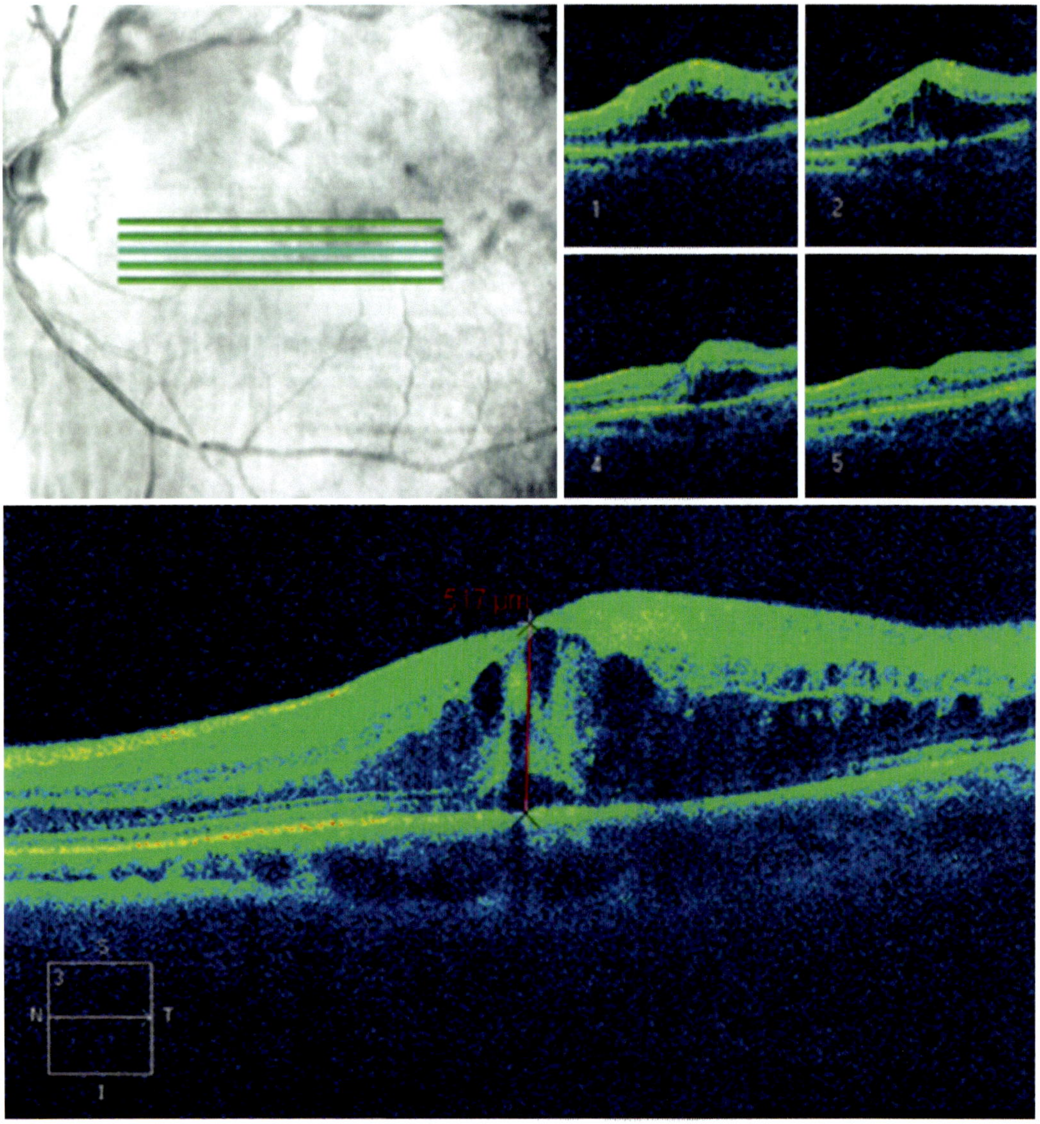

Fig. 15.3 OCT printouts of the macula. Cystoid macular edema, intraretinal fluid, inner-segment-outer-segment abnormalities, and a large cyst could be seen in the left eye

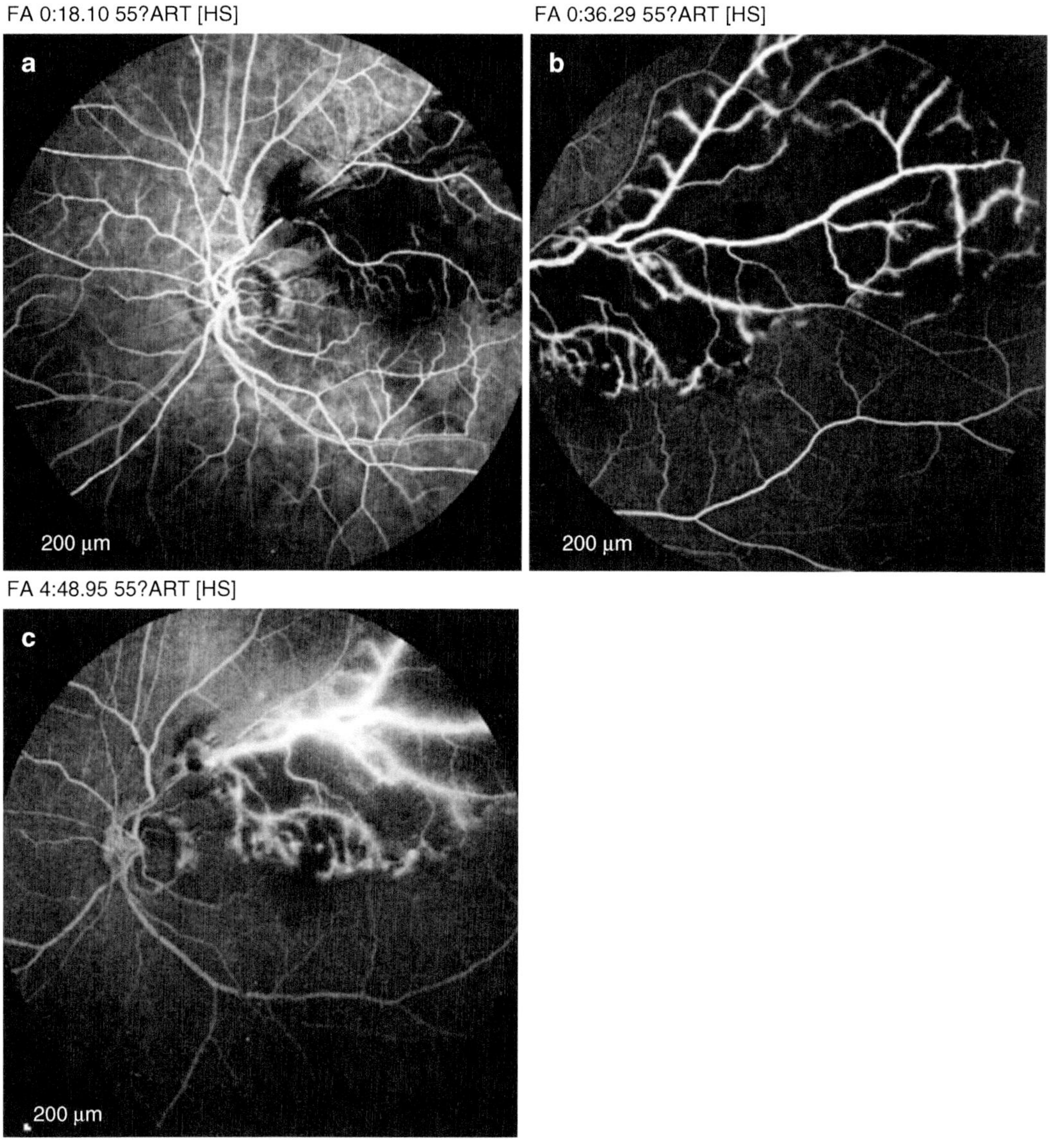

Fig. 15.4 FFA images of the left eye. FFA showed tortuous and dilated branch retinal veins, staining, and leakage in the occluded vessels, a large nonperfusion area, and involvement of the macula by the foci in the left eye. Panel a: Arteriovenous phase. Panel b: Venous phase. Panel c: Late phase

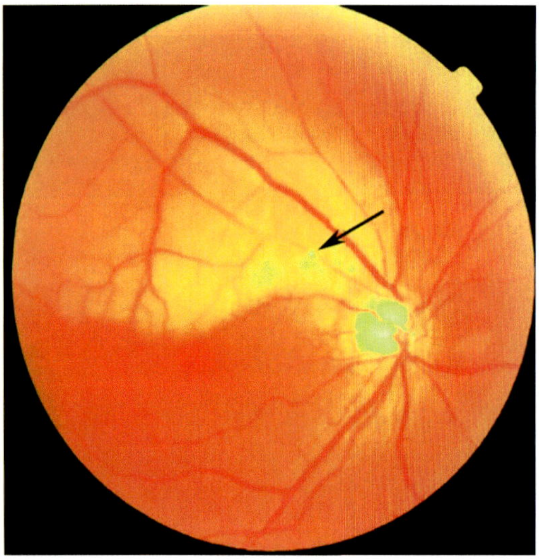

Fig. 15.5 Fundus photograph. Edematous opacification of the supratemporal retina in the distribution of the occluded vessel was shown in the right eye, and a white embolus (black arrow) could be observed in the supratemporal arcade arteriole

Visual field examination revealed inferotemporal visual field impairment delimited by the horizontal line in the right eye (Fig. 15.6) and no abnormalities in the visual field of the left eye.

Red-free fundus photography showed an embolus inside the artery, and FFA indicated fluorescence leakage of the arteriole blocked by the embolus, with macula involved by the local nonperfusion area in the superior region (Fig. 15.7).

15.2.2 Final Diagnosis

The final diagnosis was branch retinal artery obstruction in the right eye.

15.2.3 Case Review

This case is a typical case of branch retinal artery occlusion. The patient was a senior male, and edematous opacification of the supratemporal retina in the distribution of the occluded vessel could be observed at 3 days after onset. The superior macula was also involved. Red-free fundus photography and FFA showed clearly an embolus in the supratemporal arcade arteriole. The visual field manifestation was a sudden and dense visual field defect in the inferior quadrants that extends from the blind spot and is demarcated by the horizontal line.

15.3 Discussion

BRVO is frequently seen in clinical practice. The supratemporal branch is the most frequently affected part followed by the inferotemporal branch, the supranasal branch, and the inferonasal branch. A quadrantal visual field defect consistent with the drainage area of the blocked veins is often manifested. The mechanism of BRVO is as follows: vein occlusion causes edema and effusion of the retina; meanwhile, ischemia and hypoxia of the part of the retina drained by the blocked branches will result, and nonperfusion retinal capillary vessels will appear at the late stage. The consequent retinal changes will result in corresponding visual field impairment and light sensitivity reduction. Besides, blood supply deficiency in local retinal arterioles usually accompanies BRVO, which leads to visual field changes in corresponding areas. BRVO can lead to neovascular glaucoma if the treatment is not prompt [1, 2].

BRAO is less common and it's often caused by an embolus or thrombus formation. Temporal branch involvements, especially the supratemporal branch, occupy 90% of the BRAO cases. The arterioles and venules in the superior and inferior temporal retina are common sites of occlusion, and the large number of arteriovenous crossings in these quadrants is considered to be associated with such manifestation. The retinal arterioles are terminal arteries, so acute ischemia and hypoxia of retina tissues will result, which will further cause retinal edema and tissue necrosis, once they are blocked. Therefore, the visual field manifestation of BRAO is serious visual field damage (usually absolute scotomas) in the

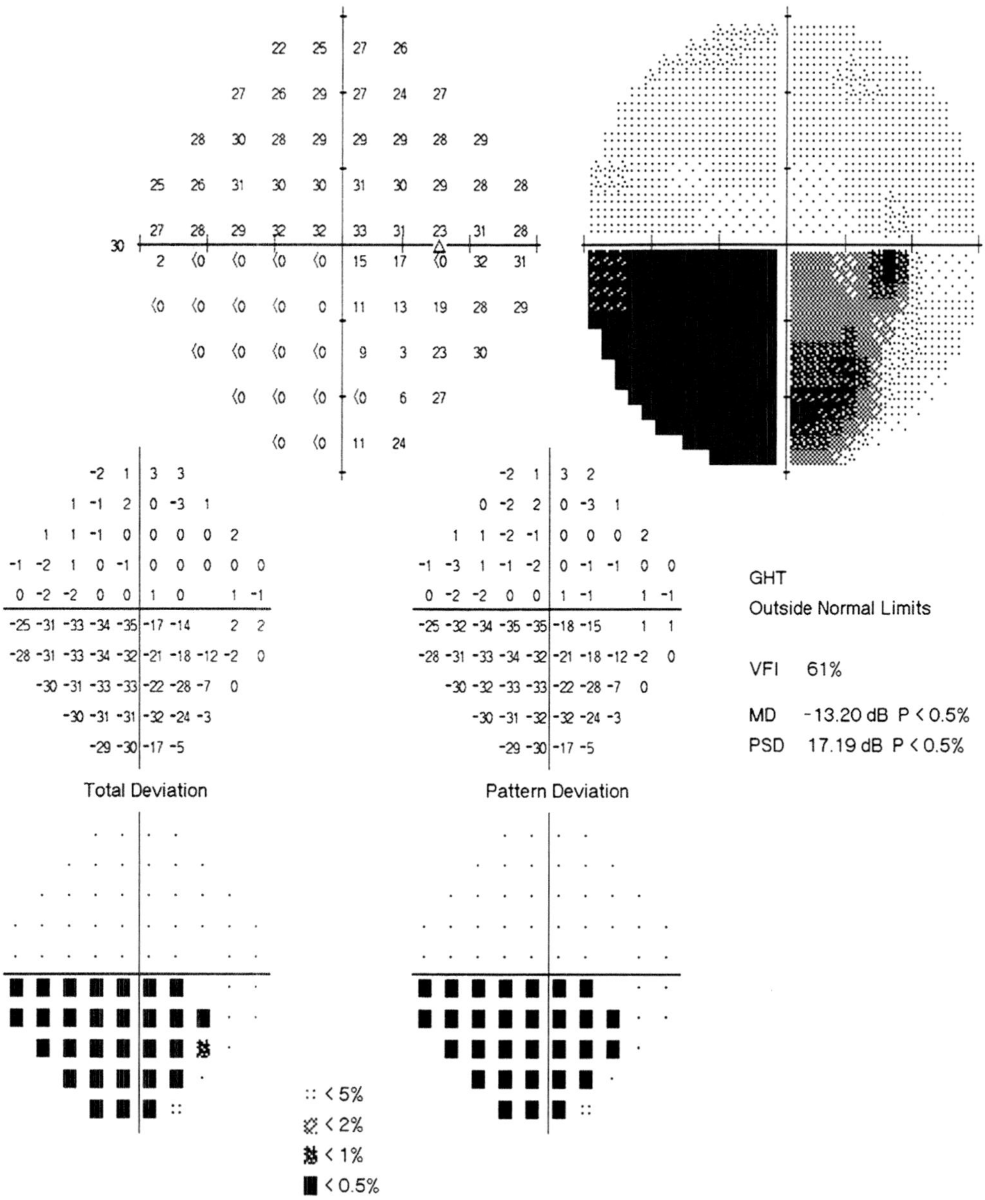

Fig. 15.6 Humphrey visual field analysis printout. Standardized automated perimetry with the 24-2 test showed inferotemporal visual field impairment in the right eye, and the impairment was sharply demarcated by the horizontal line

corresponding vessel distribution areas of the blocked arterioles [3, 4]. A study reported that the probability of developing neovascular glaucoma secondary to central retinal artery occlusion (CRAO) is about 1–2%. However, the chance of developing neovascular glaucoma secondary to BRAO is lower. Such phenomenon may be related to the fact that retinal artery occlusion causes tissue necrosis, so the retina needs less oxygen, and the stimulated production of vascular endothelial growth factors is lower [5–7].

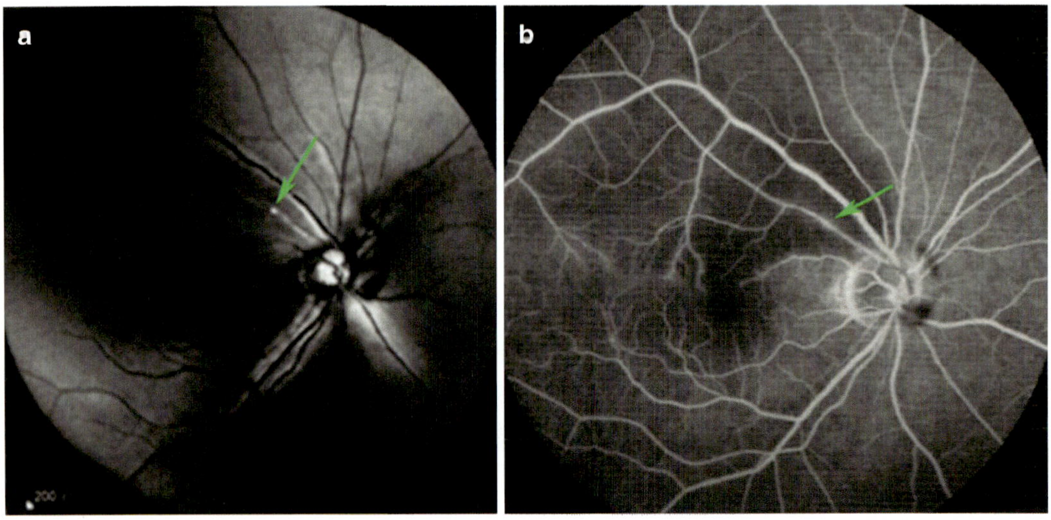

Fig. 15.7 Red-free fundus photograph and FFA image of the right eye. Panel a: Red-free fundus photography revealed an embolus (green arrow) inside the artery. Panel b: FFA indicated fluorescence leakage of the arteriole blocked by the embolus (green arrow). The macula was involved by the local nonperfusion area in the superior region

The severity of visual field impairment caused by BRVO and BRAO is determined by the nature of the blocked vessel and the site and severity of the occlusion. The severity of ischemia and hypoxia induced by BRVO is usually milder than that induced by BRAO. Therefore, the reduction of light sensitivity is also not as serious as that in BRAO. BRVO will lead to relative scotomas in the distribution area of the blocked vessels in most cases. In contrast, BRAO will result in absolute scotomas in the distribution area of the blocked vessels in most cases. A similar mechanism may explain why the total visual field damages caused by central retinal vein occlusion (CRVO) and CRAO are different in severity [6].

Combination of BRVO and BRAO in one eye, which was observed in patients with homocysteinemia, diabetes, etc., has also been reported, and visual field damages from both of them were found in such patients [6].

References

1. Zheng C. Ocular fundus diseases. 2nd ed. Beijing: People's Medical Publishing House; 2014.
2. Boyd SR, Zachary I, Chakmvarthy U, et al. Correlation for increased vascular endothelial growth factor with neovascularization and permeability in ischemic central vein occlusion. Arch Ophthalmol. 2002;120(12):1644–50.
3. Yannuzzi LA. The retinal atlas. Translated by Zhao Mingwei Tianjin. Tianjin Science & Technology Translation and Publishing Co., Ltd; 2013.
4. Bhullar PK, Grewal DS, Fekrat S. Regional changes in choroidal thickness in branch retinal artery occlusion. Ophthalmic Surg Lasers Imaging Retina. 2016;47(9):811–8.
5. An TS, Kwon SI. Neovascular glaucoma due to branch retinal vein occlusion combined with branch retinal artery occlusion. Korean J Ophthalmol. 2013;27(1):64–7.
6. Sengupta S. Combined branch retinal artery and vein occlusion in hyperhomocysteinemia. JAMA Ophthalmol. 2014;132(10):1255.
7. Yamamoto K, Tsujikawa A, Hangai M, et al. Neovascular glaucoma after branch retinal artery occlusion. Jpn J Ophthalmol. 2005;49(5):388–90.

Every Contact Leaves a Trace

16

Ning Fan, Xuyang Liu, and Jiantao Wang

When a visual field defect fails to be explained by the documented eye disease or is found even in absence of ocular system or visual pathway diseases, the abnormalities causing the visual field impairment should be figured out. Whether the process to find out the responsible reason or pathogenesis is complicated or not, or the abnormalities are curable or not, we at least get to know what truly happened to the patient.

16.1 Case 1

16.1.1 Case Presentation

A 44-year-old male patient presented with intraocular pressure (IOP) increase in both eyes for 5 years. Travoprost eye drops had been taken intermittently for IOP lowering, but the treatment was ineffective. Histories of trauma, previous eye diseases, systemic diseases, and familial diseases were denied.

On examination, the uncorrected visual acuity (UCVA) was 20/200, and the best corrected visual acuity (BCVA) was 20/25 OU. IOP by standard Goldmann applanation tonometry was measured as 22 mmHg OD and 23 mmHg OS. The central cornea thickness (CCT) was 534 μm OD and 540 μm OS. Slit-lamp examination of his anterior segments was unremarkable in both eyes. Fundus examination revealed that, in both eyes, the C/D ratio was 0.8, there was a narrowing of inferior neuroretinal rim and thinning of retinal nerve fiber at the corresponding site, and foveal reflex could be observed (Fig. 16.1).

Standardized automated perimetry showed enlargement of the blind spot in both eyes, a localized superior visual field defect in the right eye, and a superior arcuate scotoma in the left eye (Fig. 16.2).

16.1.2 Case Analysis

The clinical characteristics of the patient were as follows: (a) the IOP increased in both eyes; (b) the narrowing of inferior neuroretinal rim and thinning of retinal nerve fiber at the corresponding site were observed in both eyes; and (c) there was a localized superior visual field defect in the right eye and an superior arcuate scotoma in the left eye. Therefore, the diagnosis of primary open-angle glaucoma (POAG) was established. It is worth noting that the superior visual field defect in the right eye is a localized absolute scotoma and the location was relatively peripheral, which did not conform to the typical visual field changes in glaucoma.

N. Fan · J. Wang (✉)
Shenzhen Eye Hospital, Shenzhen University, Shenzhen, China

X. Liu
Xiamen Eye Center of Xiamen University, Xiamen, China

Shenzhen Eye Hospital, Shenzhen University, Shenzhen, China

N. Wang et al. (eds.), *Optic Disorders and Visual Field*, Advances in Visual Science and Eye Diseases 2, https://doi.org/10.1007/978-981-13-2502-1_16

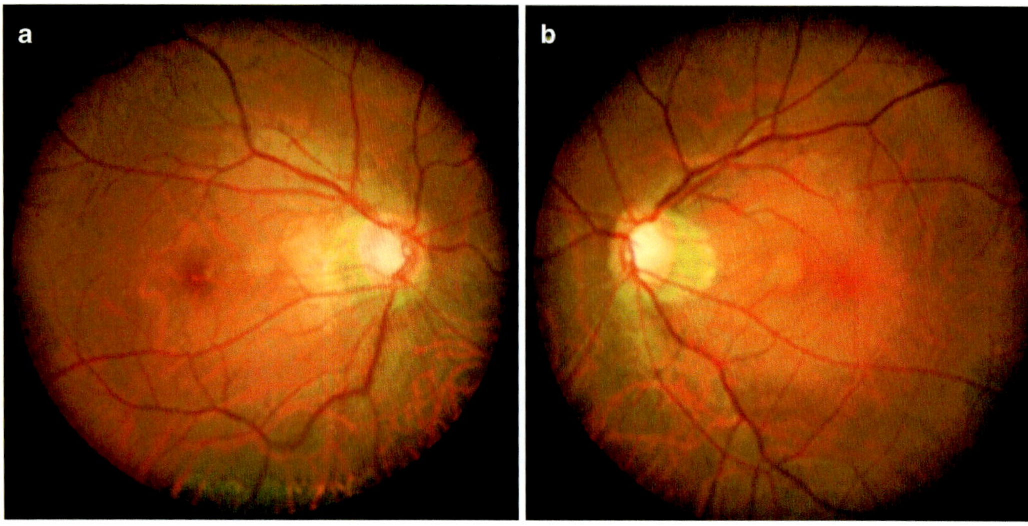

Fig. 16.1 Fundus photographs. The cup-disc ratio was 0.8. Narrowing of inferior neuroretinal rim and thinning of retinal nerve fiber at the corresponding site were exhibited. Panel a: Right eye. Panel b: Left eye

We examined the patient carefully by a video monitor in the visual field machine and did not find right eyelid ptosis during the visual field examination. Further detailed examination on the fundus after the pupils were dilated revealed a local chorioretinal atrophy focus in the inferior quadrant of the right eye (Fig. 16.3).

Fundus fluorescein angiography (FFA) and indocyanine green angiography (ICGA) revealed old retinal and choroidal foci in the inferior quadrant of the right eye (Fig. 16.4).

16.1.3 Final Diagnosis

The final diagnosis was bilateral POAG with old chorioretinopathy in the right eye.

16.1.4 Case Review

The patient in this case had glaucoma, but the visual field changes in the right eye were not typical. It was just that we always doubted whether the visual field defect was caused completely by the glaucoma, and only through careful dilated fundus examination could we find the old retinal and choroidal foci and get rid of such a doubt.

16.2 Case 2

16.2.1 Case Presentation

A 51-year-old male patient presented with shadow in the inferior visual field of the right eye for about 2 years. The defect was not progressive. Symptoms of red eye and eye pain were denied. The patient had been diagnosed with a visual field defect in the right eye for multiple times at different hospitals, but the specific cause had not been identified. The patient had myopia in both eyes and had been wearing glasses for about 30 years. He had a history of diabetes. Histories of trauma and familial diseases were denied.

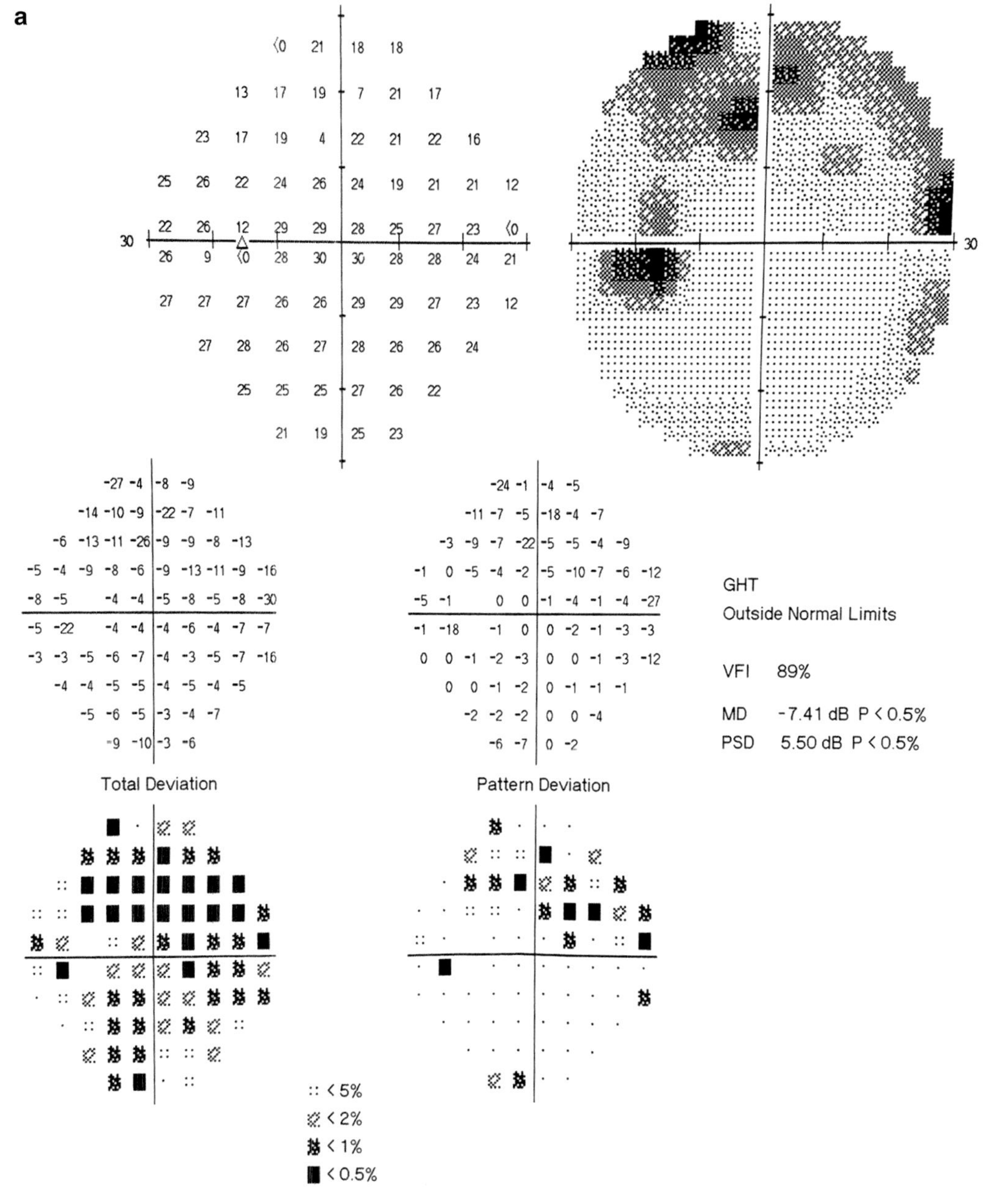

Fig. 16.2 Humphrey visual field analysis printouts. Panel a: Standardized automated perimetry with the 30-2 test showed a superior arcuate scotoma in the left eye. Panel b: A localized superior visual field defect in the right eye was seen

b

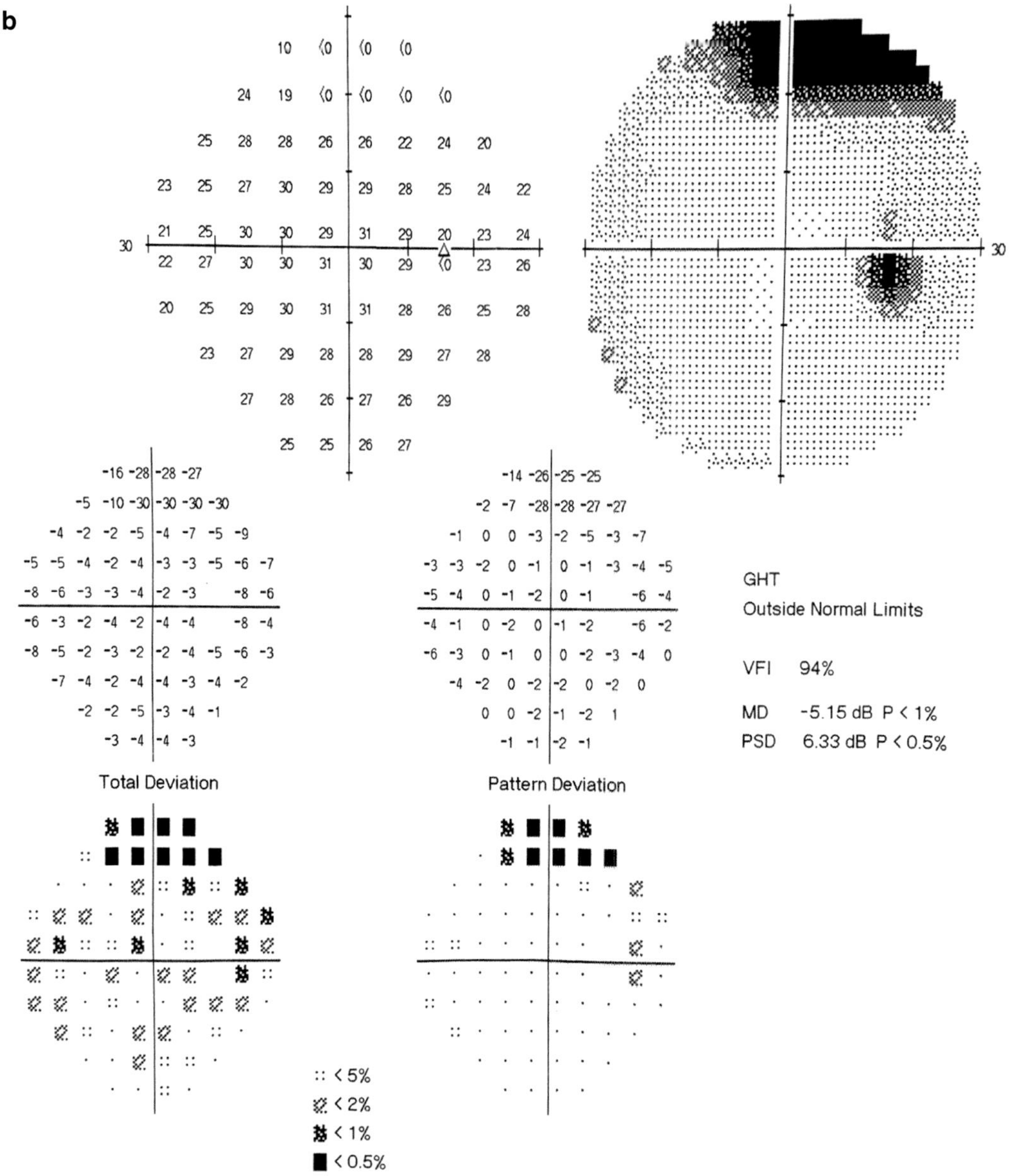

Fig. 16.2 (continued)

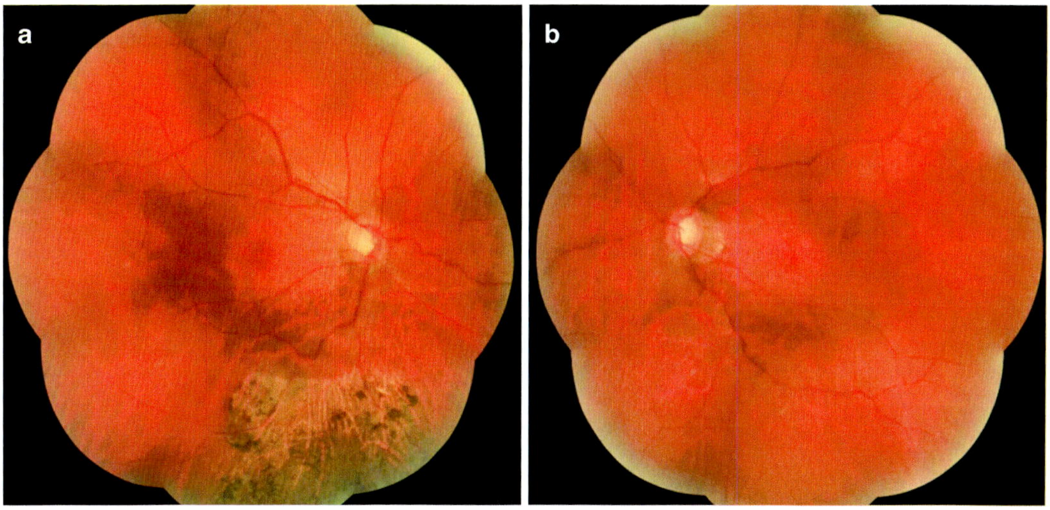

Fig. 16.3 Montage images of fundus photographs. Panel a: A local chorioretinal atrophy focus was seen in the inferior quadrant of the right eye. Panel b: No abnormality was found in the retina of the left eye

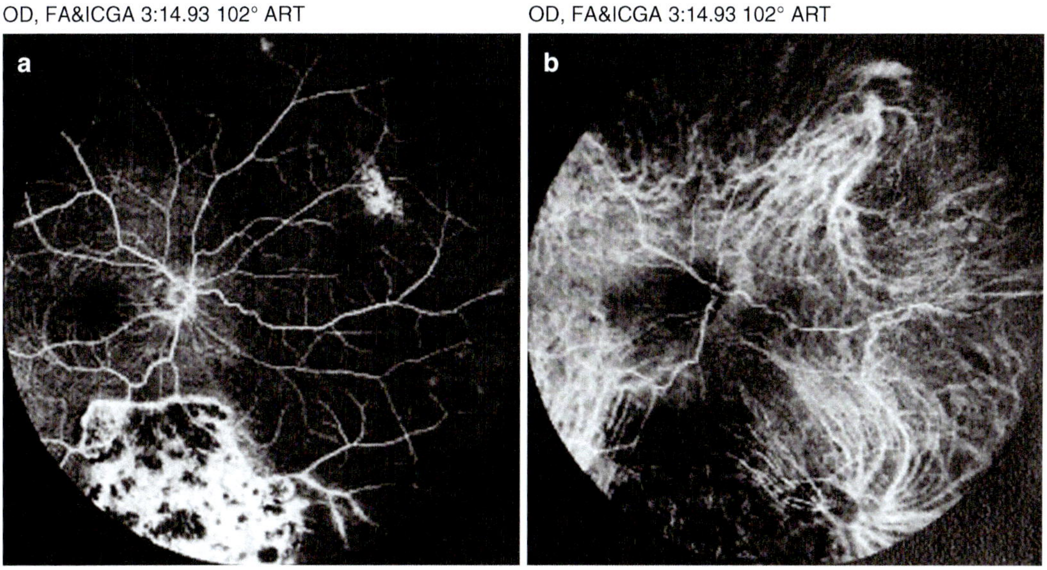

Fig. 16.4 FFA and ICGA images of the right eye. Old retinal and choroidal foci were shown in the inferior quadrant. Panel a: Fluorescein leakage during the venous phase in FFA. Panel b: Local choroid hypofluorescence in ICGA

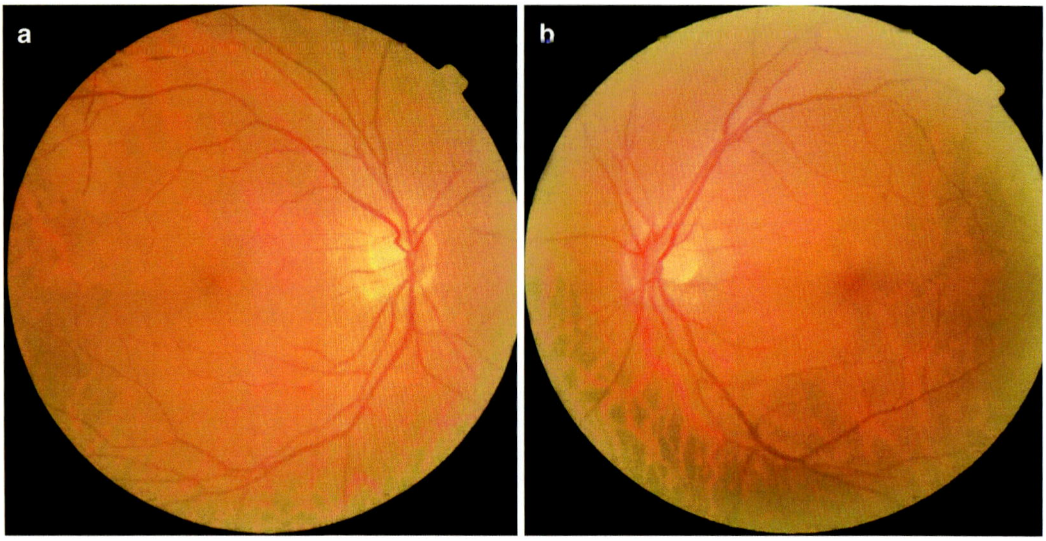

Fig. 16.5 Fundus photographs. The optic disc was pink in color with peripapillary atrophy, the C/D ratio was 0.3, and there was no abnormality in the posterior pole in both eyes. Panel a: Right eye. Panel b: Left eye

The BCVA was 20/20 with myopic correction (−4.50DS) in both eyes. The IOPs measured with Goldmann applanation tonometry were 11 mmHg OU. Slit-lamp examination of his anterior segments was unremarkable in both eyes. Fundus examination also revealed nothing remarkable at the posterior pole except that peripapillary atrophy could be observed in both eyes (Fig. 16.5).

Standardized automated perimetry showed an inferonasal relative scotoma in the right eye and a normal visual field result in the left eye (Fig. 16.6).

B-ultrasound revealed mild vitreous opacity of both eyes (Fig. 16.7).

Dilated fundus examination showed the occlusion and white sheath formation in the supratemporal branch retinal arteriole in the right eye (Fig. 16.8).

Fundus fluorescein angiography (FFA) showed complete occlusion of the supratemporal branch retinal arteriole; local inferotemporal peripheral retinal atrophy foci and avascular area could be seen, and fluorescent staining was shown in the inferotemporal peripheral retina at the late stage of angiography in the right eye (Fig. 16.9).

16.2.2 Final Diagnosis

The final diagnosis was old retinal vasculitis in the right eye.

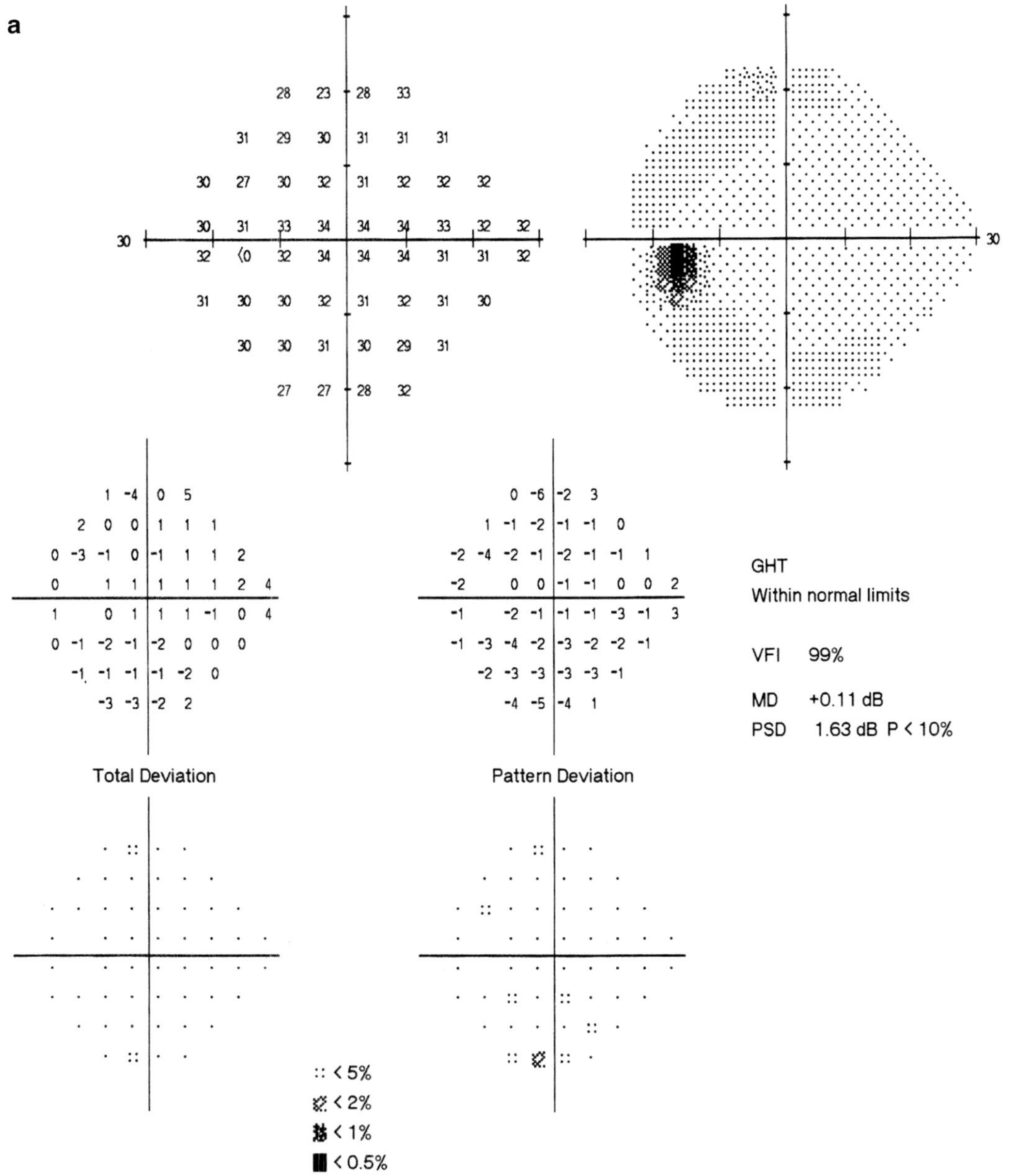

Fig. 16.6 Humphrey visual field analysis printouts. Panel a: Standardized automated perimetry with the 24-2 test showed that the left eye was normal. Panel b: There was an inferonasal relative scotoma in the right eye

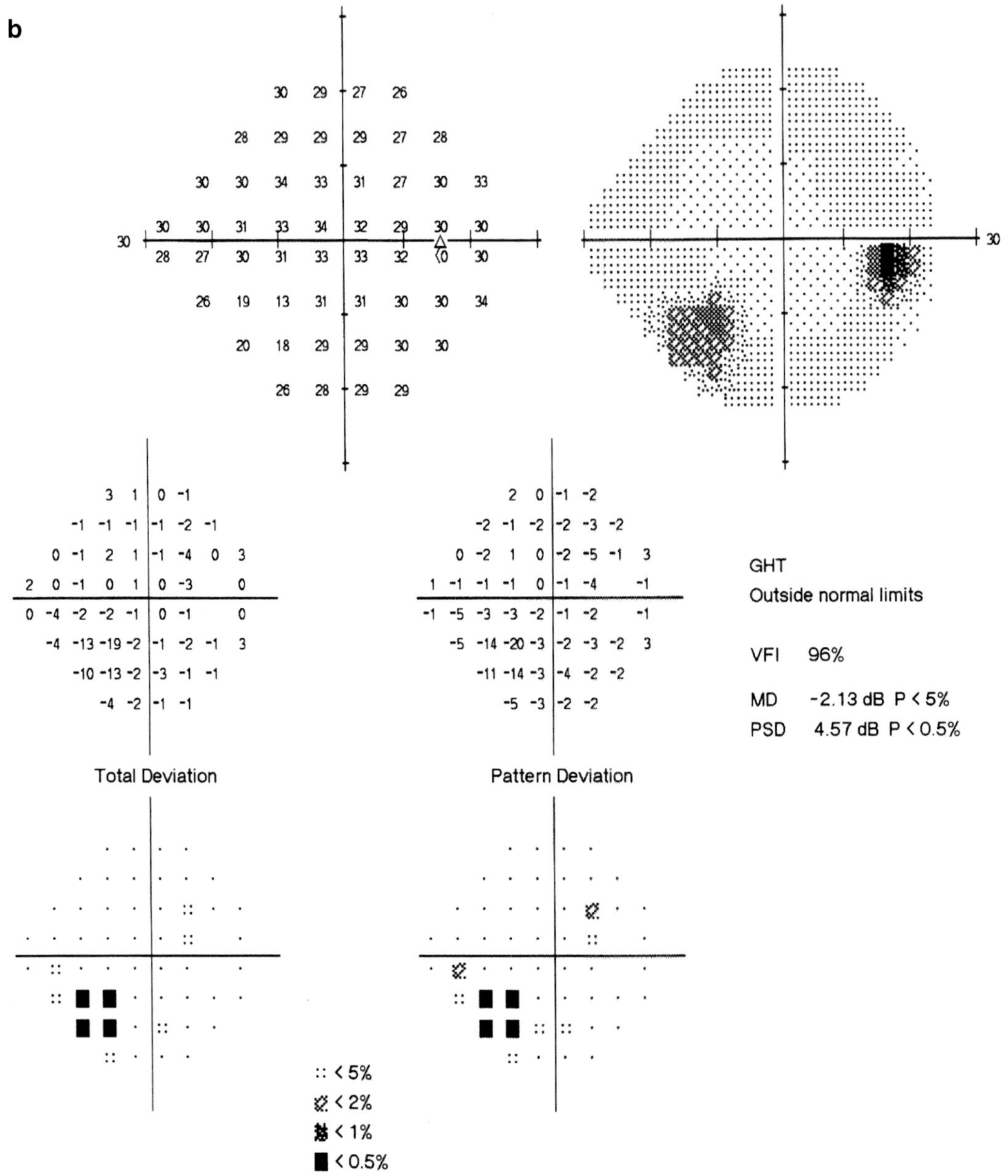

Fig. 16.6 (continued)

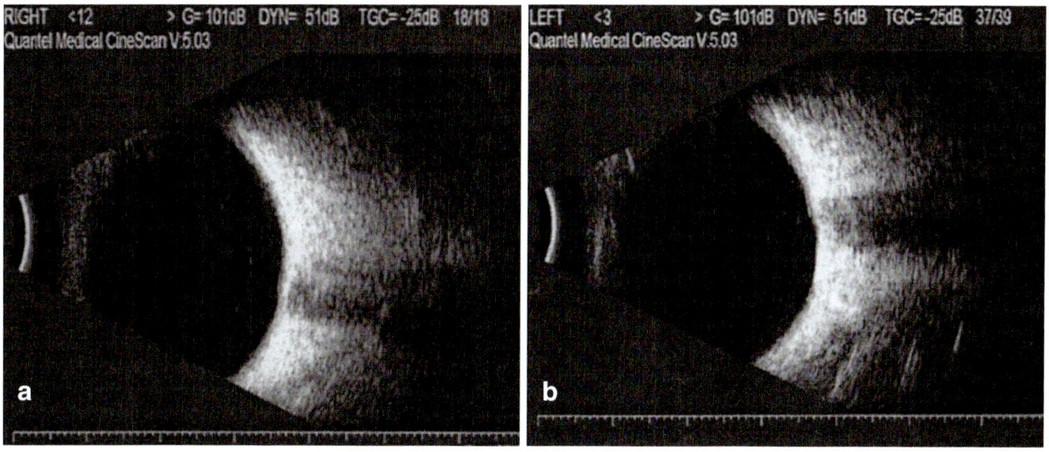

Fig. 16.7 B-ultrasound images of both eyes. Mild vitreous opacity was shown in both eyes

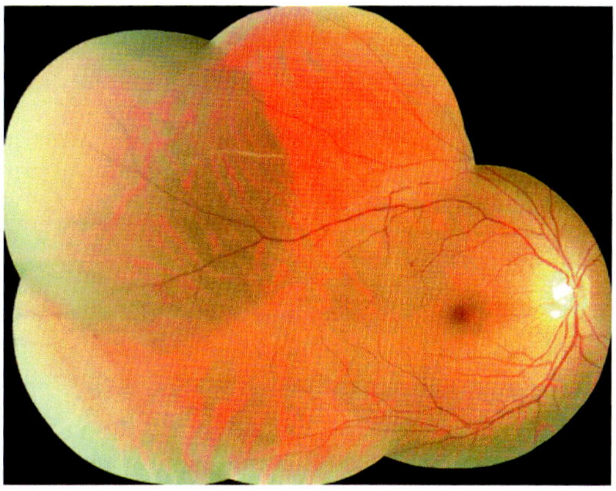

Fig. 16.8 Montage images of fundus photographs. Occlusion and white sheath formation in the supratemporal branch retinal arteriole were seen in the right eye

16.2.3 Case Review

The patient's central vision was normal in both eyes, but he always felt the shadow in the vision of the right eye. After repeated presentations to hospitals, this problem could not be satisfactorily resolved. The visual field changes suggested that there might be lesions in the supratemporal retina of the right eye. Careful fundus examination soon revealed the cause of the visual field defect, and the presence of similar lesions in other parts of the retina was also noticed. Therefore, it was speculated that the right eye had once suffered from focal retinal vasculitis. The cause of shadow in the vision of the right eye was thus explained, and the patient was then relieved gradually.

16.3 Discussion

The cause shall be explored carefully in the clinical practice when the visual field defect is difficult to explain (after exclusion of the factors such as inaccurate examination). Generally speaking, the common causes of a visual field defect resulting from eye diseases alone are

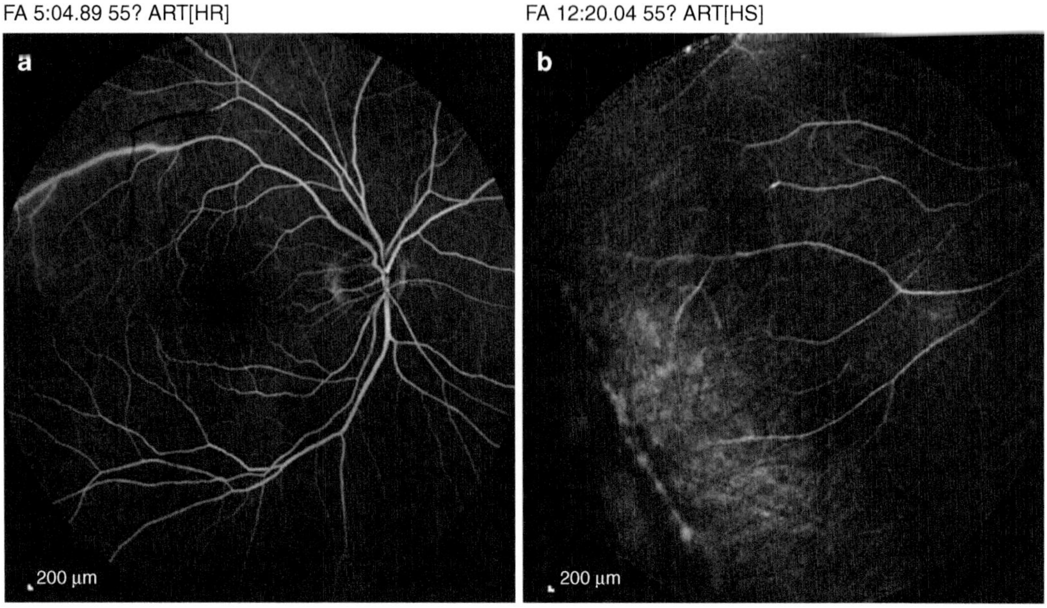

Fig. 16.9 FFA images of the right eye. Panel a: Complete occlusion of the supratemporal branch retinal arteriole was observed in the right eye. Panel b: Fluorescent staining was shown in the inferotemporal peripheral retina at the late stage of angiography. Local retinal atrophy foci and avascular area could also be seen

fundus (retina and optic nerve) diseases. Sometimes the patient can feel small changes in the visual field although the central visual acuity is good enough, so fundus lesions are probably difficult to find by undilated ophthalmoscopy examination. However, through detailed examination on the fundus after the pupils were dilated and with the help of other assistant examinations such as FFA, OCT, Amsler chart, ERG, VEP, etc., retinopathy and/or optic neuropathy corresponding to the visual field defect can usually be found. Besides, both retinopathy and optic neuropathy may accompany an intracranial visual pathway disease, and the damages to the visual field from these diseases may be manifested together. Careful differential diagnosis shall be carried out to avoid a missed diagnosis [1].

The two cases mentioned in this section are both visual field defects caused by old retinal diseases. The causes of occult retinochoroiditis are various, and they are mainly in connection with local blood circulation disorders, allergic reactions, infectious foci, endocrine disorders, etc. The treatments should mainly be symptomatic and supportive therapies.

Reference

1. Karna S. Atlas of neuro-ophthalmology. Translated by Jialiang Zhao. Beijing: Beijing Science and Technology Press; 2007.

When Rhegmatogenous Retinal Detachment Is Accompanied by Glaucoma

17

Ning Fan, Xuyang Liu, and Jiantao Wang

In general, when rhegmatogenous retinal detachment occurs, the liquefied vitreous will flow into the sub-neuroepithelium space via the retinal hole, and the intraocular pressure (IOP) usually goes down. However, the symptoms can be confused when rhegmatogenous retinal detachment (especially shallow detachment) is accompanied by ocular hypertension or glaucoma. It may bring difficulties to the diagnosis or even lead to treatment in totally wrong direction. Schwartz-Matsuo syndrome is an example of such diseases.

17.1 Case 1

17.1.1 Case Presentation

A 16-year-old male patient presented with gradual vision decrease in the left eye for over half a year. His vision decrease in the left eye had been found by chance. There were no such symptoms as distorted vision, red eyes, eye pain, and pain upon eye movement. The patient had thought that it might be caused by unsuitable glasses, and no treatment had been taken. The patient presented this time due to aggravation of vision loss in the left eye. An inquiry into the medical history revealed that the patient had once hit the left side of his head on the door frame and no treatment was given because the symptom was mild. Histories of other eye diseases, systemic diseases, and familial diseases were denied.

The uncorrected visual acuity (UCVA) was 20/125 OD and 6/240 OS, and the best corrected visual acuity (BCVA) was 20/20 with myopic correction (−1.75DS) OD and 6/120 with myopic correction (−2.25DS) OS. The intraocular pressure (IOP) measured with Goldmann applanation tonometry was 20 mmHg OD and 35 mmHg OS. In the left eye, mild conjunctival congestion could be observed, and the cornea was transparent; the anterior chamber was deep and the peripheral anterior chamber depth was 1/2CT; the aqueous cells were observed with 2+; the pupil was round with a diameter of 3 mm without adhesion; the lens was transparent; mild vitreous opacity could be observed; the cup-disc ratio was 0.8 with a narrowing and pallor neuroretinal rim; and total retinal detachment was shown without fixed wrinkles. The retinal tears were not found by the three-mirror contact lens examination (Fig. 17.1). The examination of the anterior and posterior segments of the right eye was unremarkable except that the C/D ratio was 0.6 with a normal neuroretinal rim.

N. Fan · J. Wang (✉)
Shenzhen Eye Hospital, Shenzhen University, Shenzhen, China

X. Liu
Xiamen Eye Center of Xiamen University, Xiamen, China

Shenzhen Eye Hospital, Shenzhen University, Shenzhen, China

N. Wang et al. (eds.), *Optic Disorders and Visual Field*, Advances in Visual Science and Eye Diseases 2, https://doi.org/10.1007/978-981-13-2502-1_17

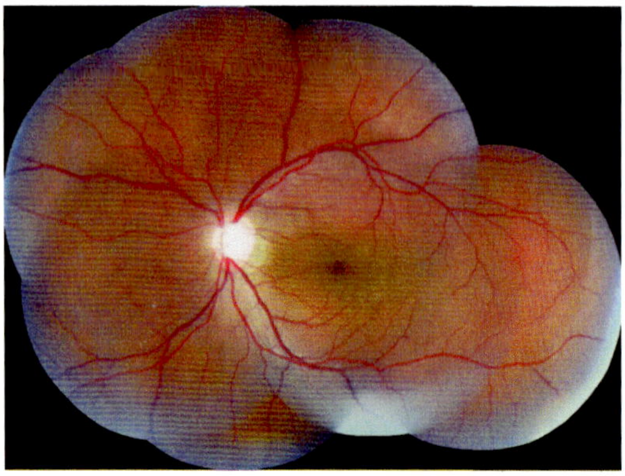

Fig. 17.1 Montage images of fundus photographs. Total retinal detachment was seen and the C/D ratio was 0.8 in the left eye

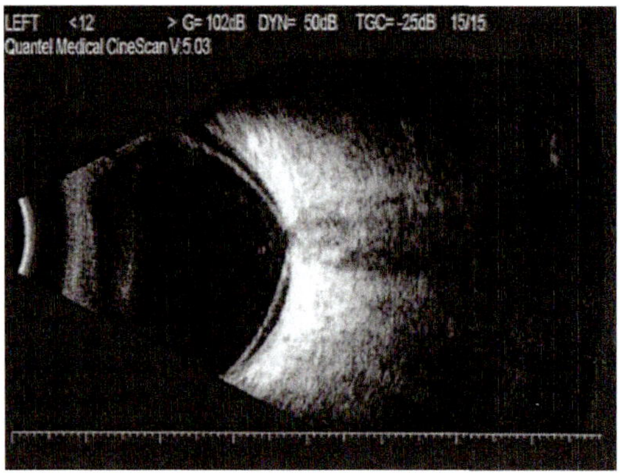

Fig. 17.2 B-ultrasound image for the left eye. Flat detachment of the total retina was seen

B-ultrasound showed flat detachment of the total retina in the left eye (Fig. 17.2).

Standardized automated perimetry with the 30-2 test revealed diffuse depression in the left eye (Fig. 17.3).

Ultrasound biomicroscopy (UBM) showed that the depth of the center anterior chamber was 3.35 mm and the anterior chamber angle was open in all quadrants of the right eye; the depth of the center anterior chamber was about 3.42 mm, echogenic dots could be found in the anterior chamber, the anterior chamber angle was totally open, and the lens was in position in the left eye (Fig. 17.4).

Three eye drop combinations such as carteolol hydrochloride + brinzolamide + brimonidine tartrate and oral administration of methazolamide tablets were given to lower the IOP in the left eye, but the pressure control was poor. Scleral buckling was then performed, and holes arranged like sieve holes in the ora serrata were observed in the peripheral retina during the operation. Pressure-lowering agents were continued after operation, and the intraocular pressure was controlled. The pressure-lowering agents were stopped after 1 month, and the intraocular pressure was normal and retinal reattachment was achieved.

17.1.2 Final Diagnosis

The final diagnosis was Schwartz-Matsuo syndrome in the left eye.

17.1.3 Case Review

Schwartz-Matsuo syndrome is usually found in young males and involves one eye. The patients may have a history of blunt trauma in the head and face. The retinal detachment was flat and serous in nature, and the tear often lies in the ora serrata or the nonpigmented epithelium of the ciliary body, which makes it uneasy to be detected. The disease had lasted for a long time

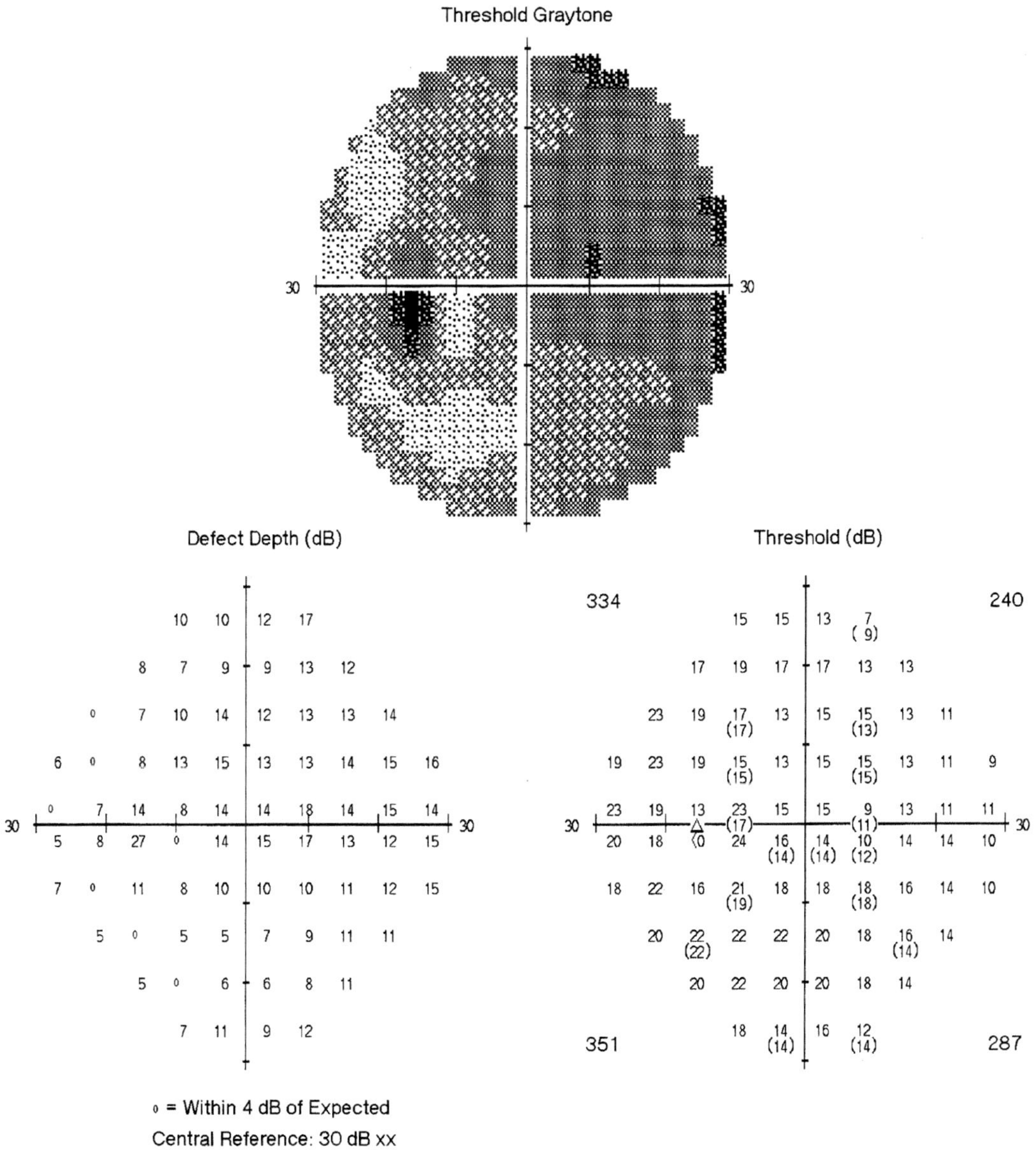

Fig. 17.3 Humphrey visual field analysis printout for the left eye. Standardized automated perimetry with the 30-2 test (a size V target was used) revealed generalized depression

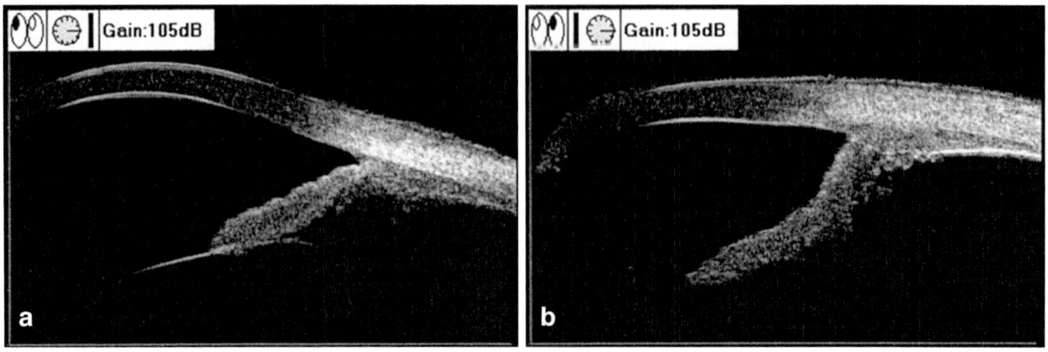

Fig. 17.4 UBM images of both eyes. Panel a: The center anterior chamber was deep, and the anterior chamber angle was totally open in the right eye. Panel b: The center anterior chamber was deep, echogenic dots could be found in the anterior chamber, the iris was posteriorly depressed, the anterior chamber angle was totally open, and the lens was in position in the left eye

in this case, and flat total retinal detachment was shown. The visual field manifestation was diffuse depression. Ocular hypotensive agents were used for intraocular pressure control for the patient before the operation, but the effect was not good. The intraocular pressure showed gradual reduction after retinal reattachment. The ocular hypotensive agents were stopped 1 month after operation, and the intraocular pressure became normal. The uveitis resolved gradually after retinal reattachment. Therefore, it's helpful to control the intraocular pressure by retinal reattachment surgery as early as possible. Please note that it's completely different from the mechanism of secondary high intraocular pressure after scleral buckling surgery.

17.2 Case 2

Zhou Wenzhong

17.2.1 Case Presentation

A 43-year-old male patient presented with the feeling of fullness in the right eye accompanied by blurred vision for 2 months. No significant trigger was observed before the disease onset. No accompanying symptoms, including red eyes, eye pain, distorted vision, pain upon eye movement, headache, etc., were present. Histories of trauma, previous eye diseases, systemic diseases, and familial diseases were denied.

The UCVA of the right eye was 20/20. The IOP of the right eye measured with Goldmann applanation tonometry was 38 mmHg. Slit-lamp examination of his anterior segment in the right eye was unremarkable except that the aqueous cells were observed. The undilated ocular fundus examination revealed nothing remarkable except that C/D = 0.4 in the right eye and no abnormality was found in the left eye.

Visual field examination showed an arc-shaped scotoma in the inferotemporal visual field of the right eye (Fig. 17.5).

17.2.2 Case Analysis

The patient was a young male and had no myopia or trauma history. One eye had high IOP and the aqueous cells were positive. No glaucomatous optic disc damage was observed. These findings were suggestive of secondary glaucoma (such as glaucoma secondary to uveitis). But the affected eye exhibited an arc-shaped scotoma in the inferotemporal visual field, which didn't conform to the typical visual field impairment of

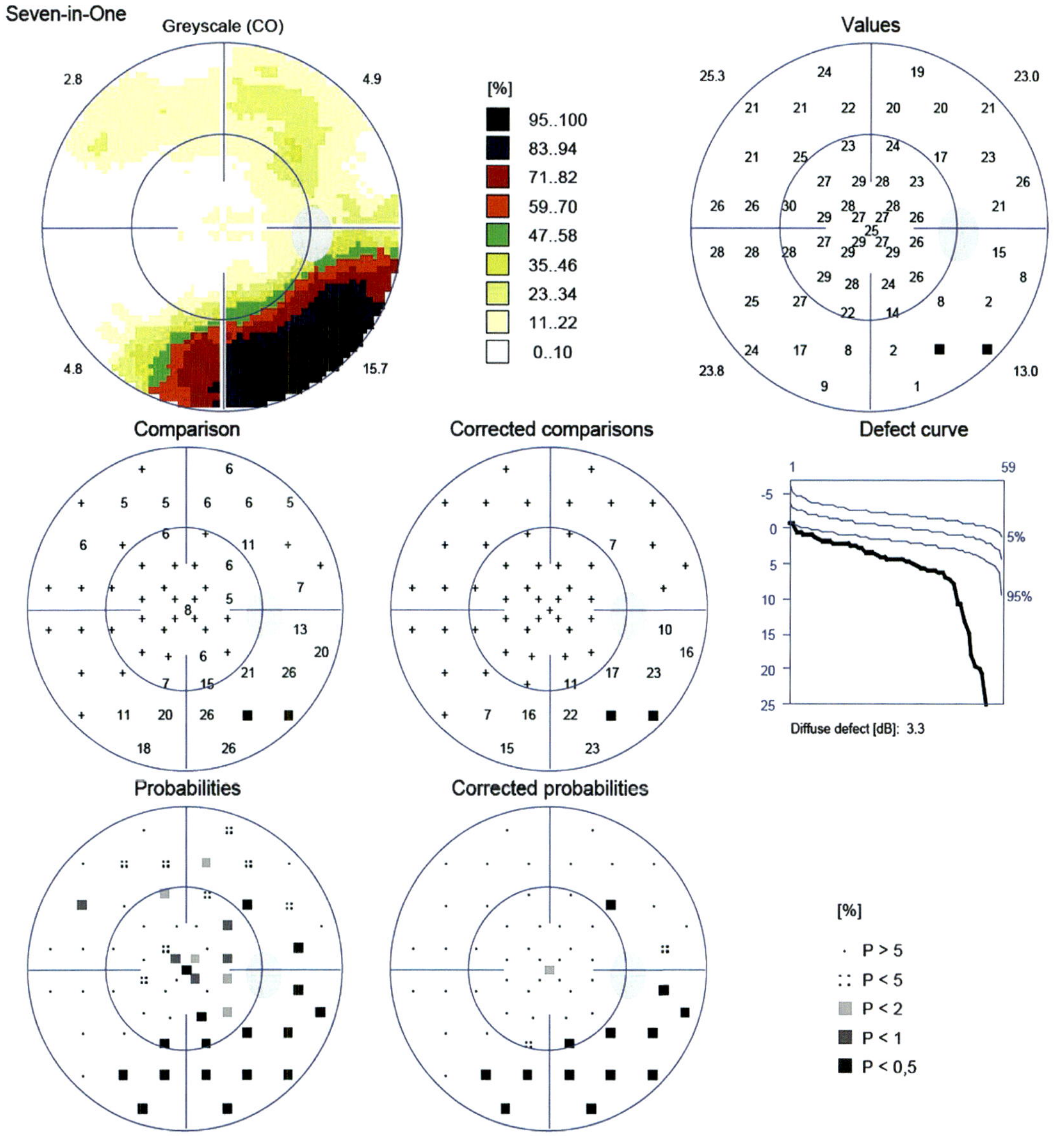

Fig. 17.5 Octopus visual field analysis printouts for the right eye. Central 30° visual field examination revealed an inferotemporal arc-shaped scotoma

glaucoma. We then carried out B-ultrasound scan and dilated fundus examination.

C-ultrasound showed flat detachment of the supranasal retina in the right eye (Fig. 17.6).

The dilated fundus examination found a localized flat detachment in the supranasal retina and a tear, which was a small round hole near the ora serrata, at the 2 o' clock position.

17.2.3 Final Diagnosis

The final diagnosis was Schwartz-Matsuo syndrome in the right eye.

The IOP was hard to control even after the eye drops of carteolol hydrochloride + brinzolamide were administered to the patient's right eye. The scleral buckling surgery was carried out. Ocular hypotensive agents were continued for 3 days after the operation, and the IOP was stably controlled within normal range, and retinal reattachment was achieved (Fig. 17.7).

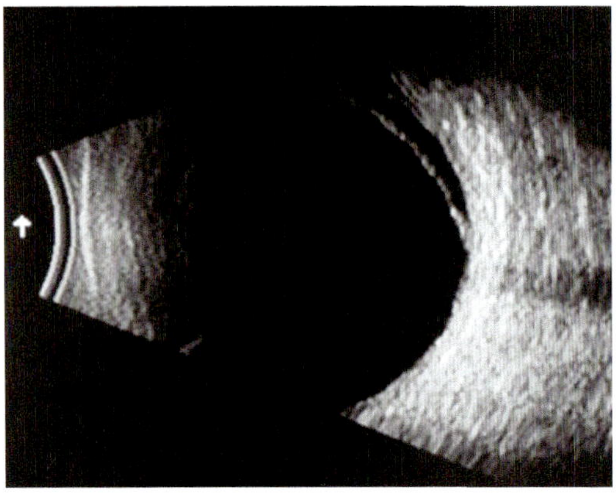

Fig. 17.6 B-ultrasound image for the right eye. Flat detachment of the supranasal retina was exhibited

17.2.4 Case Review

The retinal detachment location was the supranasal region in this case. It could be easily neglected by the patient and the doctors because of its following features: the IOP was high, the retina tear was close to the peripheral area, the retinal detachment was flat, the disease onset was occult, and the disease progression was relatively slow. The disease involved only one eye, with good central vision and increased IOP, and mild anterior uveitis was seen, so it could usually be misdiagnosed as glaucomatocyclitic syndrome or primary open-angle glaucoma. However, visual field examination indicated an arc-shaped inferotemporal scotoma, which could not be explained by the glaucoma. Dilated fundus examination found flat retinal detachment and a small tear in the peripheral area. These findings conformed to the manifestation of Schwartz-Matsuo syndrome.

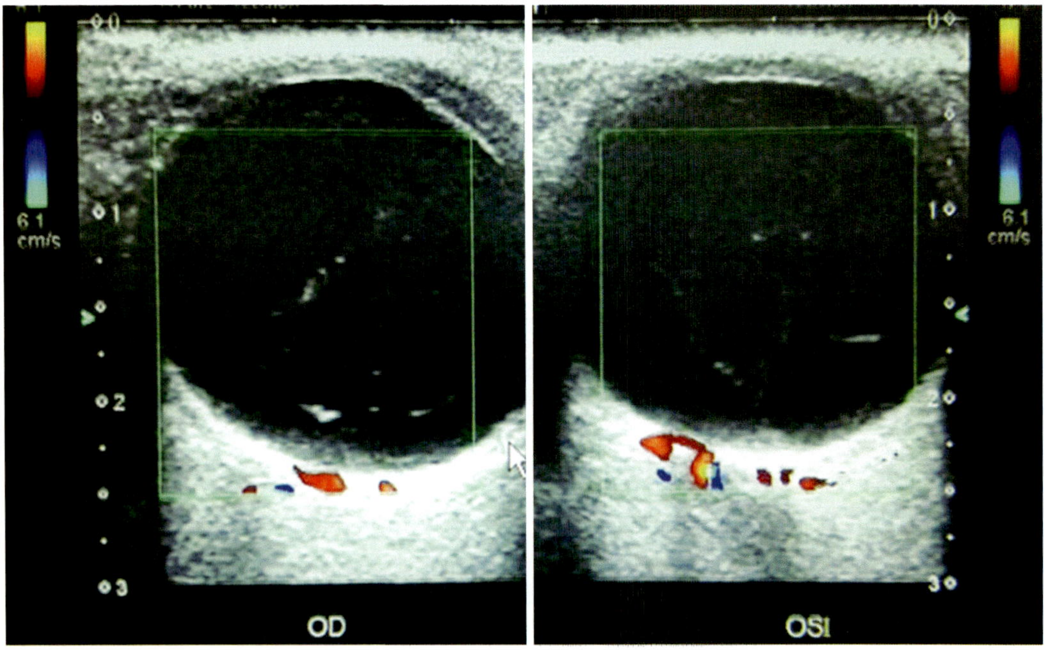

Fig. 17.7 Color ultrasound image after scleral buckling surgery of the right eye. Retinal reattachment was displayed

17.3 Case 3

17.3.1 Case Presentation

A 29-year-old male patient presented with high IOP in the right eye for 1 year and eye floaters accompanied by feeling of fullness in the right eye for 2 months. The patient had been found with high IOP in the right eye (the peak value: 35 mmHg) by chance during an examination. He had been using timolol and latanoprost eye drops irregularly. He had experienced eye floaters accompanied by feeling of fullness in the right eye in previous 2 months, which is the reason for this visit. Histories of trauma, other eye diseases, and familial diseases were denied.

The BCVA of the right eye was 6/60. The UCVA of the left eye was 20/20. The IOP measured with Goldmann applanation tonometry was 40 mmHg OD and 15 mmHg OS. Slit-lamp examination of the anterior segment of his right eye was unremarkable except that mild conjunctival congestion was shown, the diameter of the pupil was 4 mm, and the relative afferent pupillary defect (RAPD) was positive. Fundus examination of the right eye revealed that the optic disc was pallor with a C/D ratio of 0.95; the retina was attached; and there was a round hole about 1PD in size in the supranasal peripheral retina around which the retina was mildly detached. Examinations of the left eye showed no abnormality and a C/D ratio was 0.4.

Local retinal photocoagulation was then performed to seal the tear of the retina. Refer to Fig. 17.8 for the color photograph of the postoperative fundus.

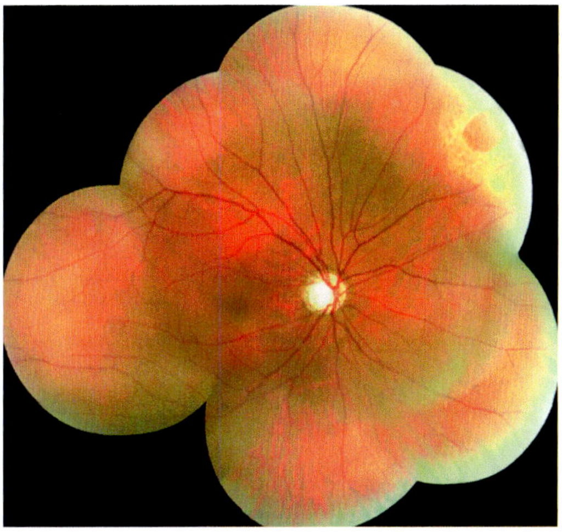

Fig. 17.8 Montage images of fundus photographs after laser treatment. The tear in the supranasal peripheral retina has been sealed and spotty laser-produced imprints could be observed in the right eye. The retina was attached. The optic disc was pallor with a C/D ratio of 0.95

17.3.2 Case Analysis

The patient was a young male with unilateral high IOP. Advanced glaucomatous optic nerve damage was found. Dilated fundus examination found a peripheral retinal tear with mild retinal detachment. Was he with juvenile glaucoma with only one eye involved? Or was it Schwartz-Matsuo syndrome? We then performed additional examinations, including visual field, central cornea thickness measurement, gonioscopy, etc.

The central cornea thickness (CCT) was 474 μm in the right eye and 490 μm in the left eye by A-ultrasound scan measurement.

Humphrey visual field examination with the 24-2 test revealed a tubular visual field in the right eye and a normal visual field in the left eye (Fig. 17.9).

Gonioscopy examination demonstrated that the anterior chamber is deep, and the angle between the iris and the surface of the trabecular meshwork was 40°, with mild pigmentation of the posterior trabecular meshwork in both eyes; a high insertion of the iris into a narrow ciliary body band with pectinate ligament attachment was observed in the right eye (Fig. 17.10); and a normal insertion of the iris into a normal ciliary body band was observed in the left eye.

a

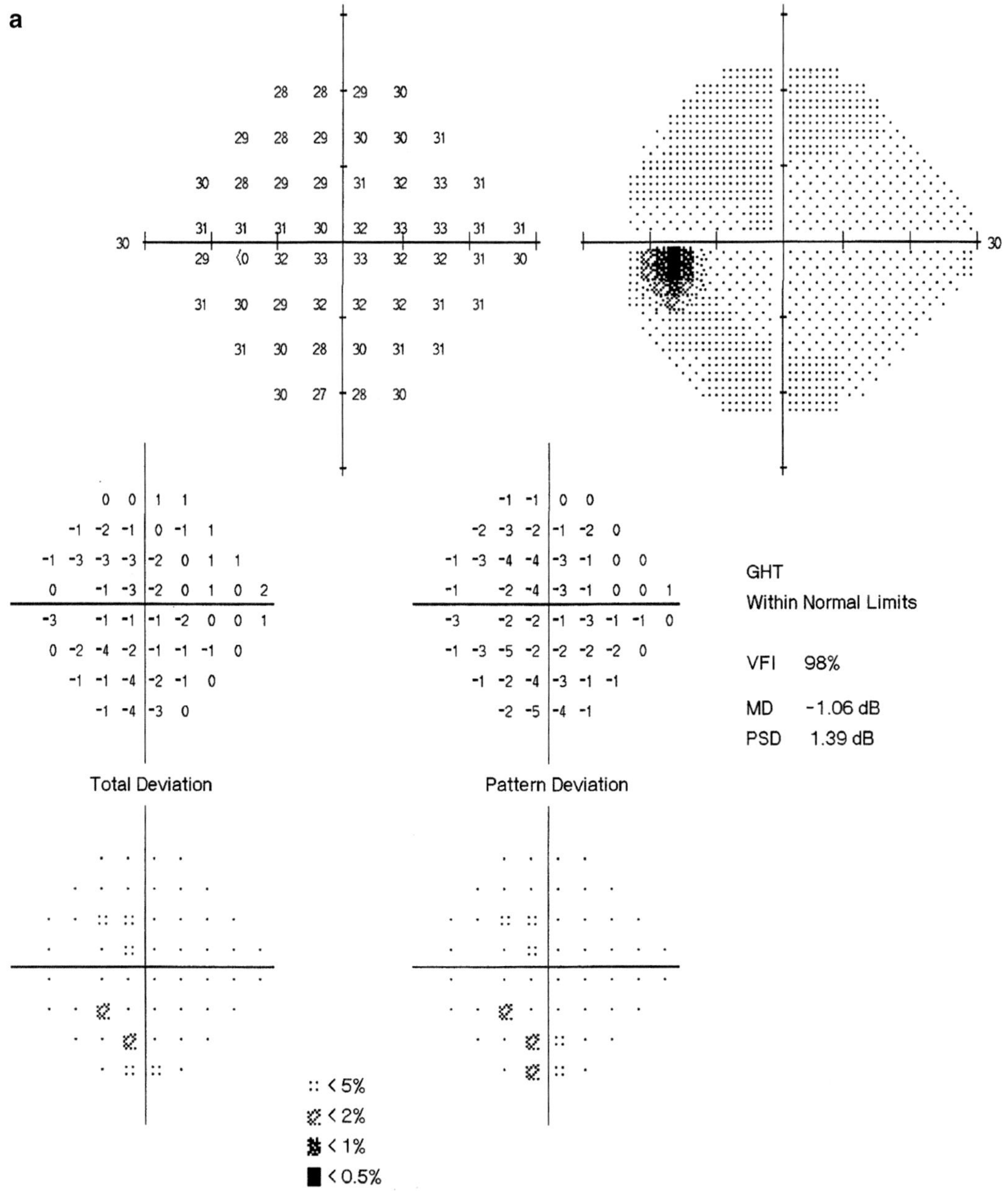

Fig. 17.9 Humphrey visual field analysis printouts with the 24-2 test. Panel a: Normal visual field in the left eye. Panel b: Tubular visual field in the right eye

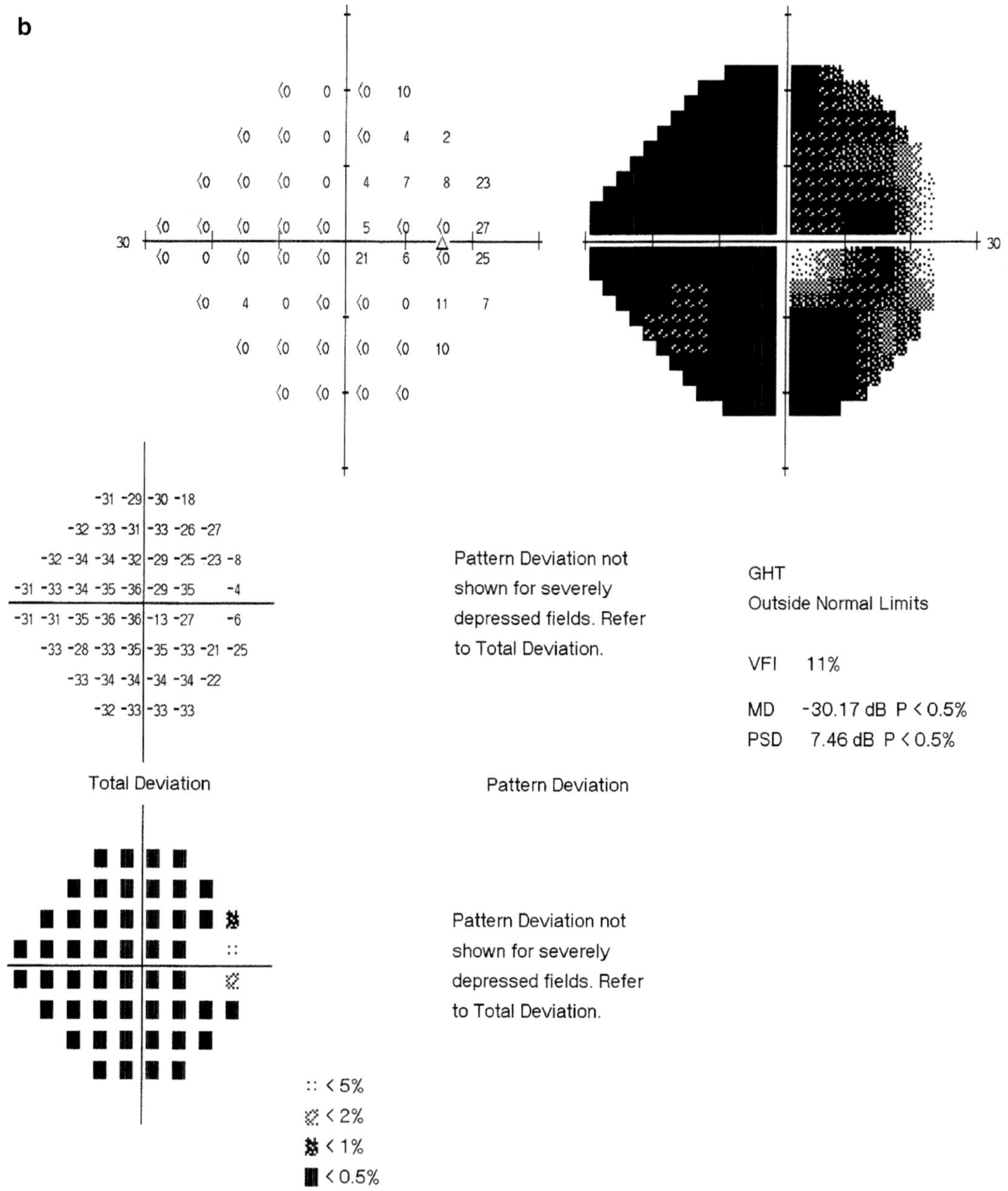

Fig. 17.9 (continued)

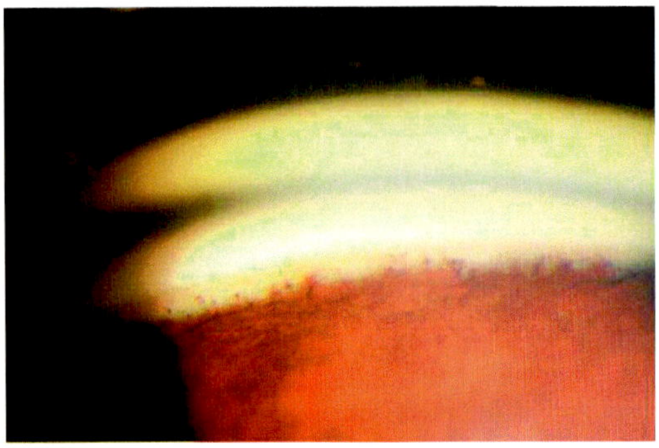

Fig. 17.10 Gonioscopic photograph of the right eye. Gonioscopic photograph showed mild pigmentation of the posterior trabecular meshwork and a high insertion of the iris into a narrow ciliary body band with pectinate ligament attachment

The manifestations of the optic disc were indicative of advanced glaucomatous damage and were consistent with the visual field impairment, so the diagnosis of juvenile glaucoma in the right eye could be established when taking also the high IOP, gonioscopic findings, and thinning CCT into consideration. The evidence found in the left eye was still not enough to make a diagnosis of glaucoma, but close follow-ups were required. Although the patient was observed with a retinal hole around which the retina was mildly detached in the peripheral region of the right eye, there was no anterior uveitis, and the IOP was not controlled after the tear was sealed. Therefore, the possibility of Schwartz-Matsuo syndrome could be ruled out.

17.3.3 Final Diagnosis

The final diagnosis was juvenile glaucoma with rhegmatogenous retinal detachment in the right eye.

The patient was given an antiglaucoma operation (glaucoma drainage implant surgery). The intraocular pressure was well controlled after the operation.

17.3.4 Case Review

The patient had concomitant juvenile glaucoma and rhegmatogenous retinal detachment in the right eye in this case, which could easily be misdiagnosed as Schwartz-Matsuo syndrome. Unilateral juvenile glaucoma is relatively rare, but its diagnosis in this case was supported by the anterior chamber angle development abnormality, IOP increase, typical glaucomatous cupping, and glaucomatous visual field impairment. The chronological sequence of intraocular pressure increase, optic nerve damage, retinal tear, and detachment didn't conform to the manifestations of Schwartz-Matsuo syndrome. The visual field change was typical advanced glaucomatous manifestation; no uveitis was found; after sealing of the retinal tear by laser treatment, the IOP was still not well controlled. With this information, it can be said that the patient had both glaucoma and rhegmatogenous retinal detachment, but they had no pathological or causal relationship.

17.4 Discussion

Schwartz-Matsuo syndrome is a condition characterized by the triad symptoms of rhegmatogenous retinal detachment, high IOP, and uveitis. It was reported and named by Schwartz in 1973. This syndrome is a rare secondary glaucoma. In addition to the clinical features of glaucoma, anterior uveitis and flat retinal detachment are usually also present. The central vision often shows no significant decrease if the macula is not involved [1, 2].

In glaucoma, paroxysmal increase can be found in the IOP. No significant symptom may be observed at the early stage, but manifestations of IOP increase, such as blurred vision, feeling of fullness, etc., will appear gradually. The anterior chamber angle is wide and open with or without mild recession (possibly associated with trauma). After retinal reattachment, the photoreceptor outer segments which have drifted into the anterior chamber will significantly decrease in number or disappear; therefore, the patient's IOP will be restored gradually.

In uveitis, the symptoms of anterior uveitis, such as aqueous flare, cells, etc., can be found, but there will be no KP or only a few pigmented KPs. No iris posterior synechiae will be observed.

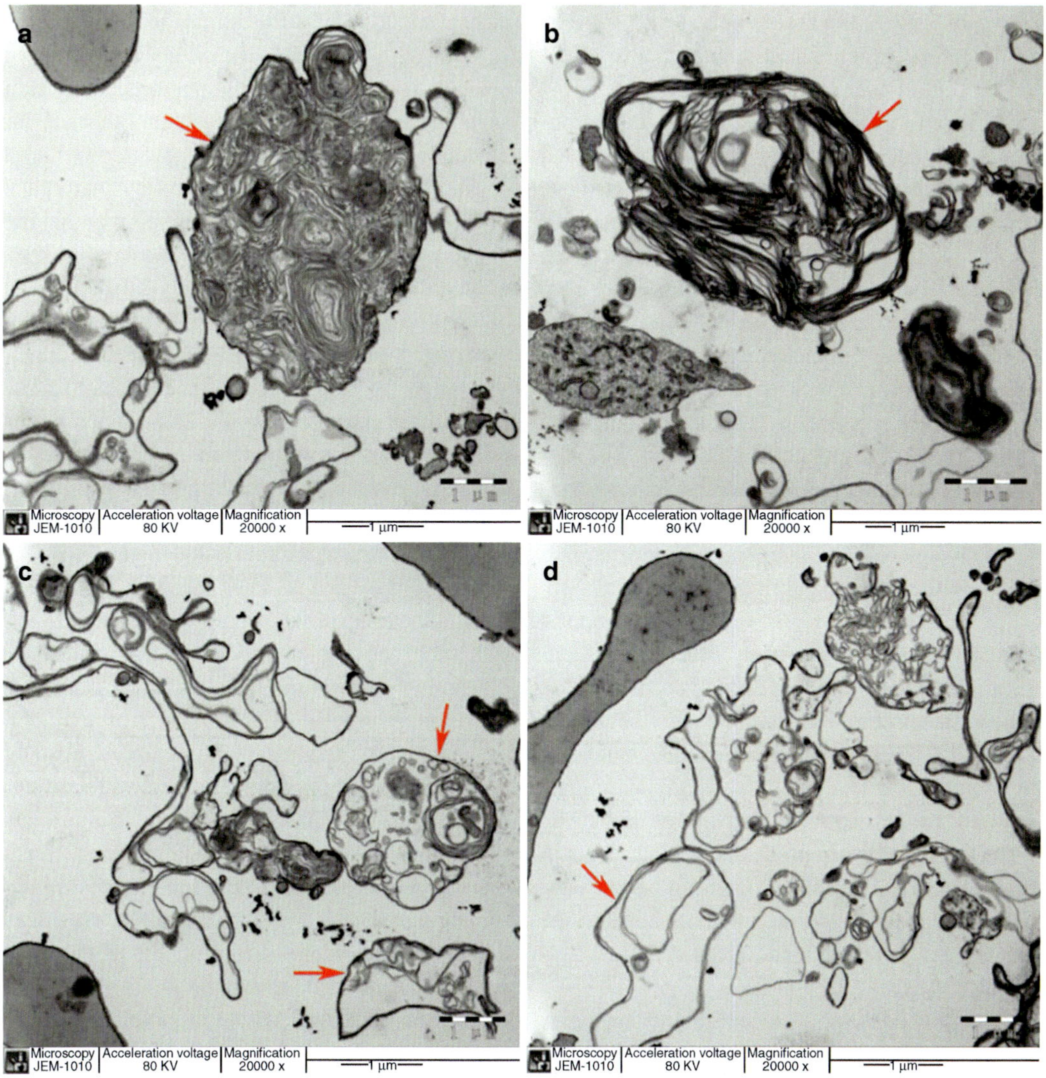

Fig. 17.11 Electron microscopy images of the photoreceptor outer segments in aqueous humor. The electron microscopy photographs showed the photoreceptor outer segments in the aqueous humor from a Schwartz syndrome patient. Panel a: Intact photoreceptor outer segment (red arrow). Panel b: Mild damaged photoreceptor outer segment (red arrow). Panel c: The pieces of photoreceptor outer segment (red arrow). Panel d: "Photoreceptor debris" (red arrow); the photographs were contributed by Dr. Qinghuai Liu

In rhegmatogenous retinal detachment, the tear is usually small and often lies in the peripheral area, such as near the ora serrata or at the ciliary pars plana, which makes it difficult to be observed. Retinal detachment is generally flat.

The pathogenesis of this disease is still unclear. The electron microscopy on the patients' aqueous humor of the anterior chamber in a study found photoreceptor outer segments in the aqueous humor. The photoreceptor outer segments can be intact or in pieces or even in the form of "photoreceptor debris" (Fig. 17.11). Studies have proved that the high IOP shown in the disease is caused by the aqueous humor outflow disorder resulting from photoreceptor outer segments that drifted into the anterior chamber via the retinal tear and covered the trabecular meshwork. The electron microscopy on the aqueous humor of the patient in Case 1 of this section carried out during the retinal reattachment operation also found photoreceptor outer segments. Besides, the UBM examination in Case 1 also supports this pathogenesis, though indirectly. The UBM showed posterior depression of the iris of the affected eye (compared with the contralateral normal eye). It's speculated to be "reverse pupillary block" caused by increased anterior chamber pressure and increased the pressure difference between the anterior and posterior chambers resulting from the trabecular meshwork covering by the photoreceptor outer segments 1. This is similar to the pathogenesis of pigmentary glaucoma. The difference between them is as follows: in Schwartz-Matsuo syndrome, the chamber angle blockage by outer segment disc membranes happens first, and then the reverse pupillary block is caused, while in pigmentary glaucoma, the temporal sequence of reverse pupillary block and chamber angle blockage by pigments is still unclear; to be more specific, it is still unclear whether the posterior depression of the iris caused by reverse pupillary block leads to the frictional contact between the iris and the suspensory ligaments of the lens which then produces free pigments or the reverse pupillary block resulting from chamber angle blockage by the pigments leads to the contact between the iris and the suspensory ligaments of the lens.

If so, why do the photoreceptor outer segments in rhegmatogenous retinal detachment generally not lead to intraocular pressure increase? Firstly, it's because of the position of the retinal tear. The detached photoreceptor outer segments will diffuse and degrade inside the vitreous chamber if the retinal tear is located posteriorly. Therefore, the outer segment disc membranes entering the anterior chamber will be too scarce to lead to aqueous humor outflow blockage in the trabecular meshwork and IOP increase even when the anterior limiting membrane of the vitreous body is not intact. When the retinal tear lies in the anterior region (such as the ciliary pars plana or even ciliary epithelium), the photoreceptor outer segments can even enter directly into the anterior chamber through local microscopic gaps without passing through the anterior limiting membrane of the vitreous body. The author believes that the above pathogenesis still cannot explain all phenomena, and further exploration on the disease causes from the perspectives of eyeball development and molecular mechanism is needed.

It is worth emphasizing that the treatment of this disease may be delayed if the diagnosis is not correct and only treatment targeting at glaucoma is given. It's a mistargeted treatment if an operation is performed to treat the glaucoma when the intraocular pressure-lowering effect is not good by drugs. The therapeutic effect on uveitis by a hormone therapy is not good, and risk of glucocorticoid-induced glaucoma may result. In contrary, the intraocular pressure will decrease gradually after retinal reattachment, and the uveitis can also subside spontaneously after the operation. This is a kind of therapeutic diagnosis. Therefore, the keys to the treatment of Schwartz-Matsuo syndrome are early diagnosis and timely operation for sealing of the retinal tear. It will facilitate the diagnosis and a deeper understanding of this disease if a small amount of aqueous humor can be taken during the operation for electron microscopy to confirm whether there are photoreceptor outer segments.

References

1. Gutiérrez C, Merayo J, Cuevas J, et al. Glaucoma related with photoreceptor outer segments in aqueous humor. Schwartz-Matsuo syndrome. Arch Soc Esp Oftalmol. 2001;76(5):315–8.
2. Fan W, Sun X, Xie P, et al. One case of Schwartz syndrome. Chin J Ophthalmol. 2015;51(9):699–700.

Ectopia of the Physiological Blind Spot

18

Ning Fan, Xuyang Liu, and Jiantao Wang

Blind spot ectopia is actually macular ectopia, which is a result of retinal dysplasia. A case of blind spot ectopia caused by retinal dysplasia is described in this section.

18.1 Case

18.1.1 Case Presentation

A 39-year-old male patient presented with poor vision in the right eye and worse vision in the left eye, which had started since childhood. He had neither made the correction by wearing glasses nor undergone diagnosis and treatment. No accompanying symptoms such as double vision, night blindness, etc. were present. Histories of trauma, systemic diseases, and familial diseases were denied. The patient was delivered normally and born full term.

The best corrected visual acuity (BCVA) was 20/63 with refractive correction (−5.25DS −1.75DC × 137) OD and 20/400 with refractive correction (−5.50DS −0.75DC × 140) OS. The intraocular pressures (IOPs) in both eyes were normal. Slit-lamp examination of his anterior segments was unremarkable. Fundus examination revealed that, in both eyes, the optic disc was pink in color with a clear boundary; the C/D ratio was 0.2; foveal reflex was absent; the distance between the optic disc and macula was large; and the arrangement of the retinal vessels was rigid (Fig. 18.1a, b). The three-mirror lens examination revealed atrophy foci and grid-like degeneration areas accompanied by pigmentation in the peripheral retina. The indirect ophthalmoscopy examination combined with scleral depression showed sudden termination of peripheral retinal vessels and presence of a definite boundary between them and the peripheral avascular area, and retinal atrophy and degeneration areas could also be seen in the peripheral area (Fig. 18.1c).

Corneal light reflex test with the patient fixating at 33 cm showed that both eyes were in normal position. The eyeball showed no movement in the alternate cover test, and the eyeball movement was normal.

Standardized automated perimetry with the 24-2 test showed that the blind spot was located temporally from its normal location in both eyes and generalized depression accompanied by peripheral visual field defect in the left eye (Fig. 18.2).

Optical coherence tomography (OCT) (Fig. 18.3) showed that the thicknesses of the

N. Fan · J. Wang (✉)
Shenzhen Eye Hospital, Shenzhen University, Shenzhen, China

X. Liu
Xiamen Eye Center of Xiamen University, Xiamen, China

Shenzhen Eye Hospital, Shenzhen University, Shenzhen, China

N. Wang et al. (eds.), *Optic Disorders and Visual Field*, Advances in Visual Science and Eye Diseases 2, https://doi.org/10.1007/978-981-13-2502-1_18

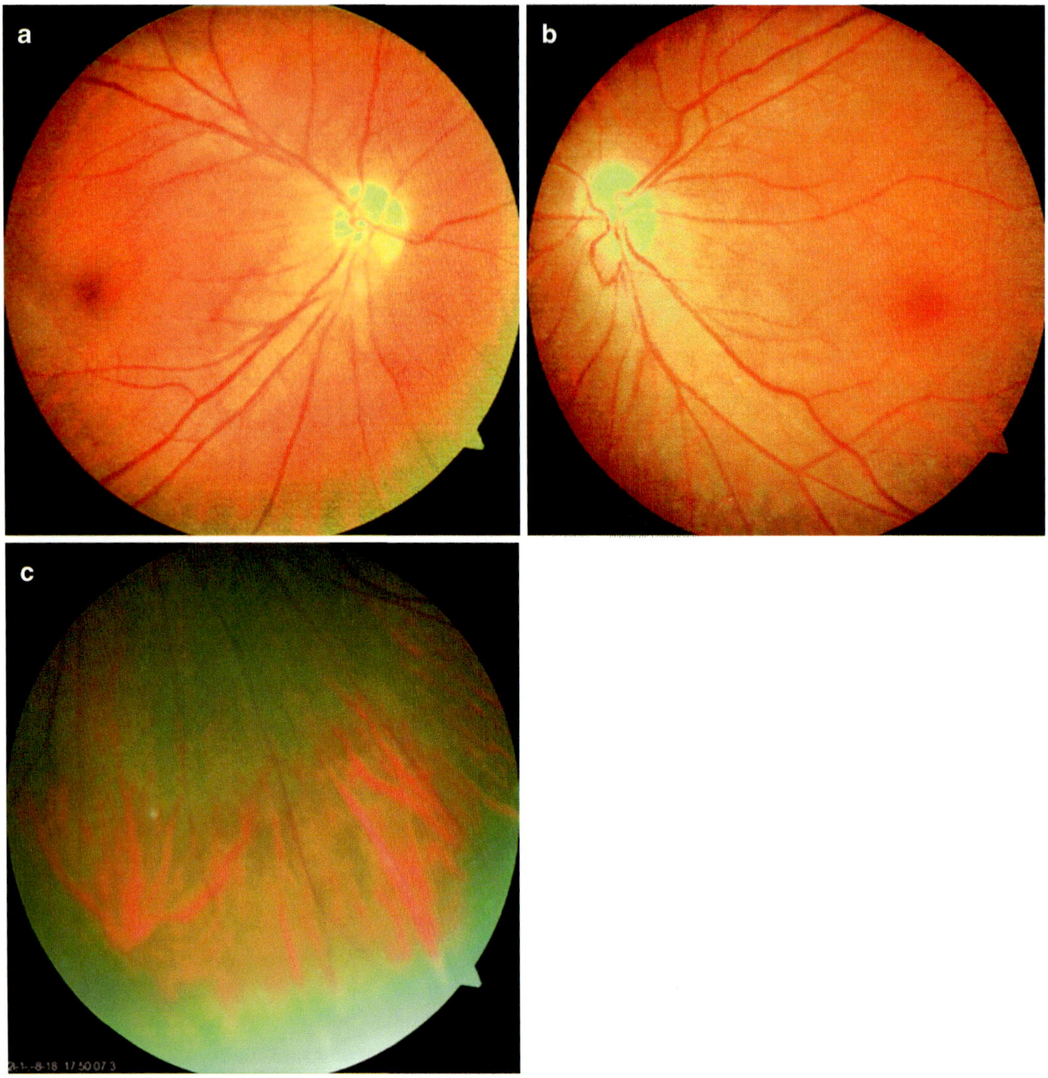

Fig. 18.1 Fundus photographs. It could be seen that the arrangement of the retinal vessels was rigid, and the macula was dislocated. Panel a: Right eye. Panel b: Left eye. Panel c: Inferotemporal peripheral area of the left eye

fovea was about 223 μm and the distance between the fovea and the temporal edge of the optic disc was about 6000 μm (the distance in normal people is about 3500 μm) in both eyes.

Fundus fluorescein angiography (FFA) showed straight retinal vessels and local atrophy foci accompanied by pigmentation at the termination of peripheral retinal vessels in both eyes (Fig. 18.4).

Electroretinography (ERG) showed normal dark adaptation and almost normal light adaptation in the right eye and moderately to severely abnormal dark adaptation and light adaption in the left eye.

a

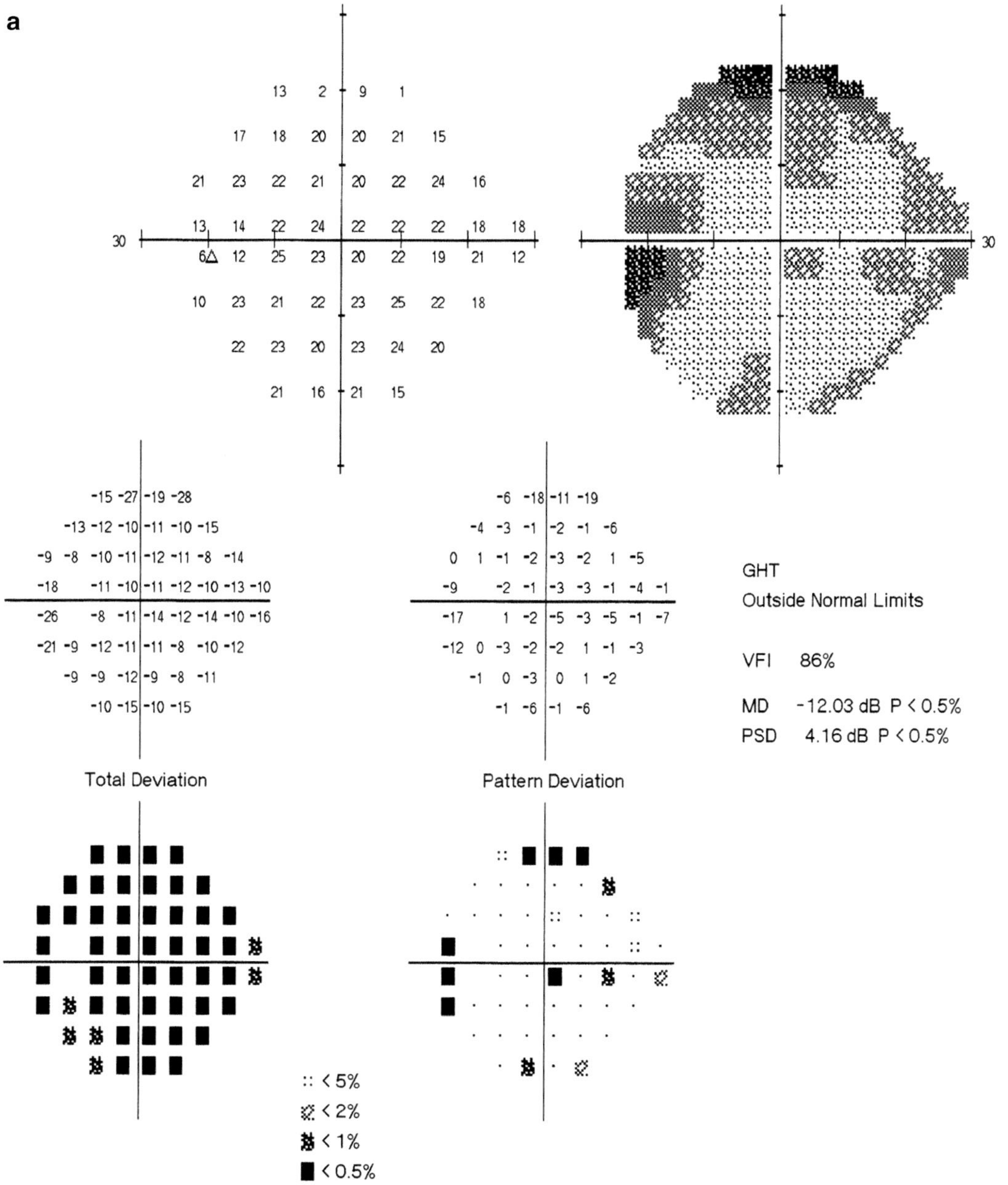

Fig. 18.2 Humphrey visual field analysis printouts. Standardized automated perimetry with the 24-2 test (a size III target was used) showed that the blind spots were located temporally from the normal location in both eyes. Panel a: Generalized depression accompanied by peripheral visual field defect was seen in the left eye (visual field reliability may be affected by the poor vision of the left eye). Panel b: The blind spots were located temporally from the normal location in the right eye

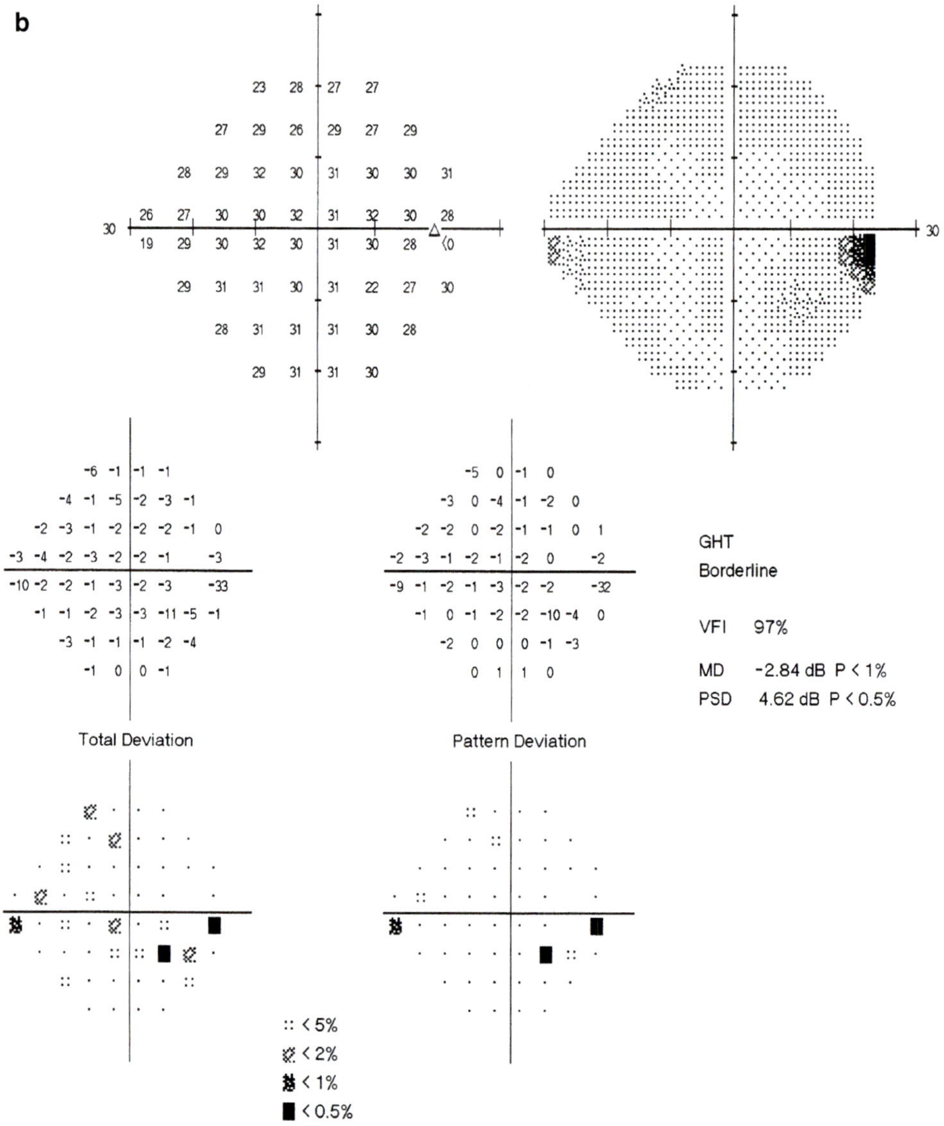

Fig. 18.2 (continued)

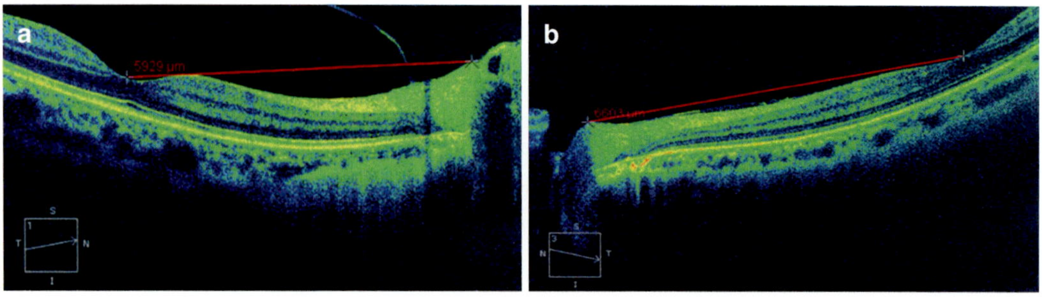

Fig. 18.3 OCT images of the retinas. Panel a: The distance between the fovea and the temporal edge of the optic disc in the right eye was about 5929 μm. Panel b: The distance between the fovea and the temporal edge of the optic disc in the left eye was about 6603 μm (length of scanning line: 9 mm)

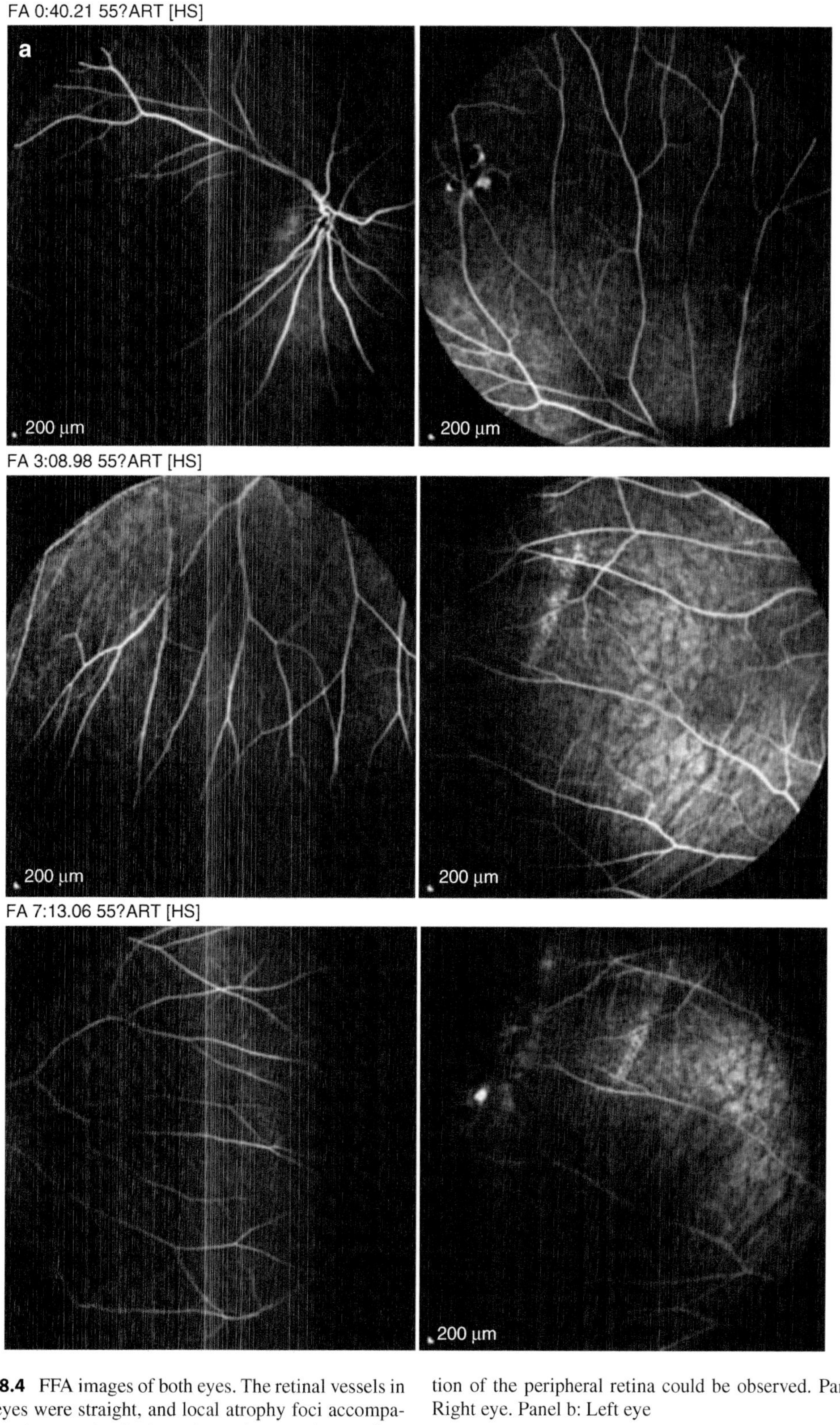

Fig. 18.4 FFA images of both eyes. The retinal vessels in both eyes were straight, and local atrophy foci accompanied by pigmentation in the retina at the vascular termination of the peripheral retina could be observed. Panel a: Right eye. Panel b: Left eye

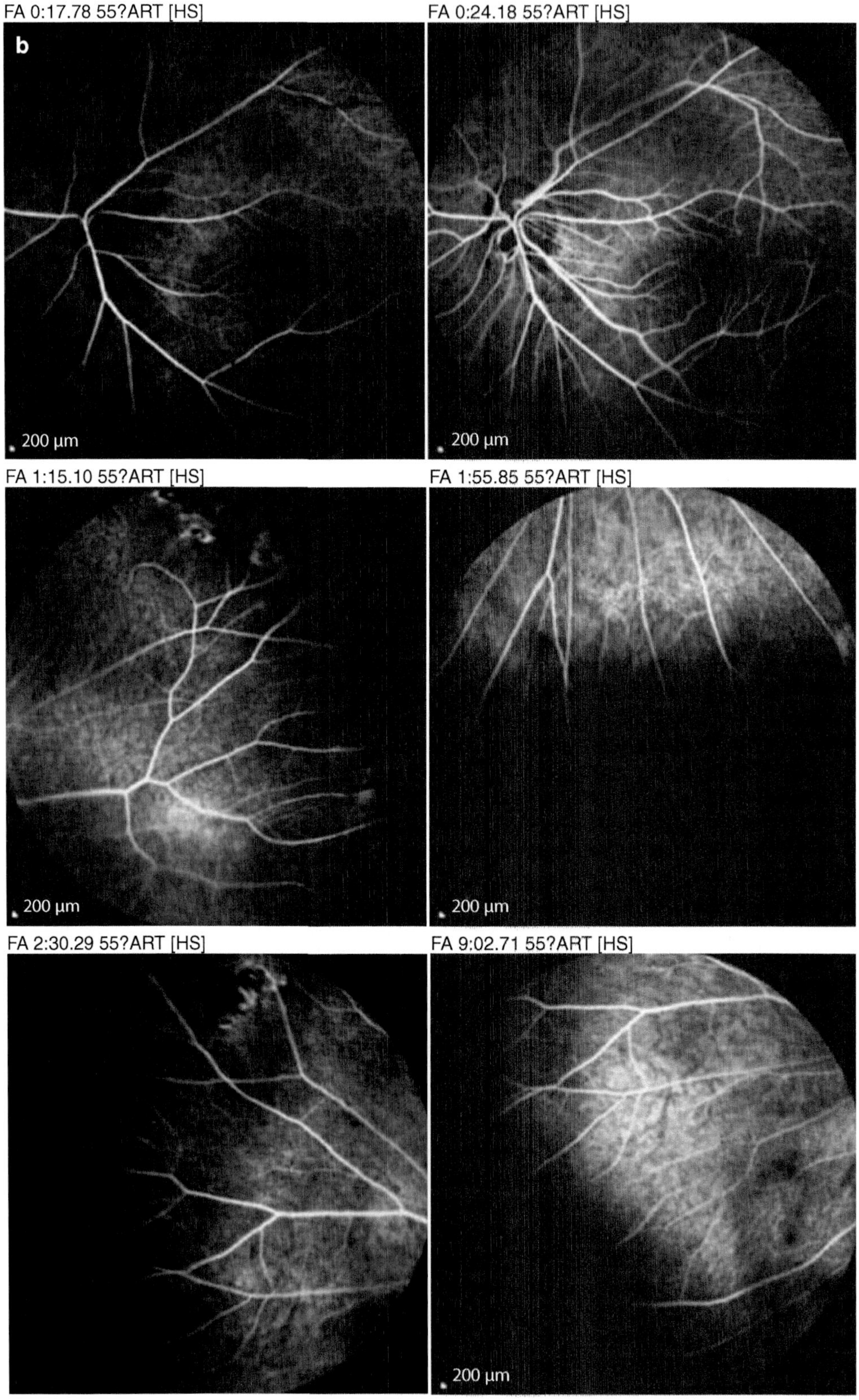

Fig. 18.4 (continued)

18.1.2 Final Diagnosis

The final diagnosis was bilateral familial exudative vitreoretinopathy with bilateral macular ectopia.

18.2 Discussion

Normally, the fovea is about 2.5PD (papilla disc) and 15–18° from inferotemporal to the optic disc, and it is already there at birth. Macular ectopia is rare and can be found in retinopathy of prematurity, familial exudative vitreoretinopathy, persistent hyperplastic primary vitreous, etc. [1–4]. This disease may result from retinal dysplasia caused by hereditary or congenital factors. Because the retina is pulled by the peripheral retinopathy, the retinal vessels run straight, and the macula is located temporally, which manifests as increased distance between the blind spot and the central region of the visual field.

Macular ectopia leads to the abnormalities of the visual axis and optical axis. The visual function is rarely spared even the macular structure is normal (or partially normal). The central vision of such patient is usually poor, and pseudostrabismus can be formed due to the increase of the angle kappa [3, 4].

No significant macroscopic eye position abnormality was shown in this case, but the central vision was poor in both eyes. Visual field examination revealed that the ectopia of the macula led to visual field abnormality (the blind spot was located temporally).

References

1. Peng X. Diagnosis and speculation of ocular fundus diseases. Beijing: People's Medical Publishing House; 2009.
2. Finis D, Stammen J, Joussen AM. Familial exudative vitreoretinopathy. Ophthalmologe. 2010;107(7):683–91.
3. Soong GP, Shapiro M, Seiple W, et al. Macular structure and vision of patients with macular heterotopia secondary to retinopathy of prematurity. Retina. 2008;28(8):1111–6.
4. He T, Zhu J, Song Y, et al. One case of persistent hyperplastic primary vitreous combined with macular ectopia. Chin J Pract Ophthalmol. 2014;32(8):1038–9.

19 Be Aware of the Mild Decibel Values Loss at Central Fixation

Ning Fan, Xuyang Liu, and Jiantao Wang

Localized decibel loss in central visual field usually suggests maculopathy. Inconsistencies between visual acuity and visual field change, between disease severity and visual field damage, or between symptoms and signs could usually be noticed, due to the complexity of the diseases in the macula. Besides, a proper visual field examination strategy is also very important for the evaluation of disease.

19.1 Case 1

19.1.1 Case Presentation

A 30-year-old female patient presented with vision decrease in the left eye for 1 month. No accompanying symptoms, including red eyes, eye pain, distorted vision, etc., were present. Histories of trauma, other eye diseases, systemic diseases, and familial diseases were denied. The patient had been diagnosed with refractive error (hyperopia) at another hospital. However, she still believed that she was not hyperopic, so she visited our hospital for treatment.

The uncorrected visual acuity (UCVA) was 20/20 OD and 20/25 OS. The best corrected visual acuity (BCVA) was 20/20 with hyperopic correction (+0.50DS) in the left eye. The intraocular pressure (IOP) was normal. Slit-lamp examination of her anterior segments was unremarkable. Fundus examination revealed that the vitreous was clear and the optic disc was pink in color with a clear boundary in both eyes; orange-red subretinal foci with irregular boundary could be observed in the posterior pole of the left eye, and the retinal vessels were still normal (Fig. 19.1).

The pattern deviation probability plot showed a relative scotoma in the center of the left eye (Fig. 19.2).

Macular optical coherence tomography (OCT) image showed the neurosensory retina and retinal pigment epithelium (RPE) were elevated and serous neuroretinal detachment in the inferonasal region (Fig. 19.3).

Fundus fluorescein angiography (FFA) showed hyperfluorescence lesion at the early stage and diffuse fluorescent staining at the late stage (Fig. 19.4).

A-ultrasound examination showed hyperechoic peak of tumor. B-ultrasound examination showed scale-like light band in the image produced by the strong reflection of the tumor. The

N. Fan · J. Wang (✉)
Shenzhen Eye Hospital, Shenzhen University, Shenzhen, China

X. Liu
Xiamen Eye Center of Xiamen University, Xiamen, China

Shenzhen Eye Hospital, Shenzhen University, Shenzhen, China

N. Wang et al. (eds.), *Optic Disorders and Visual Field*, Advances in Visual Science and Eye Diseases 2, https://doi.org/10.1007/978-981-13-2502-1_19

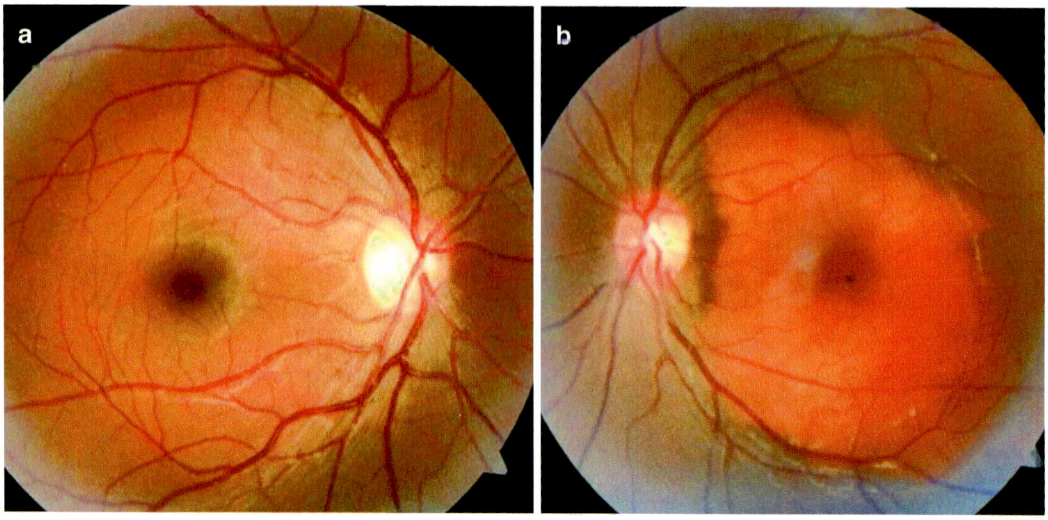

Fig. 19.1 Fundus photographs. Panel a: No abnormality was found in the right eye. Panel b: Orange-red subretinal foci with irregular boundary could be observed in the posterior pole of the left eye, and the arrangement of the retinal vessels was still normal

wave-shaped light band reflected the hilly tumor surface. The echoes of other tissues inside the eye disappeared after gain reduction, but the tumor echoes were still present (Fig. 19.5).

A high-density shadow consistent with that of the orbital bone was exhibited in the left eye during the head CT (Fig. 19.6).

19.1.2 Final Diagnosis

The final diagnosis was choroidal osteoma in the left eye.

The patient was asked to return for a follow-up visit at the outpatient department after the diagnosis was confirmed, but she was lost to follow-up for 3 years. The recent reexamination demonstrated expansion of the lesion in the left eye (Fig. 19.7).

The positron emission tomography-computed tomography (PET-CT) of the head by another hospital revealed the following results: a high-density nodular lesion was observed in the temporal side of the posterior wall of the left eyeball (Fig. 19.8); no abnormal radioactive concentration was shown, and no increase was exhibited in the glucose metabolism; and the other parts of the body showed no abnormality. The reexamination of visual field showed aggravation of the defect (Fig. 19.9). OCT and fundus fluorescein angiography (FFA) revealed significant changes (Figs. 19.10 and 19.11).

Visual field examination showed a central scotoma extending from the blind spot in the left eye. The visual field damage was more serious than that found 3 years before (Fig. 19.9).

Macular OCT images showed structural disorder and edema of the retina, neurosensory retina elevation, and abnormally high signals in the choroid of the left eye (Fig. 19.10).

The patient's macula was not affected at the first visit, and the central vision can be corrected to 20/20 then. The lesion involved the fovea, and the BCVA decreased to 20/125 when the patient

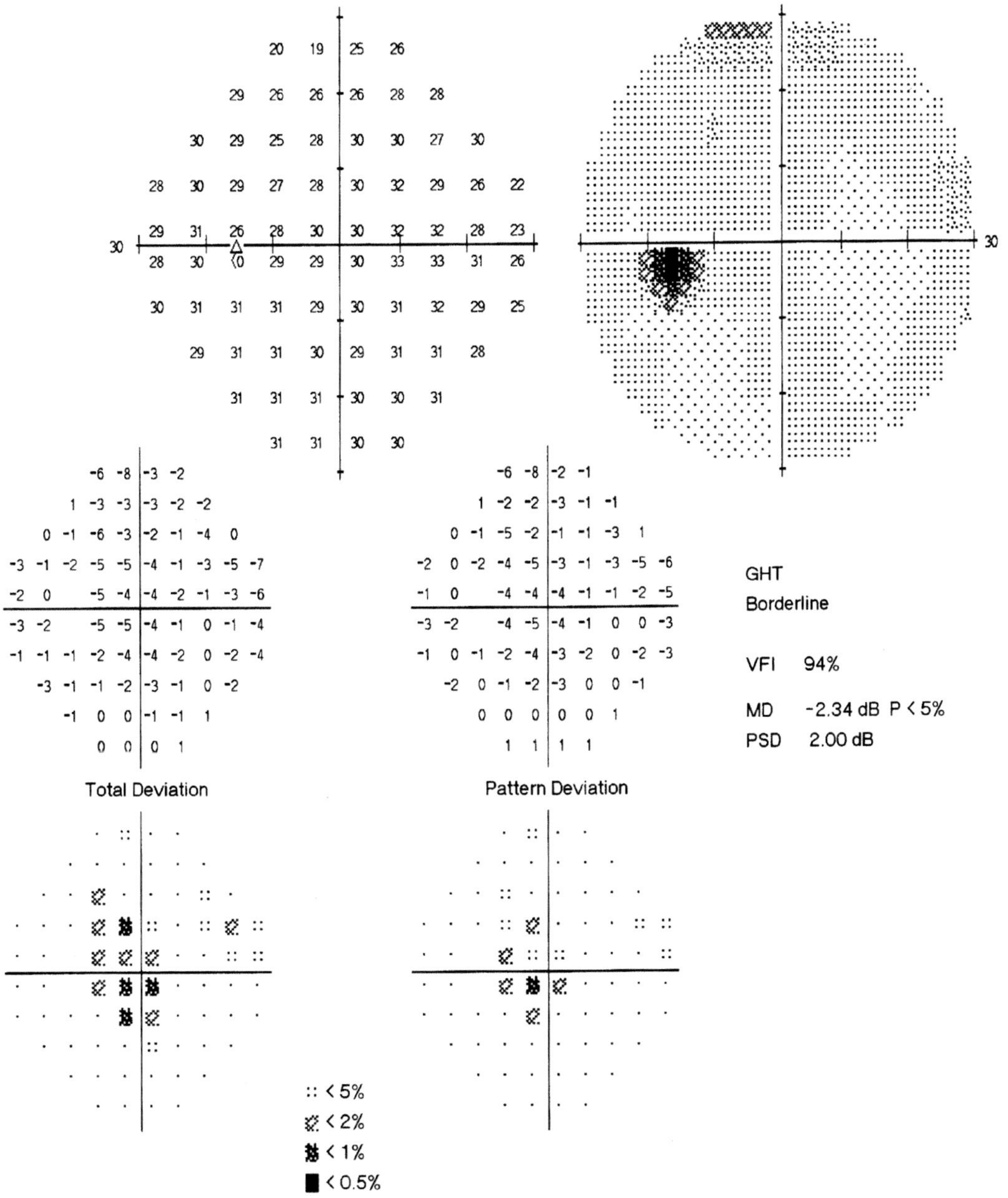

Fig. 19.2 Humphrey visual field analysis printout for the left eye. The pattern deviation probability plot showed a relative scotoma in the center of the left eye with the 30-2 test

returned for follow-up 3 years later. Meanwhile, a central scotoma extending from the blind spot occurred in the visual field.

FFA displayed patchy hyperfluorescence in the posterior pole of the left eye at the early stage. Fluorescence enhancement and fusion were shown at the late stage (Fig. 19.11).

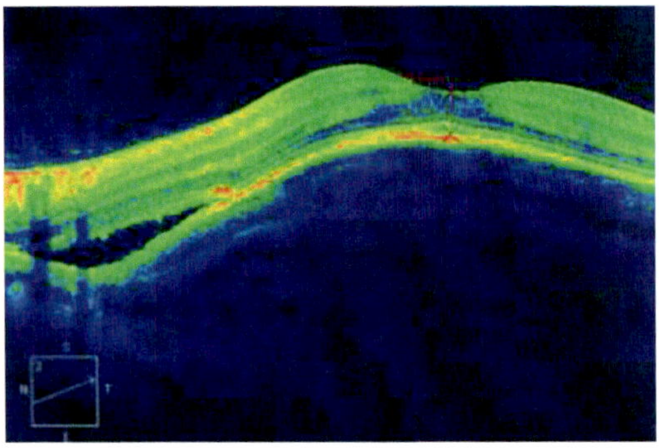

Fig. 19.3 Macular OCT image in the left eye. The neurosensory retina and RPE were elevated, and serous neuroretinal detachment in the inferonasal region could be seen

19.1.3 Case Review

Choroidal osteoma is usually observed in females aged 20–30. It typically involves one eye. The patients could be free from any symptom or experience only mild vision decrease, distorted vision, or visual field defects at corresponding tumor sites at the early stage. The patient was a young female in this case. The chief complaint was vision decrease, but the visual acuity could be corrected to 1.0 by a +0.50DS convex lens. The orange-red focus in the macula was homogeneous in color and without effusion, hemorrhage, or edema. Therefore, missed diagnosis could happen easily, and she was diagnosed with "hyperopia" by another hospital. The visual field

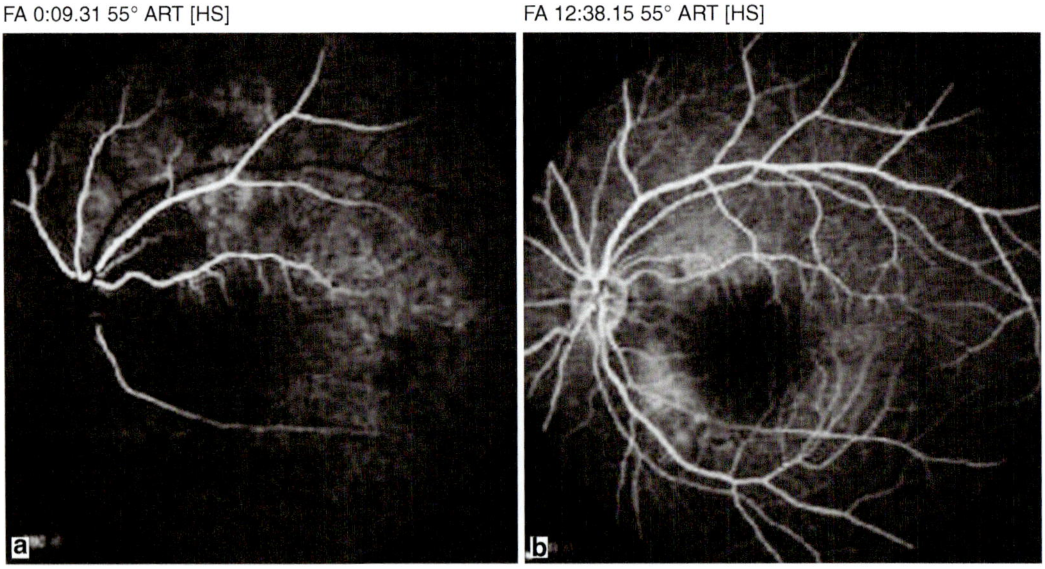

Fig. 19.4 FFA images for the left eye. Panel a: Patchy hyperfluorescence was exhibited in the lesion at the early stage. Panel b: Diffuse fluorescent staining was revealed at the late stage

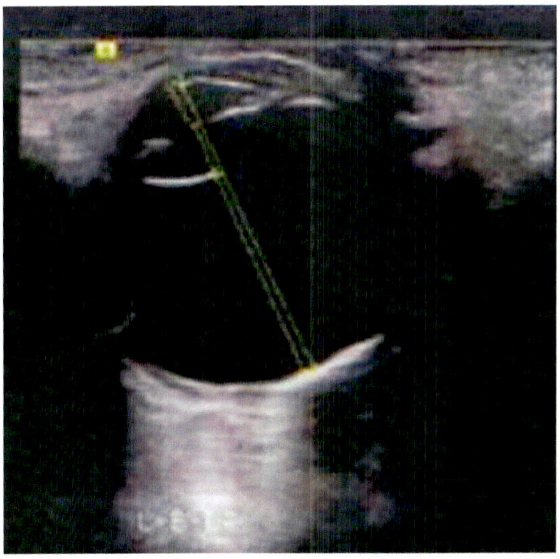

Fig. 19.5 B-ultrasound image for the left eye. The B-ultrasound revealed a hyperechoic lesion in the posterior pole, which surface showed wave-shaped light band

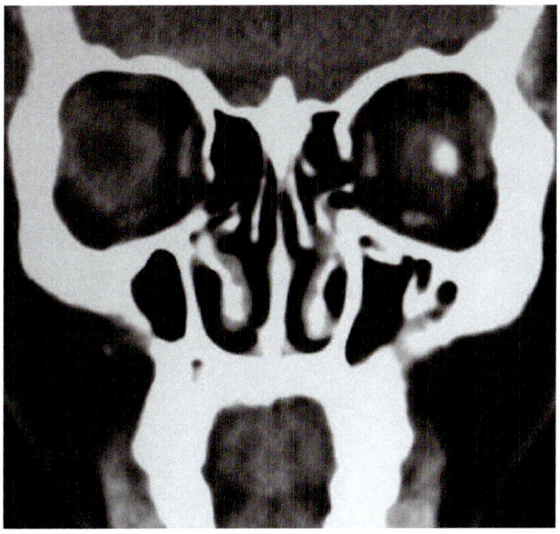

Fig. 19.6 Head CT scanning. A high-density shadow consistent with that of the orbital bone was exhibited in the left eye during the head CT

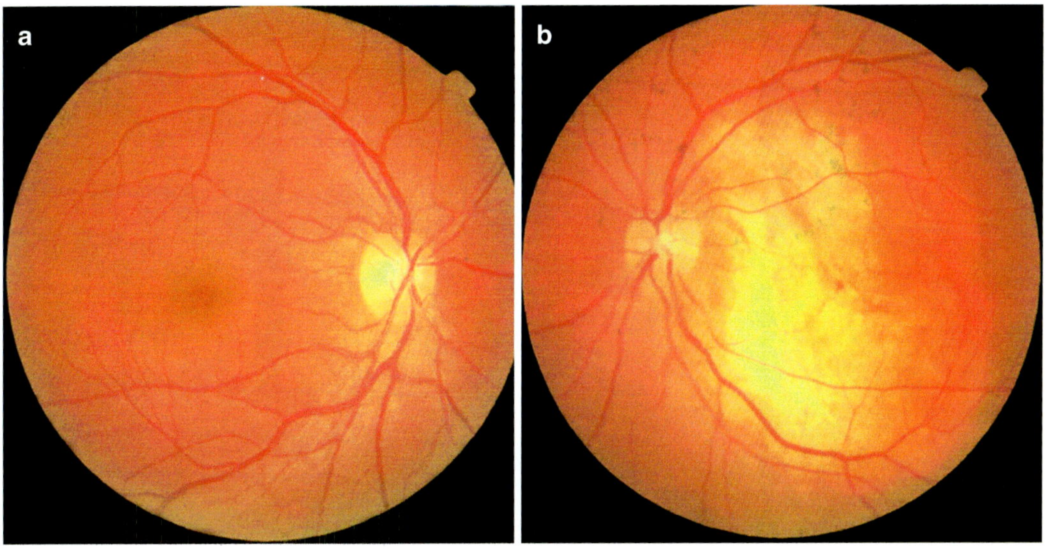

Fig. 19.7 Reexamination fundus photographs. Panel a: No abnormality was found in the optic disc and retina of the right eye. Panel b: The extent of orange-red retinal focus with irregular boundary in the posterior pole of the left eye showed significant expansion when compared with the previous findings. The arrangement of the retinal vessels was still normal

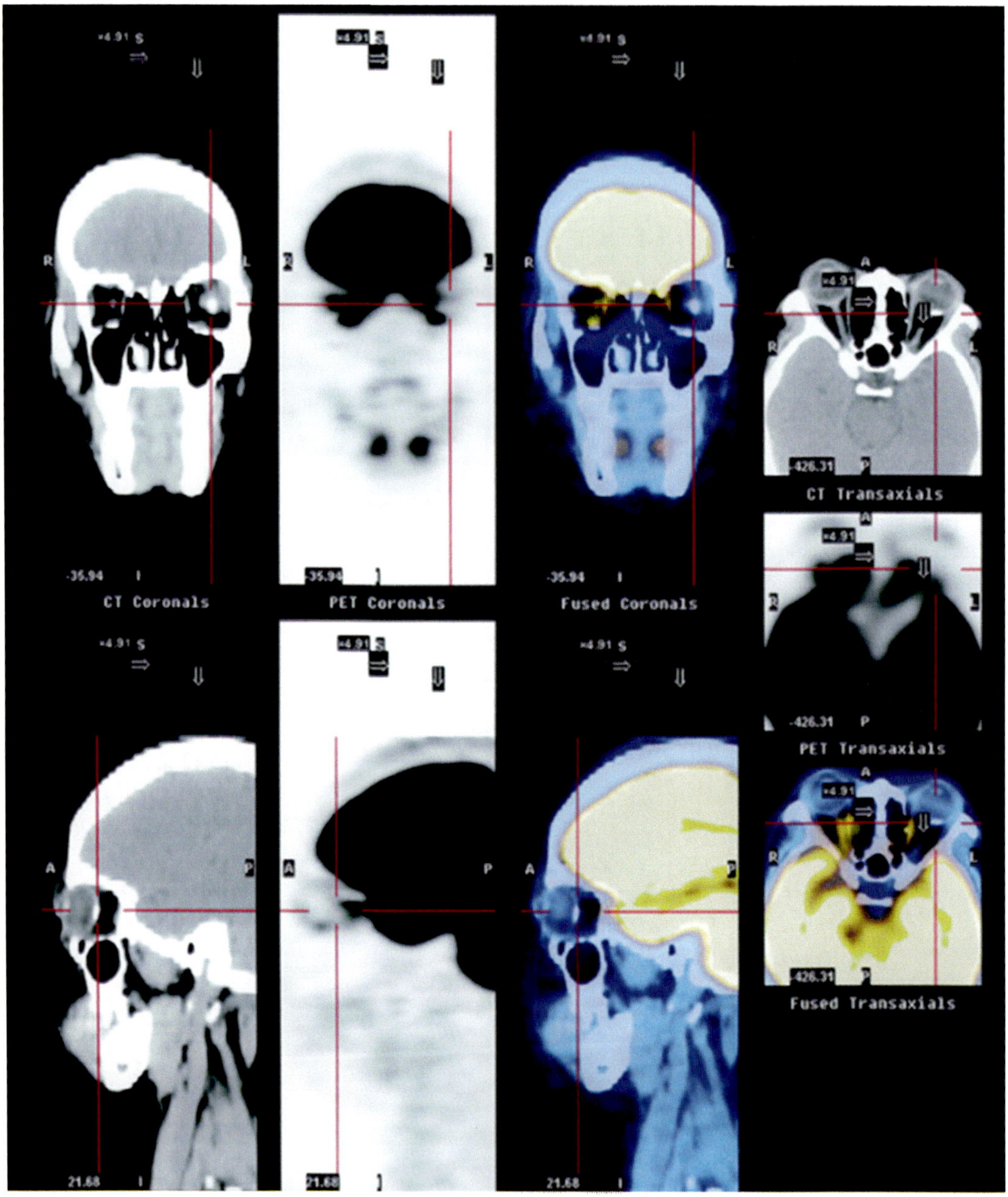

Fig. 19.8 PET-CT image. A high-density nodular lesion with a size of about 0.5 cm * 0.3 cm could be observed in the temporal side of the posterior wall of the left eyeball. The edge was clear, and no significant enhancement was shown after enhanced scanning. No abnormal radioactive concentration was shown, and no increase was exhibited in the glucose metabolism

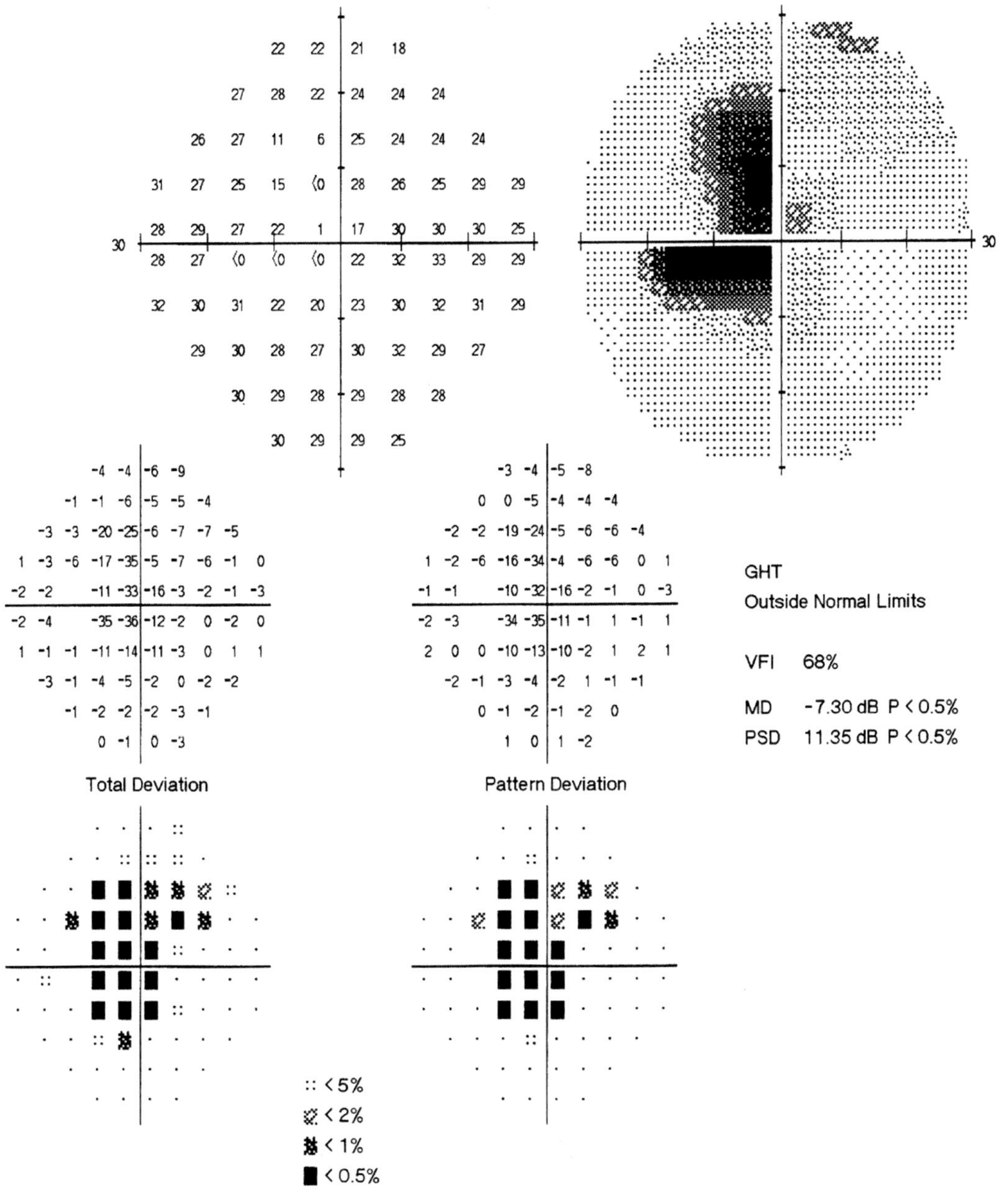

Fig. 19.9 Reexamination Humphrey visual field reexamination printout. A central scotoma extending from the blind spot was revealed by the 30-2 test in the left eye

examination showed mild reduction (only several decibels) in the central visual field, suggesting that the lesion was in the macular area. An orange-red retinal focus with irregular boundary could be observed in the posterior pole by careful fundus examination, and the diagnosis was confirmed by further examinations such as FFA, B-ultrasound, orbital CT, etc. Elevation of the full-thickness RPE layer and neuroepithelium layer could be observed in the fovea by OCT scanning. But except for the local shallow retinal detachment in the inferonasal region of the macula, the retina tissue and structure of the fovea were not significantly damaged. It could explain why the visual acuity could be corrected to 1.0 by a +0.50DS convex lens. However, mild light sensitivity reduction was revealed in the temporal side of the central visual field. The 10-2 test or even the macula test strategy can also be used to magnify the details in the central region, and this will not be discussed here.

The cause of choroidal osteoma is unclear, and the current opinion is that osteoma is a choristoma left by congenital primitive mesodermal tissues. The main complication of choroidal osteoma is neovascularization beneath the retina, causing

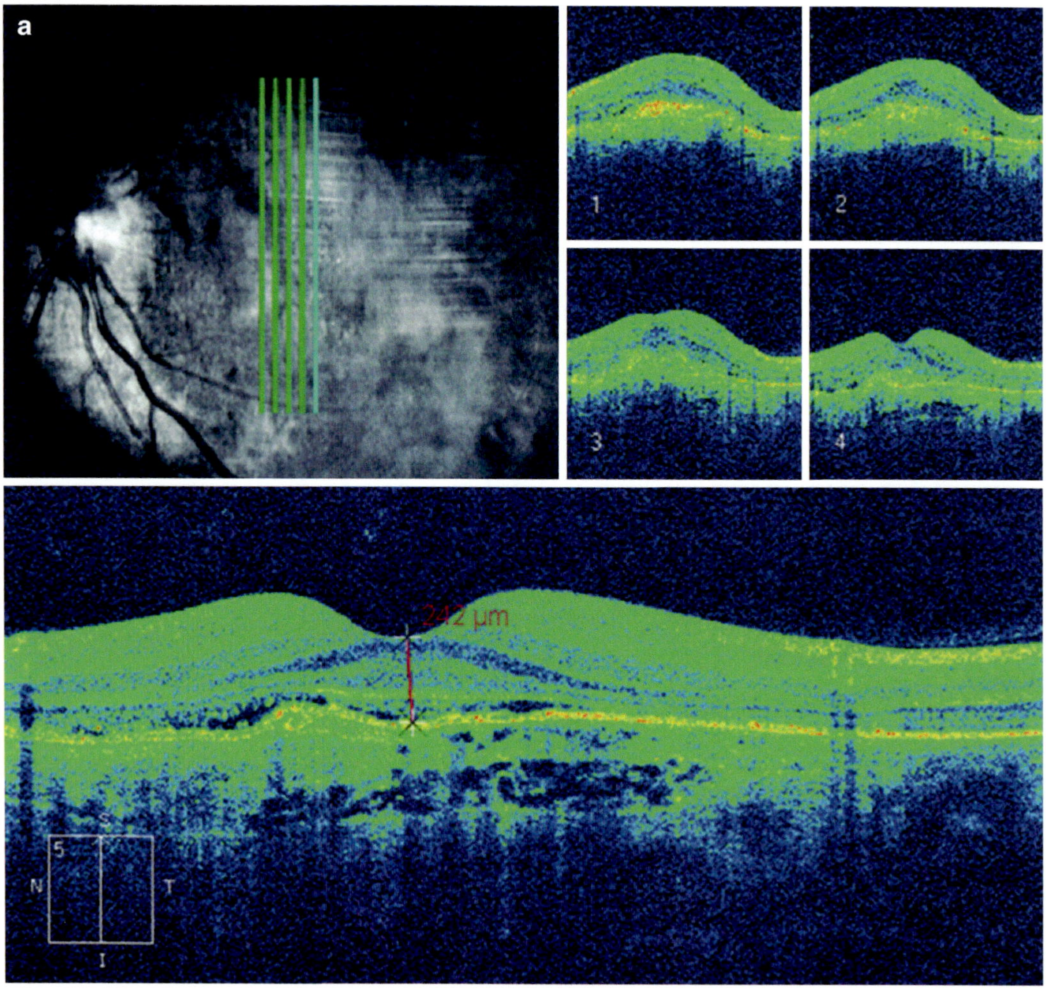

Fig. 19.10 Reexamination OCT printouts of the macula. The macular OCT images showed structural disorder and edema of the retina, neurosensory retina elevation, and abnormally high signals in the choroid in the left eye. Panel a: Horizontal linear scanning. Panel b: Vertical linear scanning

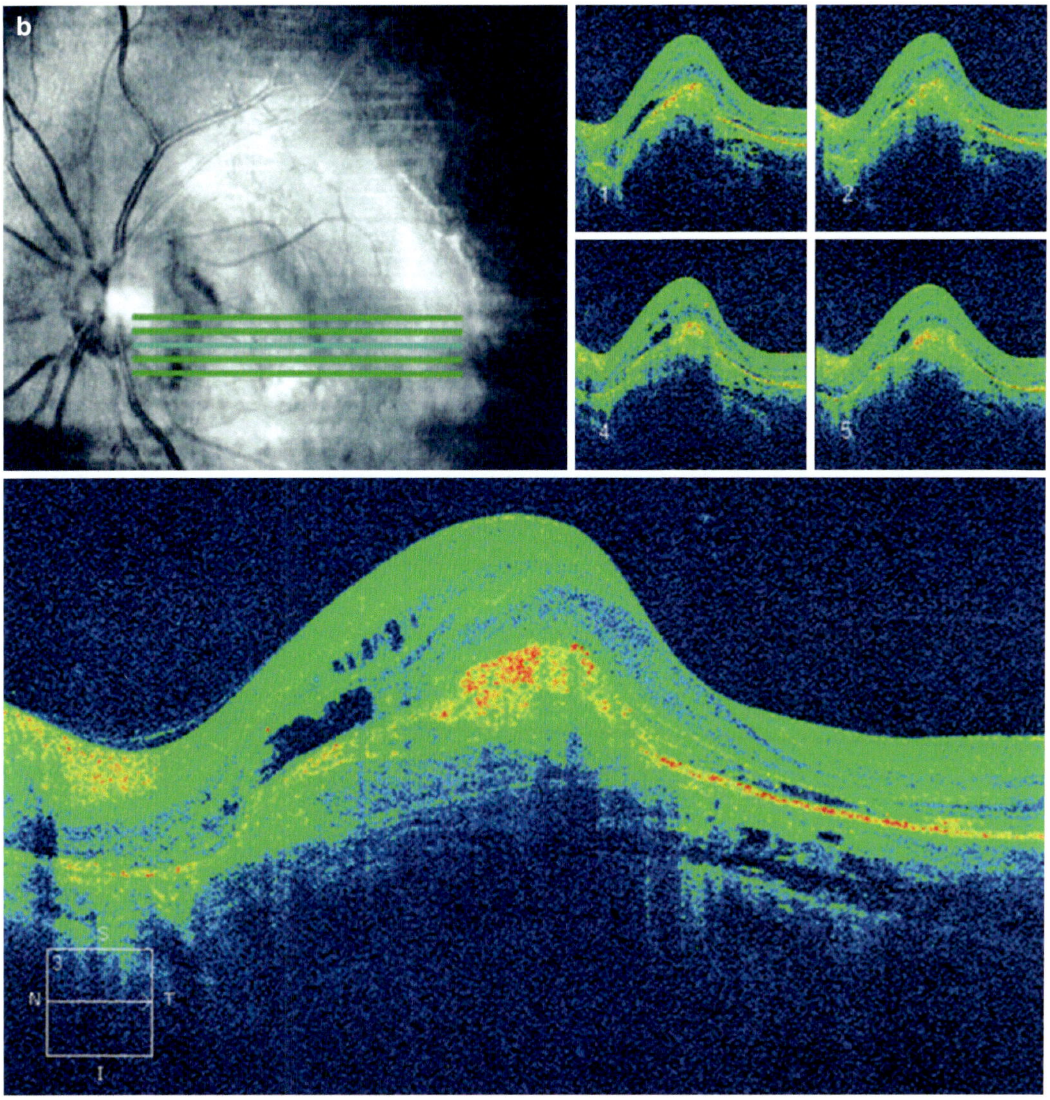

Fig. 19.10 (continued)

effusion, hemorrhage, and scars, which will seriously affect the visual acuity [1]. The patient was not observed with complication at the first visit in this case. FFA and other examinations revealed no neovascularization beneath the retina. Since the disease cause was unclear and the tumor growth was slow, no special treatment was required at the early stage, and the patient was advised to return for follow-up visits regularly so that further damage to the macula could be found in time.

The cause of the localized and mild abnormality in the center visual field should be identified. The patient was once misdiagnosed with refractive error because the BCVA was 20/20, and further examination was neglected. In general, mild refractive error will not lead to visual field defect, and whether there are other concomitant organic lesions shall be confirmed. The refractive error found in this case was secondary.

Generally, choroidal osteoma is relatively static. However, the patient was lost to follow-up for 3 years, and the disease condition aggravated in this period. With the appearance of the complications, the macula was significantly affected and

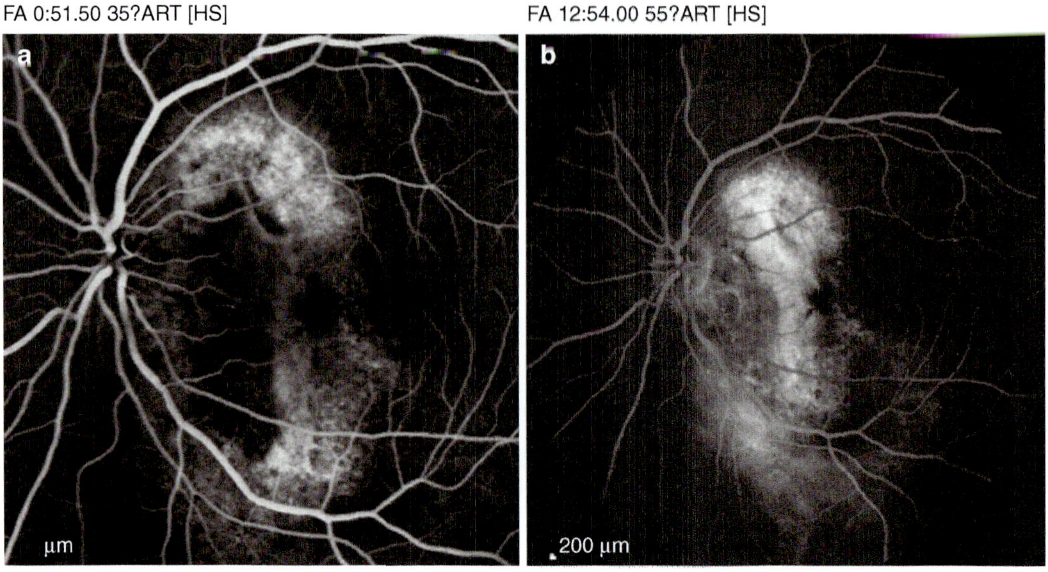

Fig. 19.11 Reexamination FFA images of the left eye. Panel a: Patchy hyperfluorescence was seen in the posterior pole at the early stage. Panel b: Fluorescence enhancement and fusion were shown at the late stage

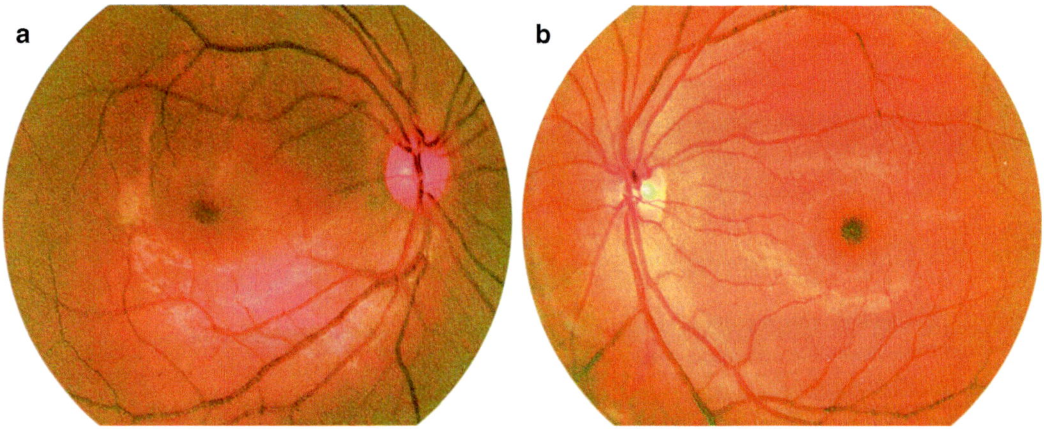

Fig. 19.12 Fundus photographs. Panel a: Serous retinal detachment could be observed in the fovea and superior region of the macula in the right eye. Panel b: No abnormality was found in the retina of the left eye

presented morphologic changes and irreversible vision decrease and visual field impairment.

19.2 Case 2

19.2.1 Case Presentation

A 34-year-old male patient presented with vision decrease in the right eye for 2 weeks. No accompanying symptoms, including red eyes, eye pain, distorted vision, etc., were present. Histories of trauma, previous eye diseases, systemic diseases, and familial diseases were denied.

The UCVA was 20/32 OD and 20/20 OS, and the BCVA of the right eye was 20/20 with hyperopic correction (+0.25DS). Slit-lamp examination of his anterior segments was unremarkable. Fundus examination also revealed nothing remarkable in either eye except serous retinal detachment in the fovea and superior region of the macula in the right eye (Fig. 19.12).

Standardized automated perimetry revealed relative scotomas in the central and inferior areas of the right eye (Fig. 19.13).

Fundus fluorescein angiography (FFA) showed a fluorescent leakage with inkblot appearance located in the superior region of the macula. Corresponding optical coherence tomogram (OCT) illustrated the subretinal fluid accumulation. Accumulation of deposits on the outer surface of the photoreceptors could be seen. The white arrow and line on the infrared reflectance imaging showed the scan location of the OCT image (Fig. 19.14).

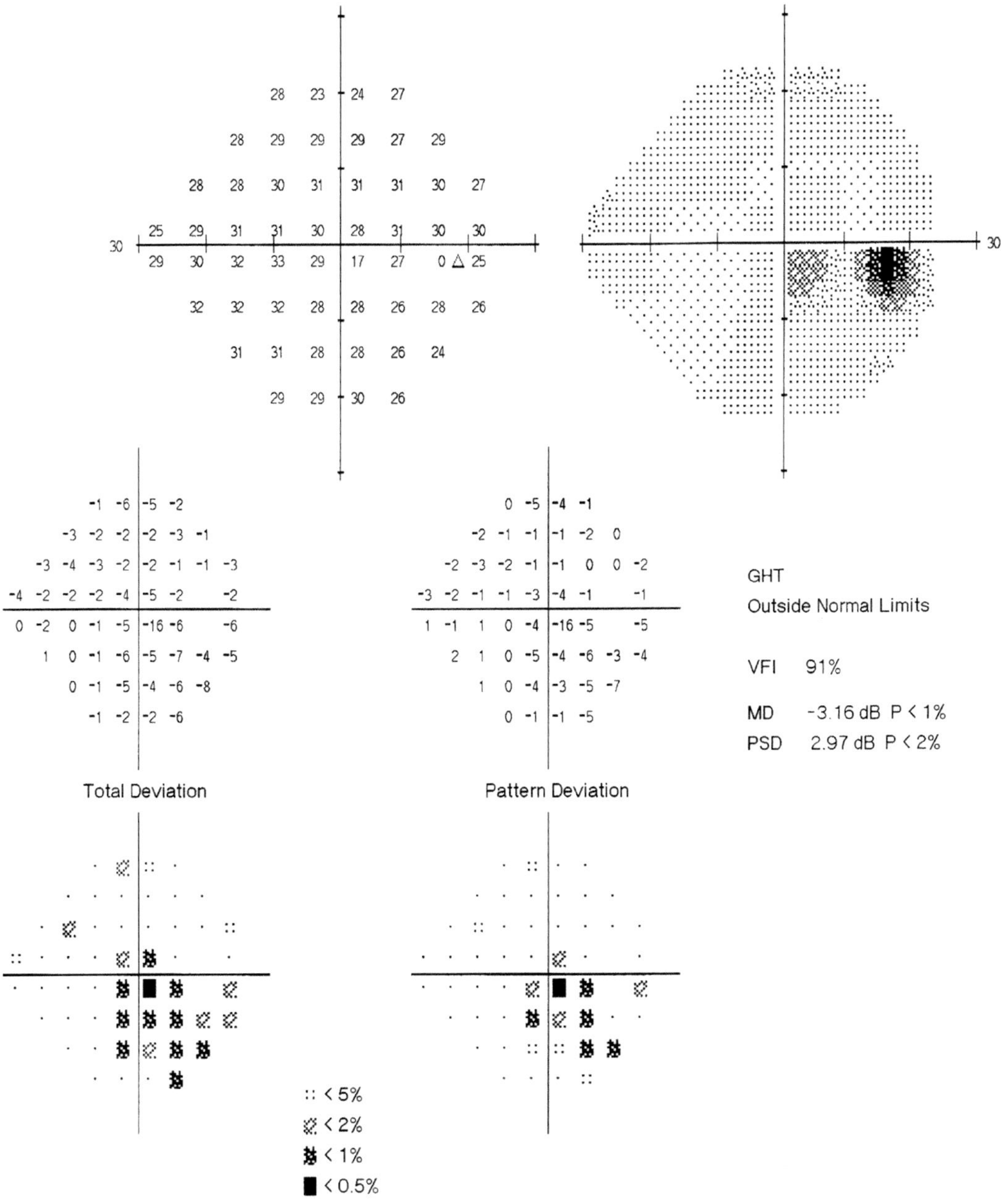

Fig. 19.13 Humphrey visual field analysis printout for the right eye. Standardized automated perimetry with the 24-2 test showed relative scotomas in the central and inferior area of the right eye

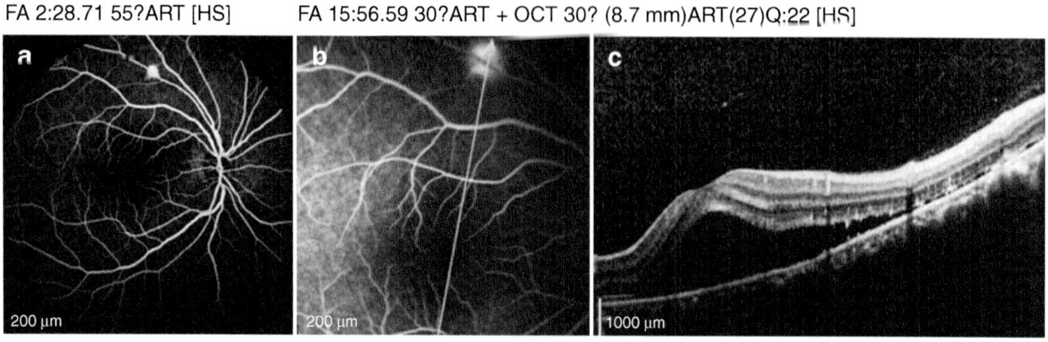

Fig. 19.14 FFA and OCT images for the right eye. Panel a and Panel b: FFA showed a fluorescent leakage with ink-blot appearance located in the superior region of the macula. Panel c: Corresponding OCT illustrating the subretinal fluid accumulation. Accumulation of deposits on the outer surface of the photoreceptors can be seen. The white arrow and line on the infrared reflectance imaging showed the scan location of the OCT image

19.2.2 Final Diagnosis

The final diagnosis was central serous chorioretinopathy in the right eye.

19.2.3 Case Review

Resulting from dysfunction of the retinal pigment epithelium layer as a barrier, the central serous chorioretinopathy is a common ocular fundus disease characterized by serous detachment of the retinal neuroepithelium layer in the macula. The visual signal is transmitted by three types of neurons from the retinal neuroepithelium, namely, photoreceptor cells, bipolar cells, and ganglion cells. The neurites of the ganglion cells (nerve fiber) will transmit the signal along the visual pathway to the visual center and finally form the vision. The central vision of patients with central serous chorioretinopathy is usually not lower than 20/40 and can be partially or completely corrected by a convex lens because the structure of the retinal neuroepithelium is not damaged. Round or oval central scotoma, which is consistent with the extent of the neuroepithelium lesion, can be observed in visual field examination. In this case, the visual acuity of the patient's right eye could be corrected to 20/20 by a convex lens. FFA showed that the leakage point was located in the superior region of the macula. Neuroepithelium detachment focus was found in the foveal and superior region of the macula. Therefore, the central scotomas revealed in the center and inferior area of the visual field were consistent with them.

However, not all the central serous chorioretinopathy patients will be observed with light sensitivity reduction in the central visual field. The severity of the lesion, neuroepithelium function, and visual field examination sensitivity are all relevant. The 10-2 or macular test strategies are more suitable for the examination of macular lesions [2].

The physiological function of the RPE is to transfer selectively the nutriments and metabolites between the choroid and the outer layer of the retina and meanwhile devour and digest the detached photoreceptor outer segment disc membranes. Long-term detachment of the RPE and neuroepithelium will lead to microenvironment changes and metabolic and functional disorders in the photoreceptors. The visual signal transmission will thus be affected, and permanent disorders of vision and visual field will result.

19.3 Case 3

19.3.1 Case Presentation

A 56-year-old female patient presented with vision decrease in the left eye for 1 month. No accompanying symptoms, including red eyes,

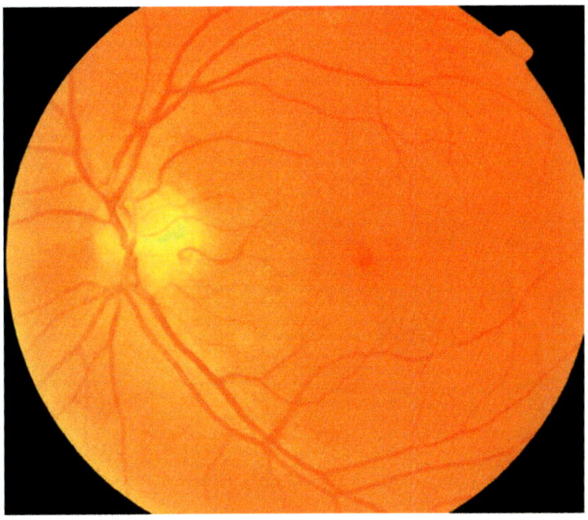

Fig. 19.15 Fundus photograph of the left eye. The optic disc was red in color with a clear boundary. A small, dark red, and round hole with a clear boundary could be observed in the macula (imaging quality was affected by the cataract)

eye pain, shadow in the vision, etc., were present. Histories of trauma, previous eye diseases, systemic diseases, and familial diseases were denied.

The BCVA was 20/25 OD and 20/200 OS. The intraocular pressure was normal in both eyes. Slit-lamp examination of her anterior segments was unremarkable except that the lens was turbid in both eyes. Fundus examination was also unremarkable except that a small dark red round hole with a clear boundary could be observed in the macular region of the left eye (Fig. 19.15).

Standardized automated perimetry indicated that the visual field of the left eye was normal (Fig. 19.16).

Optical coherence tomography (OCT) showed a full-thickness neuroepithelium defect in the fovea. Cystic retinal edema could be observed at the edge of the hole. The diameter of the hole was 272 μm. Complete posterior vitreous detachment was exhibited (Fig. 19.17).

19.3.2 Final Diagnosis

The final diagnosis was an idiopathic macular hole in the left eye.

19.3.3 Case Review

The central vision will show serious reduction in patients with idiopathic macular hole due to the neuroepithelium defect in the fovea. But why is the visual field impairment mild or even absent? It's related to the visual field examination strategy we select.

Let's take the Humphrey perimeter as an example. The examination area of the 24-2 test is the central 24° of the visual field (24° for the superior and inferior visual fields and 30° for the nasal visual field), in which 54 detection sites are arranged bilaterally in grid pattern with an interval of 6° between each site with the fixation point as the center of the meridians. The examination area of the 30-2 test is the central 30° of the visual field, in which 76 detection sites are arranged with an interval of 6° between each. Compared with the 30-2 test, the 24-2 test excludes only some peripheral detection sites. The examination area of the 10-2 test is the central 10° of the visual field, in which 68 detection sites are arranged with an interval of 2° between each, representing a significant increase in the density of detection sites. Roughly speaking, the light sensitivities at the detection sites distributed within 2.5° radius and 5° radius from the fixation represent, respectively, the light sensitivities of the fovea and its peripheral area. Therefore, for the examination of macular lesions, the 10-2 test will be more accurate, and the 24-2 or 30-2 test is very likely to be not able to detect small lesions in the fovea and its peripheral area [3]. Just as in this case, the 24-2 test failed to detect the "central light sensitivity" reduction that was consistent with the macular hole. And in the following case, normal result was obtained by the 24-2 test, but the focus in the visual field was shown when the 10-2 test was adopted.

There is no doubt that the best measure to reflect the function of the fovea is still the central vision. Visual field changes may be mistaken for mild lesions and thus be neglected. It's also worth pointing out that such patients may have no serious impairment of the central vision at the early stage (such as still above 20/40) and the symptoms are not consistent with the signs (OCT

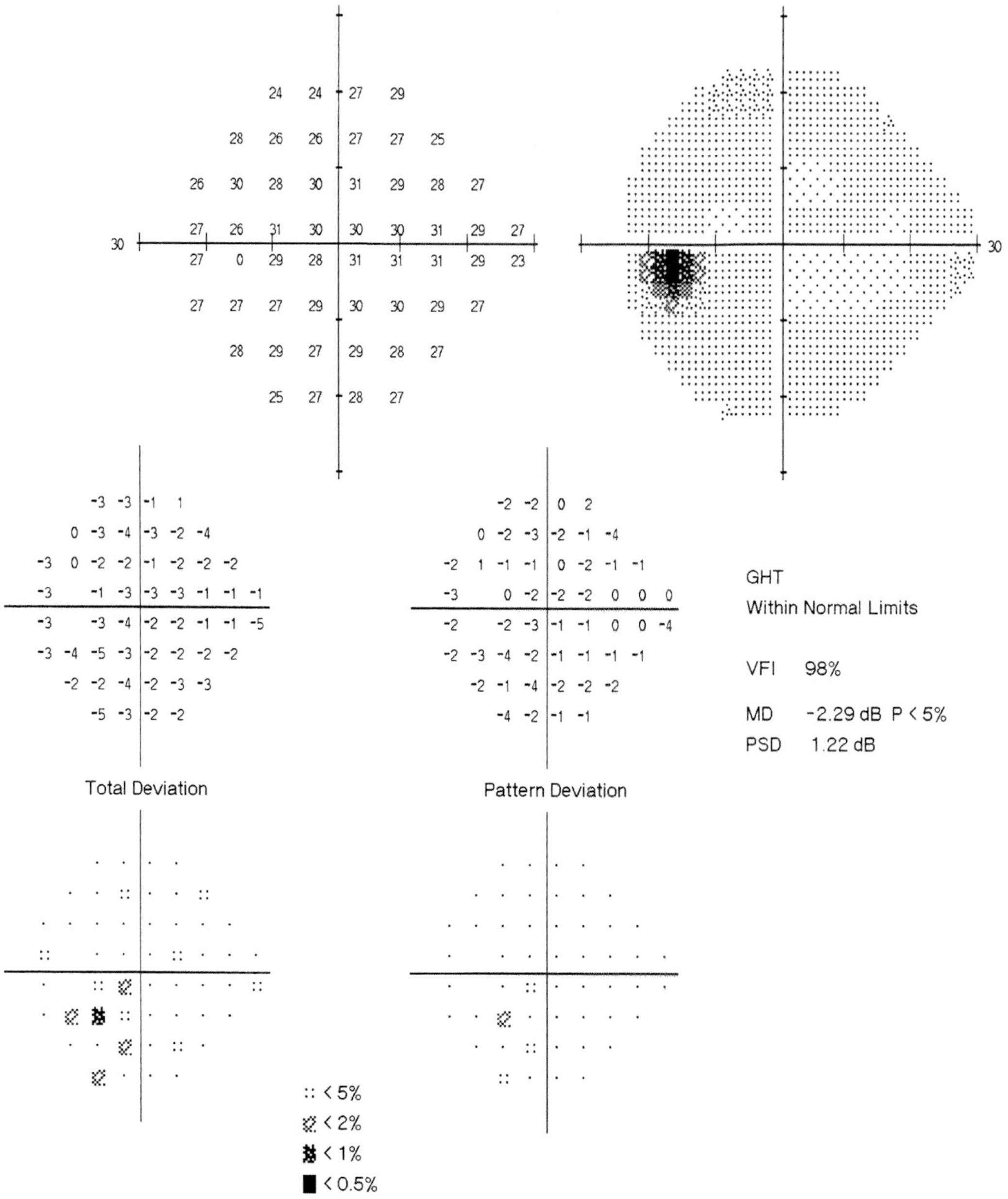

Fig. 19.16 Humphrey visual field analysis printout for the left eye. The 24-2 test showed general normal results. The mild diffuse light sensitivity reduction was considered to be an effect of cataract

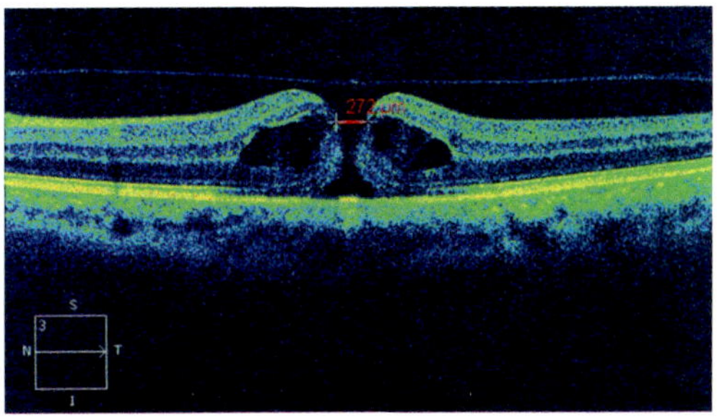

Fig. 19.17 Macular OCT image of the left eye. OCT showed a full-thickness neuroepithelium defect in the fovea. Cystic retinal edema could be observed at the edge of the hole. The diameter of the hole was 272 µm. Complete posterior vitreous detachment was exhibited

examination). It's very likely that the hole is still small and the disease is at its early stage, when partial residual function of the visual signal conduction pathway of the fovea or paracentral vision compensation is still available.

19.4 Case 4

19.4.1 Case Presentation

A 35-year-old male patient presented with distorted vision in the right eye for over a month. The patient experienced mild vision decrease without accompanying symptoms such as red eyes and eye pain. Histories of trauma, previous eye diseases, systemic diseases, and familial diseases were denied.

The BCVA was 20/25 with myopic correction (−3.75DS) OD and 20/20 with myopic correction (−4.00DS) OS. The intraocular pressure was normal in both eyes. Slit-lamp examination of his anterior segments was unremarkable. Fundus examination revealed a normal optic disc in both eyes and pigment disorder in the fovea and a yellowish-white focus in the temporal quadrant of the macula in the right eye (Fig. 19.18).

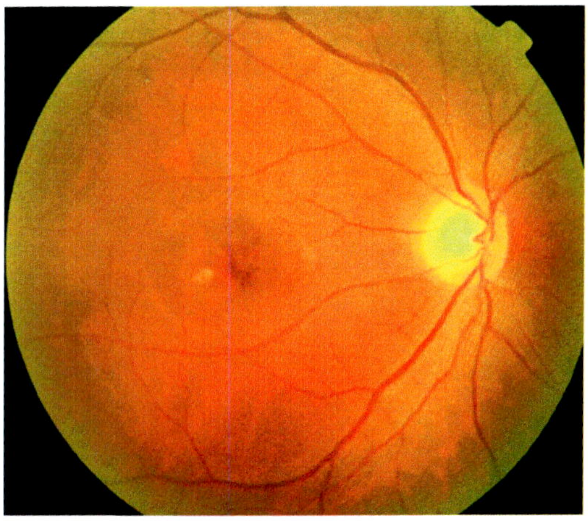

Fig. 19.18 Fundus photograph. Pigment disorder was shown in the fovea, and a yellowish-white focus was revealed in the temporal quadrant of the macula

The Humphrey field analyzer with the 24-2 test showed normal results in the right eye, and a central scotoma was revealed in the right eye with the 10-2 test (Fig. 19.19).

Optical coherence tomography (OCT) showed the local choroid bulging into the retina at the parafovea area, accompanied by RPE interruption (Fig. 19.20).

Fundus fluorescein angiography (FFA) revealed a static choroidal neovascularization (CNV) at the parafovea area in the right eye surrounded by transmitted fluorescence (Fig. 19.21).

19.4.2 Final Diagnosis

The final diagnosis was idiopathic choroidal neovascularization in the right eye.

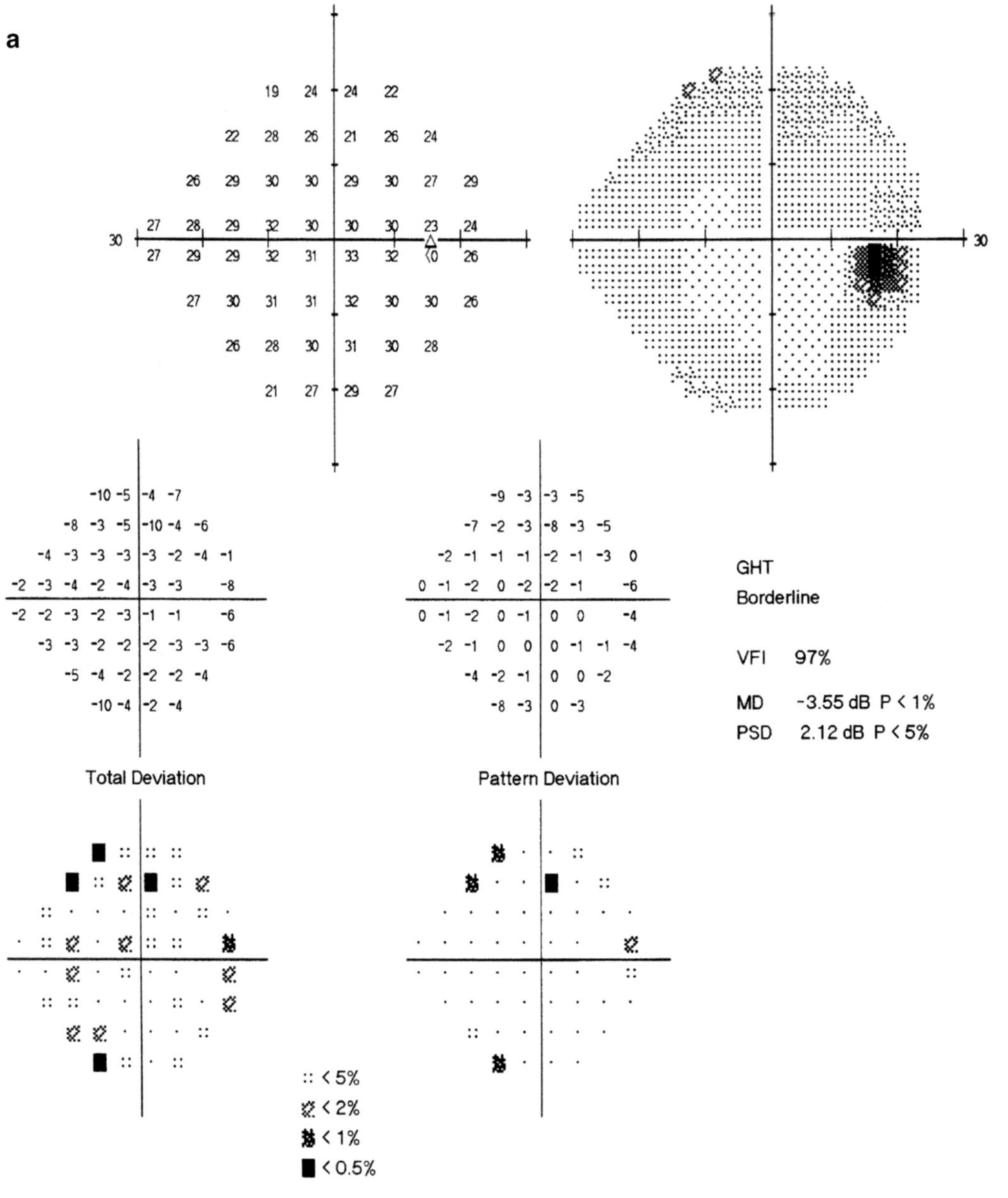

Fig. 19.19 Humphrey visual field analysis printouts for the right eye (24-2 and 10-2 test). Panel a: 24-2 Humphrey produced a normal field image. Panel b: 10-2 Humphrey showed a central scotoma

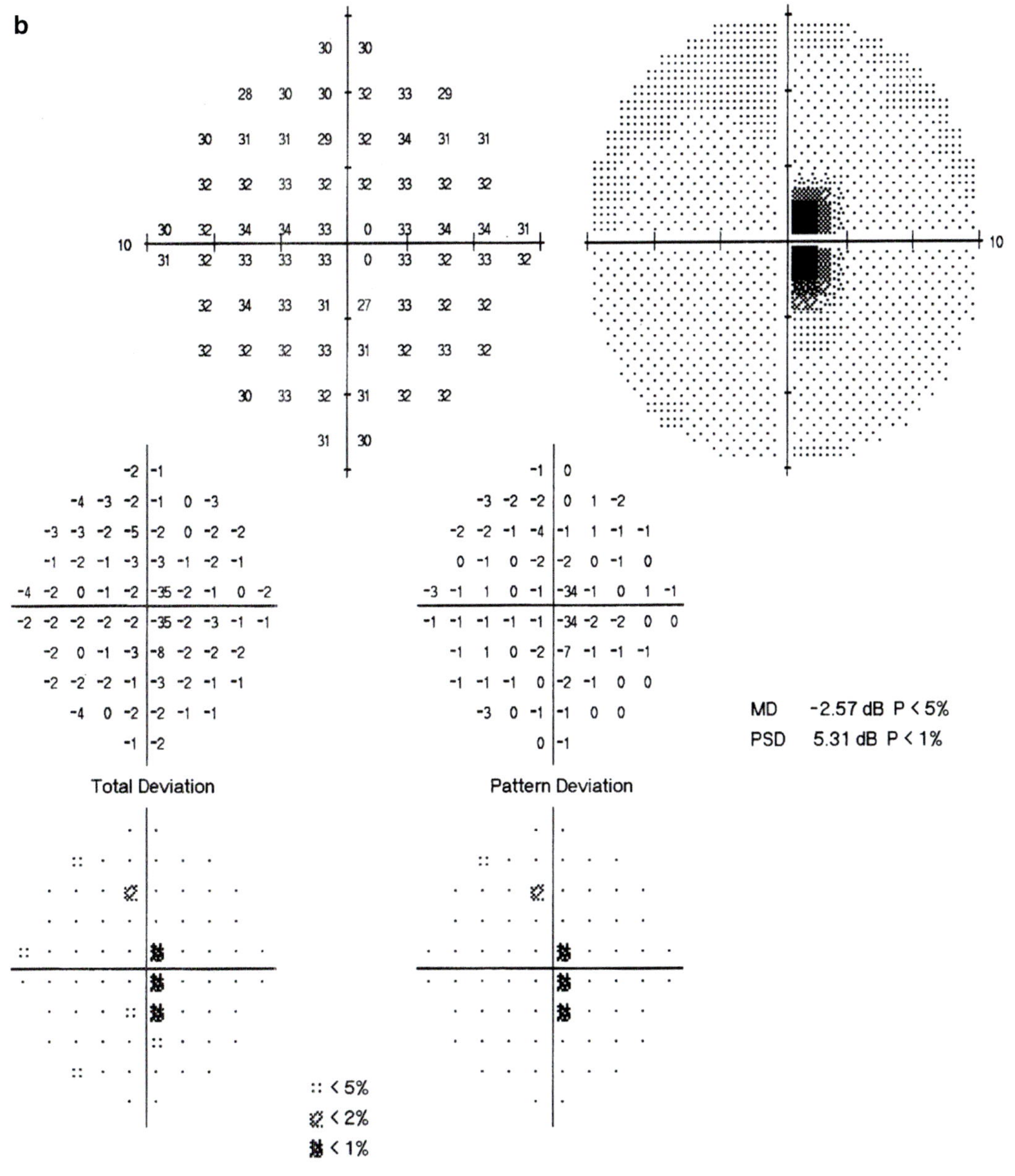

Fig. 19.19 (continued)

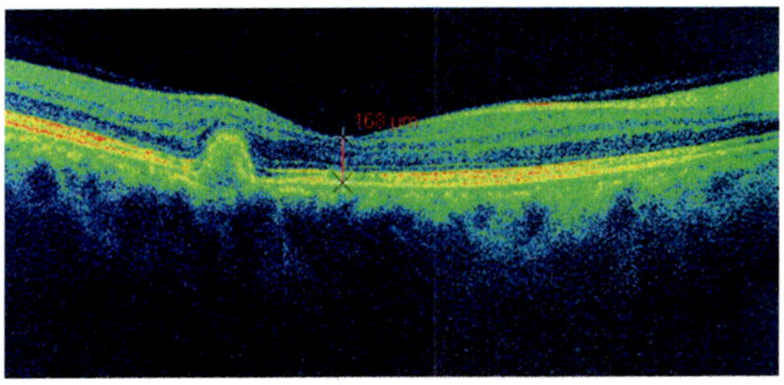

Fig. 19.20 OCT image of the macula of the right eye. OCT showed the local choroid bulging into the retina at the parafovea area, accompanied by RPE interruption

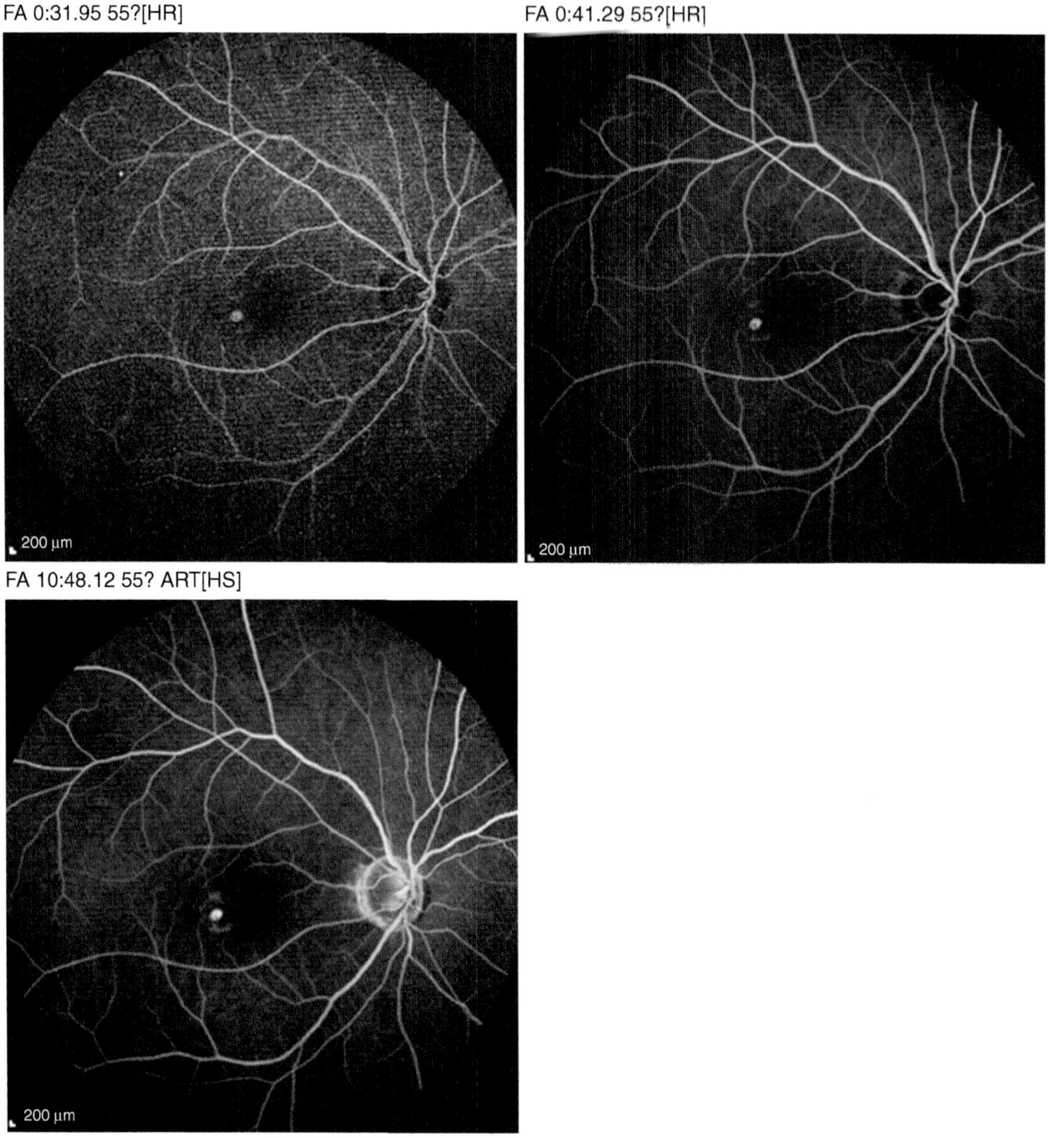

Fig. 19.21 FFA images of the right eye. FFA image showed a static choroidal neovascularization (CNV) at the parafovea area surrounded by transmitted fluorescence

19.4.3 Case Review

This disease used to be diagnosed as "central exudative chorioretinopathy," and from the prospective of visual field, we can see that its damage to the visual field is more significant and it is not self-limiting when compared with central serous chorioretinopathy. The diagnosis of central exudative chorioretinopathy has been replaced gradually by idiopathic choroidal neovascularization. The latter can better reflect the pathological characteristics of the disease.

The patient's visual field showed no significant abnormality upon examination with the 24-2 test, but visual field impairment caused by corresponding fundus lesions can be observed with the 10-2 test. This suggests that selection of visual field examination strategy has important influence on the observation, screening, and evaluation of small lesions in the macula.

19.5 Discussion

Visual acuity and visual field are the most common two measures of visual function examination. Visual acuity, or more specifically central visual acuity, reflects mainly the macular function and visual field, relatively speaking, and reflects the peripheral visual acuity. The central visual field is within 30° from the fixation point and roughly reflects the functional projection of the retina at the posterior pole within 3–4 mm radius from the macula [4]. Clinically, it is very important to choose a proper visual function examination method as per the location and size of the retinopathy because the visual function information delivered by different examination strategies is different.

The best corrected visual acuity of the patients in the first and second cases in this section could both reach 20/20, but the 24-2 visual field examination strategy showed mild localized light sensitivity reduction in the central region and suggested macular lesions. The further examinations enabled us to find the causes of the mild central visual field impairment, which were choroidal osteoma and central serous chorioretinopathy, respectively. The central vision of the patient with macular hole in the third case was very poor, but the 24-2 visual field examination strategy showed normal results. We have explained this abnormal phenomenon in terms of the principles of the visual field examination strategies. And the fourth case was a more typical case for exemplifying that different visual field results may be produced by different examination strategies. Thus, it can be seen that examination strategy selection is very important. For macular lesions, the 10-2 or macular examination strategy is more accurate and has irreplaceable advantages.

The fovea in the posterior pole of the retina, where the cone cells are densely populated, is considered to be the part with the highest visual acuity. In the fovea, one-to-one correspondence can be found between the three levels of neurons and the receptive field; the size of the receptive field is the smallest and no overlap exists, but the visual acuity, i.e., the resolving power of the eye, is the highest. In the areas outside the macular area, the cone cell density reduces gradually, and the rod cells increases with the increase of eccentricity. The connection among the three levels of the cells is not one-to-one correspondence any more but features more crossings. As a result, the receptive field and overlapping become bigger and bigger, and the visual acuity becomes lower gradually. So a very small lesion in the central region as shown in a visual field diagram will be considered as significant visual field impairment [2].

Meanwhile, as the most commonly used visual function examinations, visual acuity examination and visual field examination are both closely related to the visual information transmission at the examination sites and reflect the function of retinal ganglion cells. The combination of the two can help us diagnose correctly.

Besides, it's also noteworthy that the severity of localized visual field damage in the central region may not correspond to the lesion it represents. More attention should be paid to the situation where the visual field damage is mild but the lesion is not (especially the posterior pathway damage). This will also be discussed in other chapters and sections of this book.

References

1. Yannuzzi LA. The retinal atlas. Translated by Zhao Mingwei. Tianjin: Tianjin Science & Technology Translation and Publishing Co., Ltd; 2013.
2. Yuansheng Y, Hua Z. Modern clinical visual field examination. 2nd ed. Beijing: People's Medical Publishing House; 2015.
3. Heijl A, Patella VM. Principle for Humphrey visual field examination and analysis. Translated by Yuan Yuansheng. Beijing: People's Medical Publishing House; 2005.
4. Fan N, Huang L, Shen X, et al. Relationship between structure and function damage of retina in glaucoma patients. Chin J Exp Ophthalmol. 2015;33(3):250–4.

The Fundus Appearance of Methylmalonic Acidemia Combined with Homocystinuria

20

Ning Fan, Xuyang Liu, and Jiantao Wang

Combined methylmalonic acidemia and homocystinuria is a rare congenital disease characterized by abnormal organic acid metabolism. The cblC type is the most common clinical type of this disease, and it's a multisystem disease caused by restricted intestinal absorption of vitamin B12 resulting from transcobalamin II deficiency [1]. Its main clinical manifestations are impairments in the nervous system, the kidneys, and the blood system. Changes in the macula as a concomitant condition have not received due attention. A typical pedigree will be demonstrated in this section, and we can see the completely different prognoses resulting from different treatment timings.

20.1 Case

20.1.1 Case Presentation

A 14-year-old male patient had been observed with poor visual acuity and incapability of fixation in both eyes by his parents since childhood. Abnormalities, including hypersomnia, projectile vomiting, eczema, hematuria, etc., were found in the patient after birth, and he had been taken to multiple hospitals for treatment, but the disease causes were still unclear. Jaundice and dilated cardiomyopathy were also observed later. He was diagnosed with combined methylmalonic acidemia and homocystinuria (cblC type) after the methylmalonic acid level (in urine) and homocysteic acid level (in blood) were determined by gas chromatography-mass spectrometry at another hospital when he was 10 years old. Long-term treatment, including high caloric- and low-protein diet, intramuscular injection of vitamin B12, oral administration of L-carnitine and betaine, etc., had been given. The patient's systemic condition was stable at the time of this presentation, but the ocular condition showed no significant improvement. A history of trauma was denied.

The patient had a 6-year-old sister with suspicious histories of hypersomnia and vomiting after birth. She had been diagnosed with combined methylmalonic acidemia and homocystinuria (cblC type) by molecular genetic analysis. Her disease condition was stable after treatment. The parents didn't find abnormality in the visual acuity of her eyes. The parents and other family members had no similar systemic and eye diseases.

Eye examination of the proband demonstrated that the best corrected visual acuity (BCVA) was finger counting OD and 20/200 OS. His anterior segments were free from abnormality (Fig. 20.1). Fundus examination revealed that the optic discs

N. Fan · J. Wang (✉)
Shenzhen Eye Hospital, Shenzhen University, Shenzhen, China

X. Liu
Xiamen Eye Center of Xiamen University, Xiamen, China

Shenzhen Eye Hospital, Shenzhen University, Shenzhen, China

N. Wang et al. (eds.), *Optic Disorders and Visual Field*, Advances in Visual Science and Eye Diseases 2, https://doi.org/10.1007/978-981-13-2502-1_20

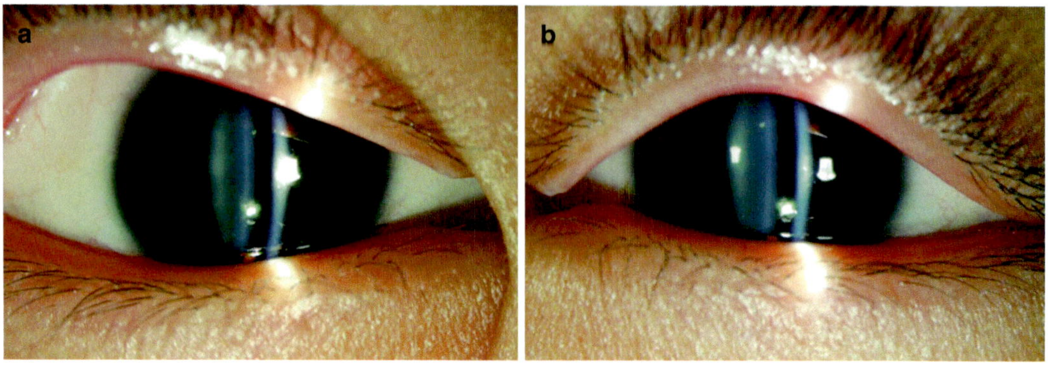

Fig. 20.1 Photographs of the anterior segments of the proband (pupil dilated pharmacologically). Panel a: Right eye. Panel b: Left eye

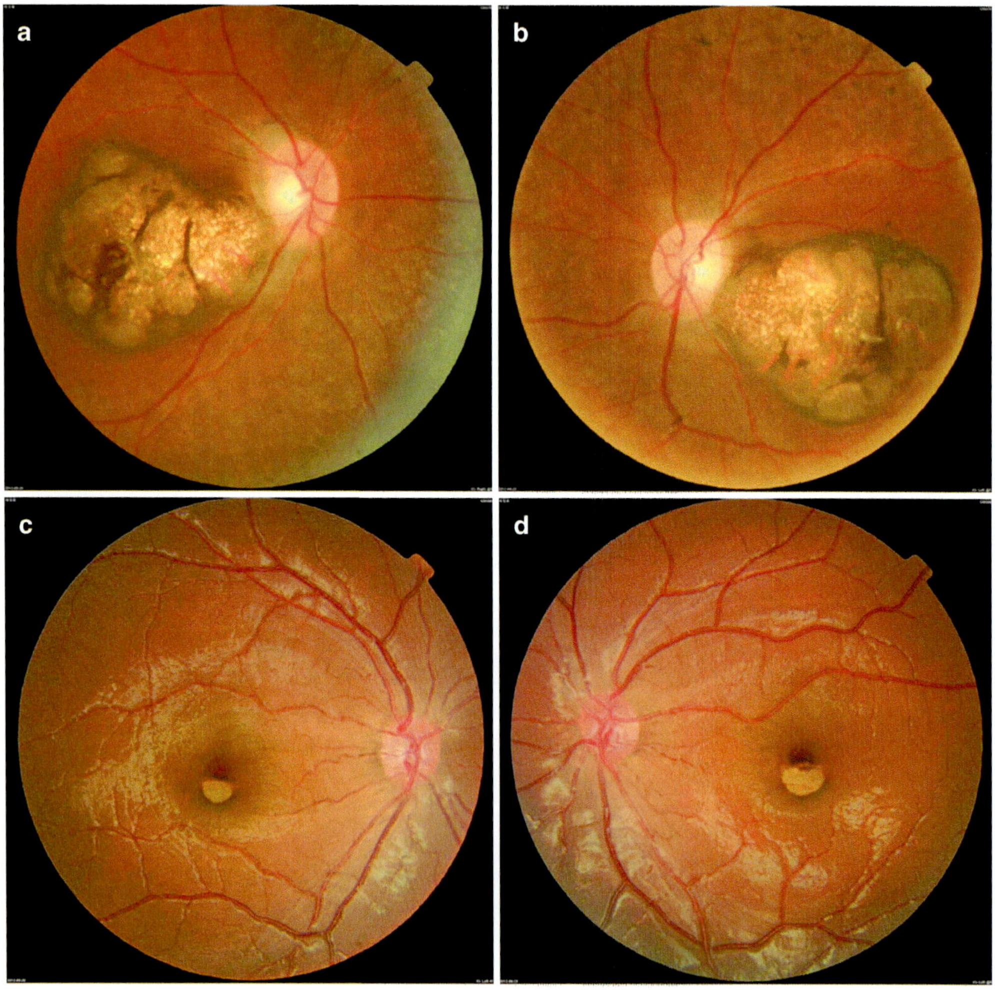

Fig. 20.2 Fundus photographs of the proband and his younger sister. Fundus examination of the proband revealed that the optic disc was pink in color; an atrophy focus with 6PD in size was shown in the macular region, and pigmentation could be observed in the peripheral retina in each eye. Panel a: Right eye of the proband. Panel b: Left eye of the proband. Fundus examination of the patient's younger sister demonstrated that the optic disc was pink in color with a clear boundary; an atrophy focus about 1/3PD in size was shown below the fovea; light reflex was present in the fovea in each eye. Panel c: Right eye of his younger sister. Panel d: Left eye of his younger sister

were pink in color. An atrophy focus about 6PD in size was shown in the macular region. Pigmentation could be observed in the peripheral retina (Fig. 20.2a, b). Poor fixations and nystagmus were revealed in both eyes.

Eye examination was also carried out for his younger sister. The UCVA of her eyes was 20/16 OU. Her anterior segments were free from significant abnormality. The optic discs were pink in color with a clear boundary. An atrophy focus about 1/3PD in size was shown below the fovea in each eye (Fig. 20.2c, d). Both the eyes were in normal position and had normal eyeball movements. The Humphrey visual field analyzer (with the 10-2 test) revealed a central scotoma in both eyes (Fig. 20.3).

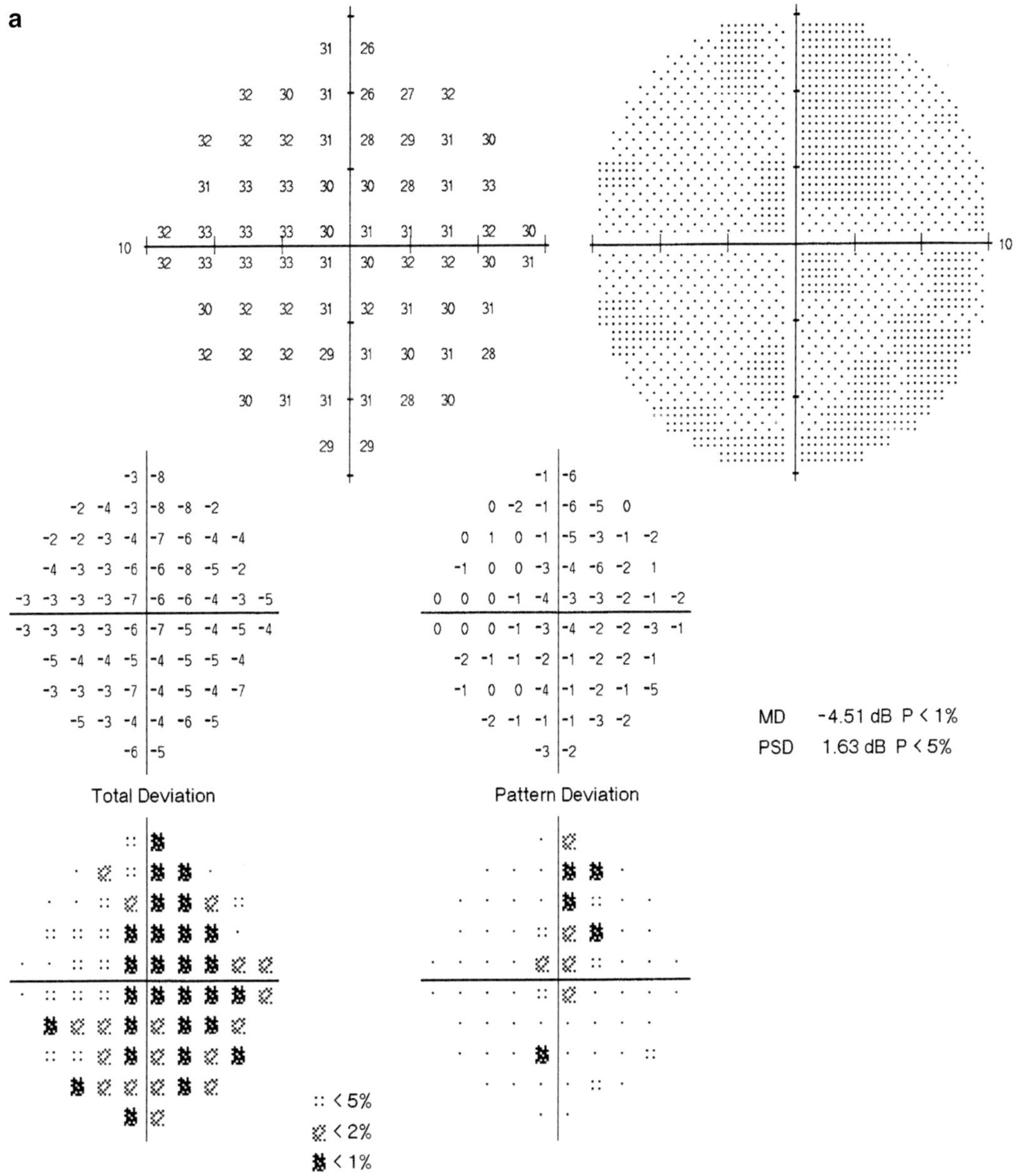

Fig. 20.3 Humphrey visual field analysis printouts for the younger sister of the proband. Humphrey visual field analysis with the 10-2 test showed central visual field defects in both eyes. Panel a: Left eye. Panel b: Right eye

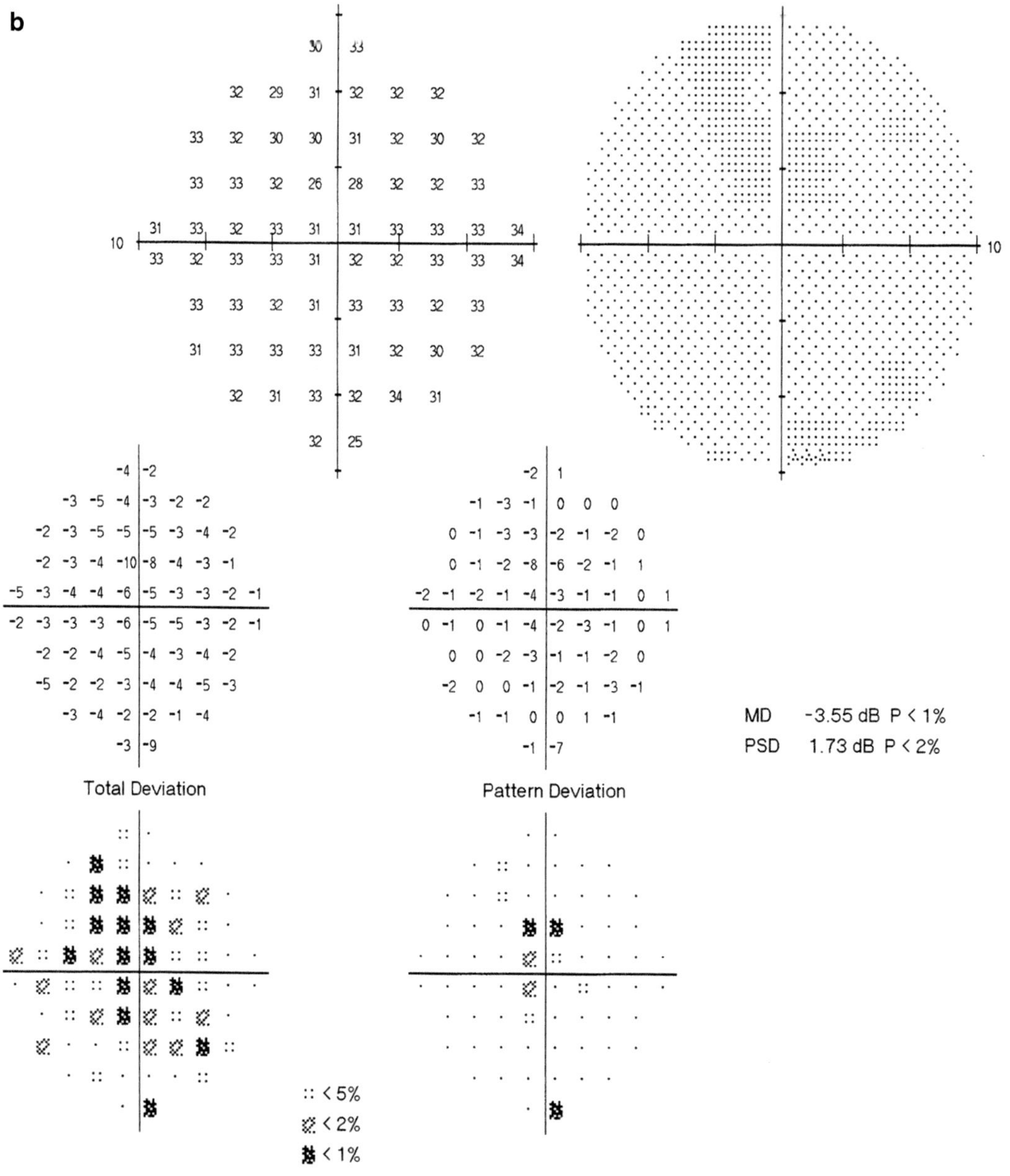

Fig. 20.3 (continued)

The eye examinations of his parents showed no abnormality (refer to Fig. 20.4 for pedigree chart).

Neither of the parents had clinical symptoms, and both their son and daughter showed clinical symptoms.

Molecular genetic studies indicated an autosomal recessive inheritance for this pedigree, and both patients were detected with disease-causing mutations. Gene sequence analysis showed that both patients had three mutations in the MMACHC gene, including heterozygous mutations c.321G > A and c.365A > T in Exon 3 and deletion mutation c.658_660delAAG in Exon 4. Among them, the c.321G > A was a synonymous mutation, which is a single nucleotide polymorphism. The heterozygous c.365A > T mutation (originated from the mother, Fig. 20.5), which leads to the conversion of the histidine at the

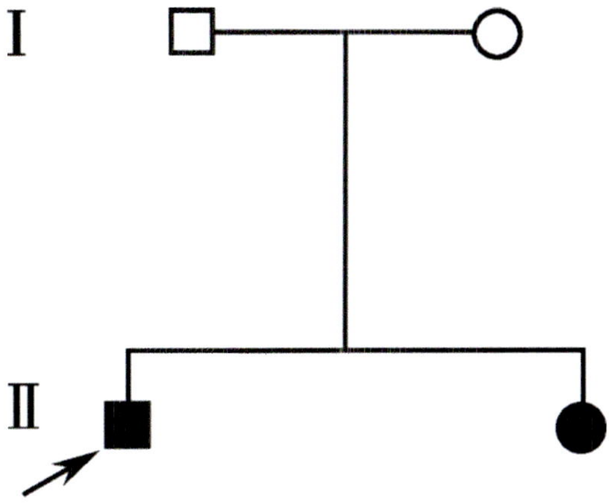

Fig. 20.4 The pedigree chart of methylmalonic acidemia combined with homocystinuria

position 122 of protein polypeptide chain into leucine (p.H122L), was located in the binding domain of cobalamin and could affect the binding of cobalamin. The c.658_660delAAG deletion mutation (originated from the father, Fig. 20.6), which leads to the deletion of lysine at the position 220 of protein polypeptide chain (p.220del Lys), was located in the C-terminal of the gene. It could change the amino acid sequence on the polypeptide chain and affect the protein function. Thus, it can be seen that the methylmalonic acidemia with homocystinuria observed in the pedigree was caused by the compound heterozygous mutations of c.365A > T and c.658_660delAAG of the MMACHC gene. Both of these heterozygous mutations occurred in highly conserved regions of homologous sequence.

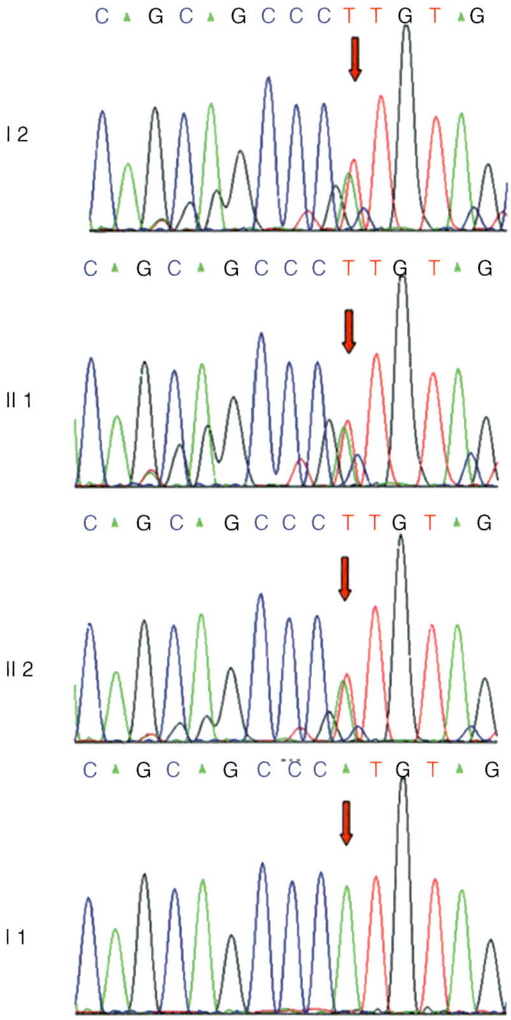

Fig. 20.5 Sequencing map of the MMACHC gene (1). A heterozygous A > T mutation could be found in the position 365 in the coding area of Exon 3. The two pediatric patients (II1, II2) and the mother (I2) had heterozygous mutation, while the father (I1) had no such mutation

20.1.2 Final Diagnosis

The final diagnosis was combined methylmalonic aciduria and homocysteinemia with bilateral macular disease.

20.2 Discussion

The biochemical phenotype of the cblC type is combined methylmalonic acidemia and homocystinuria. The clinical manifestations are complicated with large individual differences. Its onset time ranges from newbornhood to adulthood, and mild disease patient may have no symptoms for life. The disease can be divided into early-onset type and late-onset type as per the onset time. For early-onset type, the onset of the disease is usually observed before 1 year old. The clinical manifestations are multisystem damages with nervous system as the focus, and the disease can involve the skin and mucosa, liver, kidneys, gastrointestinal tract, circulation sys-

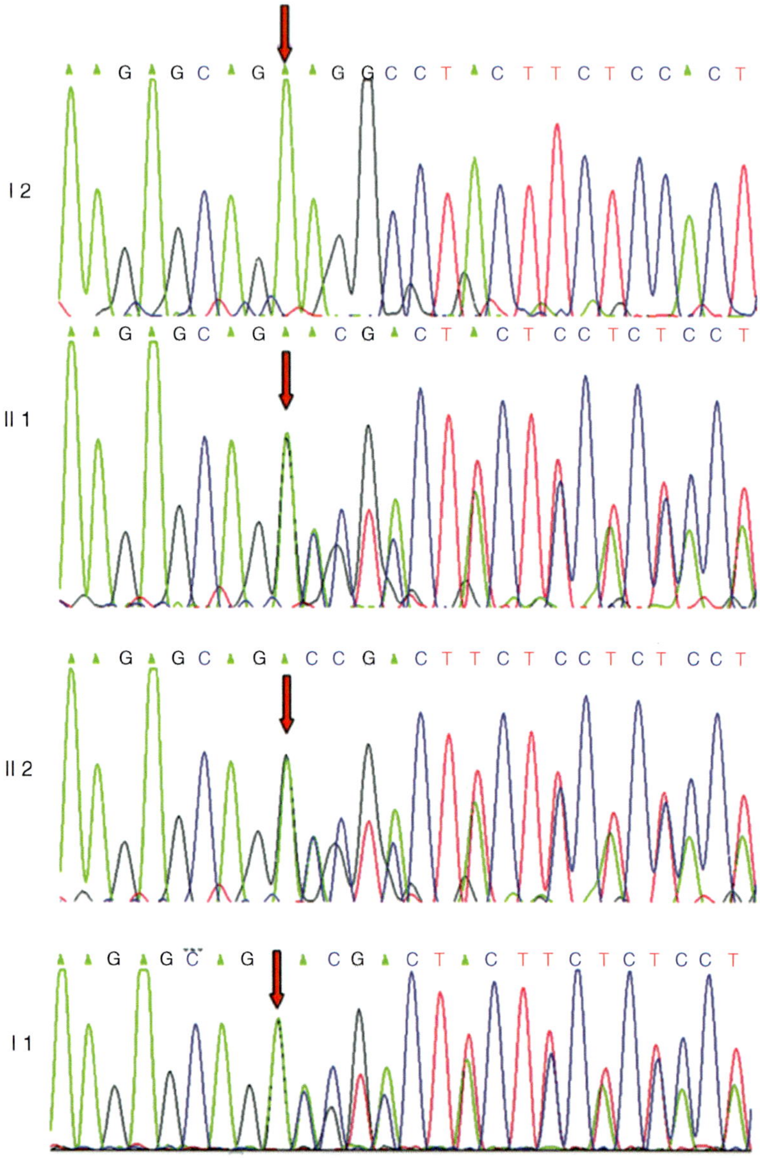

Fig. 20.6 Sequencing map of the MMACHC gene (2). Deletion of the three bases AAG could be found in the position 658_660 in the coding area of Exon 4. The two pediatric patients (II1, II2) and the father (I1) had heterozygous mutation, while the mother (I2) had no such mutation

tem, blood system, etc. Patients with concomitant eye disease are rarely reported.

The gene responsible for combined methylmalonic acidemia and homocystinuria (cblC disease) is the MMACHC gene, and over 50 mutations of the MMACHC gene have been found currently. The gene mutation sites are connected with the clinical phenotypes of cblC disease. For example, the most common mutation c.271dupA (p. R91K fsX14), which is a frameshift mutation, has an over 40% chance of causing disease. It's usually closely related with early-onset cases and c.331C>T (p. R111X) can also be found in early-onset cases. Some missense mutations, such as c.482G > A (R161Q) and nonsense mutation, such as c.394C > T (R132X), are commonly seen in late-onset cases [2]. Gene analysis on 50 cases of combined methylmalonic acidemia and homocystinuria by Wang Fei et al. found that the homozygous mutation c.609G > A was the most common mutation type (accounting for about 27%) found in Chinese early-onset patients and the compound heterozygous mutation c.609G > A and c.658_660delAAG (accounting for about 20%) was the next most common [3]. Liu Meiying et al.'s gene analysis on 79 cases of combined methylmalonic acidemia and homocystinuria found that the incidence rate of the mutation c.609G > A is the highest (about 48.1%), the next was c.658_660delAAG (about 13.9%), and the third was c.394C > T (about 5.7%) [4].

The proband's mother in our study carried the heterozygous mutation c.365A > T (p.H122L), which was rarely reported [5]. The proband's father carried the heterozygous deletion mutation c.658_660delAAG. Both the parents had no disease symptoms, and their son and daughter showed clinical symptoms with eyes involved. At the molecular level, we can see that both the pediatric patients carried the mutations c.365A > T and c.658_660delAAG. Therefore, this compound heterozygous mutation is the cause of the disease phenotype for this family. Although relevant reports on such compound heterozygous mutation are relatively rare, the present study has confirmed the pathogenicity of this mutation and is the first pedigree report on this specific mutation.

cb1C disease is a multisystem disease caused by restricted intestinal absorption of vitamin B12 resulting from transcobalamin II deficiency. The mechanism of the eye diseases, especially the retinal diseases, caused by cb1C disease is still unclear. The common eye complications of cb1C disease include macular disease, progressive retinal disease, and optic nerve atrophy. Optic nerve atrophy can also be found in patients with other types of methylmalonic acidemia (such as MMA and cb1G disease). However, retinal diseases are only observed in disease caused by transcobalamin II deficiency, which makes it clear that MMACHC gene-related proteins play specific roles in eye tissues. There are also studies pointing out that methylcobalamin (MeCbl) and *S*-adenosylmethionine (SAM) played a protective function during retinal cell cultivation. And homocysteine is one of the essential materials for the formation of SAM. Consequently, the levels of methylcobalamin and homocysteine can possibly lead to eye diseases [6]. Histological study and electron microscopy on the eyes of cblC patients found swelling and degeneration of mitochondria inside the retinal cells caused by mucopolysaccharide accumulation [7]. As a result, macular photoreceptor damage and nerve fiber loss from the macular fasciculi in the optic disc occurred. Meanwhile, glutathione reduction may also be one of the important reasons for retinal involvement by the disease. Glutathione has been proved to be an effective factor for the prevention of RPE oxidative damage, and its biosynthesis depends on methionine. cb1C disease stops the synthesis of methionine, and consequently further RPE damages resulted. We can see that the relevant factors of retinal diseases caused by cb1C disease are various and further studies are still necessary to unravel the specific mechanism.

The gene mutation types of both patients in this study were identical, but the severities of their clinical phenotypes showed significant difference. The proband (II1) showed immediate disease onset after birth. The systemic manifestations included hypersomnia, projectile vomiting, eczema, hematuria, jaundice, dilated cardiomyopathy, etc. Symptomatic treatment with vitamin B12 was not carried out until he was diagnosed with combined methylmalonic acidemia and homocystinuria at the age of 10. His younger sister (II 2) started the treatment at the early stage after the diagnosis of the disease by molecular genetic method. Less optic function impact and smaller focal extent of macular atrophy were found, and nystagmus was not observed as compared with II1. The symptoms in her eyes and whole body are milder than those found in the proband. Both the brother and sister had the same genetic background and living environment, so what's the cause of the different clinical phenotypes? We believe that the early diagnosis and treatment is the main reason for the clinical phenotype difference. Early treatment can effectively alleviate the severity of the disease. Although there are publications believing that even sufficient treatments at the early stage cannot stop the aggravation of the optic function [8], there are also publications holding the same opinion as ours, namely, early diagnosis and treatment can effectively improve the biochemical indexes and clinical symptoms of cb1C patients [9]. The study carried out by Leah et al. [10] on a pair of blood brothers found that the retinal disease of the patient receiving early treatment was milder than that of the one receiving late treatment, which was consistent with what we have found. We have followed the lineage for 3 years so far. The proband died 1 year ago, and the macular atrophy focus of his younger sister showed no enlargement. Her visual acuity was normal and the visual field impairment showed no progression.

References

1. Carrillo CN, Chandler RJ, Venditti CP. Combined methylmalonic acidemia and homocystinuria, cblC type. I. Clinical presentations, diagnosis and management. J Inherit Metab Dis. 2012;35(1):91–102.
2. Lerner-Ellis JP, Tirone JC, Pawelek PD, et al. Identification of the gene responsible for methylmalonic aciduria and homocystinuria,cb1C type. Nat Genet. 2006;38(1):93–100.
3. Wang F, Han L, Yang Y, et al. Clinical, biochemical, and molecular analysis of combined methylmalonic acidemia and hyperhomocysteinemia (cblC type) in China. J Inherit Metab Dis. 2010;33(Suppl 3):S435–42.
4. Liu MY, Yang YY, Chiang SH, et al. Mutation spectrum of MMACHC in Chinese patients with combined methylmalonic aciduria and homocystinuria. J Hum Genet. 2010;55(9):621–6.
5. Nuria CC, Charles PV. Combined methylmalonic acidemia and homocystinuria, cblC type. II. Complications, pathophysiology, and outcomes. J Inherit Metab Dis. 2012;35(1):103–14.
6. Maestro de las Casas C, Epeldegui M, Tudela C, et al. High exogenous homocysteine modifies eye development in early chick embryos. Birth Defects Res A Clin Mol Teratol. 2003;67(1):35–40.
7. Gaillard MC, Matthieu JM, Borruat FX. Retinal dysfunction in combined methylmalonic aciduria and homocystinuria (cblC) disease: a spectrum of disorders. Klin Monatsbl Augenheilkd. 2008;225(5):491–4.
8. Schimel AM, Mets MB. The natural history of retinal degeneration in association with cobalamin C (cbl C) disease. Ophthalmic Genet. 2006;27(1):9–14.
9. Andersson HC, Shapira E. Biochemical and clinical response to hydroxocobalamin versus cyanocobalamin treatment in patients with methylmalonic academia and homocystinuria (cblC). J Pediatr. 1998;132(1):121–4.
10. Leah R, Matthieu R, Isabelle IM, et al. Ocular manifestations of cobalamin C type methylmalonic aciduria with homocystinuria. J AAPOS. 2012;16(4):370–5.

21 The Ocular Manifestation of Turner Syndrome

Ning Fan, Xuyang Liu, and Jiantao Wang

Turner syndrome is a sex chromosome disease caused by abnormalities in chromosome number or structure. Ocular dysplasia can be found in such patients [1, 2]. The visual field change in a Turner syndrome case is introduced in this section, and karyotypic abnormalities and chimerism are also analyzed.

21.1 Case

21.1.1 Case Presentation

A 30-year-old female patient presented with progressive vision decrease in both eyes for over 20 years. The patient felt progressive decrease in vision from primary school, which was especially obvious under strong light. No accompanying symptoms including red eyes, eye pain, night blindness, etc. were present. Her visual acuity showed improvement after correction with myopic eyeglasses, but the corrected visual acuity decreased continuously. The right eye also developed distorted vision and abnormal color vision. The presence of family members with similar manifestations and histories of genetic diseases was denied.

Physical examination showed that the patient's body height was 147 cm and her body weight was 40 kg. She had normal intelligence and language ability. Her cranium had no deformities and her hair was dense. Much melanin pigmentation could be found on her face. She had a short and webbed neck, low-set ears, and low hairline at the back of the neck. Bilateral cubitus valgus, swollen hands, and a bulge in the wrists with normal ranges of motion could be observed (Fig. 21.1).

On examination, the uncorrected visual acuity (UCVA) was 20/200 OD and 20/63 OS, and the best corrected visual acuity (BCVA) was 20/125 (with refractive correction of −7.00DS −1.5DC × 175) OD and 20/40 (with refractive correction of −7.00DS −0.75DC × 5) OS. The intraocular pressures in both eyes were normal. Color vision test suggested dyserythrochloropsia. Epicanthus was revealed in the upper eyelids and mild ptosis was shown (Fig. 21.2); no abnormality was observed in the anterior segments. A white feather-like focus following the pattern and architecture of the retinal nerve fiber layer could be observed in both eyes. A quasi-circular macular atrophy 2–3PD in size accompanied by pigmentation in the fundus was found in both eyes (Fig. 21.3). Both eyes were in normal position and the eyeball movements were normal.

N. Fan · J. Wang (✉)
Shenzhen Eye Hospital, Shenzhen University, Shenzhen, China

X. Liu
Xiamen Eye Center of Xiamen University, Xiamen, China

Shenzhen Eye Hospital, Shenzhen University, Shenzhen, China

N. Wang et al. (eds.), *Optic Disorders and Visual Field*, Advances in Visual Science and Eye Diseases 2, https://doi.org/10.1007/978-981-13-2502-1_21

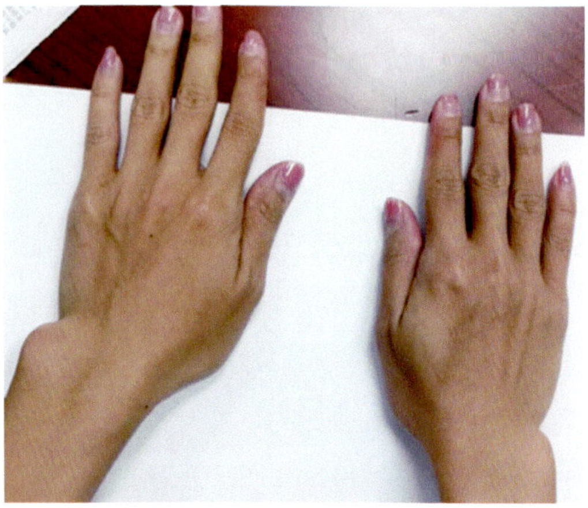

Fig. 21.1 Photograph of her wrists. Swollen hands and a bulge in both wrists could be seen, and the fingers could not be held together after straightening

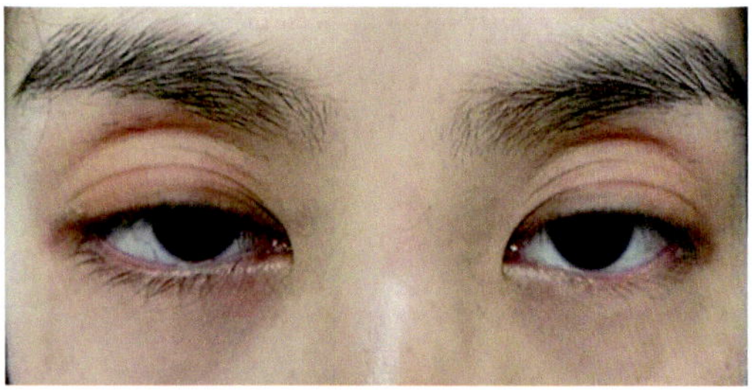

Fig. 21.2 Photograph of both eyebrows and eyes. The eyebrows were thick and bushy. Epicanthus and mild ptosis were seen. The periorbital and facial areas could be observed with much pigmentation

Visual field examination revealed bilateral central scotomas accompanied by enlargement of the blind spots (Fig. 21.4).

Optical coherence tomography (OCT) revealed significant thinning of the retina at the fovea, partial missing of the ellipsoid zone, and abnormal signals from the RPE and choroid in both eyes (Fig. 21.5).

Fundus fluorescein angiography (FFA) demonstrated annular transmitted fluorescence accompanied by punctate hypofluorescence in the macula in both eyes. Feather-like blockage in the fluorescence inferior to the optic disc in the right eye and both superior and inferior to the optic disc in the left eye was exhibited. The blockage continued to the late stage (Fig. 21.6).

Karyotype examination with peripheral venous blood carried out at another hospital revealed that the patient's karyotype was sex chromosome chimerism 45, X/46, X, ? del (X) (q21). The mitotic figure count of 45, X was 56 (56.1%) and 30 for 46, X, ? del (X) (q21) (34.9%). Refer to Fig. 21.7 for the photograph of the karyotype.

No abnormality was found in the urinary system, 3-D cardiac color ultrasound, or cardiac function examination.

Gynecology B-ultrasound showed that the uterus was in a flat position with a smaller-than-normal volume of about 36 mm * 26 mm * 32 mm. The echoes from the uterine wall were homogeneous. The endometrium line was in the middle and its thickness was

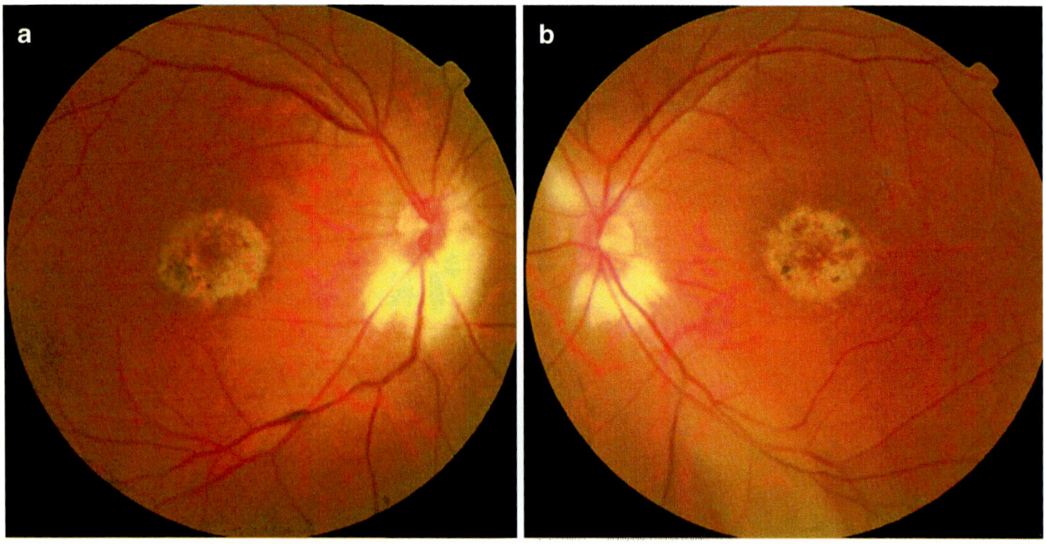

Fig. 21.3 Fundus photographs. A white feather-like focus following the pattern and architecture of the retinal nerve fiber layer and a quasi-circular macular atrophy were found in both eyes. Panel a: Right eye. Panel b: Left eye

about 4 mm. No abnormal echo was found inside the uterus. The ovaries were not displayed, and no abnormal lump-produced echo was obtained from bilateral uterine adnexa (Fig. 21.8). Endocrine examination of sex hormone, thyroid function, and pituitary hormone revealed no abnormality.

21.1.2 Final Diagnosis

The final diagnosis was Turner syndrome with bilateral macular disease, bilateral myelinated nerve fibers, and bilateral epicanthus.

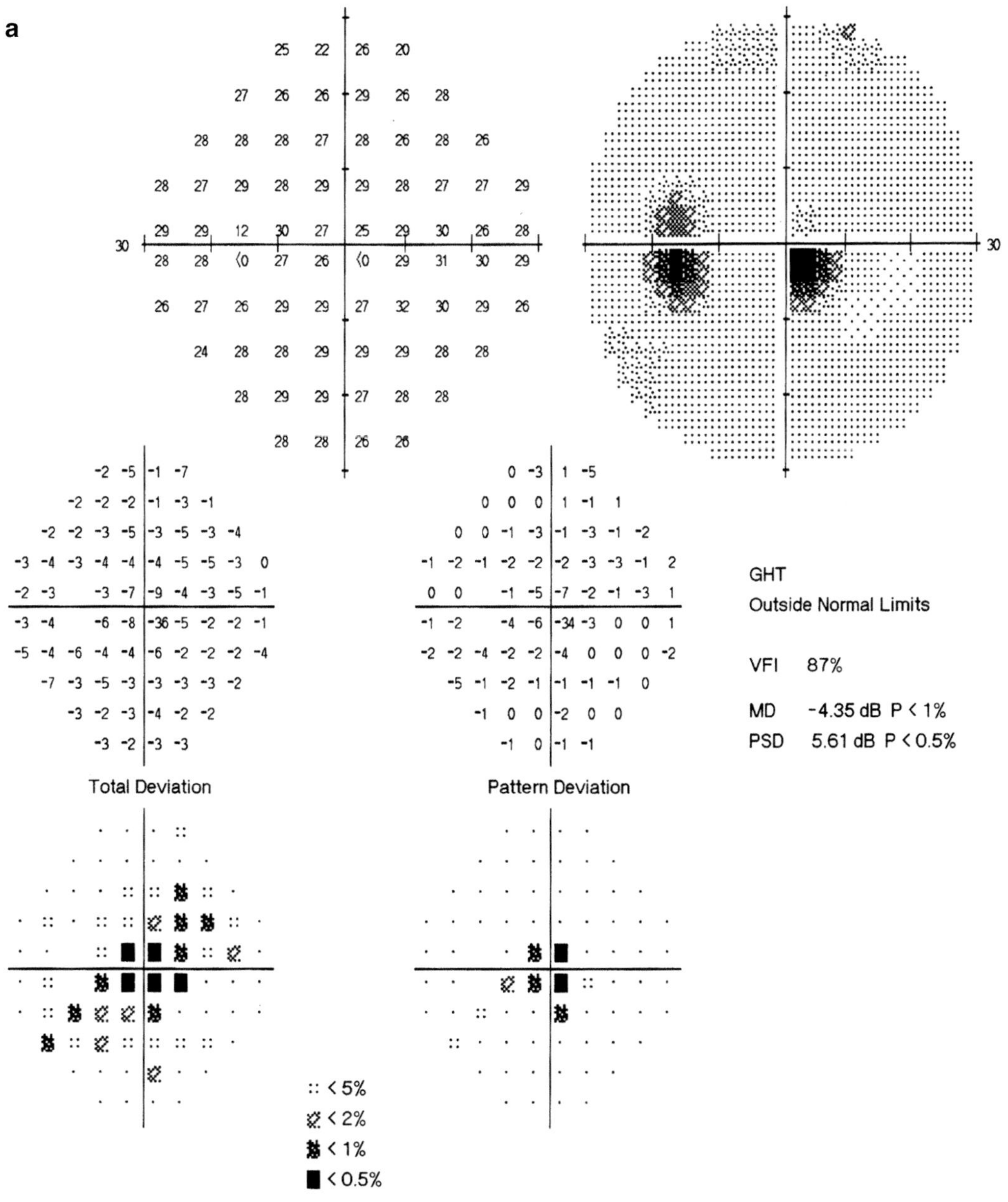

Fig. 21.4 Humphrey visual field analysis printouts. The 30-2 test showed bilateral central scotomas accompanied by enlargement of the blind spots. Panel a: Left eye. Panel b: Right eye

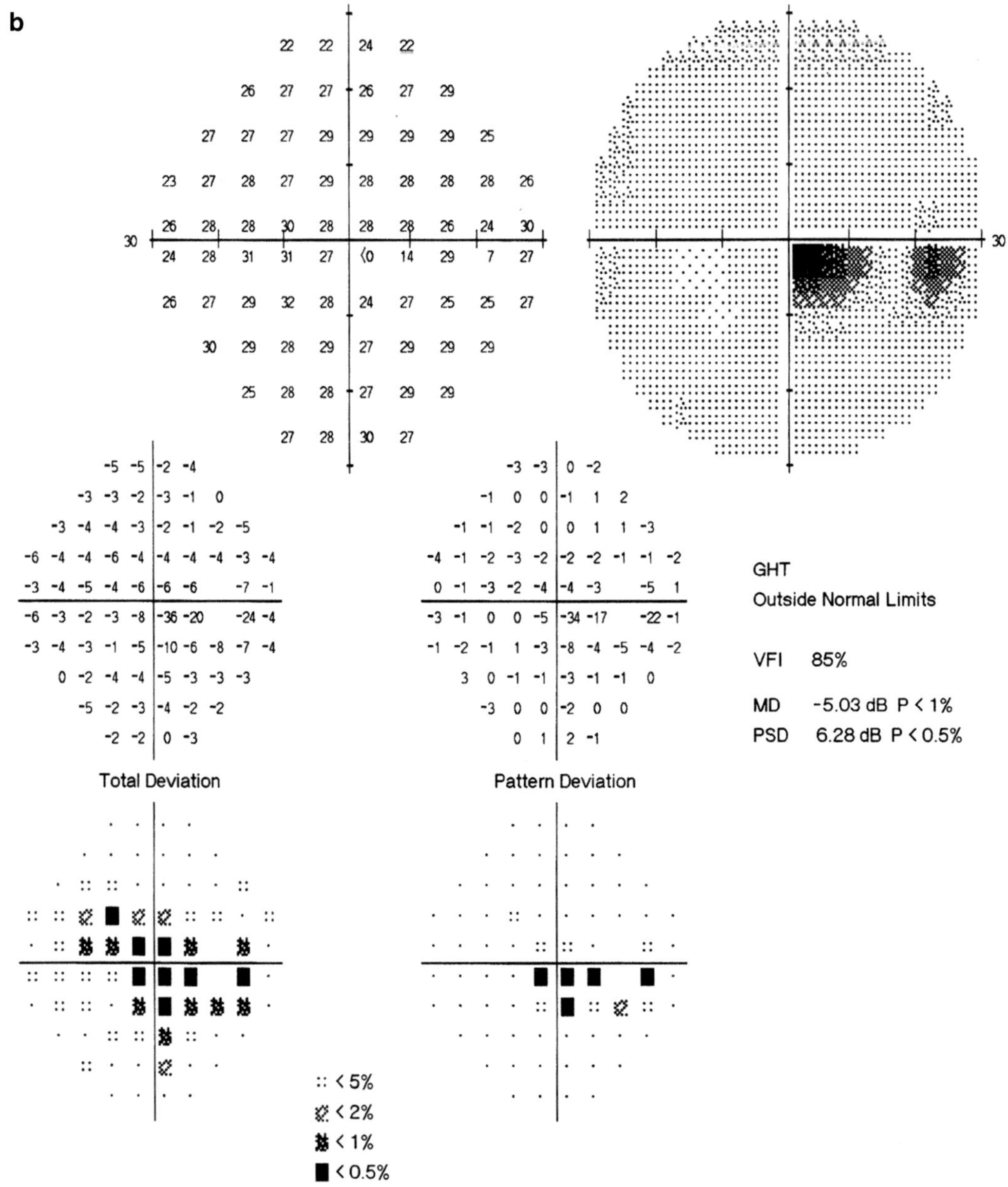

Fig. 21.4 (continued)

21.2 Discussion

The patient was a 31-year-old young female. She had once visited another hospital due to delay of menarche. Karyotype examination with peripheral venous blood revealed that her karyotype was 45, X/46, X, ? del (X) (q21) and she was diagnosed with Turner syndrome. Physical examination showed dysplasia and typical systemic malformations in Turner syndrome, such as low hairline, webbed neck, cubitus valgus, distal enlargement of the four limbs, etc. Dysplasia could be observed in the uterus and bilateral adnexa upon gynecologic ultrasound (B-mode).

Turner syndrome was firstly described in 1938 by Turner and is a sex chromosome disease caused by abnormalities in chromosome number or structure. It results from inadequate gene dosage caused by total or partial deletion of the X-chromosome. It's only found in females and affects about 1/4000 of the live births. Its clinical symptoms mainly include growth retardation, cardiovascular diseases, gonad hypoplasia, etc. [3]. In some Turner syndrome patients, there might be a normal X-chromosome and a structurally rearranged X-chromosome. By karyotype analysis on 410 Turner syndrome cases, Birkebaek et al. found that 49% of them had karyotype 45, X; 23% were chimeras with structurally abnormal X-chromosomes; 19% were 45, X/46, and XX chimera; and 9% were chimeras with a 46, XX, and a structurally abnormal X-chromosome. 45, X is a common karyotype [4]. The X-chromosome of 45, X in most of the Turner syndrome patients is from the mother, and its karyotype was a result of nondisjunction of sex chromosomes in the generative cells of one of the parents at meiosis I. The higher the proportion of 45, X karyotype is, the more remarkable the abnormal manifestations are. The structure abnormalities of X-chromosome found in Turner syndrome include deletion, repetition, insertion,

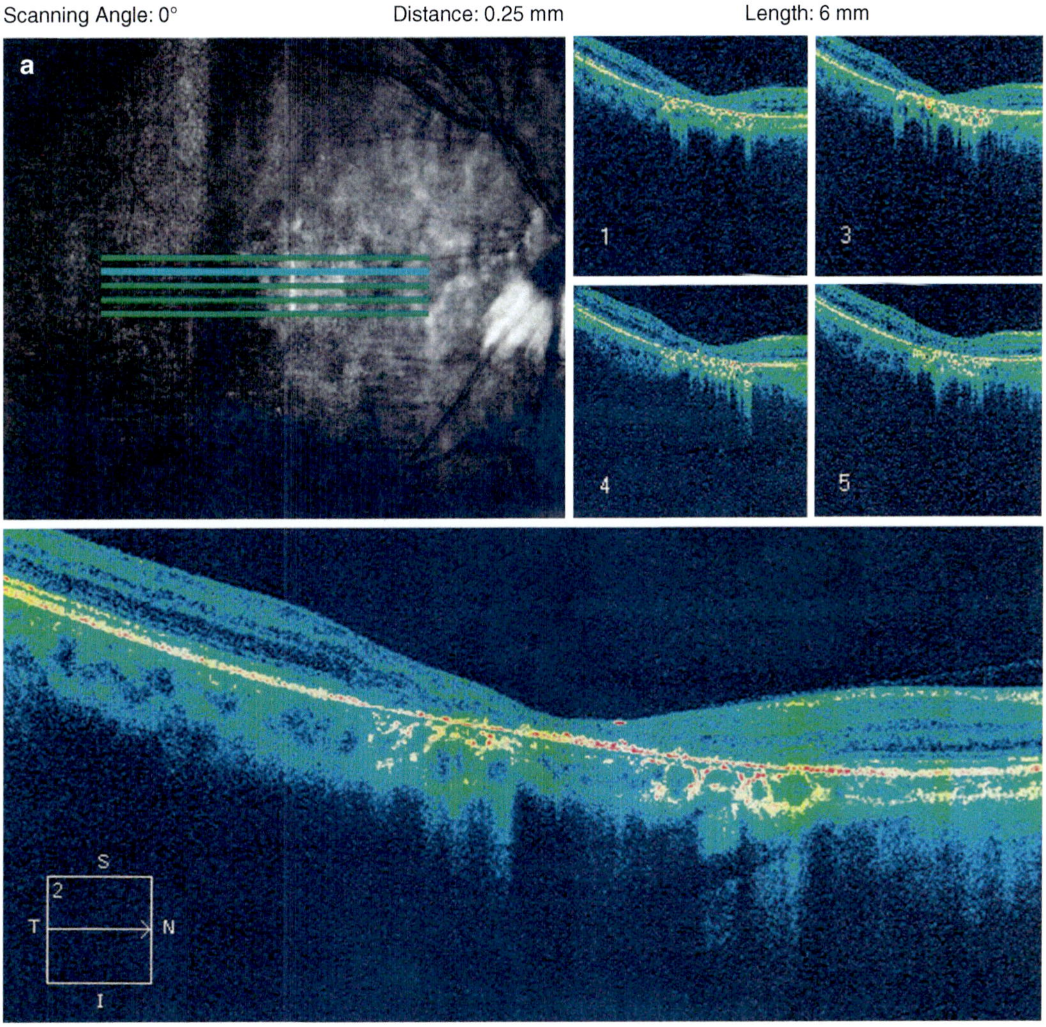

Fig. 21.5 OCT printouts of the macula. The OCT showed significant thinning of the retina at the fovea, partial missing of the ellipsoid zone, and abnormal signals from the RPE and choroid. Panel a: Right eye. Panel b: Left eye

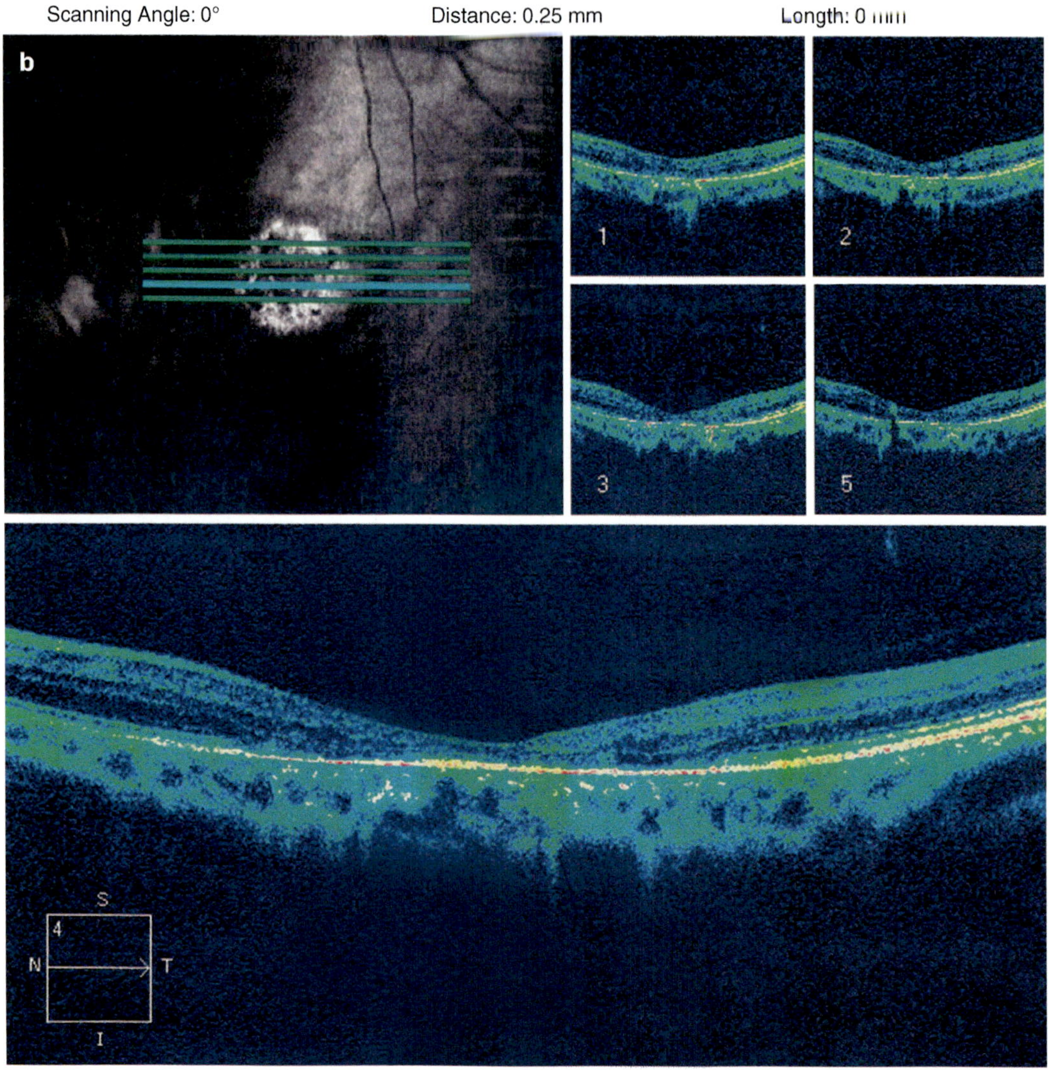

Fig. 21.5 (continued)

dicentric chromosome, translocation, annularity, etc. The karyotype of the patient in this case was chimerism 45, X [56]/46, X, ? del (X) (q21). The cause of chimerism may be the random loss of X-chromosome due to abnormality in chromosome reduplication in the first or first several cleavages of zygote or abnormality in chromosome assortment during mitosis.

In genetics, individuals with chimerism or hybridism of different genetic characters or coexistence of different karyotypes (in brief, two or more karyotypes coexist in the same organism) are chimeras, which is a type of chromosome abnormality. An individual formed by cell lines from different zygotes is called a heterologous chimera. Individual formed by cell lines that develop into different karyotypes from the same zygote is called a homologous chimera.

A systematic review carried out by AK Denniston focusing on the ocular manifestations in 274 Turner syndrome patients found that the most common eye abnormality was simple recessive strabismus (46%) followed by decreased accommodation ability and decreased conver-

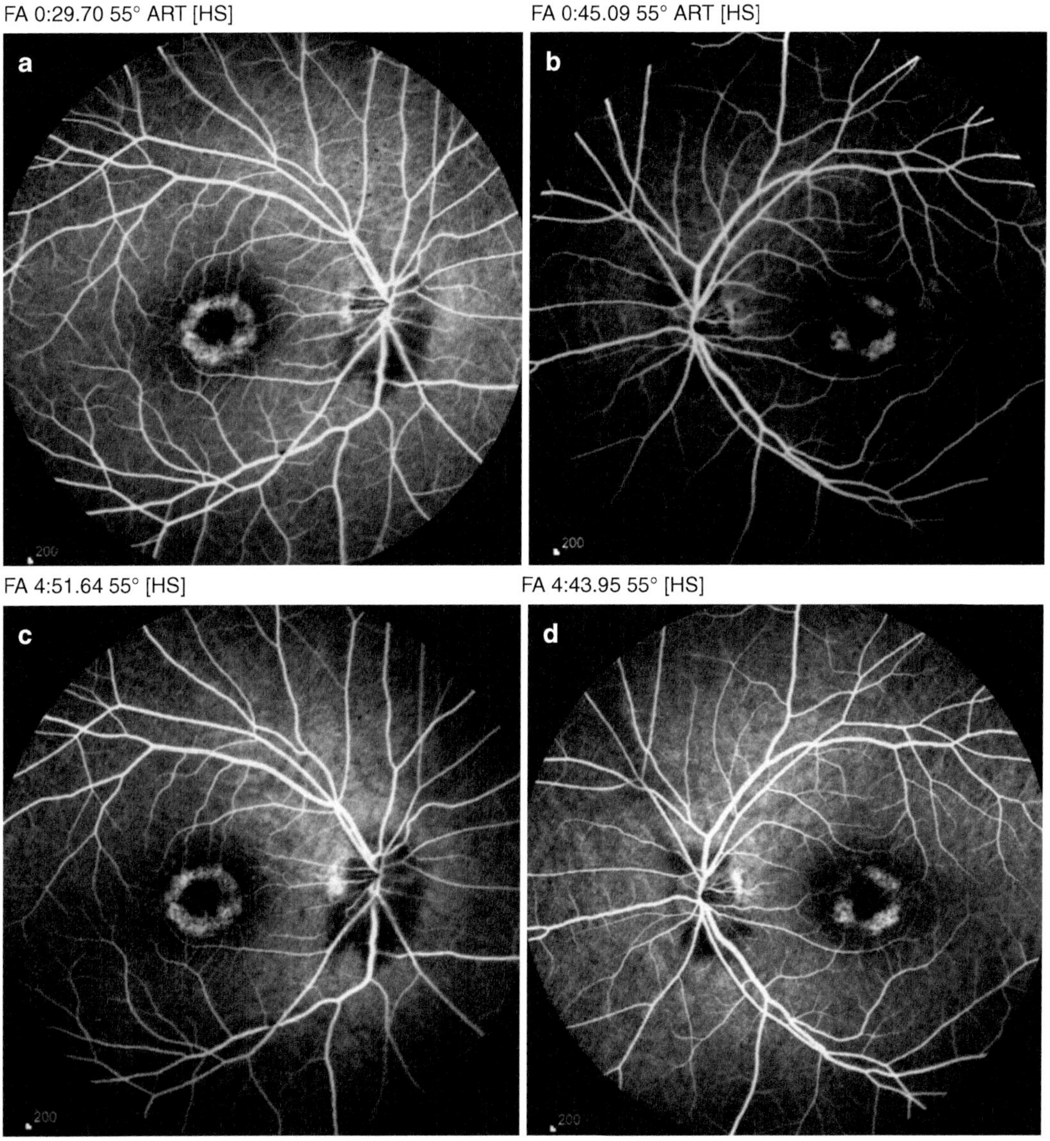

Fig. 21.6 FFA images of both eyes. Annular hyperfluorescence about 1–2PD in size accompanied by punctate hypofluorescence could be observed in the macula of both eyes. Panel a: Right eye. Panel b: Left eye. Feather-like blockage in the fluorescence inferior to the optic disc in the right eye and both superior and inferior to the optic disc in the left eye was exhibited. The blockage continued to the late stage. Panel c: Right eye. Panel d: Left eye

gence ability (both 40%). Besides, epicanthus (35%), strabismus (33%), hyperopia (27%), ptosis (21%), hypertelorism (10%), red-green color blindness (9%), blue sclera (2%), and congenital glaucoma (1%) were also observed [1]. And an eye abnormality study carried out by Beata Wikiera on 82 Turner syndrome cases showed that about 52% of Turner syndrome patients were with concomitant eye abnormalities, among which 35% were bilateral eye abnormalities, 44% were observed with visual acuity impairment, 6% had posterior segment abnormalities, and 5% had anterior segment abnormalities. Anterior segment abnormalities mainly include

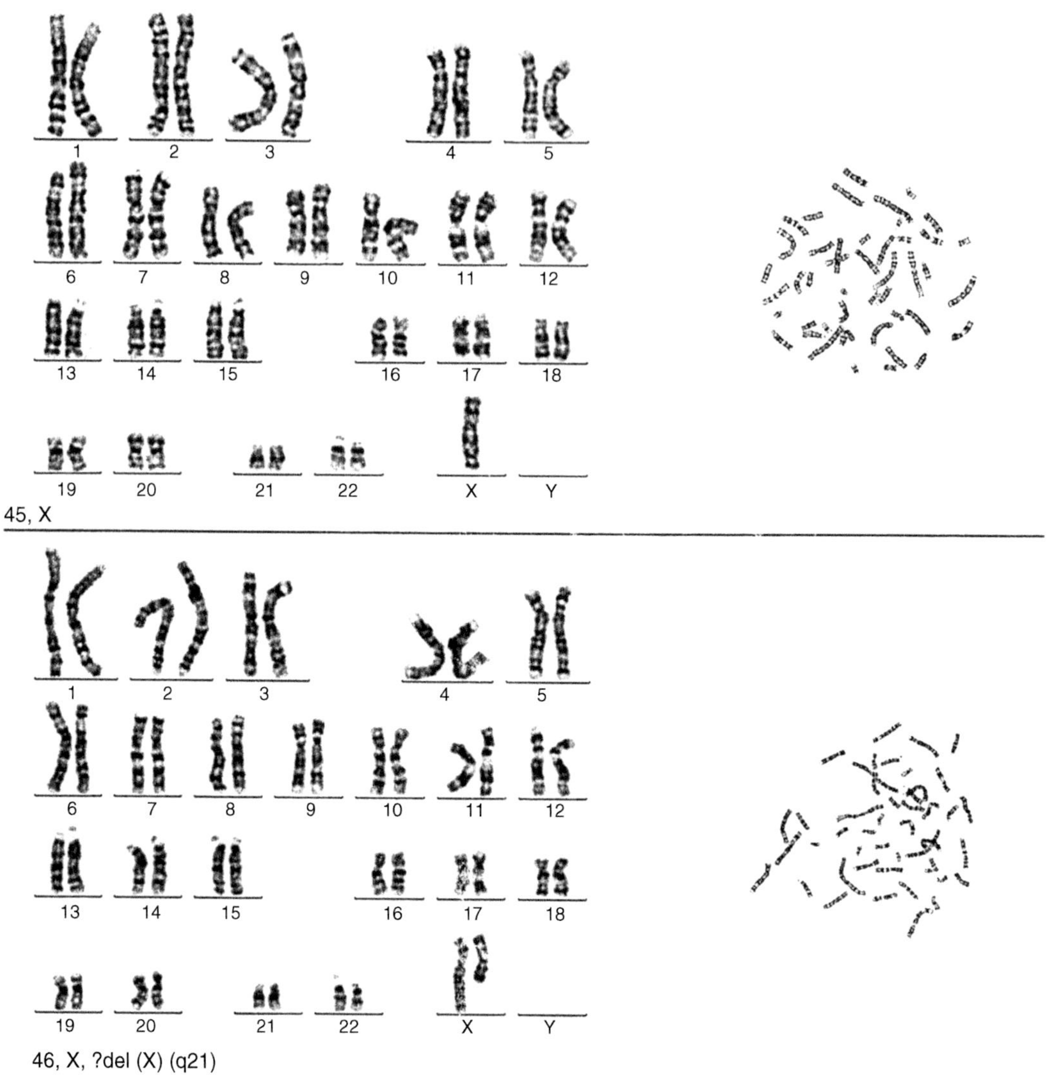

Fig. 21.7 Karyotype analysis printouts. Karyotype examination with peripheral venous blood revealed that the patient's karyotype was 45, X/46, X, ? del (X) (q21)

cornea thickening, uveal cyst, etc. And fundus abnormalities include choroidal defect, fundus vascular tortuosity, optic disc drusen, etc. [2]. The fundus diseases found in this case included myelinated nerve fiber and macular degeneration, which were rarely reported in the literature.

Bilateral central scotomas accompanied by enlargement of the blind spots were found in the visual field examination in this case, and it could be explained by the myelinated nerve fiber and macular degeneration revealed in both eyes of the patient.

It's currently believed that the systemic manifestations of Turner syndrome, especially underdeveloped physical constitution and secondary sex characters, are connected with the chromosome abnormality type and involvement degree. However, Beata Wikiera et al. carried out a correlational study on eye abnormalities and karyotype in 82 Turner syndrome cases and found that eye abnormalities were usually present in Turner syndrome patients, but there was no special correspondence pattern between the occurrence of eye abnormalities and chromosome abnormality types [2].

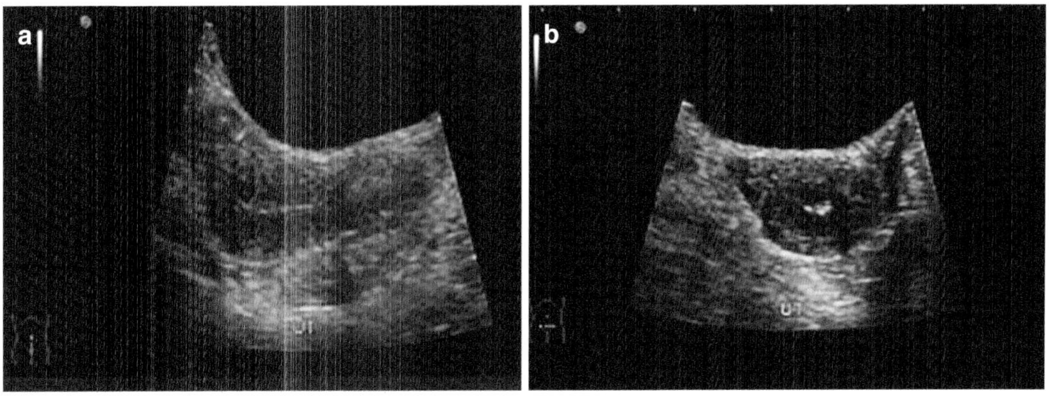

Fig. 21.8 Gynecologic ultrasound (B-mode) images. The uterus was in a flat position with a smaller-than-normal volume of about 36 mm * 26 mm * 32 mm. The echoes from the uterine wall were homogeneous. The endometrium line was in the middle and its thickness was about 4 mm. No abnormal echo was found inside the uterus. The ovaries were not displayed, and no abnormal lump-produced echo was obtained from bilateral uterine adnexa

References

1. Denniston AK, Butler L. Ophthalmic features of Turner's syndrome. Eye. 2004;18(7):680–4.
2. Wikiera B, Mulak M, Koltowska-Haggstrom M, et al. The presence of eye defects in patients with Turner syndrome is irrespective of their karyotype. Clin Endocrinol. 2015;83(6):842–8.
3. Hjerrild BE, Mortensen KH, Gravholt CH. Turner syndrome and clinical treatment. Br Med Bull. 2008;86(86):77–93.
4. Birkebaek NH, Crüger D, Hansen J, et al. Fertility and pregnancy outcome in Danish women with Turner syndrome. Clin Genet. 2002;61(1):35–9.

22 The Clinical and Genetic Analysis of Stargardt's Disease

Ning Fan, Xuyang Liu, and Jiantao Wang

Stargardt disease is also called juvenile macular degeneration, and its main ocular manifestations are bilateral vision decrease and central visual field defects. Three cases are discussed in this section, among which the patient was a descendant from consanguineous marriage in two cases. This phenomenon highlights the importance of the family planning work.

22.1 Case 1

22.1.1 Case Presentation

A 27-year-old female patient presented with painless and gradual bilateral decrease of vision for 2 years. No significant trigger for disease onset was noticed and refraction correction was useless. No accompanying symptoms including distorted vision and night blindness were present. Histories of trauma, systemic diseases, and genetic diseases were denied. No family member was observed with a similar disease. Consanguineous marriage of her parents was denied.

Upon examination, her uncorrected visual acuity (UCVA) was 20/200 OD and 20/200 OS, and her best corrected visual acuity (BCVA) was 20/160 (with refractive correction of −0.50DS −0.75DC × 20) OD and 20/200 (with refractive correction of −0.50DS −0.5DC × 165) OS. The intraocular pressure (IOP) was normal in both eyes. Slit-lamp examination of her anterior segments was unremarkable. Fundus examination revealed a small disciform area of RPE atrophy centered on the fovea, with a few tiny intraretinal crystals overlying this atrophy. There were no typical flecks in either eye (Fig. 22.1).

Visual field examinations with the 30-2 and 10-2 strategies both revealed a superior central scotoma in both eyes (Fig. 22.2).

Optical coherence tomography (OCT) revealed photoreceptor abnormalities, RPE atrophy and significant thinning of the fovea in both eyes (Fig. 22.3).

Fundus fluorescein angiography (FFA) demonstrated that the area of RPE atrophy was hyperfluorescent centered on the fovea in both eyes, with a silent and masked choroid. The hyperfluorescent foci of flecks were not found. These findings conformed to the manifestations of early Stargardt disease (Fig. 22.4).

N. Fan · J. Wang (✉)
Shenzhen Eye Hospital, Shenzhen University, Shenzhen, China

X. Liu
Xiamen Eye Center of Xiamen University, Xiamen, China

Shenzhen Eye Hospital, Shenzhen University, Shenzhen, China

N. Wang et al. (eds.), *Optic Disorders and Visual Field*, Advances in Visual Science and Eye Diseases 2, https://doi.org/10.1007/978-981-13-2502-1_22

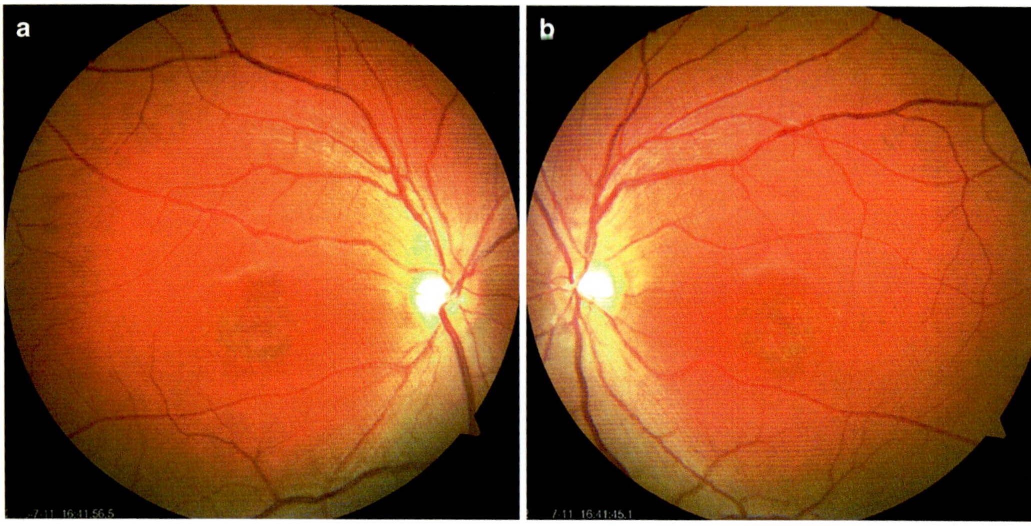

Fig. 22.1 Fundus photographs. A small disciform area of RPE atrophy centered on the fovea could be seen, with a few tiny intraretinal crystals overlying this atrophy. There were no typical flecks in either eye. Panel a: Right eye. Panel b: Left eye

22.1.2 Final Diagnosis

The final diagnosis was Stargardt disease.

22.1.3 Case Review

The patient was a young female and had been suffering from painless vision decrease in both eyes for 2 years. Fundus examination disclosed a small disciform area of RPE atrophy centered on the fovea, with a few tiny intraretinal crystals overlying this atrophy, and there were no typical flecks in either eye. OCT revealed photoreceptor abnormalities, RPE atrophy and significant thinning of the fovea in both eyes. FFA demonstrated that the area of RPE atrophy was hyperfluorescent centered on the fovea in both eyes, with a silent and masked choroid (masked choroid sign), and the hyperfluorescent foci of flecks were not found. Bilateral central scotomas corresponding to the macular lesions could be observed in visual field examination. The clinical diagnosis was Stargardt disease.

22.2 Case 2

22.2.1 Case Presentation

A 10-year-old male patient presented with poor bilateral vision since his childhood. The patient's parents found that his visual acuity was poor and correction with spectacles was useless. No accompanying symptoms including red eyes and eye pain were present. Trauma history, history of systemic diseases, and family medical history were denied. The patient was born full term thorough virginal delivery. His growth and development were normal. His parents' marriage was consanguineous.

On examination, the BCVA was 20/125 OU. The IOP was normal in both eyes. Anterior segment and fundus examinations were unremarkable except for a very subtle oval area of RPE at the fovea (Fig. 22.5).

OCT revealed foveal photoreceptor loss and RPE atrophy in both eyes (Fig. 22.6).

FFA showed hyperfluorescent foci of RPE atrophy centered on the fovea in both eyes (Fig. 22.7).

Multifocal electroretinography (mf-ERG) disclosed amplitude decrease in the center of the macula in both eyes (Fig. 22.8).

Visual field examination demonstrated a central visual field defect in both eyes (Fig. 22.9).

22.2.2 Final Diagnosis

The final diagnosis was Stargardt disease.

Detail review on the patient's family history was carried out, and the pedigree chart was drawn (Fig. 22.10). The review found that the patient's

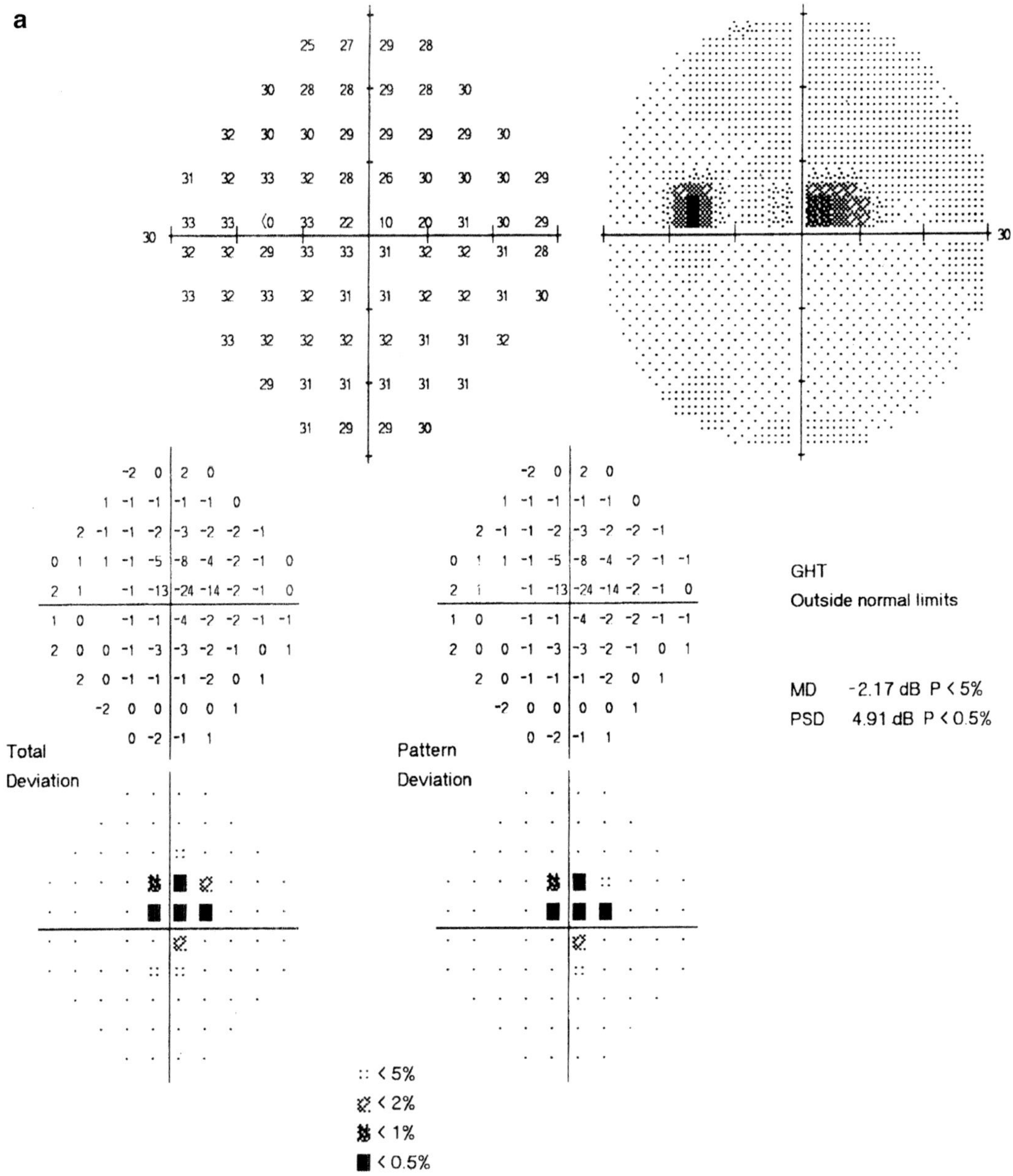

Fig. 22.2 Humphrey visual field analysis printouts. Bilateral central scotomas were shown: 30-2 test (Panel a: Left eye. Panel b: Right eye); 10-2 test (Figure c: Left eye. Panel d: Right eye)

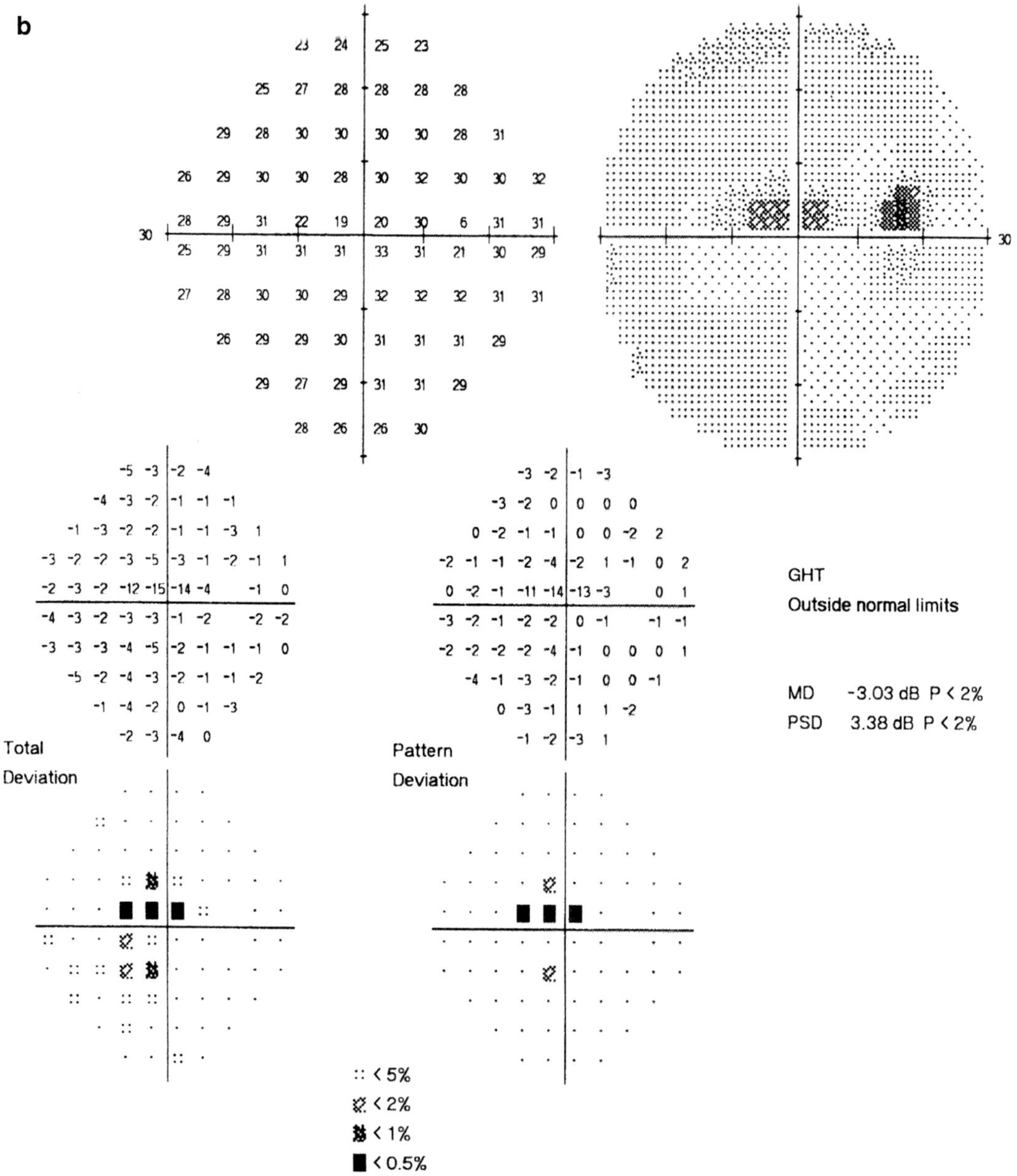

Fig. 22.2 (continued)

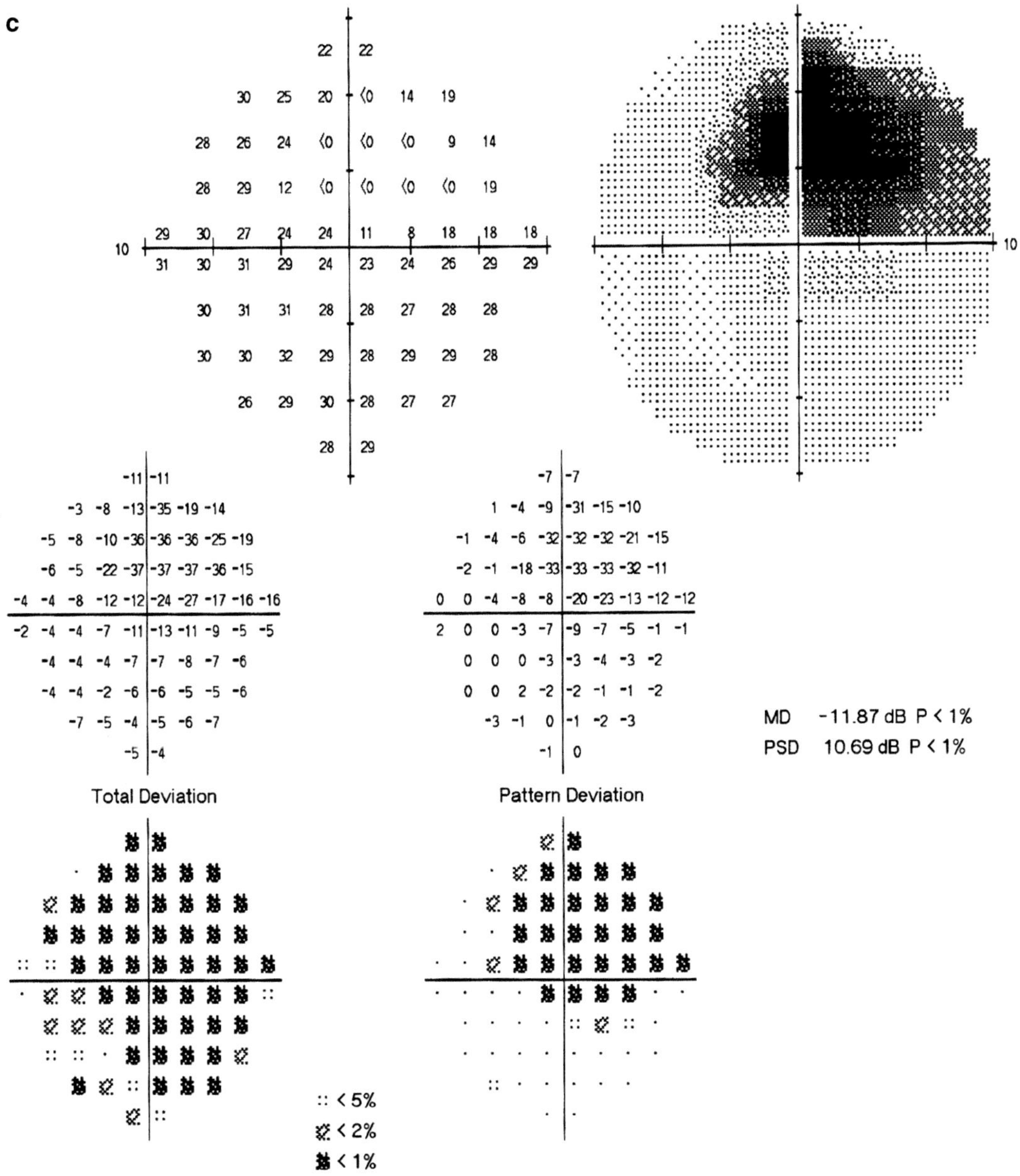

Fig. 22.2 (continued)

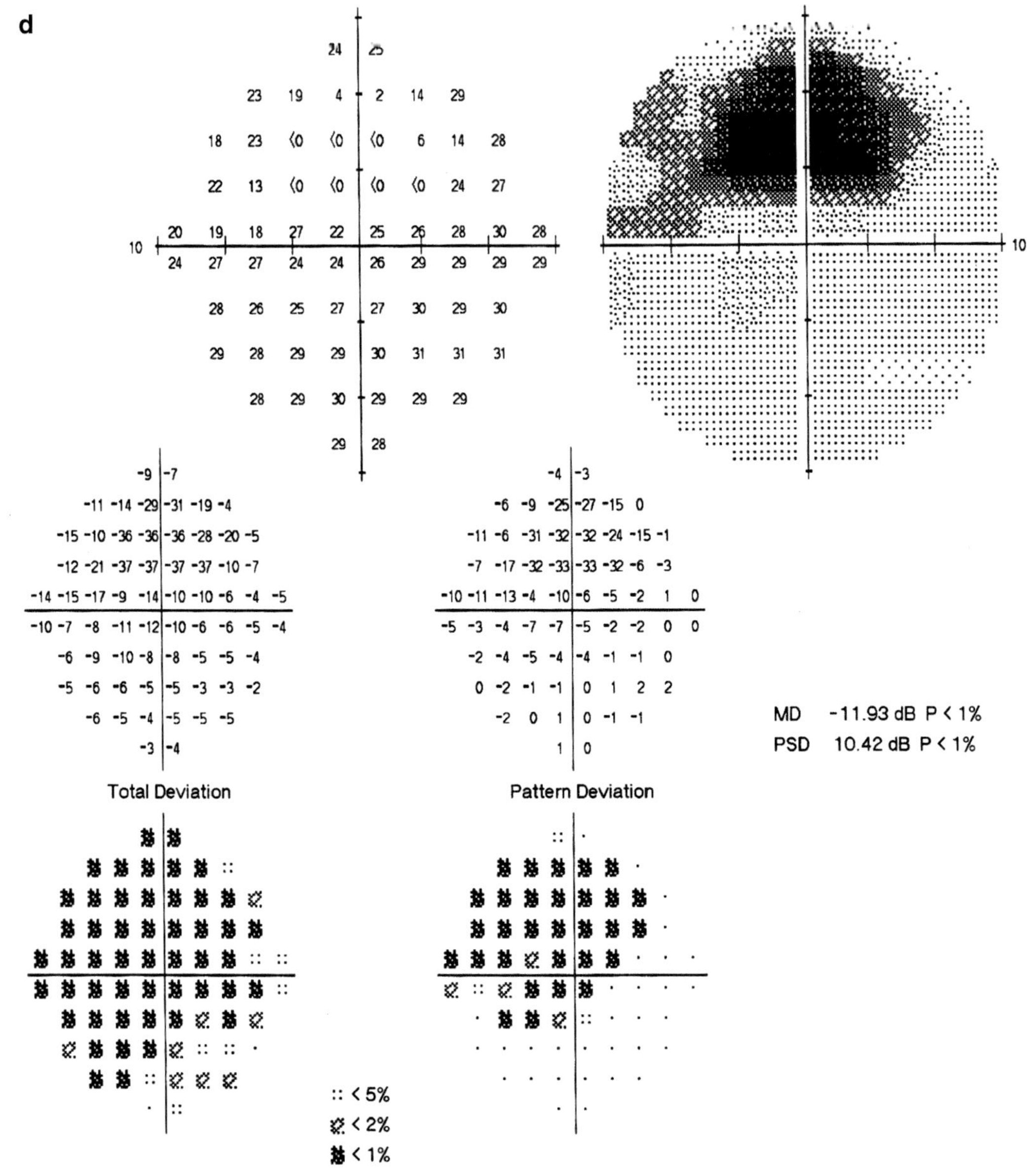

Fig. 22.2 (continued)

parents had a consanguineous marriage and no similar eye manifestation was observed in other family members.

The parents had a consanguineous marriage. The disease was not found in the parents and their elder son but was found in their second son.

22.2.3 Case Review

The patient was 10 years old and had been suffering from poor bilateral vision for years in this case. The clinical manifestations conform to those of Stargardt disease. Bilateral central scotomas corresponding to the macular disease could be observed in visual field examination. The damages to the cone and rod cells precede the visible macular lesions in Stargardt disease, and ERG can earlier and more sensitively reveal the damages.

22.3 Case 3

22.3.1 Case Presentation

A 33-year-old male patient presented with progressive vision decreases in both eyes for about 20 years. No significant trigger was observed before disease onset. No accompanying symptoms, including red eyes, eye pain, etc., were present. Histories of trauma and systemic diseases were denied. Family history was admitted and his parents' marriage was consanguineous.

On examination, the BCVA was hand motion OU. The IOP was normal in both eyes. The refracting media of both eyes were transparent. There were numerous flecks in the posterior pole and a reticular network of RPE atrophy with some clumps of dark pigment in the atrophic lesion (Fig. 22.11).

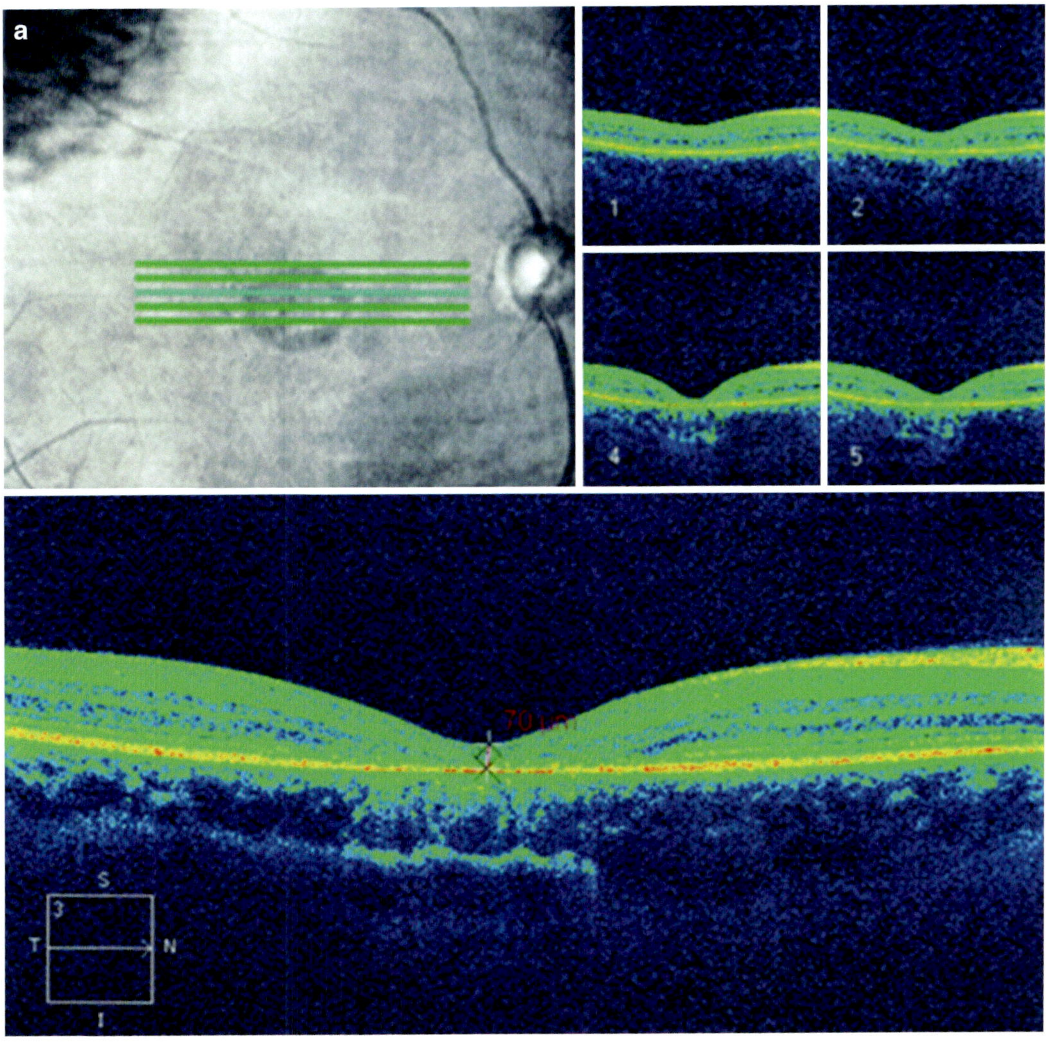

Fig. 22.3 OCT printouts of the macula. Photoreceptor abnormalities, RPE atrophy and significant thinning of the fovea could be seen in both eyes. Panel a: Right eye. Panel b: Left eye

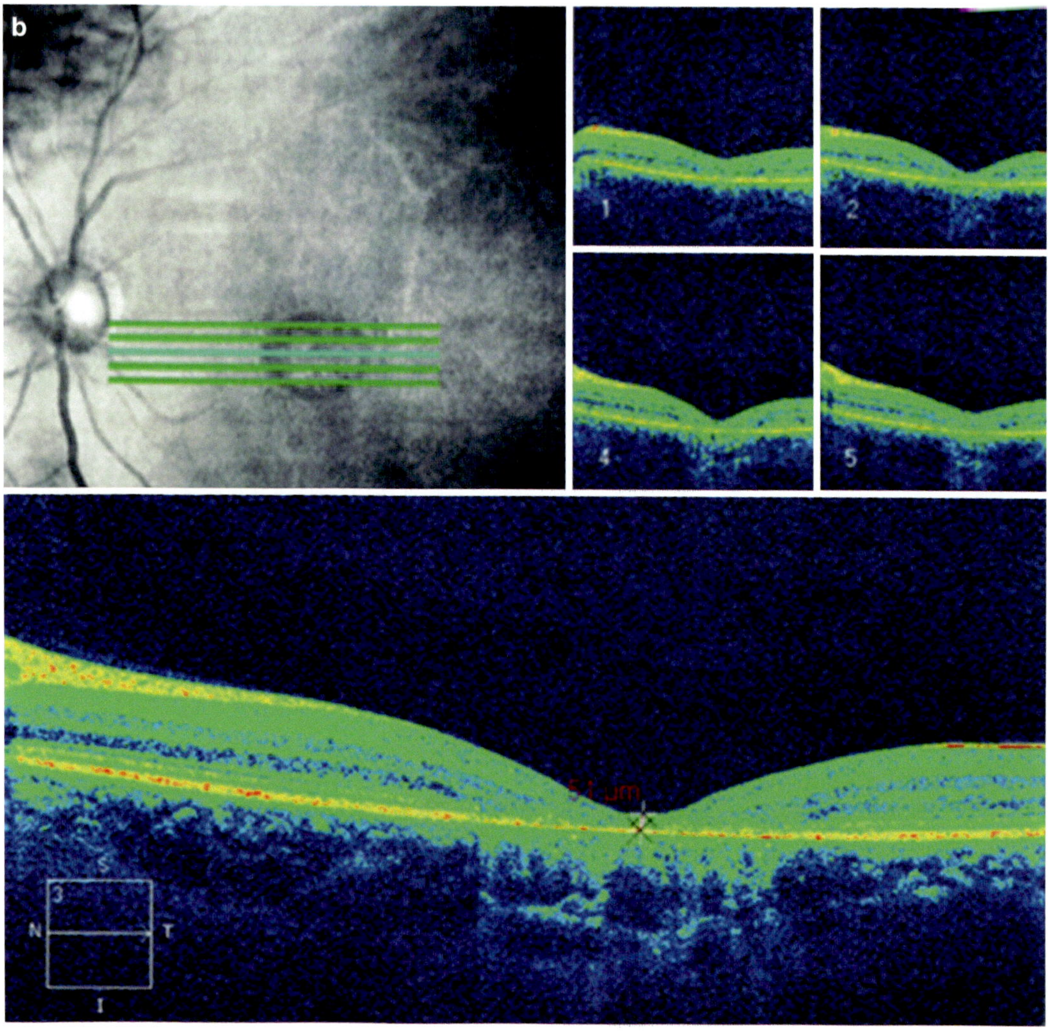

Fig. 22.3 (continued)

OCT of the macula showed an abnormal and atrophic fovea with the loss of photoreceptor and RPE layers (Fig. 22.12).

Examinations were carried out on the other members in the pedigree. Except another consanguineous descendant who also had this disease, no abnormality was shown in the other members of this pedigree.

Genetic tests of Stargardt disease were carried out on the peripheral blood of the proband, and the family members after permission were obtained. By candidate gene screening, we found that the proband had homozygous mutation c.4773 + 1g > t and three SNPs (H423R, M1209T, and T1428M) of the ABCA4 gene (refer to Fig. 22.13 for the sequencing results). This disease was not observed in his parents, and both of them carried heterozygous mutation c.4773 + 1g > t of the ABCA4 gene. However, his brother had no such disease and mutation, which conformed to the pattern of autosomal recessive inheritance (Fig. 22.14).

22.3.2 Final Diagnosis

The final diagnosis was Stargardt disease.

The patient was diagnosed with Stargardt disease with the medical history, fundus mani-

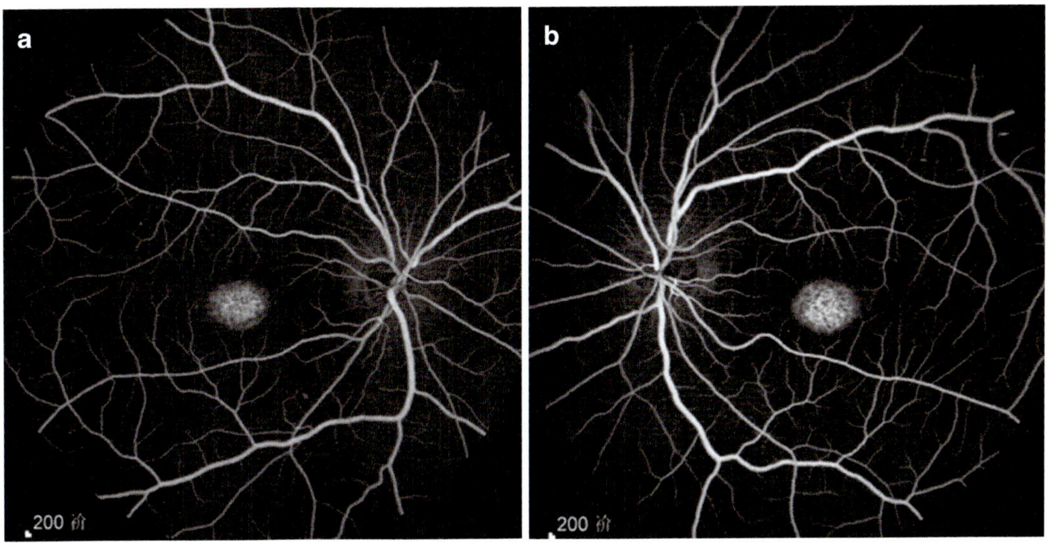

Fig. 22.4 FFA images. FFA demonstrated that the area of RPE atrophy was hyperfluorescent centered on the fovea in both eyes, with a silent and masked choroid. The hyperfluorescent foci of flecks were not found. Panel a: Right eye. Panel b: Left eye

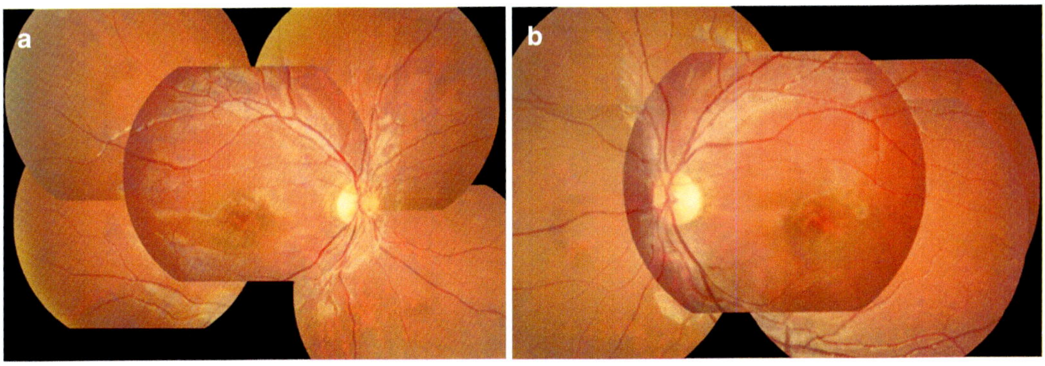

Fig. 22.5 Montage images of fundus photographs. A very subtle oval area of RPE could be seen at the fovea. Panel a: Right eye. Panel b: Left eye

festations, and gene detection results all taken into consideration. The parents of another patient in the pedigree also had a cross-cousin marriage.

22.3.3 Case Review

The disease duration of the patient was long and the fundus manifestations conformed to those of advanced Stargardt disease. The genetic tests showed that the proband of the pedigree harbored homozygous c.4773 + 1g > t mutation of the ABCA4 gene. The disease was not observed in the patient's parents but they were carriers. The disease was not found in the younger brother of the proband, and the mutation site was also not detected. The findings demonstrated co-segregation of the clinical manifestations of Stargardt disease and the ABCA4 gene mutation and that Stargardt disease is inherited in an autosomal recessive pattern.

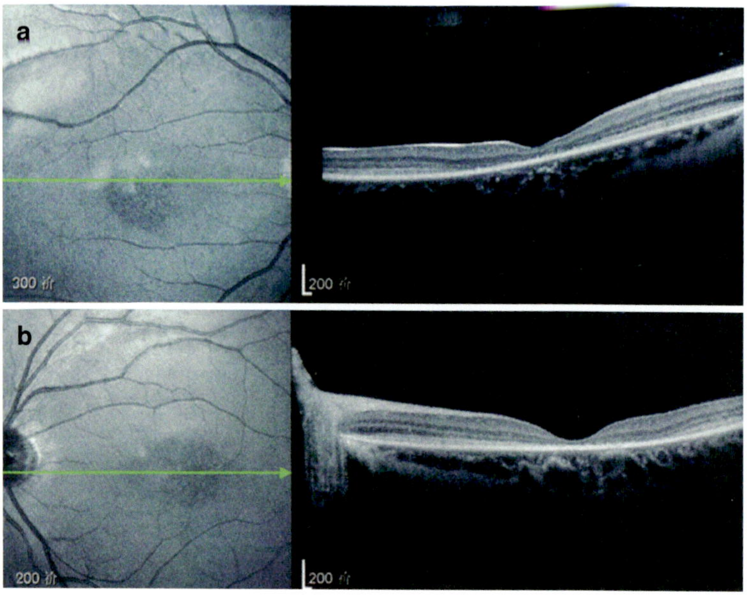

Fig. 22.6 OCT images of the macula of both eyes. OCT showed foveal photoreceptor loss and RPE atrophy in both eyes. Panel a: Right eye. Panel b: Left eye

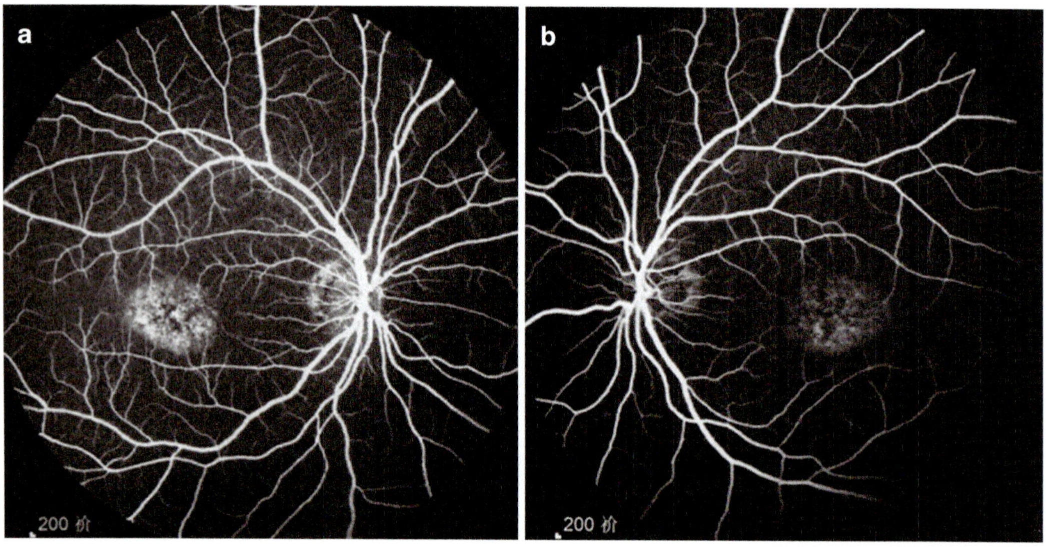

Fig. 22.7 FFA images. FFA showed hyperfluorescent foci of RPE atrophy centered on the fovea in both eyes. Panel a: Right eye. Panel b: Left eye

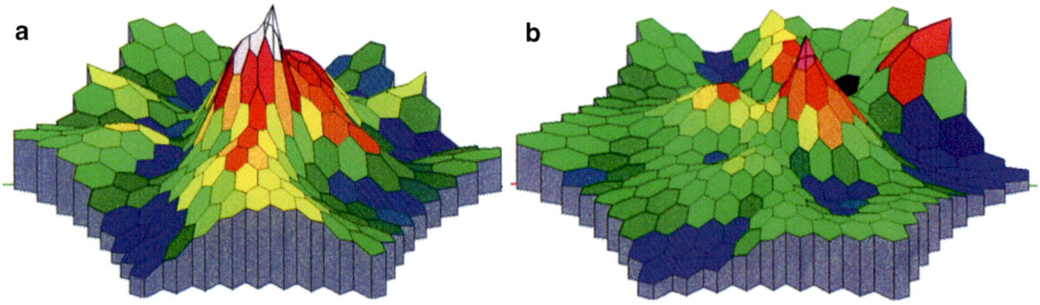

Fig. 22.8 mf-ERG images. Amplitude decrease was shown in the center of the macula in both eyes. Panel a: Right eye. Panel b: Left eye

22.4 Discussion

All the three patients in this section suffered from Stargardt disease.

Stargardt disease is a common hereditary macular dystrophy disease. It is also called juvenile macular degeneration and was first reported by Stargardt in 1909. Most of Stargardt disease cases have autosomal recessive inheritance. Autosomal dominant inheritance or X-linked inheritance can also be found in some cases. Most of the patients' parents have a consanguine-

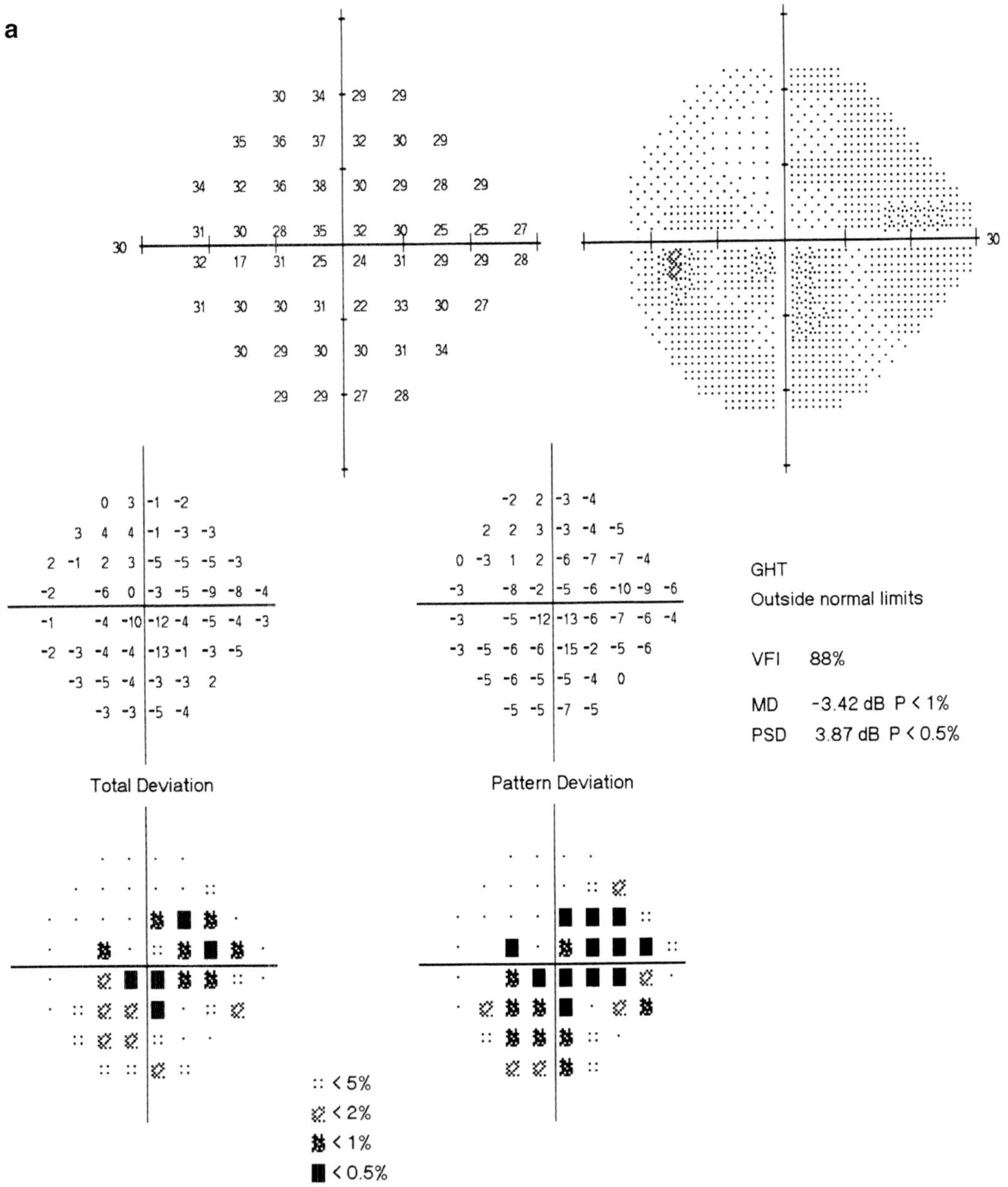

Fig. 22.9 Humphrey visual field analysis printouts. The 24-2 test showed a central visual field defect in both eyes. Panel a: Left eye. Panel b: Right eye

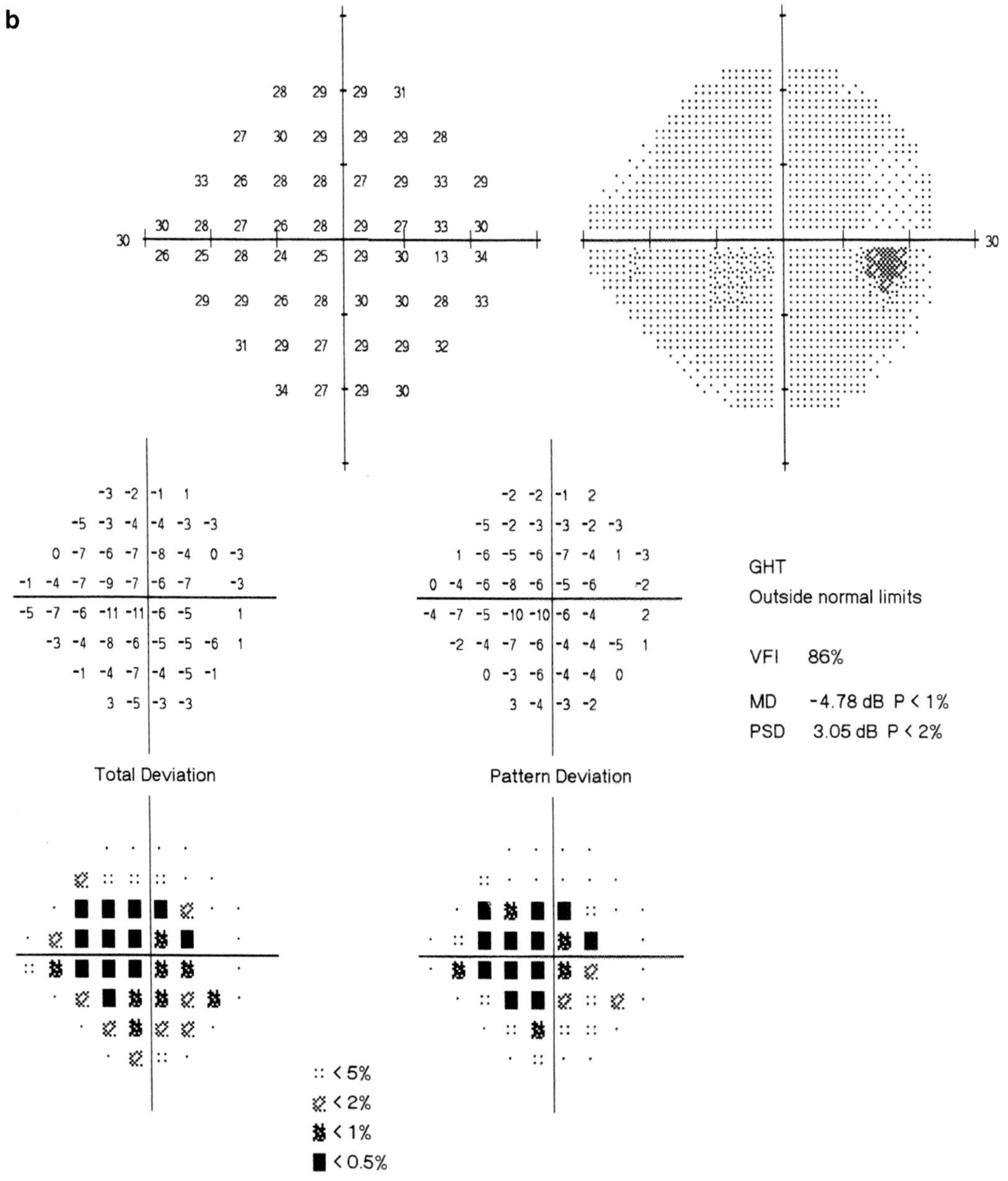

Fig. 22.9 (continued)

ous marriage. The onset of this disease is found at young ages and the patients are 6–20 years old. Its incidence is about 1/10,000.

Most of Stargardt disease patients will experience loss of bilateral visual acuity that will gradually decrease to 20/200 and, in some cases, even to light perception. Eye examination shows no significant positive signs at the initial stage of the disease, and it's usually misdiagnosed as amblyopia. However, central visual field damage can be found in visual field examination, and retinal function abnormality can also be found in ERG examination. Case 2 is a typical case for such phenomenon. With the progression of the disease, a very subtle oval area of RPE at the fovea and flecks can be found against a gray-yellow background. Some scholars described such appearance as a "beaten-bronze" appearance. Hyperfluorescent foci of RPE atrophy and flecks, accompanied by pigmentation, as seen in case 3, can be observed in the fundi of patients with advanced Stargardt disease. FFA examination of early Stargardt disease may not disclose any abnormality or only spot-like hyperfluorescence in the macula. With the progression of the disease, symmetrical elliptical-speckled hyperfluorescence, i.e., bull's-eye sign, will be exhibited in the macula in the two eyes. Meanwhile, the background fluorescence of the choroid will be blocked, weakened, or even disappear due to lipofuscinosis inside the RPE cells, and the retinal capillaries will become more visible as a result. This phenomenon is called "masked choroid sign." Scattered spot-like hyperfluorescence can be observed at sites corresponding to those flecks in the retina at late stages. These signs have been observed in all of the above three cases.

In summary, Stargardt disease has specific symptoms and signs, and it's not difficult to diagnose clinically with the help of the examinations such as visual field examination, FFA, OCT, ERG, etc. [1].

The pathogenesis of Stargardt disease is still unclear so far. The reported disease-causing genes for Stargardt disease include ABCA4, PROM1, VMD2, ELOVL4, PRPH2, etc. These gene mutations are considered to be possible

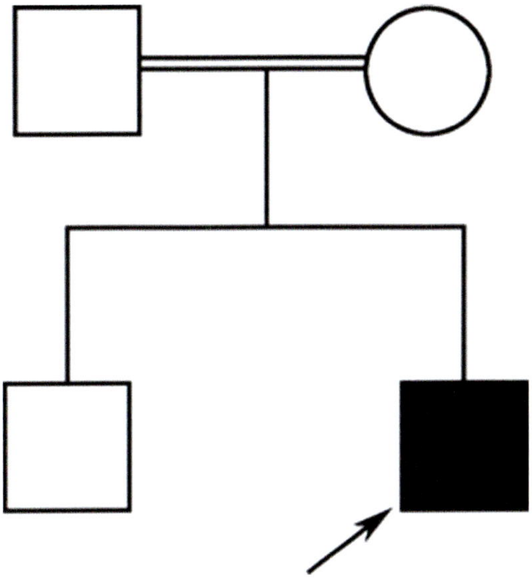

Fig. 22.10 The pedigree chart of Stargardt disease

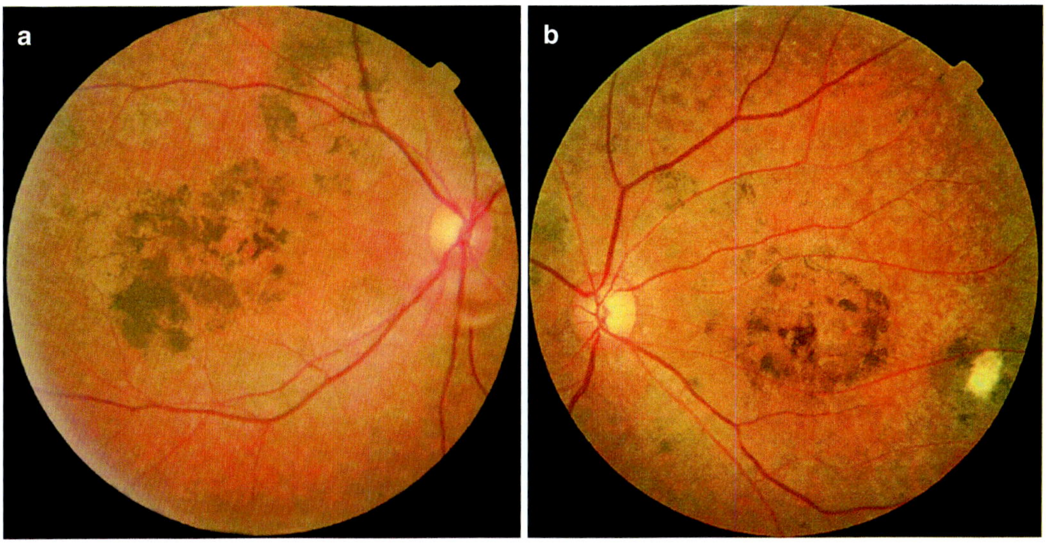

Fig. 22.11 Fundus photographs. It could be seen that there were numerous flecks in the posterior pole and a reticular network of RPE atrophy with some clumps of dark pigment in the atrophic lesion. Panel a: Right eye. Panel b: Left eye

causes of retinal dystrophy, which can finally damage the photoreceptor cells, RPE, etc. These genes have also been reported in cone-rod cell dysplasia, retinitis pigmentosa, age-related macular degeneration, etc. Further studies are still required for their specific action mechanisms.

Among the abovementioned genes, the ABCA4 gene is the fourth member of the subtype A of the ATP-binding cassette (ABC) family. It encodes the specific ABC transporter proteins in the retina. It was found as early as 1997 to be the disease-causing gene for autosomal recessive Stargardt disease (STGD 1). After that, ABCA4 has been found to be related to other retinal degeneration diseases, such as cone-rod cell dysplasia, primary retinal pigmentary degeneration, etc. Over 500 mutation sites have been identified in the encoding regions of the gene, and these

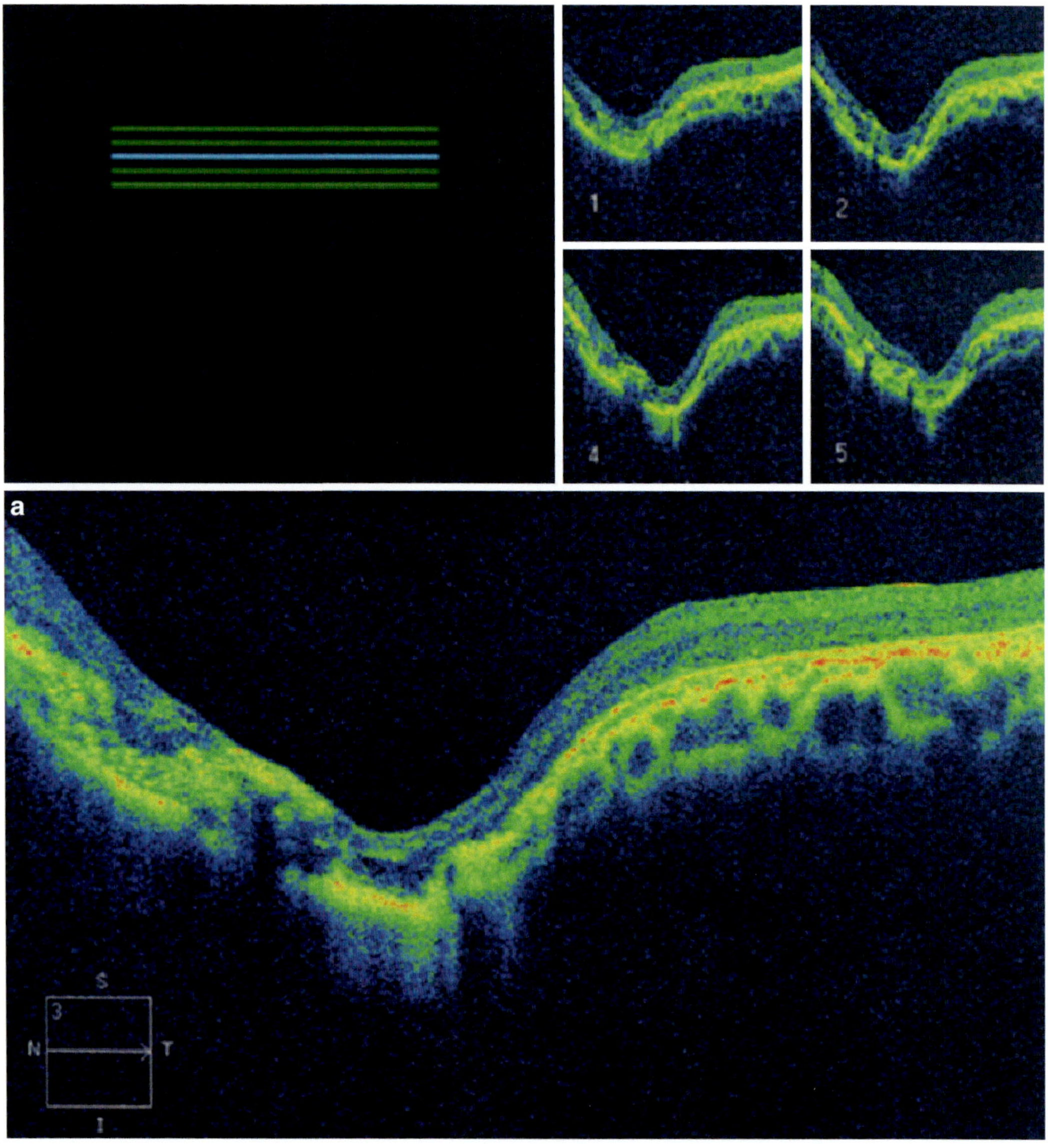

Fig. 22.12 Macular OCT images of both eyes. OCT showed an abnormal and atrophic fovea with the loss of photoreceptor and RPE layers. Panel a: Right eye. Panel b: Left eye (Note: The examination was affected by the patient's poor bilateral visual acuity and fixation)

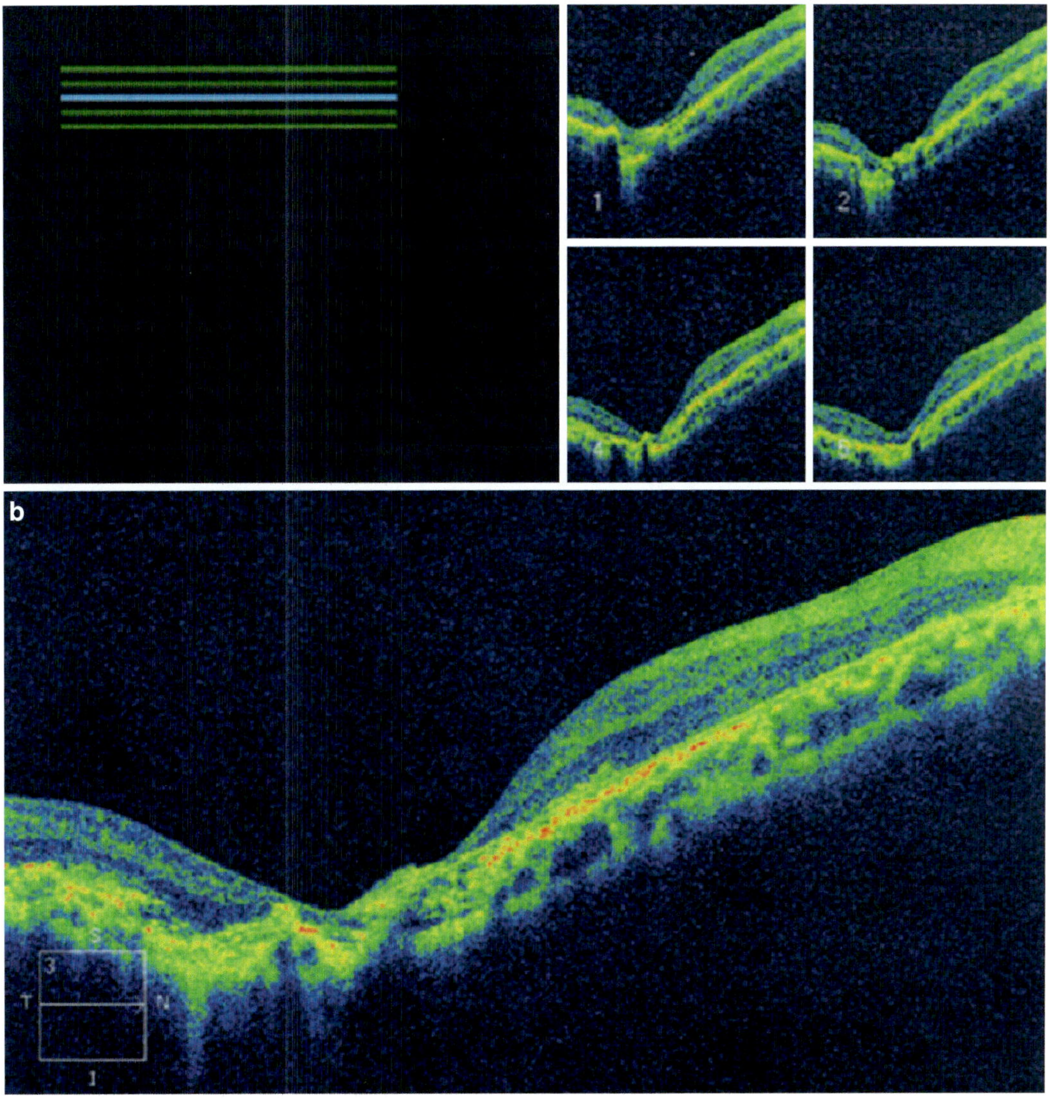

Fig. 22.12 (continued)

mutations are associated with the spectrum of retinal degenerative diseases that follow Mendelian inheritance patterns. Relevant gene therapy research has made big progresses with the continuous deepening of the research on the functions of this gene (including its mutations) in recent years [2, 3]. The introduction of its wild type to add a protein function is expected to restore certain visual acuity of the patient because nearly all of the ABCA4-related diseases are inherited in a recessive manner and caused by homozygous mutation. Meanwhile, the retinal cell degenerations in these diseases are comparatively slow, which creates opportunities for intervention with a gene therapy. What's worth expecting is that subretinal injection of wild-type ABCA4 expression vector mediated by lentivirus has entered the clinical trial stage, and other vectors, such as adeno-associated virus, adenovirus, etc., are also being studied. This disease mainly involves the macula, and therefore, an effective therapeutic concentration at the focal area can be easily reached by subretinal injection of relevant vectors. These research findings have made the

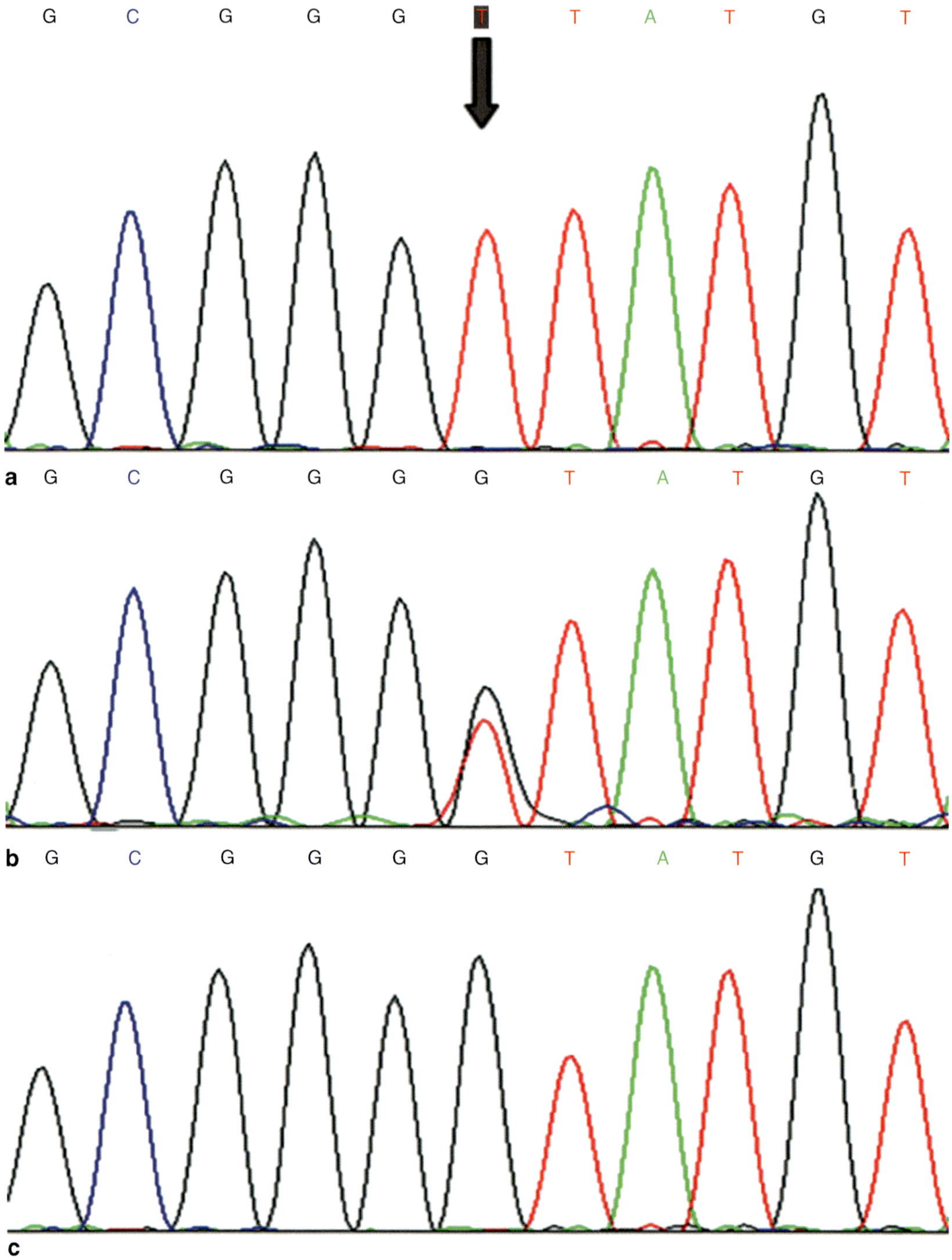

Fig. 22.13 Sequencing printouts for the ABCA4 gene. Homozygous c.4773 + 1g > t mutation in the first position of intron 33. Panel a: The patient harbored a homozygous mutation. Panel b: The father/mother harbored a heterozygous mutation. Panel c: The younger brother had no such mutation

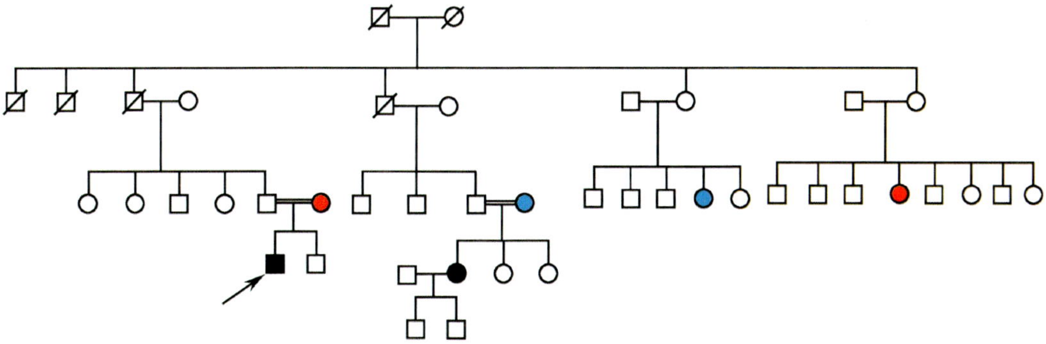

Fig. 22.14 The pedigree chart of Stargardt disease

gene therapies for Stargardt disease and other ABCA4-related diseases no longer far away from us but just around the corner.

It should be noted that the patient was a descendant of consanguineous marriage in two of the three cases in this section, and there was another patient whose parents had a consanguineous marriage in the pedigree presented in case 3. Consanguineous marriage can still be found now and then in the long-term molecular genetic research carried out by the author; therefore, it's still very important to strengthen the education on healthy marriage and family planning.

References

1. Walia S, Fishman GA. Natural history of phenotypic changes in Stargardt macular dystrophy. Ophthalmic Genet. 2009;30(2):63–8.
2. Riveiro-Alvarez R, Lopez-Martinez M-A, Zernant J, et al. Outcome of ABCA4 disease-associated alleles in autosomal recessive retinal dystrophies: retrospective analysis in 420 Spanish families. Ophthalmology. 2013;120(11):2332–7.
3. Auricchio A, Trapani I, Allikmets R. Gene therapy of ABCA4-associated diseases. Cold Spring Harb Perspect Med. 2015;5(5):a017301.

23 Syphilis: The "Great Imitator"

Ning Fan, Xuyang Liu, and Jiantao Wang

Syphilis is a chronic sexually transmitted disease caused by *Treponema pallidum*. It can invade any structure of the eyes, and its clinical symptoms are complicated and variable. The manifestations of the disease can be similar with those of many other diseases, and therefore it's usually called "the great imitator" [1]. The disease can lead to various damages to the visual field, and careful differentiations are required. Three syphilis cases are introduced in this section, and they are special cases with different fundus manifestations and visual field impairments.

23.1 Case 1

23.1.1 Case Presentation

A 39-year-old female patient presented with painless vision loss in the left eye for 2 weeks. No significant trigger had been found before disease onset. Distorted vision, shadow in the vision, and systemic symptoms were denied. Histories of previous eye diseases, trauma, and familial diseases were denied.

On examination, the best corrected visual acuity (BCVA) was 20/20 OD and 20/40 OS. The intraocular pressure (IOP) was 12 mmHg OD and 13 mmHg OS. Remarkable findings of the anterior segment and fundus examinations of the left eye include positive RAPD, disc edema and hemorrhage, intraretinal hemorrhage with nerve fiber layer infarct, Roth spots, and venous congestion (Fig. 23.1). No abnormality was detected in the examinations of the anterior and posterior segments of the right eye.

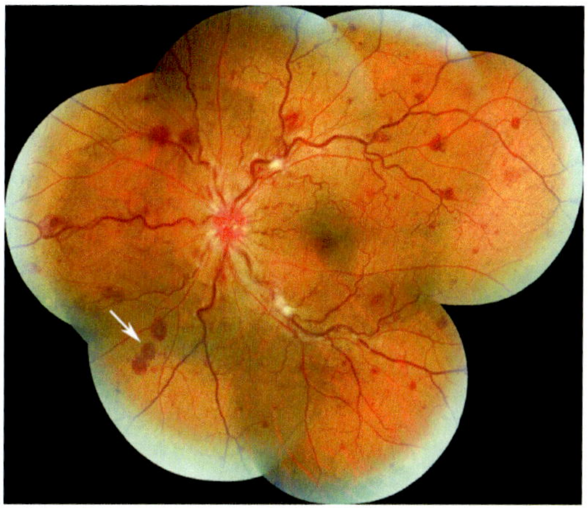

Fig. 23.1 Montage images of fundus photograph. Disc edema and hemorrhage, intraretinal hemorrhage with nerve fiber layer infarct, Roth spots (white arrow), and venous congestion were present in the left eye

N. Fan · J. Wang (✉)
Shenzhen Eye Hospital, Shenzhen University, Shenzhen, China

X. Liu
Xiamen Eye Center of Xiamen University, Xiamen, China

Shenzhen Eye Hospital, Shenzhen University, Shenzhen, China

N. Wang et al. (eds.), *Optic Disorders and Visual Field*, Advances in Visual Science and Eye Diseases 2, https://doi.org/10.1007/978-981-13-2502-1_23

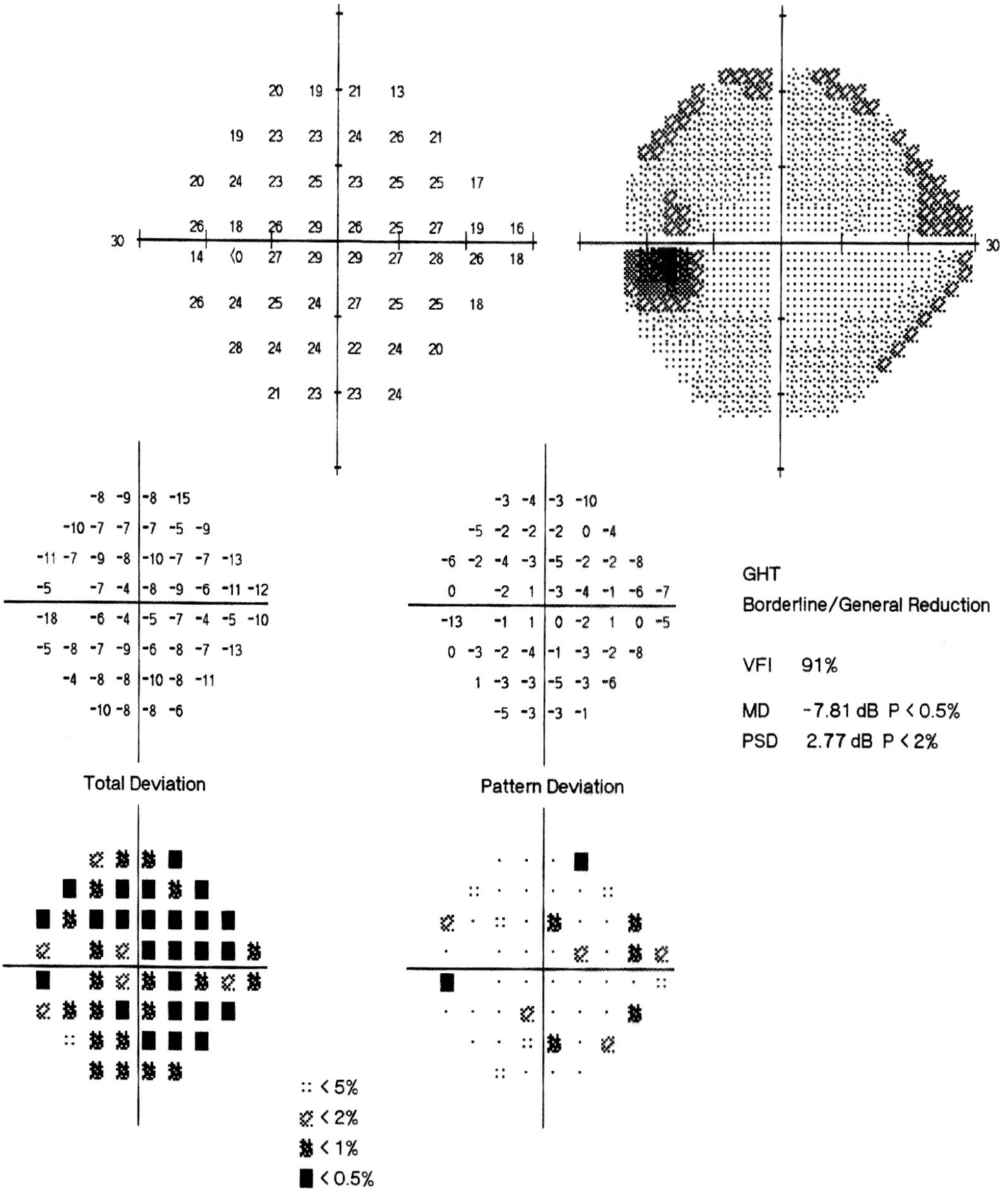

Fig. 23.2 Humphrey visual field analysis printout for the left eye. Diffuse light sensitivity decrease accompanied by enlargement of the blind spot could be found

Visual field examination showed generalized sensitivity decrease accompanied by enlargement of the blind spot in the left eye (Fig. 23.2). The visual field of the right eye was normal.

Pattern visual evoked potential (P-VEP) examination demonstrated normal latency and significantly reduced (compared with the right eye) amplitude of the P100 wave in the left eye. The latency and amplitude of the P100 wave were both normal in the right eye (Fig. 23.3).

Fundus fluorescein angiography (FFA) revealed that the normal filling of the retinal arteries in the left eye at the early stage of the angiography. Significant fluorescein leakage from the retinal vessels, especially the veins, could be observed at the late stage of the angiography (Fig. 23.4).

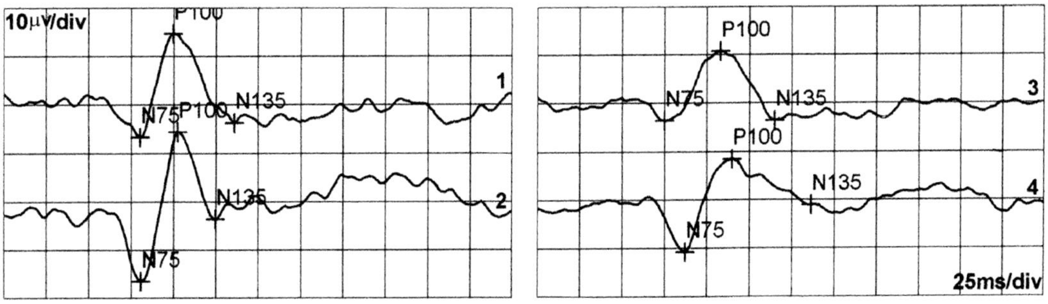

Channel	N75 [ms]	P100 [ms]	N135 [ms]	N75-P100	P100-N135
1 R-1 1,0	80	100	136	21.4µV	18.4µV
3 L-1 1,0	75	108	140	14.4µV	14.4µV
2 R-1 0,15	81	103	125	30.9µV	18µV
4 L-1 0,15	87	115	161	19.2µV	9.61µV
Normals	-	90-117-90-117	-	-	-

Channel	Stimulus	Ampl., Range, Filter
1 R-1 1,0	MON Patt. Rev. CB, 1?Full Field, Ctr:97% 1.5Hz, Avg:25	1, +/-100µV 1-50Hz
2 R-1 0,15	MON Patt. Rev. CB, 0?5' Full Field, Ctr:97% 1.5Hz, Avg:29	1, +/-100µV 1-50Hz
3 L-1 1,0	MON Patt. Rev. CB, 1?Full Field, Ctr:97% 1.5Hz, Avg:29	1, +/-100µV 1-50Hz
4 L-1 0,15	MON Patt. Rev. CB, 0?5' Full Field, Ctr:97% 1.5Hz, Avg:32	1, +/-100µV 1-50Hz

Fig. 23.3 P-VEP printouts. The latency and amplitude of the P100 wave were both normal in the right eye. Normal latency and significantly reduced (compared with the right eye) amplitude of the P100 wave were observed in the left eye

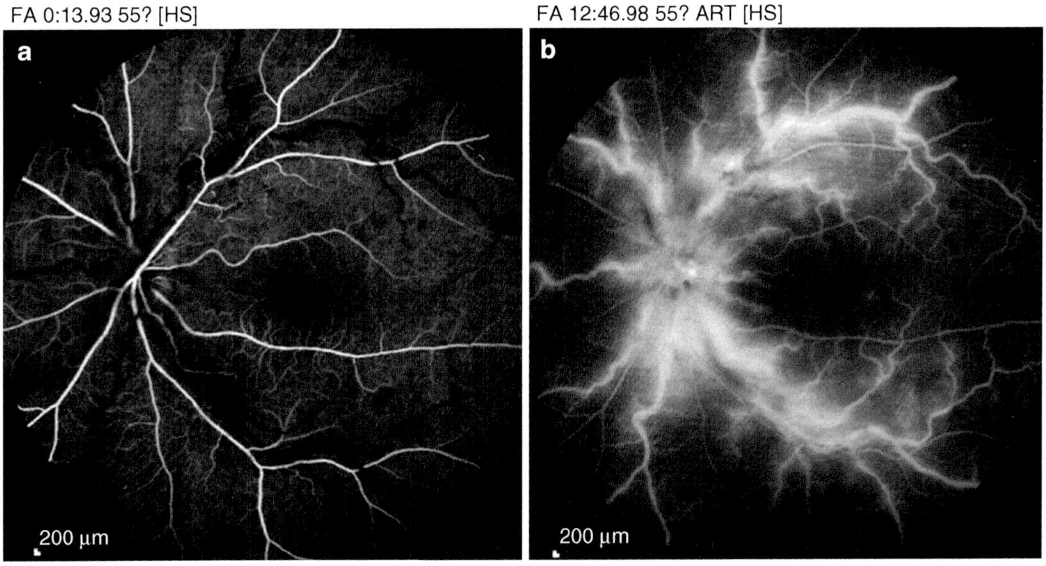

Fig. 23.4 FFA printouts for the left eye. Panel a: The filling of the retinal arteries was fine at the early stage of the angiography. Panel b: Significant fluorescein leakage from the retinal vessels, especially the veins, could be observed at the late stage of the angiography

Serological tests for syphilis (TP-Ab, TPPA, TRUST) showed positive results and were all indicative of infectivity.

Blood system and immune parameters tests showed that erythrocyte sedimentation rate (ESR), C-reactive protein (CRP), anti-neutrophil cytoplasmic antibodies (ANCA), and autoantibody to nuclear antigen (ANA) were normal.

No abnormality was observed in the color ultrasound examinations of the abdomen and the heart.

23.1.2 Final Diagnosis

The final diagnosis was concomitant syphilitic retinal vasculitis and optic neuritis in the left eye.

Oral prednisone in addition to antisyphilitic treatment was given to the patient. The patient's visual acuity of the left eye increased and the symptoms were improved.

23.1.3 Case Review

The patient's chief complaint was moderate unilateral vision loss. Retinopathy and optic neuropathy were observed after the examinations. The main manifestation of retinopathy found in the patient was vasculitis: widely spread intraretinal hemorrhage with Roth spots and venous congestion could be observed. FFA revealed significant vascular leakage (mainly the veins). Due to the vasculitis, edema and hemorrhage of retina resulted after the blood-retinal barrier was damaged and the plasma and blood cells exuded out of the blood vessels. The occlusion of the capillary vessels and arterioles led to impaired axoplasmic flow and microinfarction (nerve fiber layer infarct). Roth spots, which were oval retinal hemorrhage spots with a white center and usually found in subacute infective myoendocarditis and blood system-related diseases, were also found in the patient. The Roth spots might be the result of capillaritis or microembolism. The abovementioned diseases were excluded for the patient, and syphilitic retinal vasculitis could explain the signs. The specific mechanism will be illustrated in the discussion part. The main manifestations of optic neuritis found in the patient were edema, hemorrhage, and effusion in the optic disc. Positive RAPD, enlargement of the blind spot, and amplitude reduction of the P100 wave were shown. Unilateral retinal vasculitis, optic neuritis, rare Roth spots, etc. found in the patient reflect the diversity of syphilis, the great imitator, in lesion position and manifestation.

23.2 Case 2

23.2.1 Case Presentation

A 53-year-old male patient presented with progressive and painless vision loss in both eyes for 8 months. There were no accompanying red eyes or eye pain. Night blindness was denied, and histories of previous eye diseases, trauma, and familial diseases were denied.

On examination, the BCVA was 20/40 OD and light perception OS. Light projection of the left eye was accurate. The IOP was normal in both eyes. RAPD was positive and pupil light reflex was blunt in the left eye. In both eyes, the lens was opaque, lacquer cracks on the fundus were revealed, a wax yellow optic disc with a clear boundary and narrowed retinal arteries were seen, the C/D ratio was about 0.4, and the arteriolar-venular ratio was about 1:3. No significant effusion or hemorrhage or osteocyte-like pigmentation was revealed in either eye (Fig. 23.5).

Visual field examination showed that there remained only a superior central tubular visual field in the right eye (Fig. 23.6). The visual acuity of the left eye was too poor for the routine visual field examination.

Optical coherence tomography (OCT) revealed significant and diffuse thinning of the peripapillary retinal nerve fiber layer (RNFL) and structure distortion in the photoreceptor and the RPE layers at the macula in the right eye (Fig. 23.7).

Flash visual evoked potential (F-VEP) examination showed moderate to severe F-VEP abnormalities in both eyes (Fig. 23.8).

The VEP examination revealed latency delay and mild reduction of amplitude for all F-VEP waveforms at low frequencies. Normal latency and serious reduction of amplitude were shown for all F-VEP waveforms at high frequencies.

Full-field electroretinography (ERG) showed that the light and dark adaptions of the right eye were moderately abnormal. The dark adaption of the left eye showed mild abnormality (Fig. 23.9).

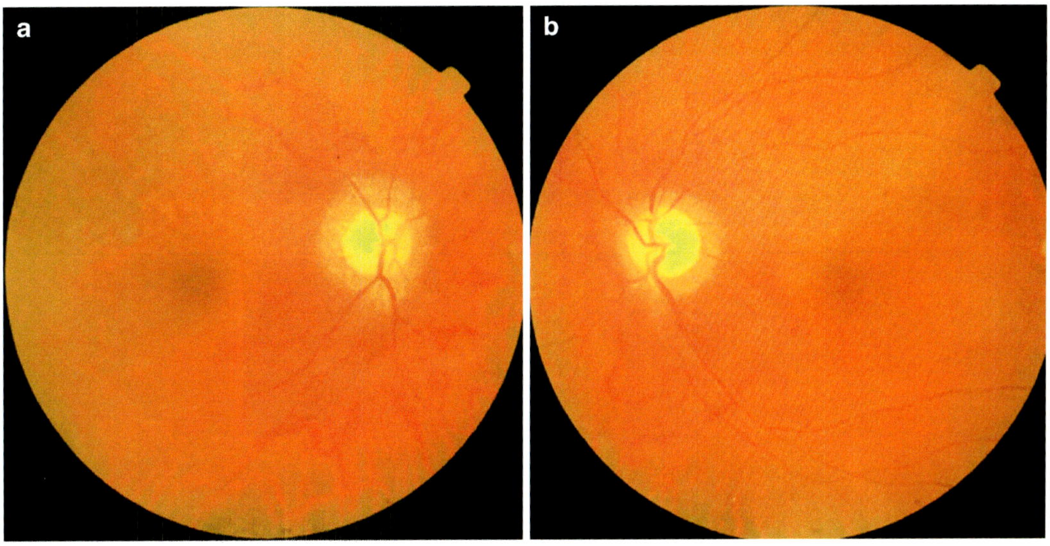

Fig. 23.5 Fundus photographs. The optic disc was wax yellow in color and the arteries were narrow in both eyes. Panel a: Right eye. Panel b: Left eye (Note: Imaging quality was affected by the lens opacity found in both eyes)

Autofluorescence examination showed sheet-like hyperfluorescence in the posterior pole of the right eye (Fig. 23.10); the left eye was normal.

FFA disclosed delayed filling and thinning of the retinal arteries and veins and persistent hyperfluorescence with a salt-and-pepper appearance in both eyes. Hypofluorescence in the optic disc was shown at the early stage, and its edge staining was seen at the late stage in both eyes (Fig. 23.11).

The serological syphilis tests (TP-Ab, TPPA, TRUST) all showed positive results and suggested infectivity. Antisyphilitic treatment was carried out after the patient was transferred to the department of infectious disease, but the reexamination of bilateral visual function showed no significant improvement.

23.2.2 Final Diagnosis

The final diagnosis was bilateral syphilitic neuroretinopathy.

23.2.3 Case Review

Different from the situation in the above case, the visual function damages resulting from the bilateral syphilitic neuroretinopathy were very serious in this case. The right eye only had a tubular visual field, and the visual acuity of the left eye was only light perception. Optic nerve atrophies were shown in both eyes. A wax yellow optic disc and thinning of the arteries were seen in both eyes. The FFA revealed delayed filling and thinning of the arteries and veins and persistent hyperfluorescences with a salt-and-pepper appearance in both eyes. The findings were similar to the manifestations of primary retinal pigmentary degeneration. But the patient's fundi were not observed with bone spicule-like pigmentation, histories of night blindness and familial disease were denied by the patient, and the full-field ERG results didn't support the diagnosis of primary retinal pigmentary degeneration. The optic neuropathy and retinopathy caused by syphilis found in the patient in this case had lasted for a long time, and they should be differentiated from the bilateral optic nerve atrophy and primary retinal pigmentary degeneration caused by other reasons (such as toxicosis, ischemia, compression, etc.). Serum etiology is helpful for the definitive diagnosis of this disease. The patient's visual function showed no improvement after antisyphilitic treatment, which suggests the importance of early intervention for a good prognosis.

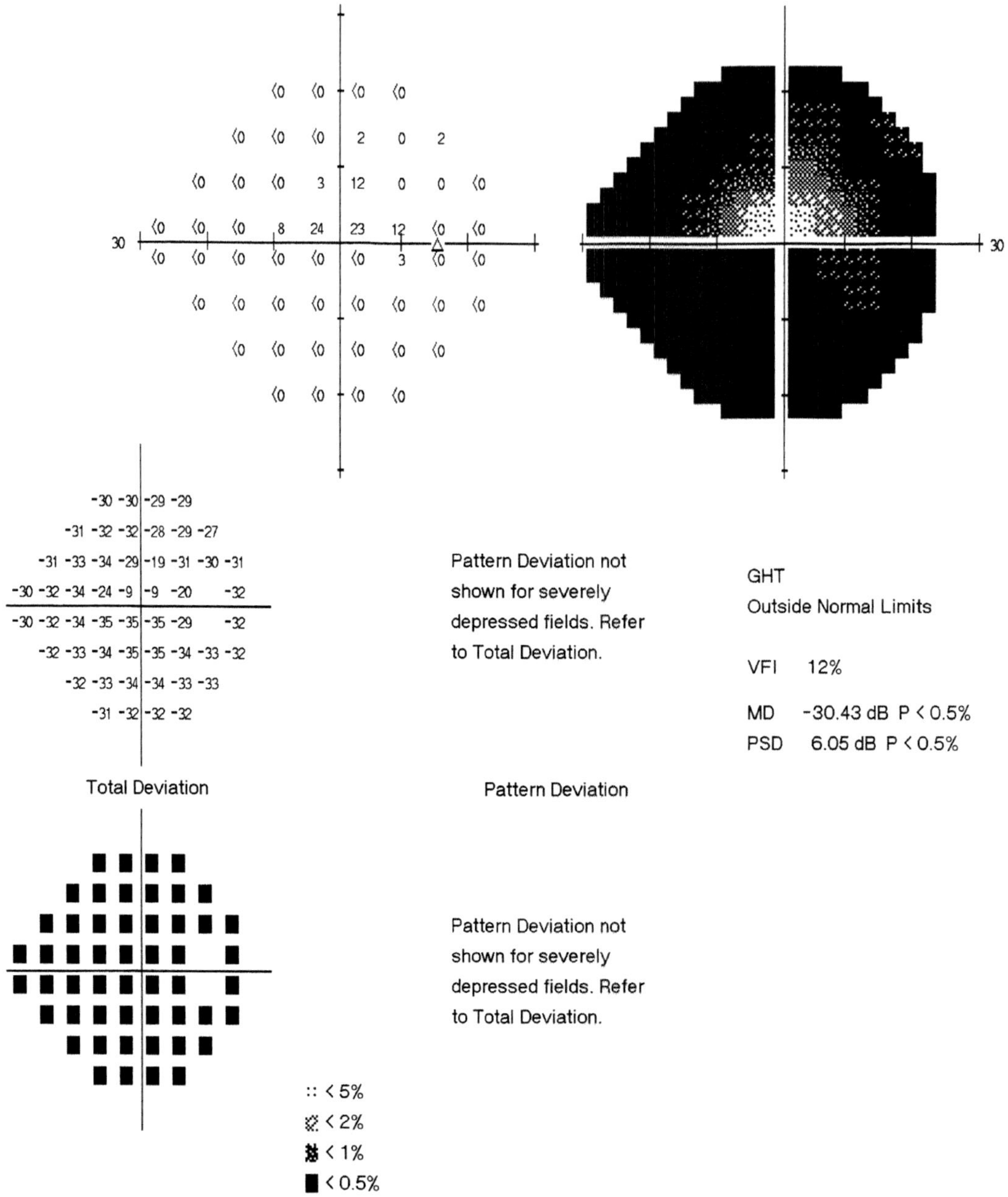

Fig. 23.6 Humphrey visual field analysis printout for the right eye. It could be seen that there remained only a superior central tubular visual field in the right eye

23.3 Case 3

23.3.1 Case Presentation

A 72-year-old male patient presented with sudden sluggishness in action and speech for 1 month and blindness in the left eye for 1 week without any significant trigger. No limb motion disorder was present. He had been diagnosed with cerebral infarction in the department of neurology at another hospital after head MR. The symptoms showed no alleviation after anticoagulation and neuro-nutrition treatments. His left eye became blind suddenly 1 week before this presentation, and the symptom of sluggishness in action and speech showed no aggravation. No headache, dizziness, or limb motion disorder had been observed. Histories of previous eye diseases, trauma, and familial diseases were denied. The patient had a history of diabetes and hypertension. The disease control was fine by oral medications.

On examination, the BCVA was 20/125 OD and 20/2000 OS. Light projection was accurate in both eyes. The IOP was normal in both eyes. Slit-lamp examination of his anterior segments revealed that the corneas were transparent, the anterior chambers were clear, the pupils were round with diameters of 2.5 mm and 2.0 mm in the right and left eyes, respectively, direct pupil light reflex was blunt in both eyes (pupil dilation by

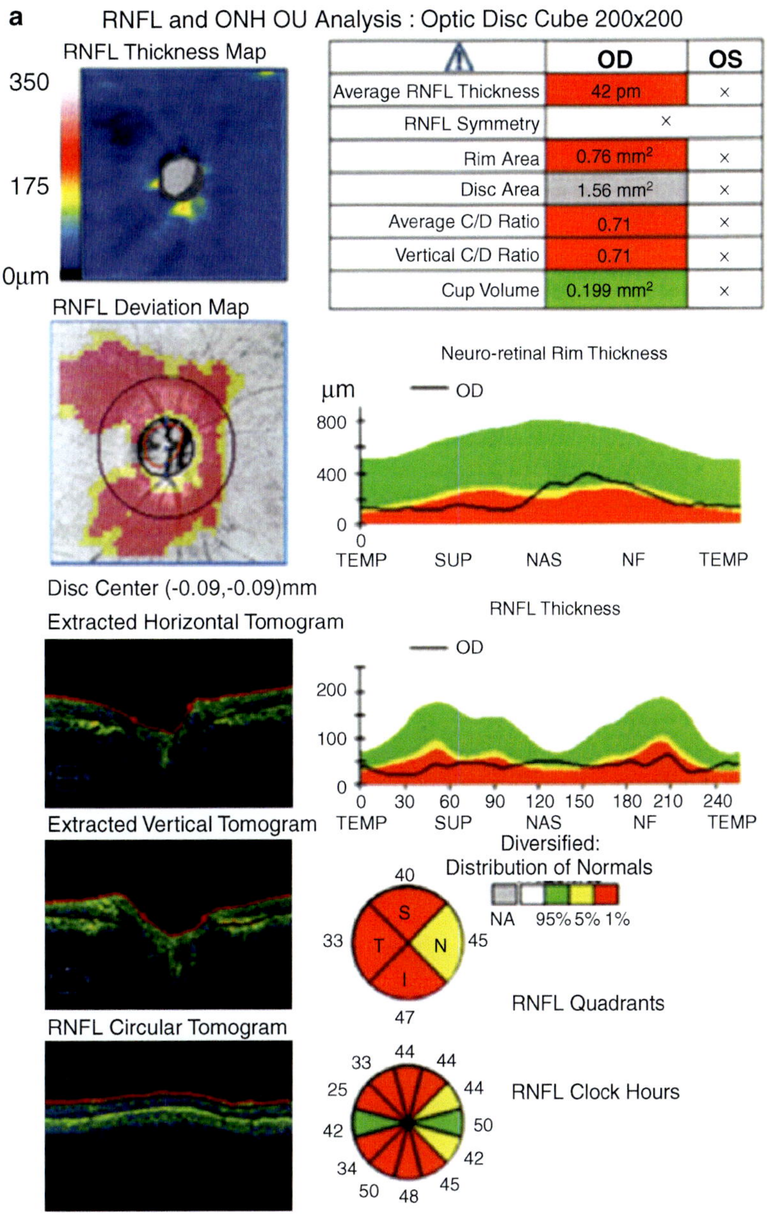

Fig. 23.7 RNFL thickness measurement and OCT scanning of the macula for the right eye. Panel a: Significant thinning of the peripapillary RNFL was seen. Panel b: Structure distortion in the photoreceptor and the RPE layers was present at the macula

Fig. 23.7 (continued)

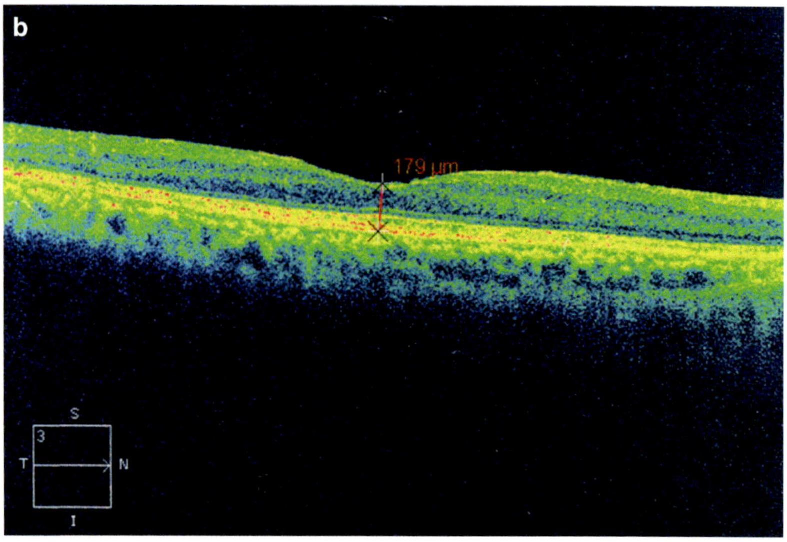

Flash-VEP 1,2 Hz

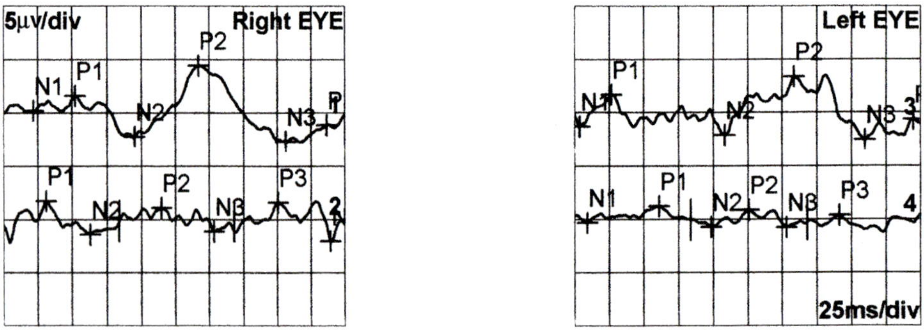

Channel	N1 [ms]	P1 [ms]	N2 [ms]	P2 [ms]	N3 [ms]	P3 [ms]	N1-P1	N2-P2	N3-P3
1 R-1 1,2 Hz	22	52	95	142	207	237	1.44µV	6.65µV	1.57µV
3 L-1 1,2 Hz	4	27	109	159	210	245	3.02µV	5.47µV	1.9µV
2 R-1 12 Hz	240	31	63	115	154	201	3.78µV	2.46µV	2.73µV
4 L-1 12 Hz	9	61	99	126	154	192	1.53µV	1.61µV	1.11µV
Normals	-	-	-	-	-	-	-	-	-

Channel	Stimulus	Ampl., Range, Filter
1 R-1 1,2 Hz	GF LED Flash 0dB (2,00 cds/m? 1.199Hz, Avg:65	1, +/-100µV 0.5-50Hz
2 R-1 12 Hz	GF LED Flash 0dB (2,00 cds/m? 11.905Hz, Avg:100	1, +/-100µV 0.5-50Hz
3 L-1 1,2 Hz	GF LED Flash 0dB (2,00 cds/m? 1.199Hz, Avg:71	1, +/-100µV 0.5-50Hz
4 L-1 12 Hz	GF LED Flash 0dB (2,00 cds/m? 11.905Hz, Avg:100	1, +/-100µV 0.5-50Hz

Fig. 23.8 VEP examination printouts of both eyes. The VEP examination revealed latency delay and mild reduction of amplitude for all F-VEP waveforms at low frequencies. Normal latency and serious reduction of amplitude were shown for all F-VEP waveforms at high frequencies

compound tropicamide was difficult), the lenses were opaque, and the vitreous was mildly opaque in both eyes. Fundus examination showed that the optic disc was pink in color with a clear boundary, the C/D ratio was about 0.6, the arteriolar-venular ratio was about 1:2, and the blood vessels were slightly tortuous in the right eye; disc hemorrhage and edema could be found, the arteriolar-venular ratio was about 1:2, and the blood vessels were slightly tortuous in the left eye (Fig. 23.12).

Visual field examination demonstrated diffuse light sensitivity reduction and a dominant tempo-

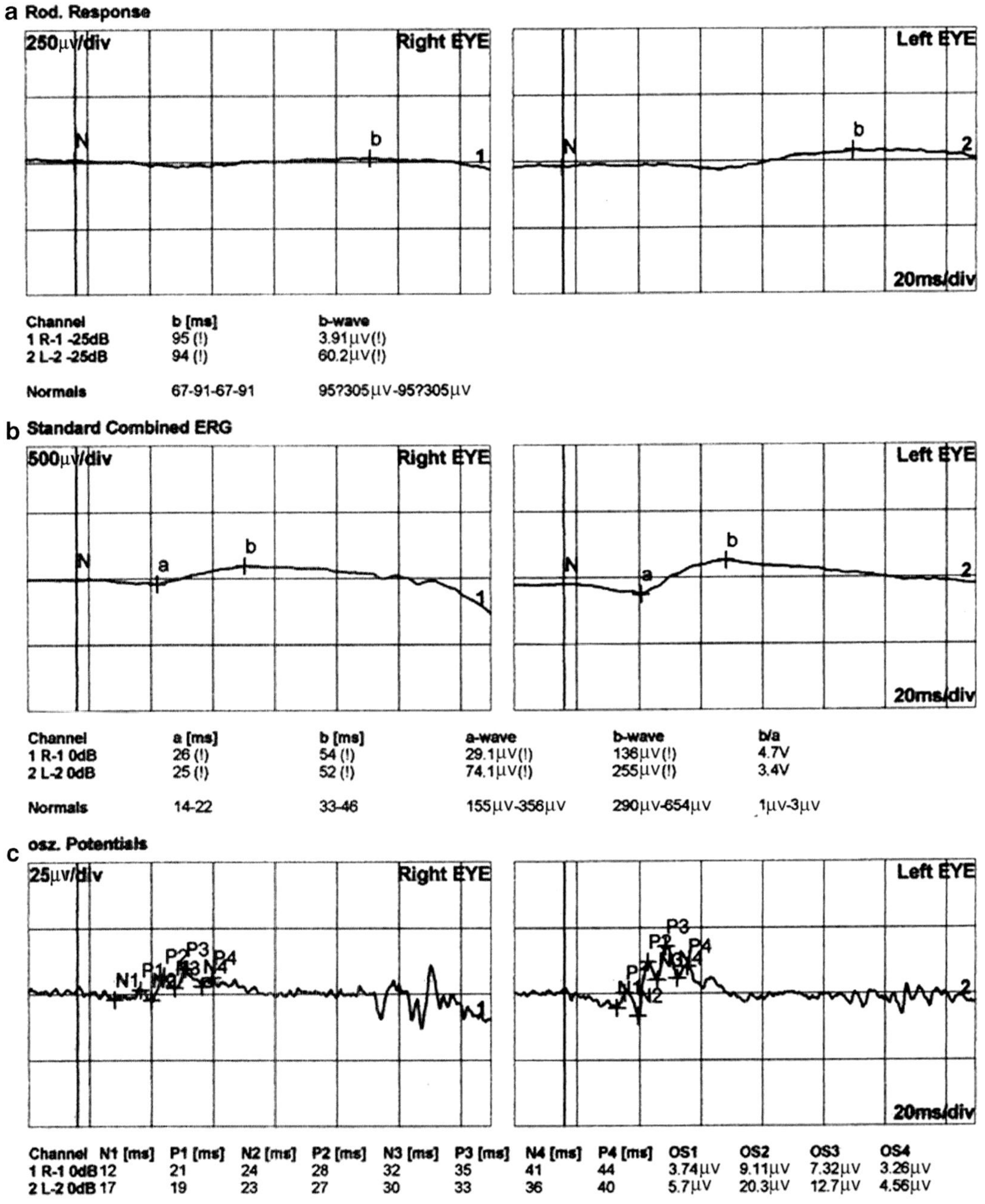

Fig. 23.9 Full-field ERG printouts of both eyes. Panel a: Rod cell response under a scotopic condition. Mild delay of the b-wave latency was seen in both eyes, and reduced b-wave amplitude was seen in the right eye. Panel b: Mixed rod-cone responses under a scotopic condition. Delayed latency and reduced amplitude were seen for the a, b-waves in both eyes, and amplitude reduction was more serious in the right eye. Panel c: Oscillatory potentials (OPs) under a scotopic condition. Reduced number of groups and significant amplitude reduction were shown for OPs waves in both eyes. Panel d: Cone cell response to a single photopic flash. Slight delay of latency and significant amplitude reduction were observed for the a, b-waves in the right eye. Figure e: Cone cell response to photopic-flicker stimulation. Amplitude of the b-wave showed reduction in the right eye and was normal in the left eye

d phot. Response

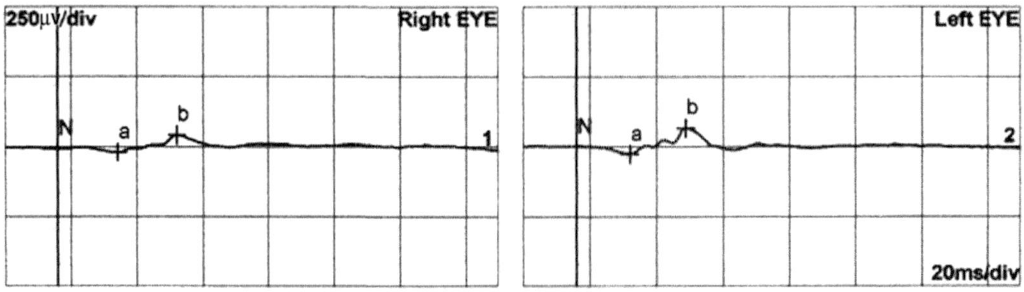

Channel	a [ms]	b [ms]	a-wave	b-wave
1 R-1 0dB	18 (!)	36 (!)	12.4µV(!)	61.5µV(!)
2 L-2 0dB	16 (!)	33	27.8µV	95.2µV(!)
Normals	13-16	29-33	26µV-62µV	103µV-250µV

e 30Hz Flicker

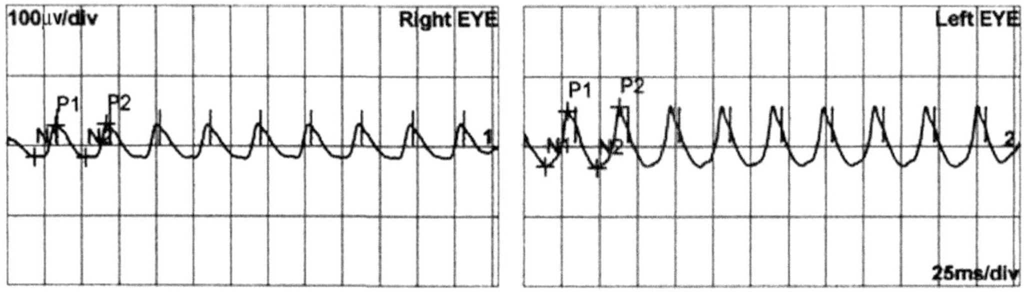

Channel	N1 [ms]	P1 [ms]	N2 [ms]	P2 [ms]	N1-P1	N2-P2	30Hz Amp
1 R-1 0dB	19	33 (!)	53	67	45.9µV(!)	48.3µV	21.5µV
2 L-2 0dB	14	29 (!)	48	63	79.5µV	87µV	35.4µV
Normals	-	58-64	-	-	57µV-223µV	-	-

Fig. 23.9 (continued)

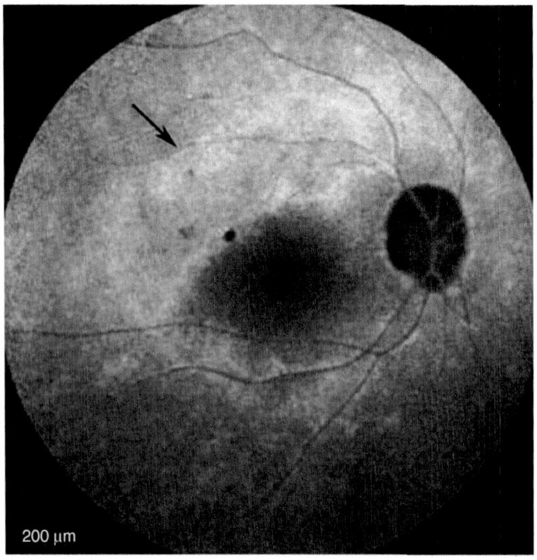

Fig. 23.10 Autofluorescence photograph of the right eye. Sheet-like hyperfluorescence could be observed in the posterior pole of the right eye (black arrow)

ral visual field defect in the right eye (impact of refracting medium opacity) and nearly total blindness in the left eye (poor central vision affected the examination results) (Fig. 23.13).

OCT revealed neuroepithelium edema and detachment at the macula in the left eye (Fig. 23.14). The OCT scanning on the macula of the right eye found no abnormality. The RNFL thickness of the right eye measured by OCT was normal.

FFA showed hypofluorescence of the optic disc at the early stage and uneven hyperfluorescence with unclear boundary of the optic disc at the late stage in the left eye (Fig. 23.15). No abnormalities were detected in the right eye.

Head MRI revealed multiple softening foci in the parietal lobe, temporal lobe, and occipital lobe of the left side and in bilateral cerebellar

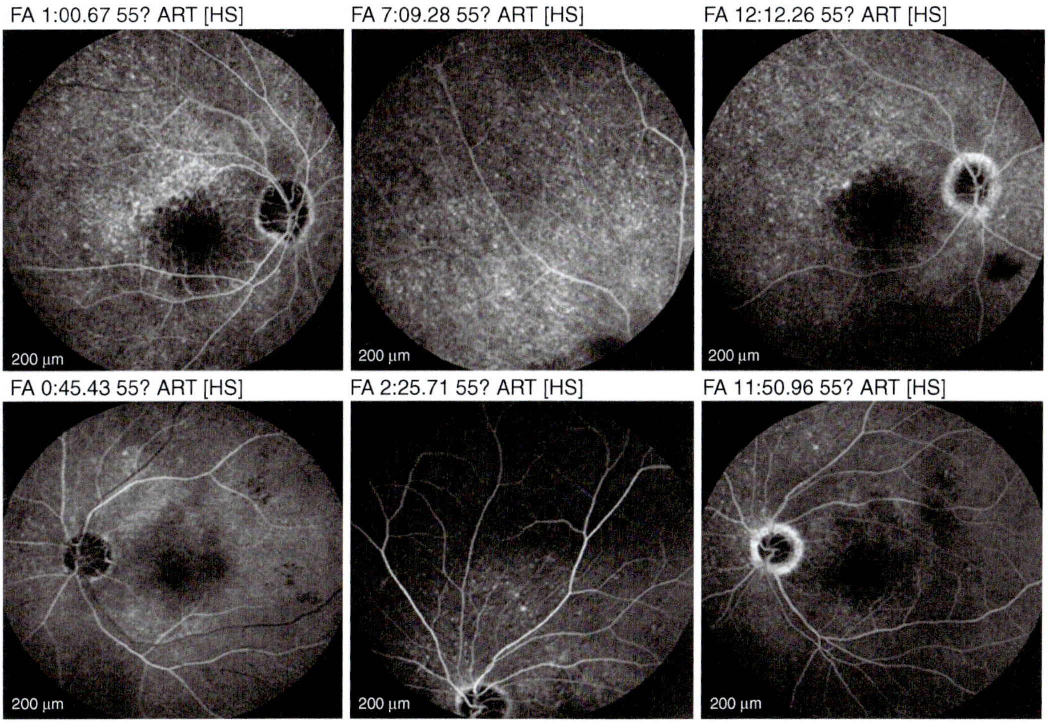

Fig. 23.11 FFA images. FFA disclosed delayed filling and thinning of the retinal arteries and veins and persistent hyperfluorescence with a salt-and-pepper appearance in both eyes. Hypofluorescence in the optic disc was shown at the early stage, and its edge staining was seen at the late stage in both eyes

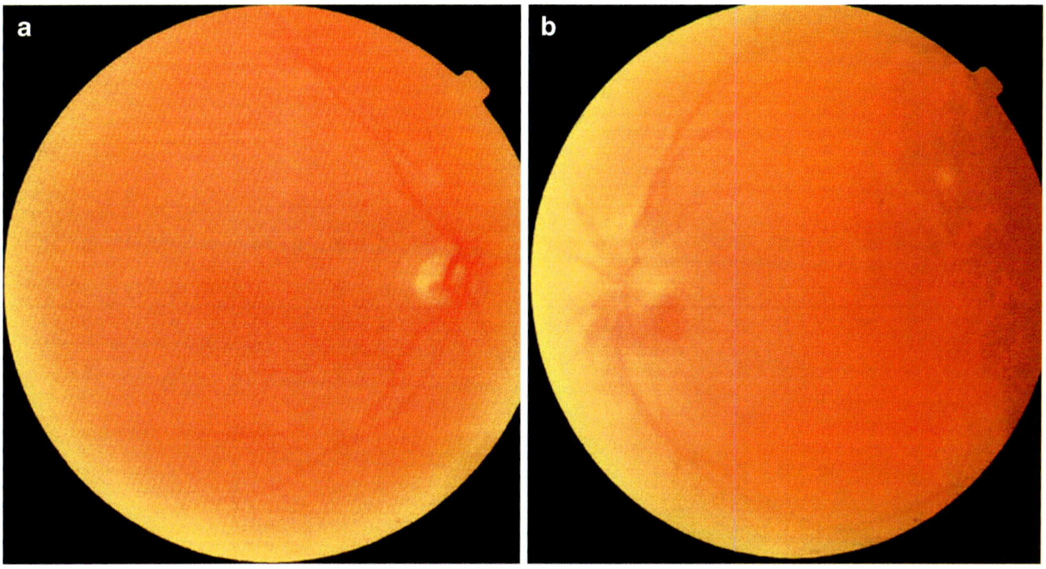

Fig. 23.12 Fundus photographs. Panel a: The optic disc was pink in color with a clear boundary, the C/D ratio was about 0.6, the arteriolar-venular ratio was about 1:2, and the blood vessels were slightly tortuous in the right eye. Panel b: Disc hemorrhage and edema could be found, the arteriolar-venular ratio was about 1:2, and the blood vessels were slightly tortuous in the left eye (imaging quality was affected by the refracting medium opacity)

hemispheres. Multiple lacunar ischemia and infarction foci were shown in both cerebral hemispheres (Fig. 23.16).

Serological syphilis tests (TP-Ab, TPPA, TRUST) all showed positive results and suggested infectivity.

Lumbar puncture showed a cerebrospinal fluid (CSF) pressure of 167 mmH2O (80–180 mmH2O). In the routine CSF tests, Perthes test was positive, the total cell count was 114 × 106/L [(0–8) × 106/L], the WBC count was 80 × 106/L, the proportion of apocytes was 5% and that of monocyte was 76%, *Treponema pallidum* hemagglutination test (TPHA) was positive, and toluidine red unheated serum test (TRUST) for syphilis screening was positive (1:8).

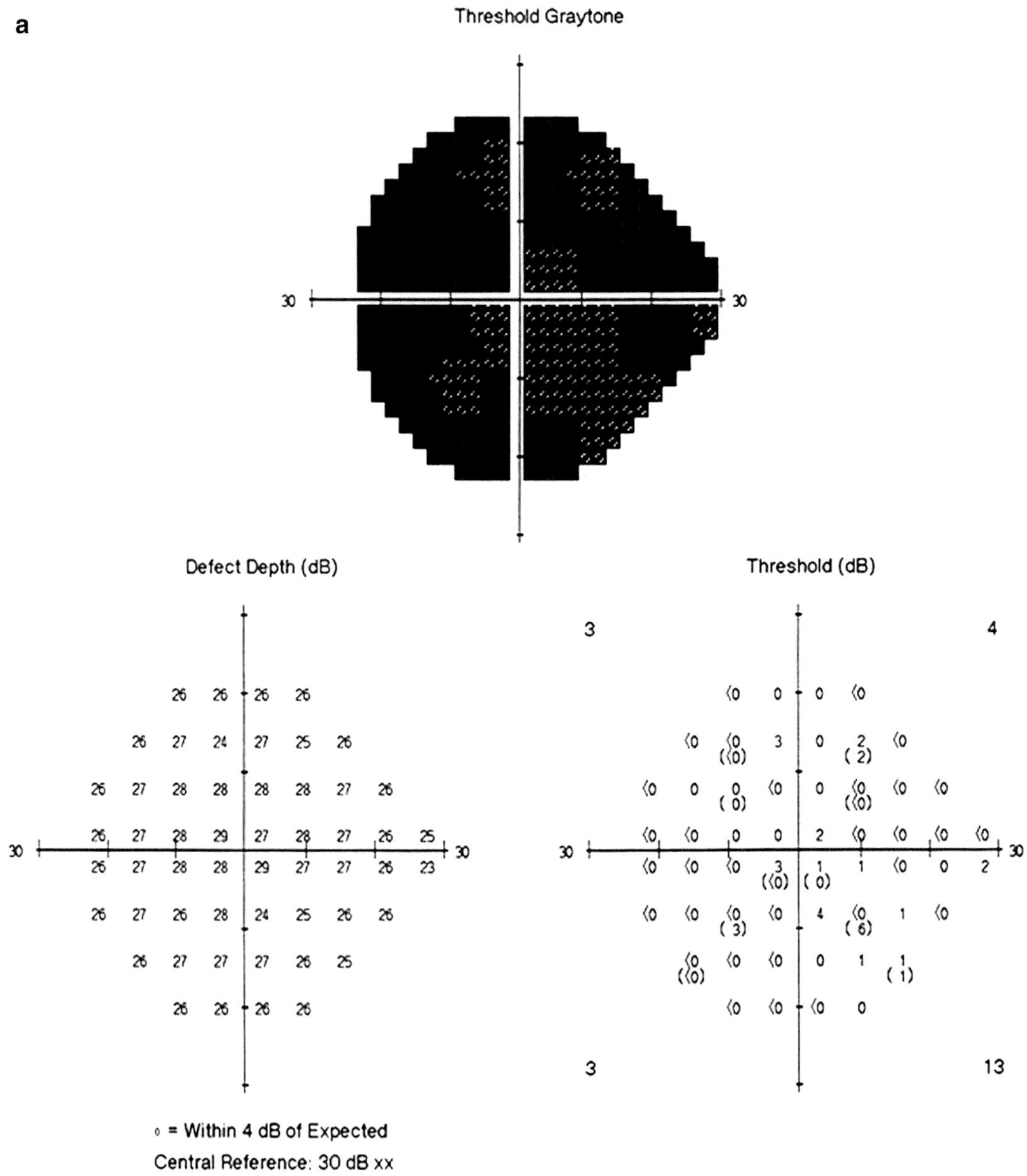

Fig. 23.13 Humphrey visual field analysis printouts. Panel a: Nearly total blindness was shown in the left eye (with a size V target). Panel b: Generalized sensitivity decrease and a dominant temporal visual field defect were shown in the right eye

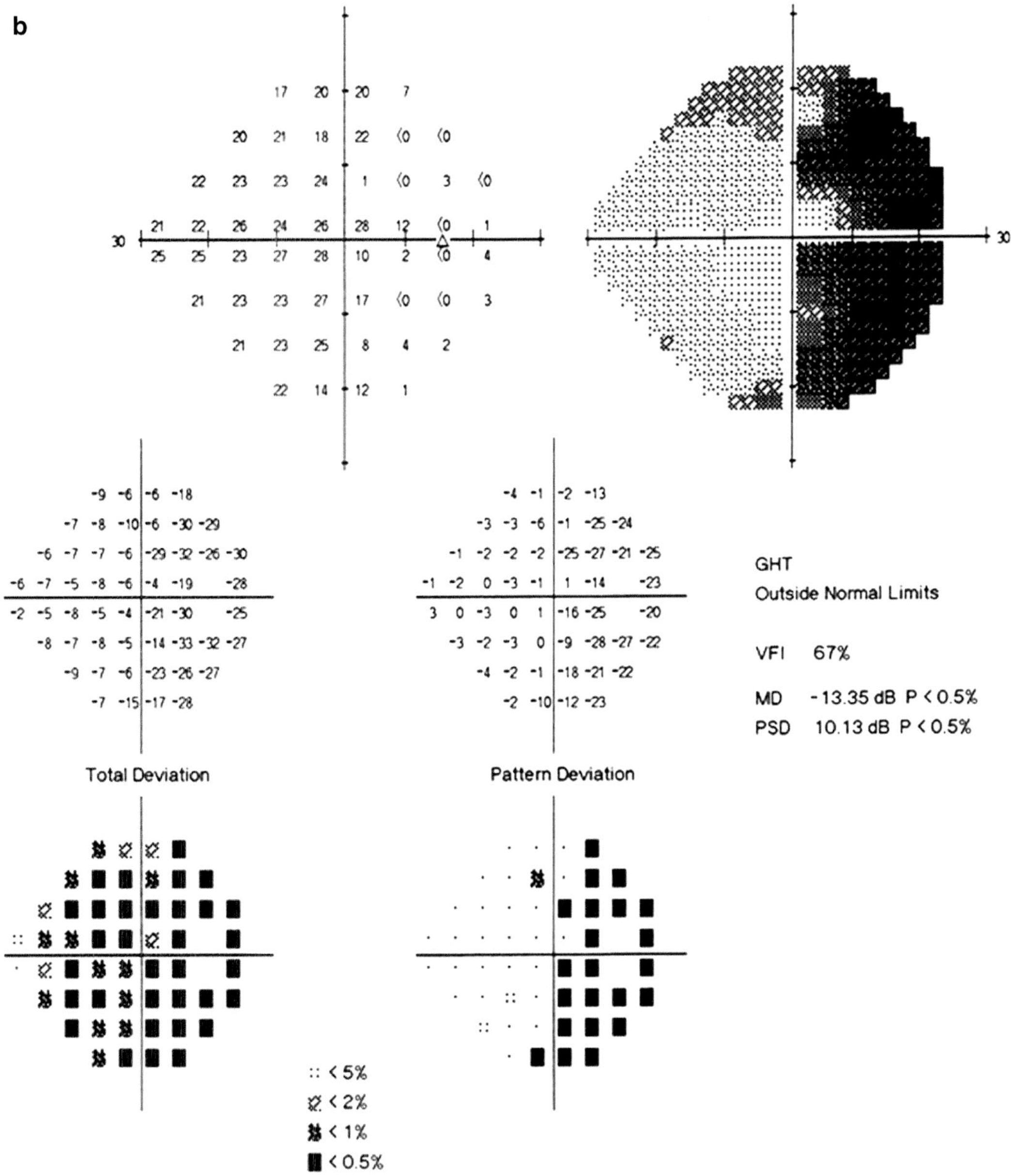

Fig. 23.13 (continued)

23.3.2 Final Diagnosis

The final diagnosis was syphilitic neuroretinopathy and neurosyphilis in the left eye.

Antisyphilitic treatment, oral vascular dilation treatment, and oral neuro-nutrition treatment were carried out. The patient's action and speech showed significant improvement, and bilateral visual functions were also improved after 1 week of treatment.

23.3.3 Case Review

The patient was a senior male, and the initial symptoms were sudden sluggishness in action

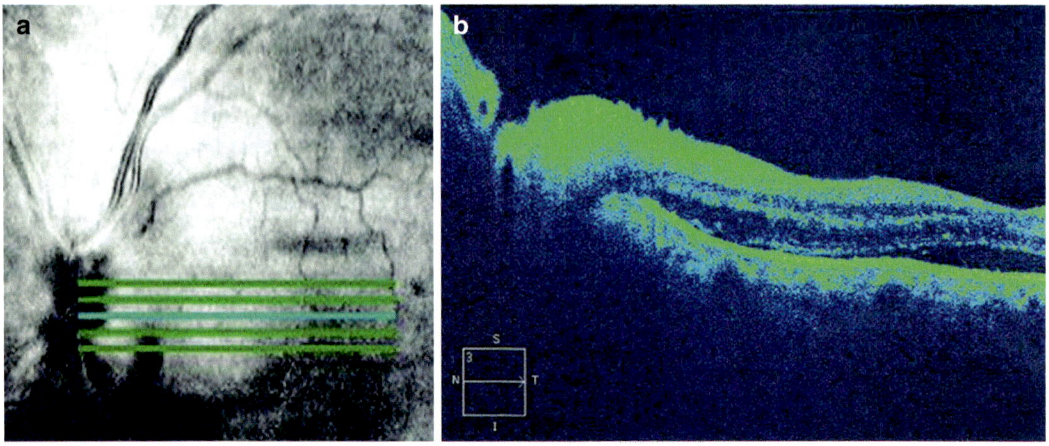

Fig. 23.14 Linear OCT images of the optic disc and macula of the left eye. Panel a: The blue line on the infrared reflectance imaging showed the scan location of the OCT image. Panel b: Neuroepithelium edema and detachment were present in the left eye

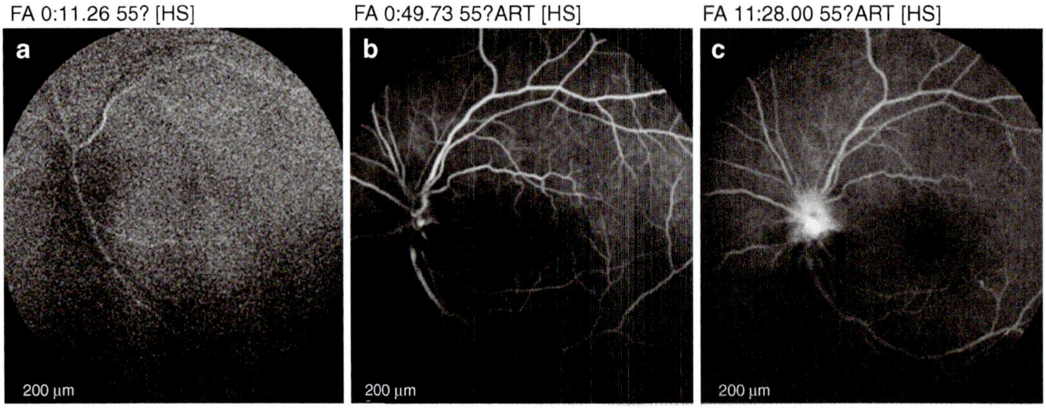

Fig. 23.15 FFA images of the left eye. Panel a, b: Hypofluorescence of the optic disc was seen at the early stage. Panel c: Uneven hyperfluorescence with unclear boundary of the optic disc was seen at the late stage

and speech. The patient was diagnosed with cerebral infarction by the department of neurology of another hospital based on systemic clinical manifestations and head MRI. Symptomatic and supportive treatments were given at that hospital, but the patient's symptoms showed no improvement until the patient's left eye became blind and resorted to the department of ophthalmology. The patient's optic disc of the left eye showed edema and hemorrhage, which were similar to the manifestations of ischemic optic neuropathy. The left eye was nearly total blind and temporal hemianopia was observed in the right eye. Head MRI revealed multiple infarction foci in the parietal lobe, temporal lobe, and occipital lobe of the left side, which could explain the visual field change of bilateral hemianopia. Serum and cerebrospinal fluid tests were then completed. The diagnosis of active neurosyphilis was confirmed. The patient's nervous system symptoms alleviated significantly, and the bilateral vision showed improvement after anti-syphilis treatments.

The neurosyphilis manifestations in this case were occult, and the eye manifestations were similar to those of ischemic optic neuropathy. However, there were still some differences: the

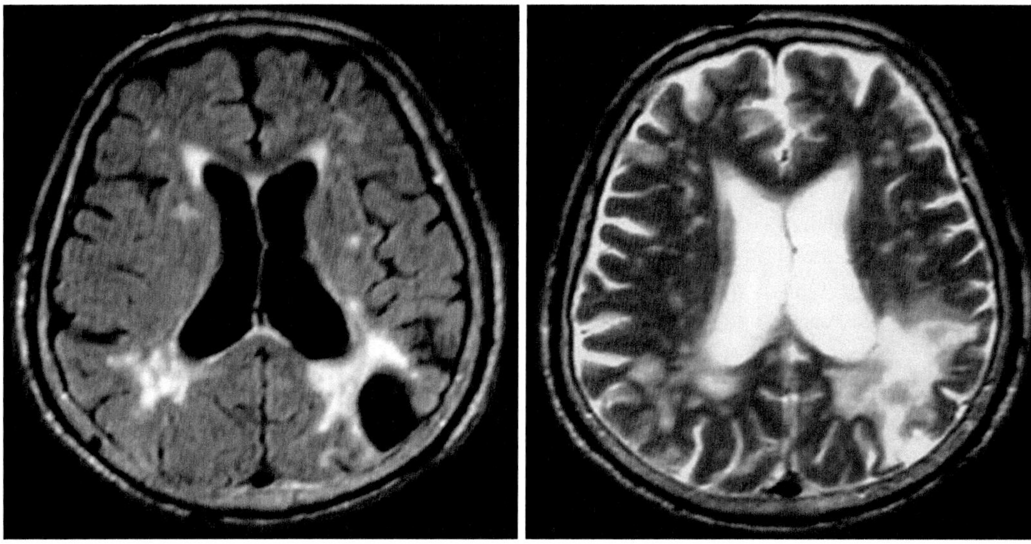

Fig. 23.16 Head MR images. Multiple softening foci were seen in the parietal lobe, temporal lobe, and occipital lobe of the left side and in bilateral cerebellar hemispheres. Multiple lacunar ischemia and infarction foci were shown in bilateral cerebral hemispheres

pupil was small and difficult to be dilated in both eyes; the RAPD was not significant in the left eye; anterior ischemic optic neuropathy (AION) seemed to be present in the left eye, but this was not supported by the fact that the C/D ratio was large and RNFL thickness normal in the right eye; temporal hemianopia was observed in the right eye and nearly total blindness in the left eye, suggesting possible posterior visual pathway lesions; MRI revealed multiple softening foci in the parietal lobe, temporal lobe, and occipital lobe of the left side and in bilateral cerebellar hemispheres; multiple lacunar cerebral ischemia and infarction foci were shown in bilateral cerebral hemispheres. Syphilitic neuroretinopathy and neurosyphilis, whose pathological mechanisms were associated with vascular damages, could explain all the clinical manifestations found in this patient.

23.4 Discussion

Syphilis is a chronic infectious disease caused by *Treponema pallidum*, and it can lead to serious systemic damages. The basic pathological changes caused by syphilis are endangiitis and periangitis. Syphilis invades the skin and mucosa at the early stages, and the tissues and organs of the whole body can be involved at the late stages. It's called neurosyphilis if the nervous system is invaded. Syphilis has three typical clinical stages: Stage I syphilis (occurs in 2–4 weeks after infection), Stage II syphilis (occurs in 7–10 weeks after infection), and Stage III syphilis (occurs in 2 years after infection). Stage I and II syphilis have strong infectivity, while Stage III syphilis has weaker infectivity. Different ocular manifestations, such as conjunctivitis, interstitial keratitis, uveitis, optic neuritis, neuroretinitis, retinal vasculitis, retinal detachment, neurosyphilis, etc., can be found in all the three stages of the syphilis [2–4].

The main pathogenic factor of syphilis is the mucinase on its surface. The *Treponema pallidum* attaches to the vascular wall through mucinase and meanwhile decomposes the mucoitin of the cell membrane on the inner wall of blood vessels to supply its synthesis of pallidum capsule. Mucoitin is an important component of vascular wall framework, so the vascular wall will be damaged after the mucoitin is decomposed by

Treponema pallidum. Vascular occlusion and collapse will be caused, and occlusive arteritis, periarteritis, arterionecrosis, or arterial ulcer will result.

Neurosyphilis is a chronic infectious disease of the central nervous system caused by invasion of *Treponema pallidum* into the meninx and brain parenchyma, and it can be found at any stage of syphilis infection. Only cerebrospinal fluid change will be observed at the initial stage of neurosyphilis, and damages to the meninges, blood vessels, brain, and spinal cord will be found gradually at the later stages. The progression of neurosyphilis was slow, and the symptoms were complicated and diverse. It's easily misdiagnosed.

The mechanisms of eye involvement and vision damages by syphilis are various. It can damage the optic nerves or involve multiple parts, including the retina, choroid, etc. Therefore, various visual field changes, which are related to the involved parts and the severity of involvement, can be observed, but none of them has specificity.

Syphilis infection should be considered when some specious nontypical intraocular inflammations are found clinically.

References

1. Davis JL. Ocular syphilis. Curr Opin Ophthalmol. 2014;25(6):513–8.
2. Balaskas K, Sergentanis TN, Giulieri S, et al. Fluorescein and indocyanine-green angiography in ocular syphilis: an exploratory study. Graefes Arch Clin Exp Ophthalmol. 2012;250(5):721–30.
3. Shen J, Feng L, Li Y. Ocular syphilis: an alarming infectious eye disease. Int J Clin Exp Med. 2015;8(5):7770–7.
4. Moradi A, Salek S, Daniel E, et al. Clinical features and incidence rates of ocular complications in patients with ocular syphilis. Am J Ophthalmol. 2015;159(2):334–43.

24 "With the Skin Gone, to What Can the Hair Attach Itself": When Optic Nerve Atrophy Occurs, What Will Happen to the Medullated Fibers?

Ning Fan, Xuyang Liu, and Jiantao Wang

Myelinated retinal nerve fiber layers (MRNFLs) are caused by myelinated nerve fibers that grow beyond the lamina cribrosa and appear on the surface of the optic disc and/or retina due to dysplasia of optic nerve fiber sheaths. They can be localized or generalized. The visual field and visual acuity may be damaged in serious cases. MRNFLs are usually static. But under what circumstances will they change?

24.1 Case 1

24.1.1 Case Presentation

A 58-year-old female patient was observed with a suspected lesion in the left fundus during a physical examination. The patient denied symptoms including vision loss, distorted vision, shadow in the vision, etc. in the left eye. The patient had a history of cataract and myopia in the left eye. No treatment had been carried out. Histories of systemic diseases, trauma, and familial diseases were denied.

N. Fan · J. Wang (✉)
Shenzhen Eye Hospital, Shenzhen University, Shenzhen, China

X. Liu
Xiamen Eye Center of Xiamen University, Xiamen, China

Shenzhen Eye Hospital, Shenzhen University, Shenzhen, China

Upon examination, the uncorrected visual acuity (UCVA) was 20/25 OD and 20/125 OS, and best corrected visual acuity (BCVA) was 20/20 with refractive correction (+0.5DC × 50) OD and 20/125 with refractive correction (−2.50DS −1.00DC ×80) OS.

The cornea was transparent and the pupil was round in both eyes. The density of the lens of the right eye showed increase, and the lens of the left eye showed mild opacity. Fundus examination revealed no abnormality in the right eye; in the left eye, a white feather-like focus following the pattern and architecture of the retinal nerve fiber layer could be observed, which nearly involved the whole optic disc, and the retinal vessels underneath it could not be seen clearly. The retina outside the focus showed no abnormality (Fig. 24.1).

Visual field examination showed enlargement of the blind spot and bundle-like visual field impairment in the left eye (Fig. 24.2).

24.1.2 Final Diagnosis

The final diagnosis was MRNFLs in the left eye.

24.1.3 Case Review

This case was a typical MRNFLs case. One eye was affected, and the visual field impairment was manifested as enlargement of the blind spot.

N. Wang et al. (eds.), *Optic Disorders and Visual Field*, Advances in Visual Science and Eye Diseases 2, https://doi.org/10.1007/978-981-13-2502-1_24

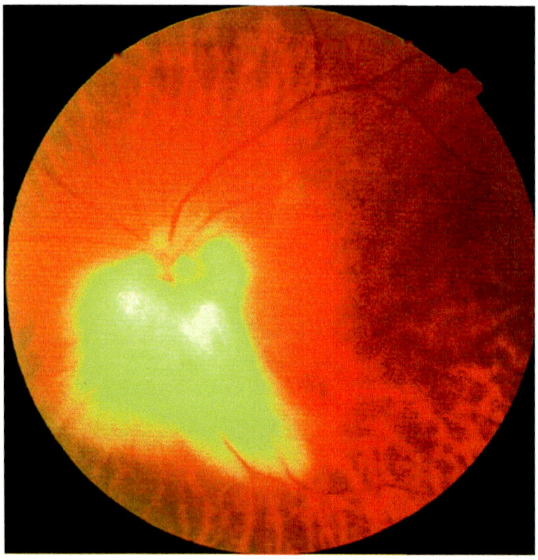

Fig. 24.1 Fundus photograph. A white feather-like focus following the pattern and architecture of the retinal nerve fiber layer could be observed, which nearly involved the whole optic disc, and the retinal vessels underneath it could not be seen clearly in the left eye. The retina outside the focus showed no abnormality (imaging quality was affected by the cataract)

There was a site of significant decibel reduction superior to the blind spot and another such site temporal to the blind spot. They were considered to be caused by the relatively serious parts of the focus inferior and nasal to the optic disc. MRNFLs are usually static. But under pathological circumstances, the sheath will disappear spontaneously. The following two cases embody such phenomenon.

24.2 Case 2

Li Jianjun and Tang Xin

24.2.1 Case Presentation

A 10-year-old male patient returned for reexamination after congenital cataract operation. The patient had received cataract extraction combined with intraocular lens implantation at another hospital 5 years before due to congenital cataract in both eyes. Increased intraocular pressure (IOP) was observed in both eyes soon after the operation, and the highest pressure was up to 38 mmHg in the right eye and 42 mmHg in the left eye. Three to four kinds of IOP-lowering eye drops had been used to control the IOP, but the IOP was still not stable.

At the first visit, fundus examination showed that the patient's optic disc was pink in color with a normal neuroretinal rim, and a white feather-like focus following the pattern and architecture of the retinal nerve fibers could be observed above the optic disc (Fig. 24.3a). During the 1.5 years of follow-up after initiation of medication, the patient's IOP was well controlled by the drugs, and no significant change was revealed in the white focus and optic disc (Fig. 24.3b–d). At 2 years and 3 years of follow-up, the patient's IOP was not well controlled, the white focus shrank gradually and finally disappeared, and the cup-to-disc ratio increased and neuroretinal rim gradually narrowed which were observed in the left eye, due to failure to take the drugs and pay return visits regularly (Fig. 24.3e, f).

24.2.2 Final Diagnosis

The final diagnosis was MRNFLs and secondary glaucoma in the left eye.

24.2.3 Case Review

In this case, the retinal nerve fibers where the sheath was located were damaged due to the secondary glaucoma found in the affected eye, and the sheath degraded and disappeared as a result.

24.3 Case 3

24.3.1 Case Presentation

A 52-year-old male patient presented with gradual vision decrease in the left eye for over 2 years and symptom aggravation for half a year. No significant trigger had been observed before disease onset in the left eye 2 years before. No accompa-

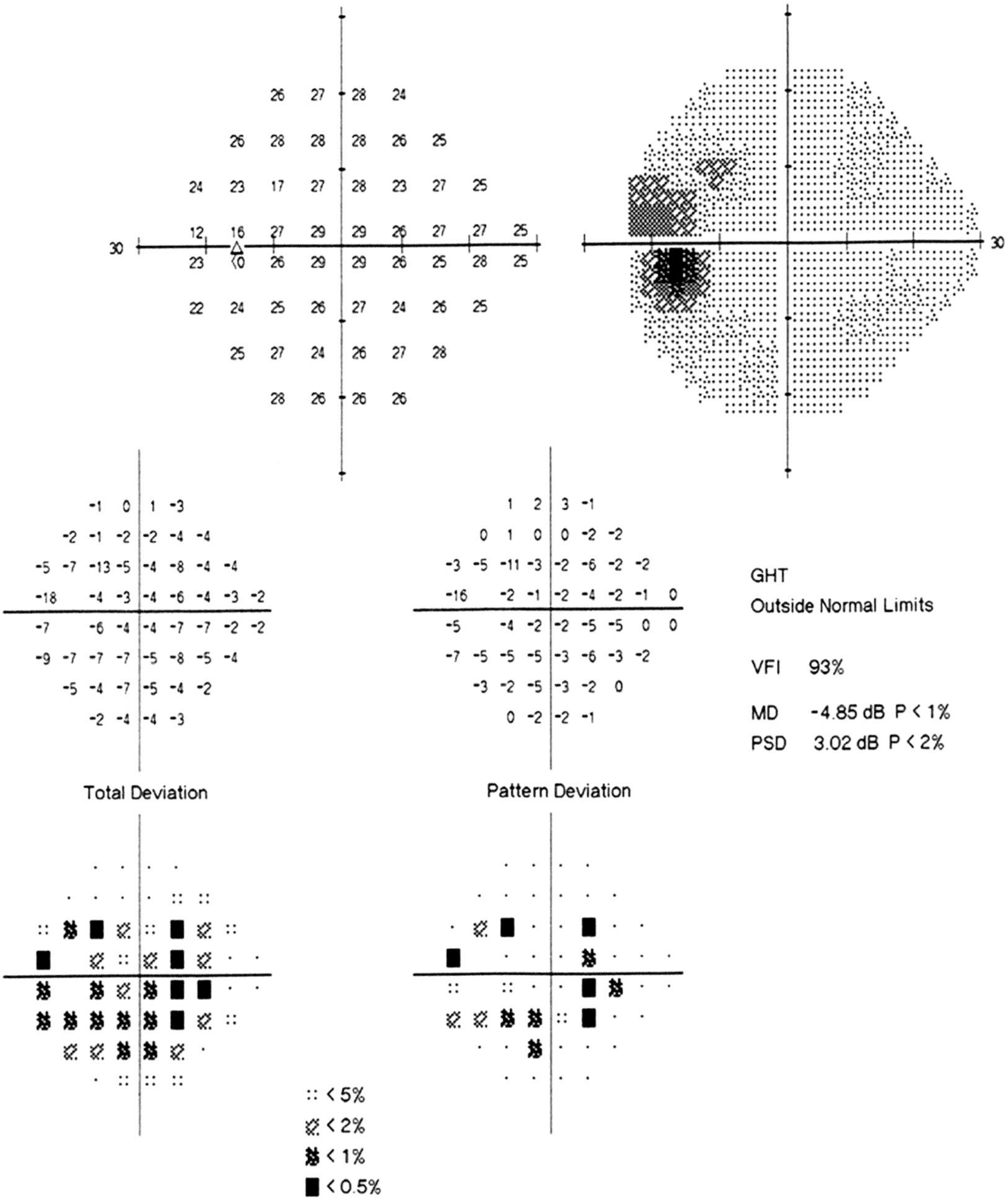

Fig. 24.2 Humphrey visual field analysis printout. Standardized automated perimetry with the 24-2 test showed enlargement of the blind spot and bundle-like visual field impairment in the left eye

nying symptoms, including red eyes, eye pain, etc., were present. Vision decrease had aggravated half a year before, and iridescent vision had been experienced occasionally. The patient's left eye had suffered from blunt trauma more than 10 years before, and drugs had been given for treatment (details unknown).

On examination, the UCVA was 20/25 OD and 20/125 OS, and the BCVA was 20/20 with refractive correction (−1.00DS) OD and 20/100 with refractive correction (−3.50DC × 60) OS. The IOP measured with standard Goldmann applanation tonometry was 12 mmHg OD and 35 mmHg OS. In the right eye, slit-lamp exami-

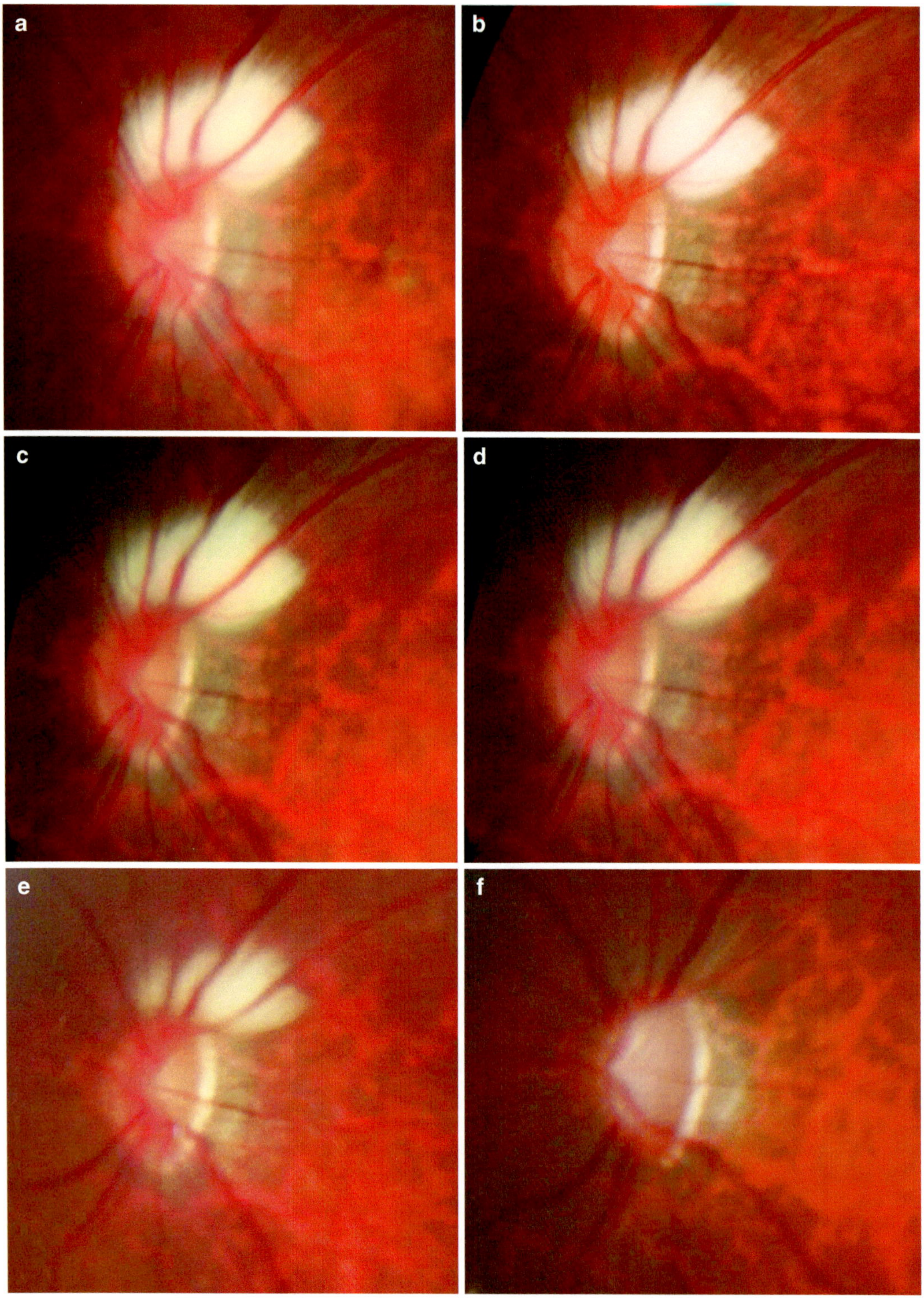

Fig. 24.3 Fundus photographs of the left eye. Panel a: A white feather-like focus following the pattern and architecture of the retinal nerve fibers could be observed above the optic disc. The appearance of the neuroretinal rim was normal. Panel b–d: These photographs were taken during the 1.5 years of follow-up after initiation of medication, which showed no significant change in the white focus and optic disc. Figure e, f: These photographs were taken at 2 years and 3 years of follow-up, which showed that the white focus shrank gradually and finally disappeared, the cup-to-disc ratio increased, and the neuroretinal rim gradually narrowed

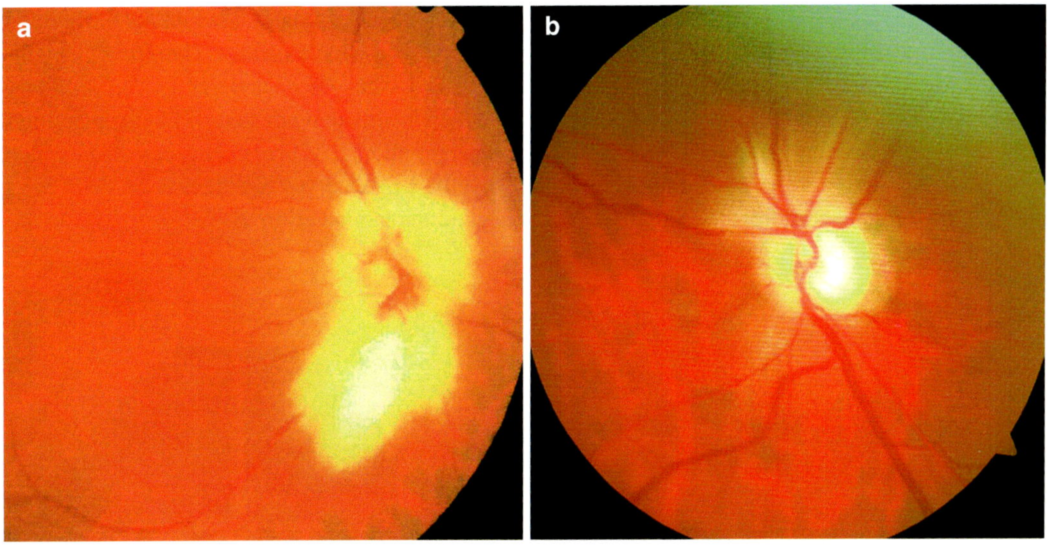

Fig. 24.4 Fundus photographs. Panel a: A white feather-like focus could be seen in the right eye. Panel b: In the left eye, the C/D ratio of the optic disc was 0.9, and a residual white feather-like focus can be seen indistinctly (Note: The imaging quality was affected by the refracting medium opacity in the left eye)

nation of his anterior segment revealed no abnormality, and fundus examination revealed a white feather-like focus with high reflection in the optic disc and following the pattern and architecture of the retinal nerve fiber layer (Fig. 24.4a). In the left eye, slit-lamp examination of his anterior segment revealed mild conjunctival congestion, mild cornea edema, multiple pigmented KPs, a deep anterior chamber, clear aqueous humor, peripheral anterior chamber about 1/2CT depth in thickness, a pupil 3.5 mm in diameter, depigmented iris (especially significant in the supratemporal area), and an opacity lens. Fundus examination revealed a C/D ratio of 0.9 and an indistinct white feather-like focus (Fig. 24.4b).

Visual field examination showed enlargement of the blind spot in the right eye and a diffuse visual field defect in the left eye (Fig. 24.5).

24.3.2 Final Diagnosis

The final diagnosis was MRNFLs in the right eye and secondary glaucoma in the left eye.

24.3.3 Case Review

Fundus photographs of the patient's left eye with MRNFLs before the occurrence of glaucoma were not collected. But the right eye had the typical manifestations, and a residual MRNFL could be observed in the left eye with advanced glaucoma. Therefore, we believed that the situation was the same as that in Case 2. The retinal nerve fibers, where the sheath was located, were damaged due to the secondary glaucoma, and the sheath then disappeared as a result.

24.4 Discussion

An axon is composed of neurofibrils originating from the neuron cytoplasm, and most of them are myelinated nerve fibers. A small number of axons, such as the nerve fibers for pain conduction or some sympathetic nerve fibers, are without sheath, and they are called unmyelinated nerve fibers. Some of the myelinated nerve fibers, such as optic nerve fibers, have no sheath only in a certain segment. Nerve fiber sheaths are formed by the interactions between neurons and their supporting cells [1].

The formation of the sheaths of optic nerve fibers and the nerve fibers at the optic chiasm starts from the lateral geniculate body when the fetus is 5 months old, and the sheaths will extend to the level of the lamina cribrosa where it terminates after birth. Therefore, the intraocular segments of the retinal nerve fibers and optic nerves are without sheaths, but the segments beyond the lamina cribrosa have sheaths. Therefore, the lamina cribrosa can be considered as the boundary between myelinated optic nerve fibers and unmyelinated optic nerve fibers. This can also explain why the optic nerves are thicker at their parts beyond the lamina cribrosa.

a

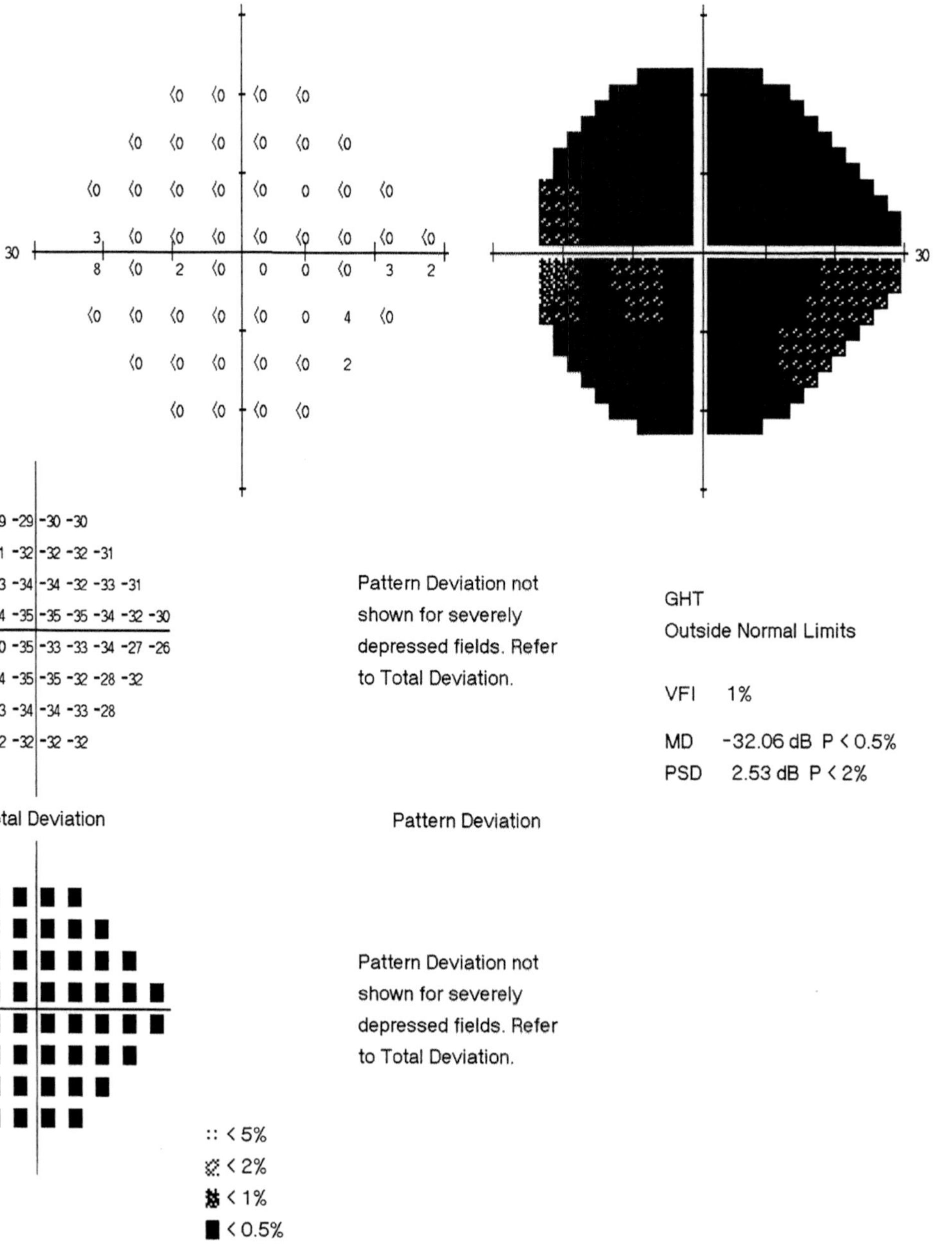

Fig. 24.5 Humphrey visual field analysis printouts. Panel a: Standardized automated perimetry with the 24-2 test showed a diffuse visual field defect in the left eye. Panel b: Enlargement of the blind spot was shown in right eye

b

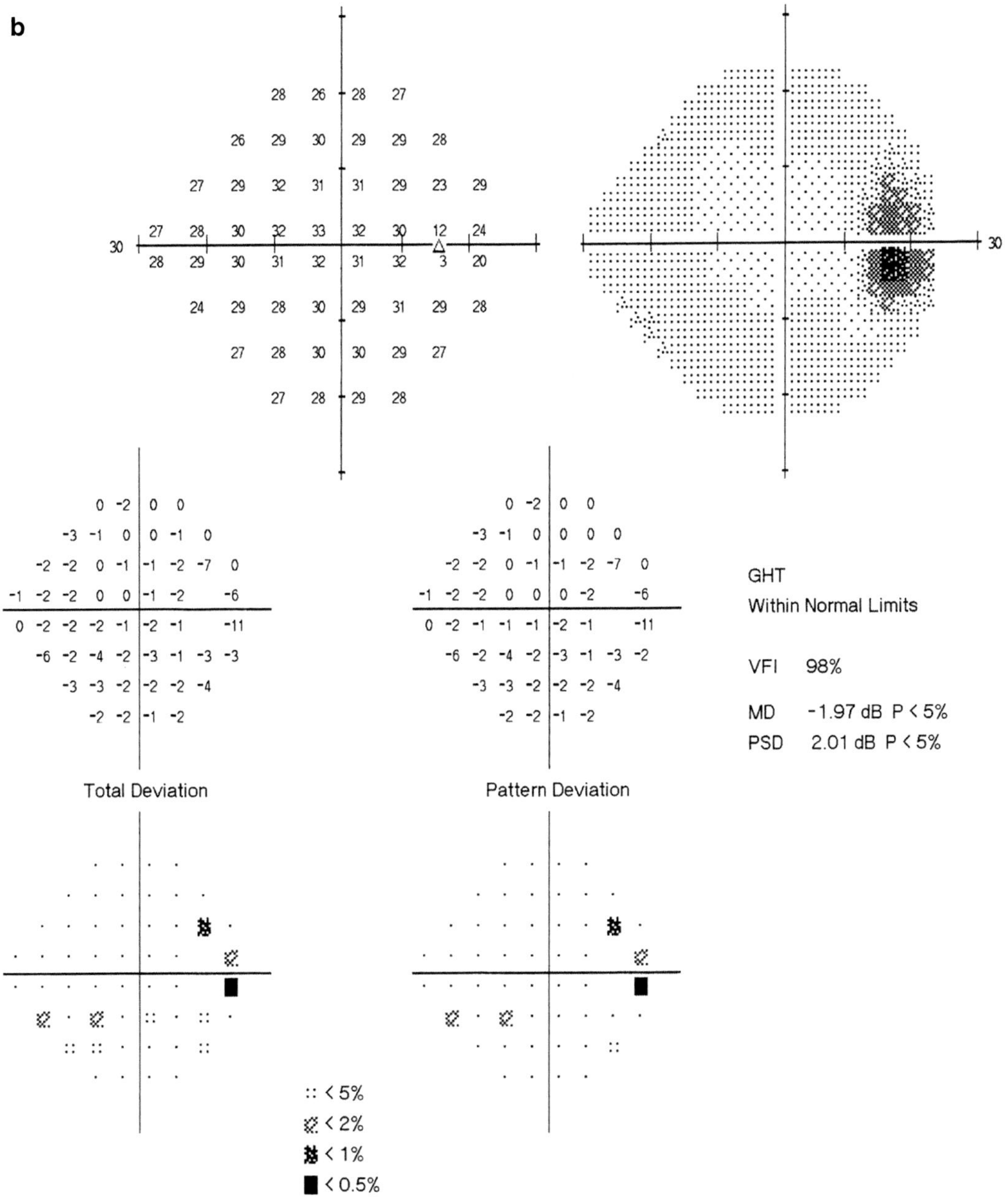

Fig. 24.5 (continued)

MRNFLs are experienced if the nerve fibers in the retinal nerve fiber layer are observed with sheaths. They were first reported by Virchow in 1856, and their fundus manifestation is a yellowish-white feather-like focus with high reflection.

The pathogenesis of MRNFLs may be connected with lamina cribrosa dysplasia and ectopia of oligodendrocytes, which produce nerve fiber sheaths, from the optic nerves to the retina. The incidence of MRNFLs is 1%, and simultaneous involvement of both eyes can be found in about 20% of the patients [2].

Myelinated nerve fibers are rarely found at the macular area. Therefore, the central vision is usually not affected. The focus can usually be observed in the retina and/or the surrounding area of the optic disc. It's distributed along the running of the nerve fibers. The common visual field impairments are enlargement of the blind spot and occurrence of scotomas. The mechanism of visual field impairment resulting from MRNFLs is still inconclusive. It may be related to light transmission blockage and weakened stimulation of visual information on the retinal photoreceptor cells caused by densely populated nerve fibers. This can explain the consistency in severity and position between MRNFLs and visual field impairment.

An interesting phenomenon is that the sheaths of the myelinated nerve fibers can disintegrate and disappear gradually as a result of nerve fiber atrophy. The Chinese old saying "with the skin gone, to what can the hair attach itself" vividly illustrates the relationship between them. The relationship between axons and sheathes is very close. Both of them have shared pathogenic factors, and the damage to sheaths is usually more serious than that to axons. As is the case with other myelinated nerve fibers, the damage to the optic nerve, whatever the cause, will lead to nerve fiber degeneration and consequent degeneration, fracture, and dissociation of the sheaths. And then, the granular fragments from the collapse and degeneration will be absorbed and finally disappear completely, leaving no trace [3].

Therefore, sheath disappearance can be observed in all other diseases that can cause nerve fiber injury, such as primary demyelinated optic neuritis, ischemic optic neuropathy, optic nerve atrophy, etc.

References

1. Straatsma BR, Foos RY, Heckenlively JR, et al. Myelinated retinal nerve fibers. Am J Ophthalmol. 1981;91(1):25–38.
2. Renaud D, Karim H, Maryam A, et al. Acquired myelinated nerve fibers in association with optic disk drusen. J AAPOS. 2010;14(14):544–7.
3. Joseph WS, Michelle JN. Regression of myelinated retinal nerve fibers in a glaucomatous eye. Optom Vis Sci. 2013;90(7):e218–20.

25 A Case with Unilateral Superior RNFL Defect and Inferior Arcuate Scotoma

Ning Fan, Xuyang Liu, and Jiantao Wang

The patient was a middle-aged male with a unilateral superior RNFL thinning accompanied by an inferior arcuate scotoma. He had once been diagnosed with normal tension glaucoma (NTG), ischemic optic neuropathy, etc. In this section, the diagnosis process for this patient is introduced.

25.1 Case

25.1.1 Case Presentation

A 52-year-old male patient presented with vision decrease in the right eye for over 10 years. He had a history of high myopia in the right eye. The myopia could be corrected by wearing glasses, but the patient still felt blurred vision. No accompanying symptoms, including red eyes, eye pain, distorted vision, night blindness, etc., were present. Histories of trauma, previous eye diseases, systemic diseases, and familial diseases were denied.

Upon examination, the uncorrected visual acuity (UCVA) was 20/2000 OD and 20/20 OS. The best corrected visual acuity (BCVA) of the right eye was 20/25 with refractive correction (−6.25DS −0.75DC × 180). The intraocular pressure (IOP) was normal in both eyes (the diurnal IOP curve showed that the IOP fluctuated between 12 and 15 mmHg in both eyes). Slit-lamp examination of his anterior segments was unremarkable. Fundus examination showed that, in the right eye, the optic disc was tilted and horizontal oval-shaped with inferior peripapillary atrophy, the C/D ratio was 0.45, and reflection from the superior retinal nerve fibers disappeared; in the left eye, the optic disc was round with a C/D ratio of 0.55, and the rim and reflection from the RNFL showed no abnormality (Fig. 25.1).

Central cornea thickness (CCT) was 514 μm OD and 518 μm OS. Axial length was 27.57 mm OD and 24.26 mm OS.

Visual field examination revealed a normal central visual field in the left eye and an inferior arcuate scotoma extending from the blind spot in the right eye (Fig. 25.2).

Optical coherence tomography (OCT) demonstrated diffuse thinning of the RNFL in the superior quadrant of the right eye (Fig. 25.3).

B-ultrasound disclosed posterior scleral staphyloma and mild opacity in the vitreous with posterior vitreous detachment in the right eye (Fig. 25.4).

N. Fan · J. Wang (✉)
Shenzhen Eye Hospital, Shenzhen University, Shenzhen, China

X. Liu
Xiamen Eye Center of Xiamen University, Xiamen, China

Shenzhen Eye Hospital, Shenzhen University, Shenzhen, China

N. Wang et al. (eds.), *Optic Disorders and Visual Field*, Advances in Visual Science and Eye Diseases 2, https://doi.org/10.1007/978-981-13-2502-1_25

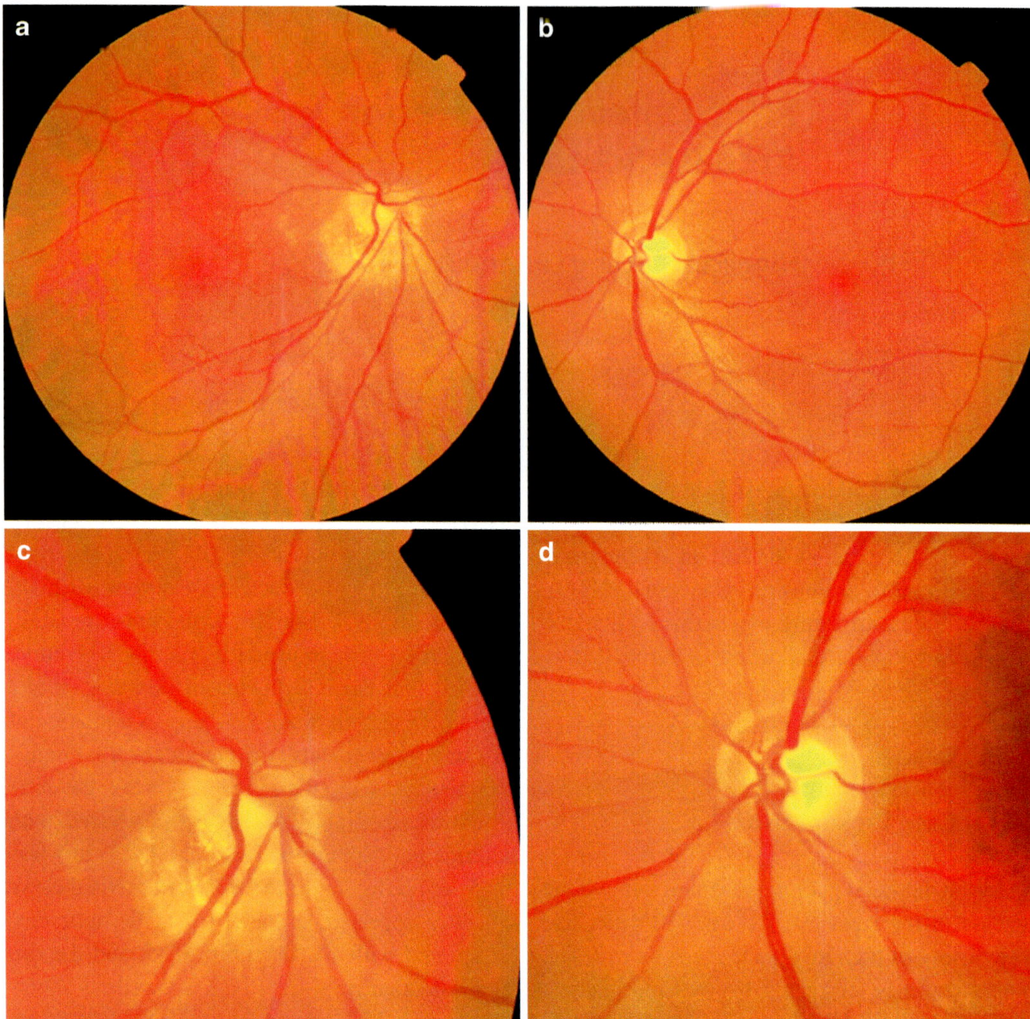

Fig. 25.1 Fundus photographs. Panel a, c: The optic disc in right eye was tilted and horizontal oval-shaped (C/D = 0.45). Reflection from superior retinal nerve fibers disappeared. Panel b, d: The optic disc in the left eye was round (C/D = 0.55) with normal retinal nerve fiber reflection

25.1.2 Case Analysis

The patient was a 54-year-old male complaining of blurred vision in the right eye. Examination revealed that his right eye had high myopia and the left eye was emmetropic. Anisometropia was revealed and the BCVA of the right eye was 20/25. An inferior arcuate scotoma in the lower area of the right eye, which corresponded exactly to the superior RNFL defect in location, could be observed in visual field examination. So, did the findings conform to the diagnosis criteria for glaucoma? Although the patient's IOP was normal, CCT was thinner than normal, and systemic diseases were denied, unilateral normal tension glaucoma (NTG) was still possible.

We then focused on the left eye. In light of the normal fundus manifestation, IOP, and CCT, glaucoma in the left eye could be basically excluded. And meanwhile, the optic disc in the left eye was not a small crowded "disc at risk" but rather had a physiologic macrocup, which didn't conform to the manifestation of a contralateral normal eye in ischemic optic neuropathy.

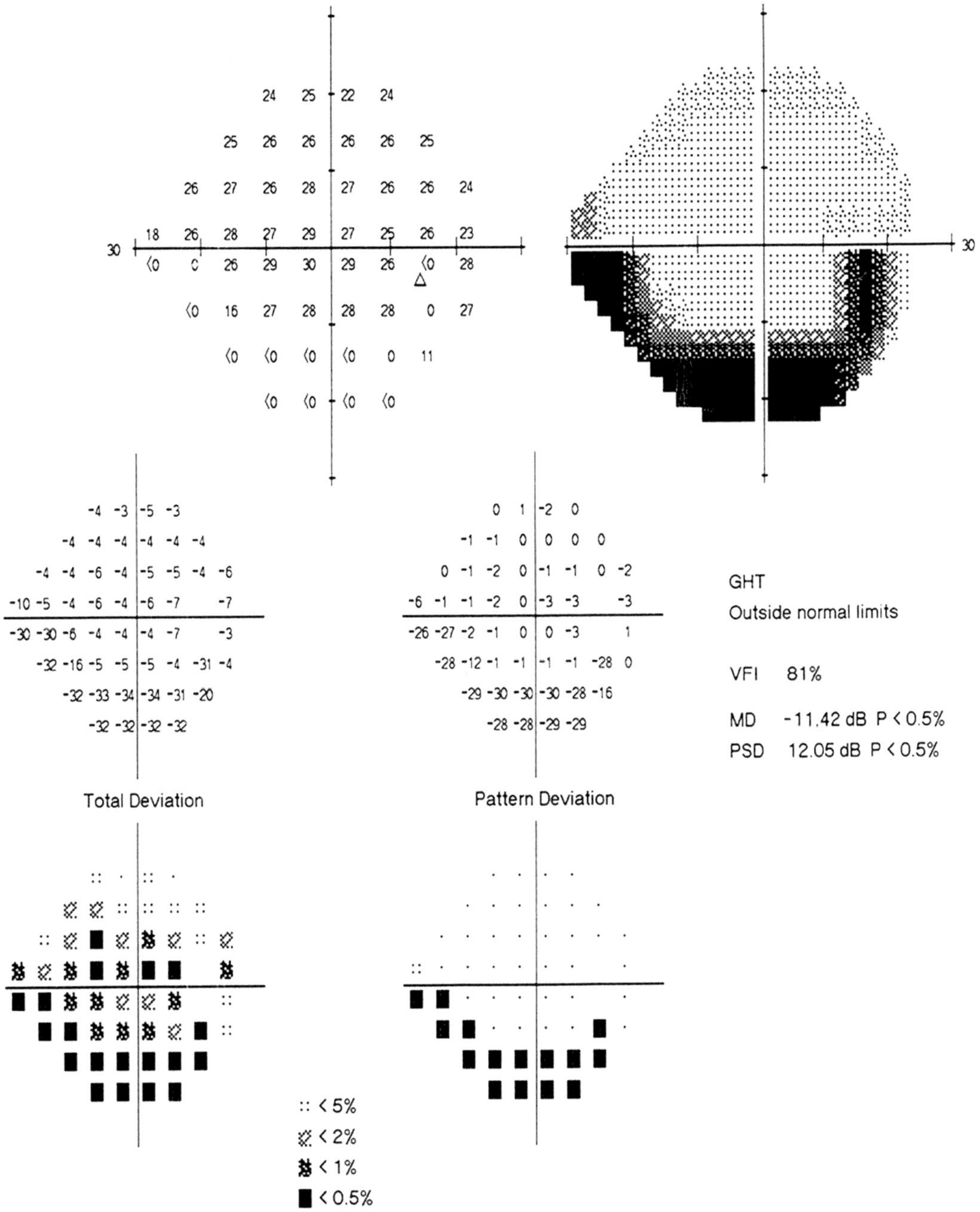

Fig. 25.2 Humphrey visual field analysis printout. An inferior arcuate scotoma extending from the blind spot was observed with the 24-2 test in the right eye

The patient's medical history was then repeatedly inquired into, and he denied previous eye diseases in the right eye, such as acute vision decrease, shadow in the vision, etc. Therefore, the assumption that the local RNFL atrophy was caused by previous retinal vascular lesions and optic neuropathy was not supported.

Besides, it could be judged from the axial lengths and refractive powers of both eyes that the patient's right eye had axial myopia rather

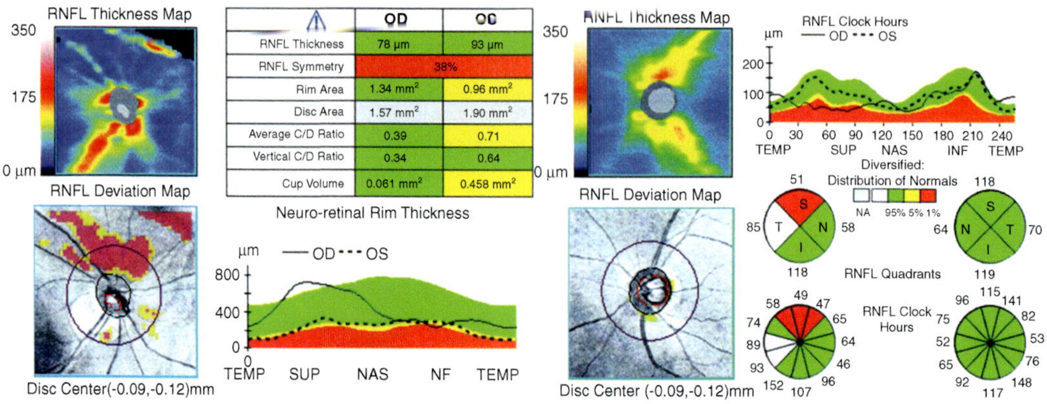

Fig. 25.3 OCT measurement printout for the RNFL thickness in both eyes. Diffuse thinning of the RNFL was revealed in the superior quadrant of the right eye. The RNFL thickness was normal in the left eye

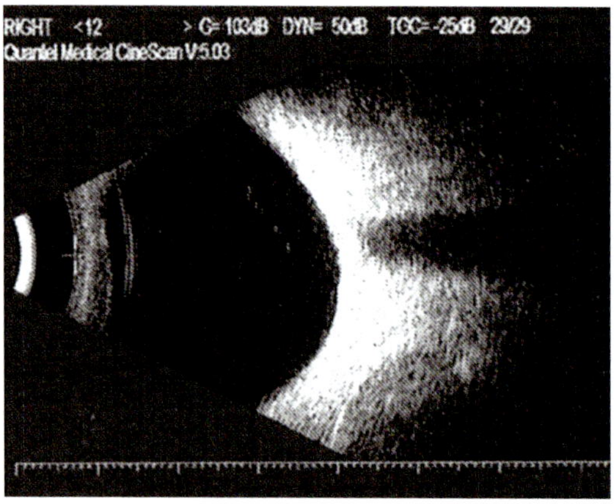

Fig. 25.4 B-ultrasound image for the right eye. Posterior scleral staphyloma was observed in the right eye. Mild opacity was shown in the vitreous, accompanied by posterior vitreous detachment

than lens-induced myopia. B-ultrasound examination suggested posterior scleral staphyloma in the right eye.

The patient's optic disc of the right eye was carefully observed. The color and width of the neuroretinal rim were normal. The superior RNFL defect was wide and large, and no concomitant superior neuroretinal rim thinning was observed, which was inconsistent with the characteristics of optic nerve atrophy caused by NTG and anterior ischemic optic neuropathy (AION). The visual field examination showed that the absolute arcuate scotoma was big, and the damages in the nasal and temporal sides were almost symmetrical in pattern and far from the fixation (not completely in the Bjerrum area). The findings were not completely in accordance with the characteristic visual field changes of common glaucoma.

The right eye has high myopia, which could explain the oval-shaped and tilted optic disc and the temporal peripapillary atrophy. However, how to explain the inconsistency between the changes in the neuroretinal rim and the RNFL? Was it possible that a drusen was buried in the optic disc and masked the changes of the disc rim? Was there any abnormality in the other layers of the retina accompanying the RNFL thinning? We decided to perform a high-resolution OCT scan on the local retina and optic disc of the patient's right eye with a view to finding the answers to the above two questions.

OCT with vertical linear scanning at the nasal peripapillary area in the right eye revealed that the neuroepithelial layer of the superior retina (at the site of the focus) was thinner compared with that of the inferior normal retina, but the RPE layer was normal, while the OCT scanning in the left eye at the same location revealed that the neuroepithelial layer and the RPE of the superior and inferior retina were symmetrical with normal shape and thickness (Fig. 25.5). The optic disc scanning excluded the possibility of buried optic disc drusen (Fig. 25.6).

The OCT excluded buried optic disc drusen and revealed that the thinning could be observed in the neuroepithelial layer of retina, rather than being localized in the RNFL, at the site of the

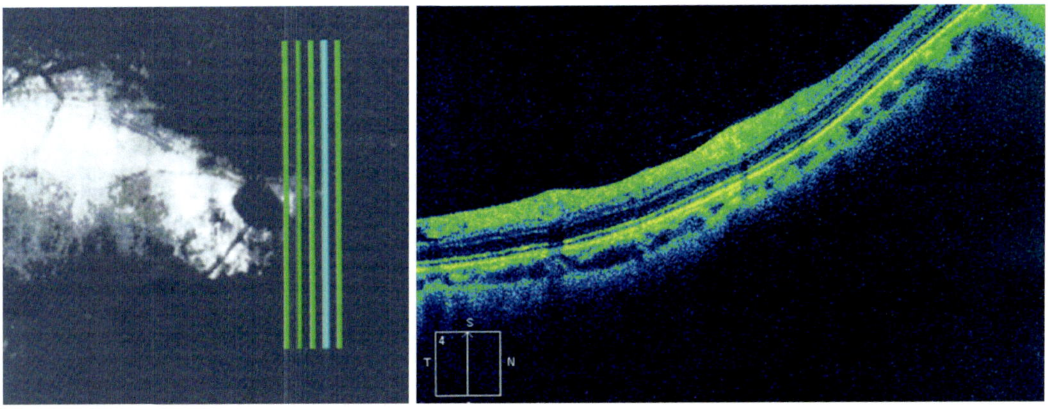

Fig. 25.5 OCT image of the peripapillary retina of the right eye. The neuroepithelial layer of the superior retina (at the site of the focus) was thinner compared with that of the inferior normal retina, but the RPE layer was normal

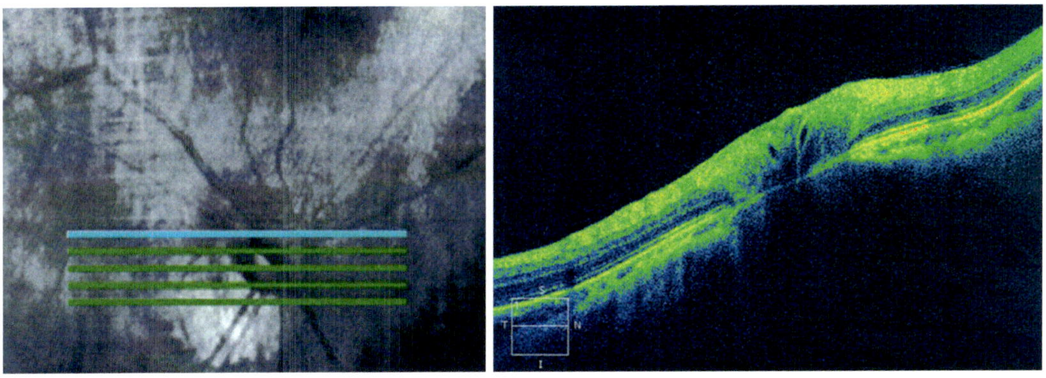

Fig. 25.6 OCT image of the optic disc of the right eye. The structures of the optic disc and neuroretinal rim in the right eye were normal

focus. Therefore, the diagnosis of optic nerve fiber atrophy caused by NTG and AION was rejected.

The analysis on the examination results obtained from multiple hospitals in the previous 5 years showed no significant change in the visual field, RNFL thickness measured by OCT, and the optic disc and retina in the color photographs of the fundus of the right eye. Therefore, we considered congenital dysplasia of the retina (the neuroepithelial layer of retina) to be the diagnosis for the patient's right eye. The site of the focus could explain the size of the visual field defect. High myopia could be found in the right eye but the BCVA was fine. The tilted optic disc was considered to be caused by expansion and stretch of the posterior pole and oblique entering of the optic nerves. Other fundus manifestations of high myopia include lacquer cracks on the fundus, inferior peripapillary atrophy, etc., which could exclude the tilted disc syndrome as a possible diagnosis.

25.1.3 Final Diagnosis

The final diagnosis was dysplasia of the retina (the neuroepithelial layer of retina) in the right eye.

25.1.4 Case Review

In this case, the disease lasted a long time, and the visual field manifestations in the right eye resembled glaucomatous damages. But the disease condition had remained stable in the previous 5 years, and no glaucomatous rim damage was shown. The possibility of glaucoma could therefore be excluded. The OCT examination revealed that the neuroepithelial layers of retina showed thinning at the site of the focus. These findings supported the diagnosis of dysplasia of the retina (the neuroepithelial layer of retina).

25.2 Discussion

The patient in this case was not young (54 years old). The IOPs were not high and the right eye had high myopia. The examination revealed a superior RNFL defect and an inferior arcuate scotoma. Therefore, he had been once diagnosed with NTG and secondary optic nerve atrophy. But some special manifestations in the patient drew our attention. For instance, the RNFL defect in the superior quadrant of the affected eye was significant, but no neuroretinal rim damage corresponding to the RNFL defect was observed; the visual field defect was an absolute arcuate scotoma, and the damages found in the nasal and temporal sides were symmetrical and far from the fixation (not completely in the Bjerrum area). These manifestations didn't conform to the characteristics of glaucomatous damages. Meanwhile, long-term follow-up revealed no disease progression.

Secondary RNFL atrophy (including ischemic optic neuropathy, branch retina vessel occlusion, etc.) was also excluded after repeated inquiry into the patient's medical history, observation on the contralateral eye and careful differential analysis of the optic disc and retina of the affected eye. We considered the possibility of congenital dysplasia because of the tilted optic disc, anisometropia resulting from the difference in axial lengths, etc. Through the OCT examination, buried optic disc drusen was excluded first, and it was confirmed that the neuroepithelial layers of the retina had dysplasia at the site of the focus which was consistent with the site of the visual field defect. The right eye was observed with high myopia, but the BCVA was fine, which can explain the abnormalities, including lacquer cracks on the fundus, tilted optic disc, inferior peripapillary atrophy, etc., which could exclude the tilted disc syndrome as a possible diagnosis [1, 2]. Dysplasia of the retina (the neuroepithelial layer of retina) was a descriptive diagnosis, and its relationship with the high myopia and tilted optic disc found in this patient was still unclear [3].

References

1. Liu Q, Fang Y. Optic disc diseases. Beijing: People's Medical Publishing House; 2015.
2. Hertle RW, David B. Pediatric eye disease color atlas and synopsis. Translated by Zhang Mei, Liu Zuguo. Guangzhou: Guangdong Science and Technology Press; 2003.
3. Lanning BK, Rod F. Optic nerve disorders. Translated by Xu Jun, Yang Qingsong, Ma Kai. Beijing: People's Medical Publishing House; 2014.

26 A Young Patient with Unilateral Superior Altitudinal Visual Field Defect

Ning Fan, Xuyang Liu, and Jiantao Wang

Shared in this section is a case in which a young female had superior altitudinal hemianopia with normal central vision in one eye. Was it optic nerve atrophy caused by optic neuritis or normal tension glaucoma (NTG), etc.? Or was it congenital optic nerve hypoplasia? The visual field findings gave us important clues.

26.1 Case

26.1.1 Case Presentation

A 24-year-old female patient presented with visual field narrowing without progression in the left eye for 3 years. The patient found her visual field narrowing in the left eye during a physical examination 3 years before. Histories of night blindness, trauma, previous eye diseases, systemic diseases, and familial diseases were denied. The patient had been diagnosed with optic nerve atrophy in the left eye for multiple times at different hospitals in the past.

N. Fan · J. Wang (✉)
Shenzhen Eye Hospital, Shenzhen University, Shenzhen, China

X. Liu
Xiamen Eye Center of Xiamen University, Xiamen, China

Shenzhen Eye Hospital, Shenzhen University, Shenzhen, China

On examination, the best corrected visual acuity (BCVA) was 20/20 with myopic correction (−1.75DS) OD and 20/20 with myopic correction (−2.00DS) OS. The intraocular pressure (IOP) was 14 mmHg in both eyes. Slit-lamp examination of her anterior segments was unremarkable. Fundus examination showed that the vitreous was clear in both eyes; the optic disc was red in color with a clear boundary, the C/D ratio was 0.5, foveal reflex was shown, and the retinal vessels exhibited no abnormality in the right eye; the optic disc was pallor in color with a clear boundary, the C/D ratio was 0.7 with a narrowing inferior neuroretinal rim, and the reflection of inferior retinal nerve fibers disappeared, and foveal reflex could be observed in the left eye (Fig. 26.1).

Visual field examination demonstrated superior visual field loss delimited by the horizontal line in the left eye and normal visual field in the right eye (Fig. 26.2).

RNFL thickness measurement by optical coherence tomography (OCT) showed diffuse thinning of the RNFL in the inferior and temporal quadrants of the left eye (Fig. 26.3).

An orbit CT scan at another hospital revealed slight thinning of the optic nerve at the left side when compared with that in the right side.

Fundus fluorescein angiography (FFA) at another hospital revealed the following results: in the left eye, hypofluorescence in the inferior optic disc was shown, and deep capillary vessels inside the cup could be observed at the early stage, and

N. Wang et al. (eds.), *Optic Disorders and Visual Field*, Advances in Visual Science and Eye Diseases 2, https://doi.org/10.1007/978-981-13-2502-1_26

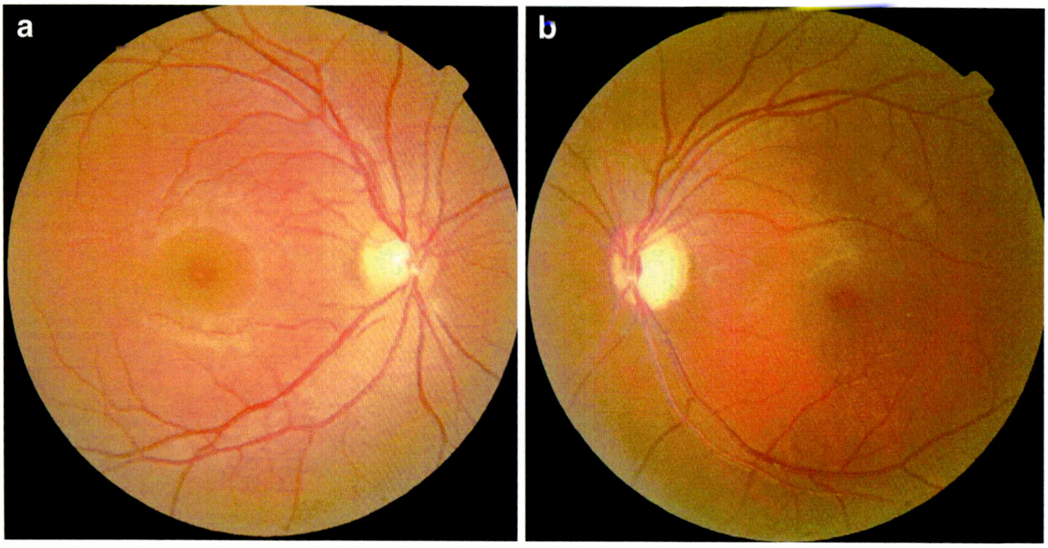

Fig. 26.1 Fundus photographs. Panel a: The optic disc of the right eye was red in color with a clear boundary and the C/D ratio was 0.5. Panel b: The optic disc was pallor in color with a clear boundary, the C/D ratio was 0.7 with a narrowing inferior neuroretinal rim, and the light reflection of inferior retinal nerve fibers disappeared in the left eye

hypofluorescence could still be observed at this site at the middle and late stages; in the right eye, the findings were normal at all the stages (Fig. 26.4).

26.1.2 Case Analysis

The patient was a young female with one diseased eye. The central vision was not involved. Loss of the superior visual field delimited by the horizontal line was manifested, which was in accordance with the RNFL defect. The inferior neuroretinal rim showed narrowing, which was consistent with the RNFL damages. An orbit CT scan revealed thinning of the left optic nerve. Was the diagnosis optic atrophy? If so, what was the cause? Or was it neuritis, NTG, retinal vascular occlusion, or anterior ischemic optic neuropathy (AION)?

Careful analysis on the visual field disclosed that the light sensitivity was zero at nearly all the test points in the superior half of the visual field with a clear horizontal boundary. This finding didn't conform to the characteristics of visual field changes caused by retinal nerve fiber bundle damage in glaucoma, AION, retinal venous occlusion, etc. The supratemporal branch retinal artery seemed to be naked with high light reflection due to the retinal nerve fiber layer (RNFL) atrophy in the inferior retina. No vessel sheathing was observed, so branch retinal artery occlusion might be excluded, and further FFA examination confirmed this and excluded other retinal vascular diseases. The relative afferent pupillary defect (RAPD) of the affected eye was negative. No pain upon eye movement was felt, and the central vision was normal, which did not support optic neuritis. The patient was young and healthy and the optic cup was big in both eyes, so there was no potential risk factor of AION.

What was the cause? The affected eye of the patient had been observed by accident with visual field narrowed 3 years before, and the disease condition showed no progression in the 3 years. We first considered the possibility of congenital optic nerve dysplasia. The hypoplasia of the retinal nerve fibers in the inferior area could explain the light sensitivity being zero in the superior area, diffuse thinning of the inferior RNFL, and the changes in the rim. This should be confirmed through the examinations of OCT, electroretinogram (ERG), and visual evoked potential (VEP) combined with analysis. OCT scan of the retina could clarify the structure of the RNFL and the other layers of the retina. Electrophysiological examination could help to locate the retinopathy from the function, and the expected results should be an abnormal pattern visual evoked potential (P-VEP) with normal ERG in the whole retina in the left eye if the disease was localized just in the RNFL.

OCT with vertical linear scanning showed that the signals from the inferior RNFL temporal to the optic disc disappeared but normal signals from the superior RNFL temporal to the optic disc could be obtained in the left eye (Fig. 26.5); normal signals could be observed from both the

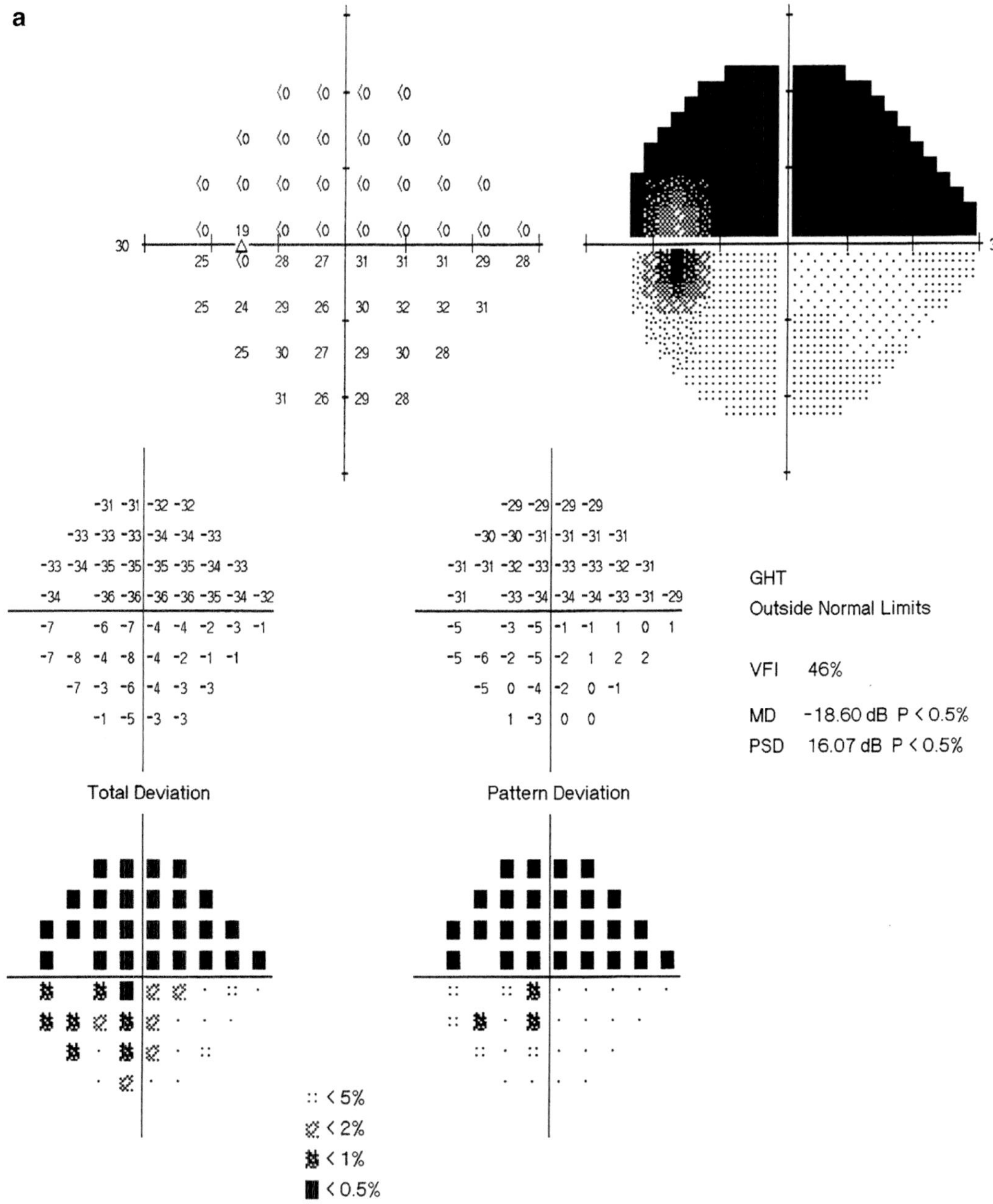

Fig. 26.2 Humphrey visual field analysis printouts. Panel a: Perimetry with the 24-2 test showed superior visual field loss delimited by the horizontal line in the left eye. Panel b: The visual field was normal in the right eye

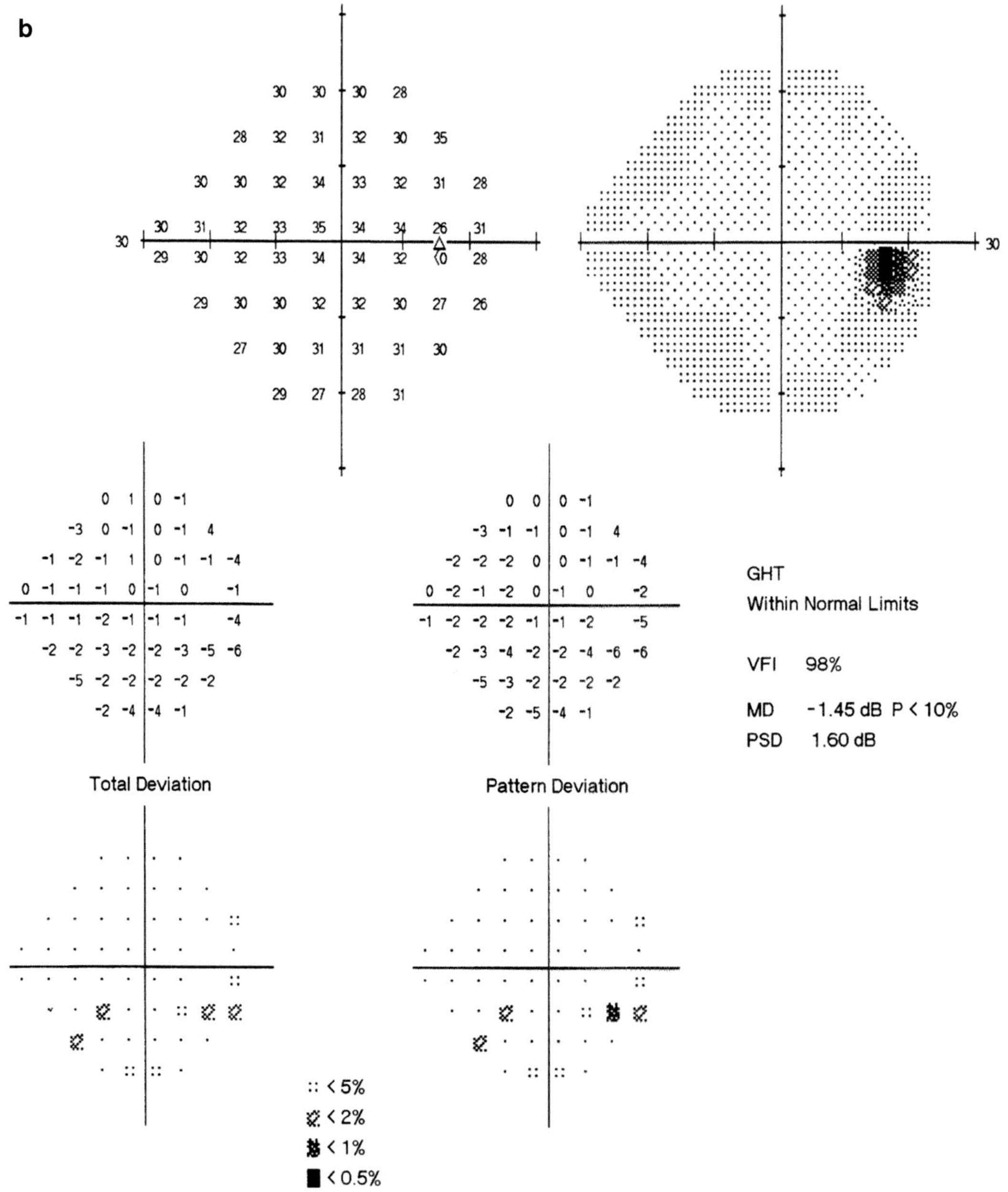

Fig. 26.2 (continued)

superior and inferior RNFL temporal to the optic disc in the right eye (Fig. 26.6).

P-VEP showed significantly reduced amplitude and normal latency of the P100 wave in the left eye and normal amplitude and latency of the P100 wave in the right eye (Fig. 26.7).

ERG demonstrated that, in both eyes, the ERG was normal in the whole visual field; the waveform, amplitude, and latency of the b-wave in the rod response were normal (Fig. 26.8); the waveforms, amplitudes, and latencies of a- and b-waves were all normal in maximal mixed response (Fig. 26.9); the amplitude of OPs wave (oscillatory potentials) showed no abnormality (Fig. 26.10); the waveforms, amplitudes, and latencies of a- and b-waves in the cone response

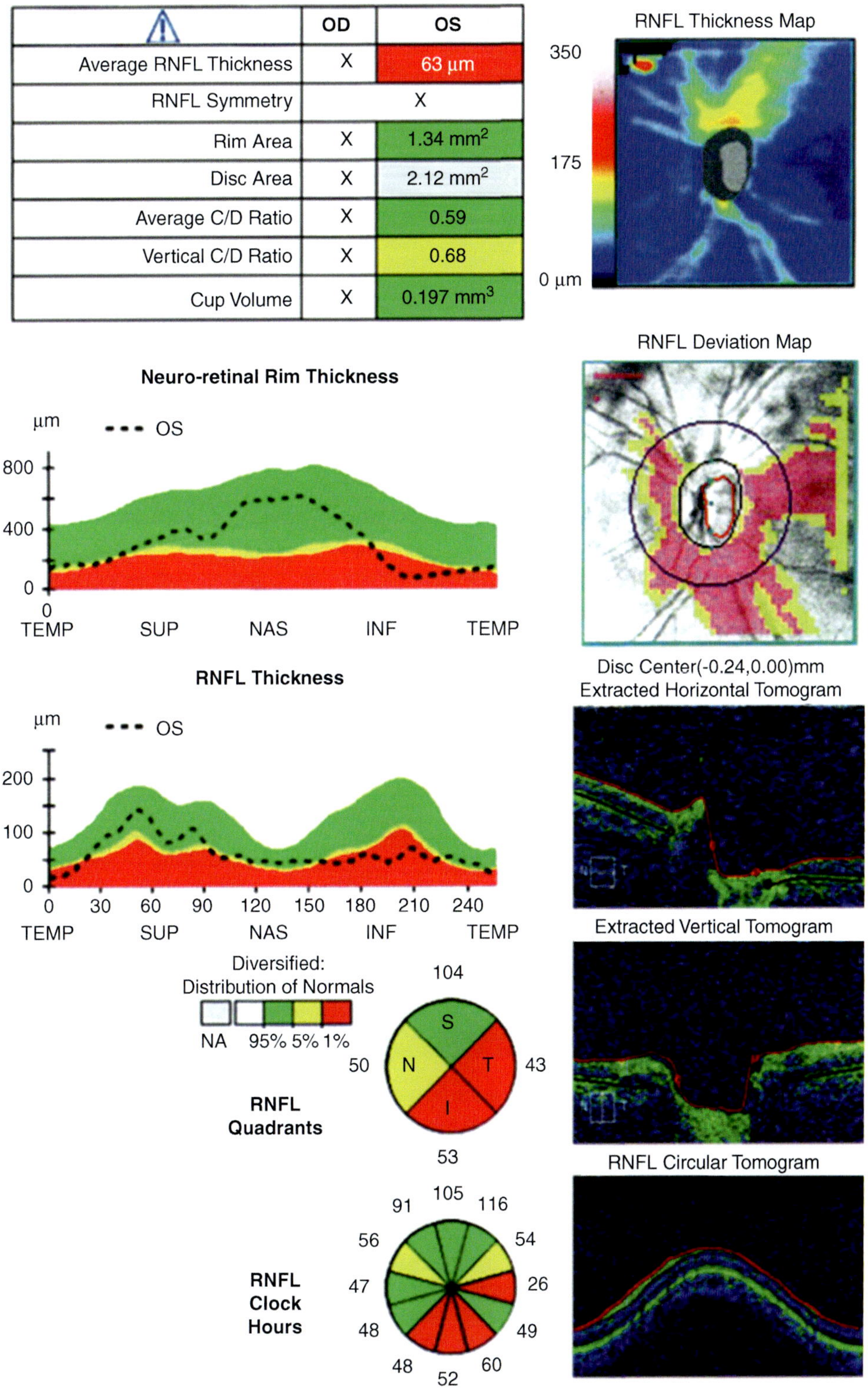

Fig. 26.3 OCT measurement of peripapillary RNFL thickness. OCT revealed RNFL thinning in the inferior and temporal quadrants of the left eye

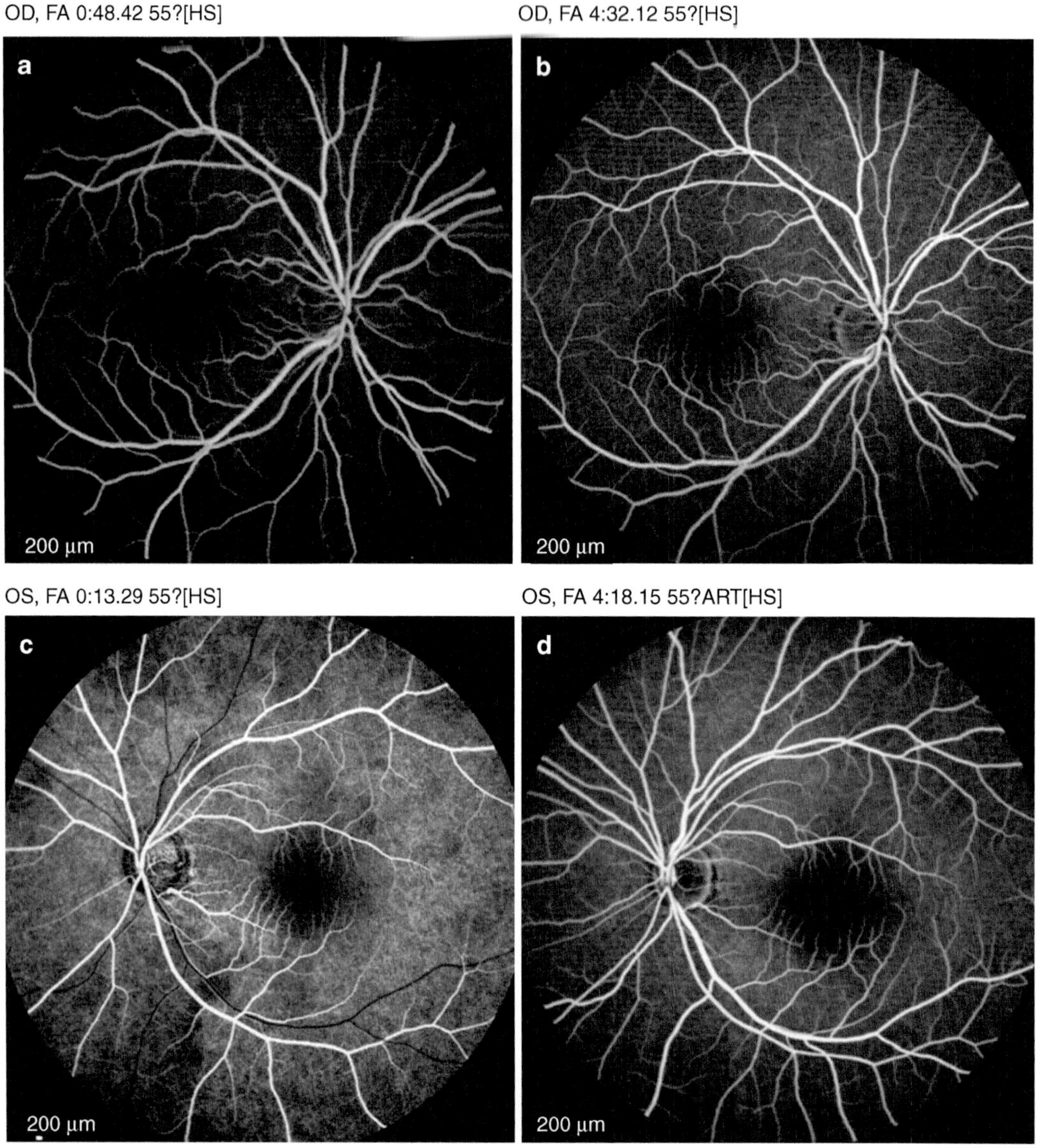

Fig. 26.4 FFA images. Panel a, b: The findings were normal at all stages in the right eye. Panel c: Hypofluorescence in the inferior optic disc was shown, and deep capillary vessels inside the cup could be observed at the early stage in the left eye. Panel d: Hypofluorescence could still be observed at this site at the middle and late stages

showed no abnormality (Fig. 26.11); and the response to 30 Hz flickering light was normal (Fig. 26.12).

26.1.3 Final Diagnosis

The final diagnosis was optic nerve hypoplasia in the left eye.

26.2 Discussion

The patient was a young female, and her chief complaint was loss of half of the visual field in one eye. The fundus examination and OCT revealed inferior RNFL thinning. She had been diagnosed with optic nerve atrophy and suspected with optic neuritis, NTG, etc. by multiple hospi-

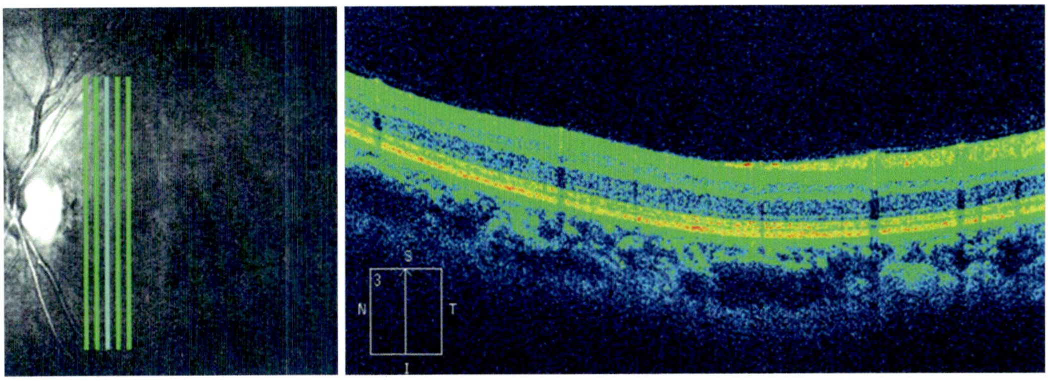

Fig. 26.5 OCT image of the retina temporal to the optic disc in the left eye. Vertical linear scanning of the area temporal to the optic disc showed that the signals from the inferior RNFL disappeared but the normal signals from the superior RNFL could be obtained

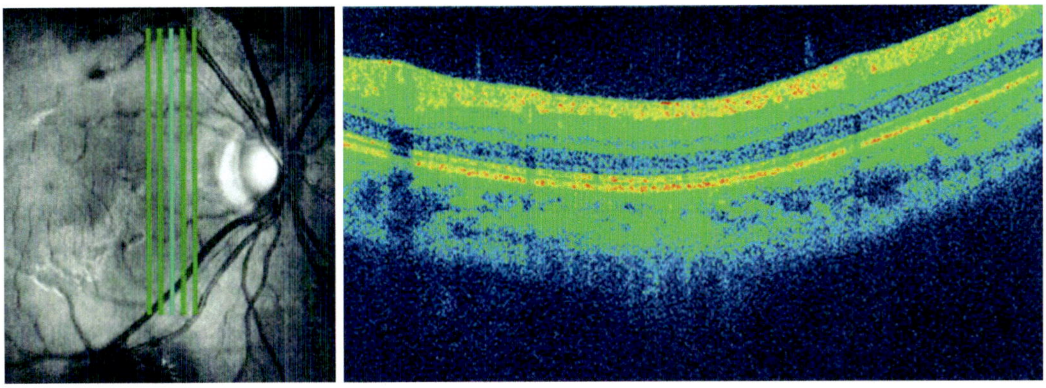

Fig. 26.6 OCT image of the retina temporal to the optic disc in the right eye. Normal signals could be observed from both the superior and inferior RNFL

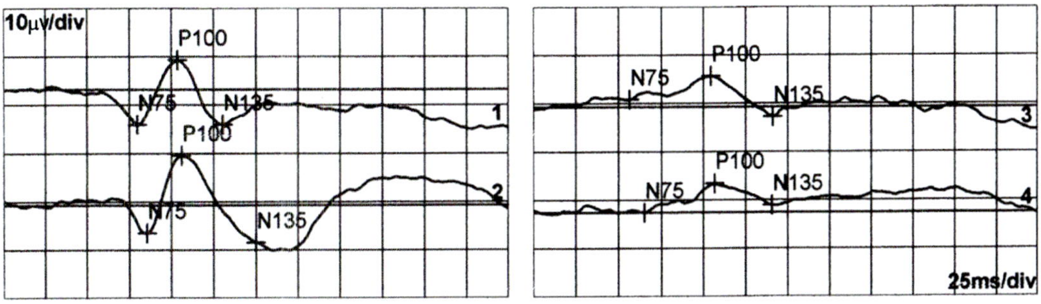

Channel	N75 [ms]	P100 [ms]	N135 [ms]	N75-P100	P100-N135
1 R-1 1,0	80	104	131	13.3µV	13.3µV
3 L-1 1,0	56	105	141	4.89µV	8.42µV
2 R-1 0,15	86	106	150	16.1µV	18µV
4 L-1 0,15	65	107	141	5.97µV	4.46µV
Normals	-	90-116-90-116	-	-	-

Channel	Stimulus	Ampl., Range, Filter
1 R-1 1,0	MON Patt. Rev. CB, 1?Full Field, Ctr:97% 1.5Hz, Avg:100	1, +/-100µV 1-50Hz
2 R-1 0,15	MON Patt. Rev. CB, 0?5' Full Field, Ctr:97% 1.5Hz, Avg:100	1, +/-100µV 1-50Hz
3 L-1 1,0	MON Patt. Rev. CB, 1?Full Field, Ctr:97% 1.5Hz, Avg:100	1, +/-100µV 1-50Hz

Fig. 26.7 P-VEP analysis printouts. A normal P100 wave was shown in the right eye; significantly reduced amplitude and normal latency of the P100 wave were shown in left eye

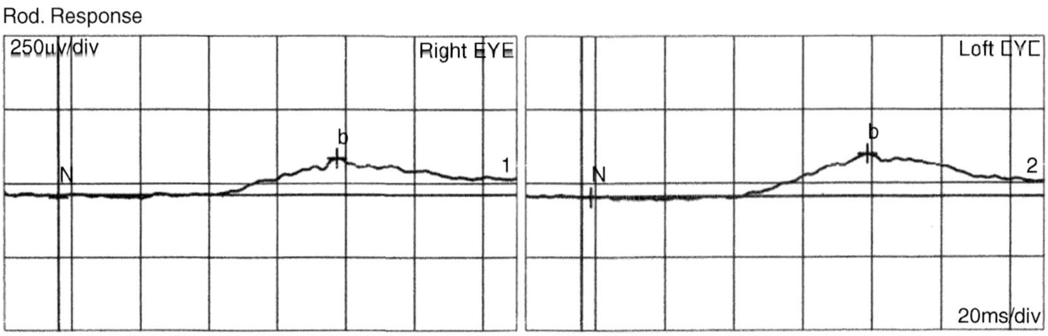

Fig. 26.8 Rod response wave in both eyes in ERG examination. The waveform, amplitude, and latency of the b-wave in the rod response showed no abnormality in either eye

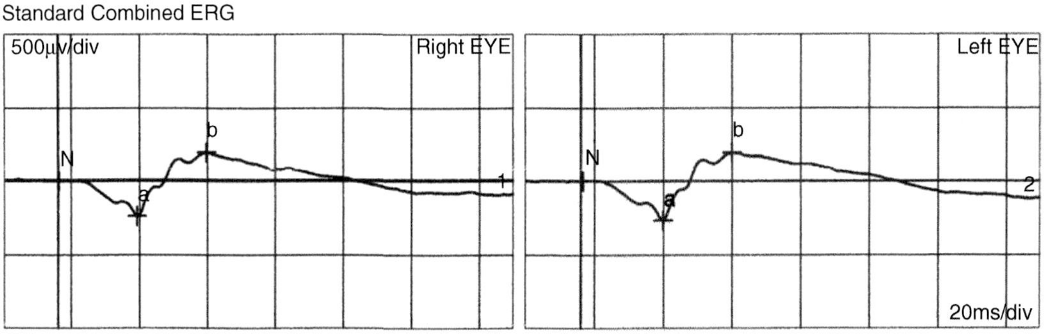

Fig. 26.9 Maximal mixed response waves in both eyes in ERG examination. The waveforms, amplitudes, and latency of a- and b-waves showed no abnormality, suggesting that the rod and cone cells were normal

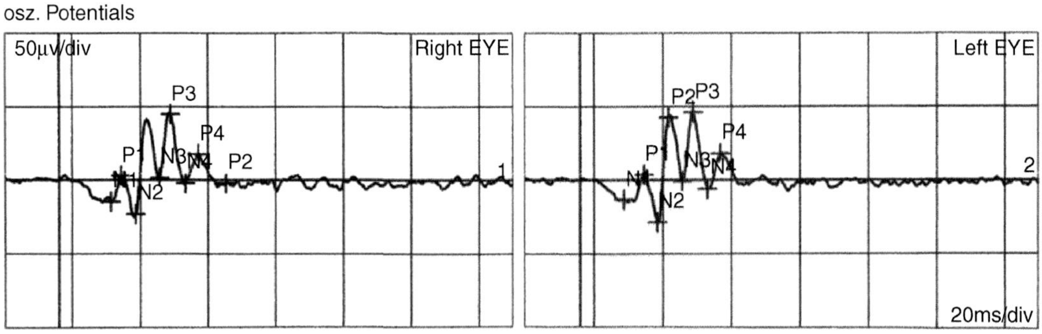

Fig. 26.10 Oscillatory potentials in both eyes in ERG examination. The amplitude of the OPs wave in ERG examination showed abnormality in both eyes, suggesting that the function of the internal layers of the retina had no abnormality

tals in the previous 3 years, which had made her suffer from great psychological burden.

Careful differential analysis of the visual field gave us important notes. The light sensitivity was zero at nearly all the test points in the superior half of the visual field with a clear horizontal boundary. This finding didn't conform to the characteristics of visual field changes caused by retinal nerve fiber bundle damage in glaucoma, AION, branch retinal vein occlusion

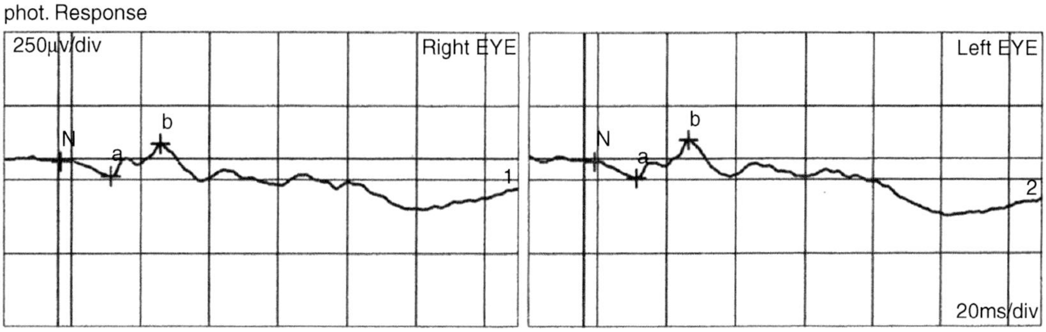

Fig. 26.11 Cone response waves in both eyes in ERG examination. The waveforms, amplitudes, and latencies of a- and b-waves in the cone response showed no abnormality

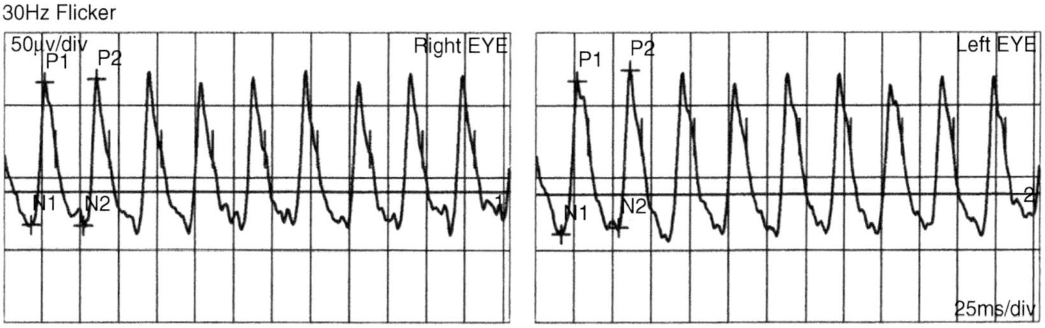

Fig. 26.12 Response to 30 Hz flickering light in both eyes in ERG examination. The amplitude of the sine wave P1 wave was free from any abnormality, suggesting that the peripheral cone cell function had no abnormality

(BRVO), etc. BRAO could be excluded in light of the medical history, fundus manifestation, and FFA. Congenital dysplasia was hence the most likely diagnosis. The OCT and electrophysiological examinations located the disease in the inferior RNFL from the perspective of structure and function, respectively. The hypoplasia of the inferior retinal nerve fibers caused the overall weakening of P-VEP and the amplitude reduction of the P100 wave. But the latency of the P100 wave was normal, which meant that most of the normal nerve fibers were preserved and the neuropotential conduction velocity was not influenced significantly.

As a nonprogressive congenital fundus dysplasia, optic nerve hypoplasia is caused by disrupted differentiation of retinal ganglion cells (RGCs) at the 13th–17th week of embryonic development. Optic nerves develop from the optic stalk whose early development takes places in a depression on the optic vesicle and in the diencephalon ventricle. The early-stage RGCs form the nerve fibers at the sixth week of embryo development. The nerve fibers will connect to the brain through the optic stalk, form sheath, and stretch to the lamina cribrosa via cerebral tissues [1].

Optic nerve dysplasia is a type of optic disc dysplasia, and significant differences could be found in its clinical manifestations depending on its severity. Superior optic nerve hypoplasia is usually seen in patients with insulin-dependent diabetes mellitus, and its clinical manifestations include the following: the position of central retinal arteries running out of the optic disc is superiorly shifted; the color of the superior optic disc is pale; halo can be observed in the peripheral area of the superior optic disc; the superior RNFL becomes thinner; and inferior visual field defects which can be very mild and are not be perceived by the patient in some cases can be found. In serious cases, the optic nerves may be absent (coloboma of the optic disc), and the affected eye has no light sensitivity.

The patient in this case denied histories of systemic diseases including diabetes. She was delivered vaginally and born full term. Her mother was healthy according to her own account. The patient's clinical manifestation was unilateral inferior optic nerve hypoplasia, which is very rare clinically. But the patient was diagnosed with congenital dysplasia after the symptoms, signs, and assistant examination results were all considered. The patient's psychological stress was alleviated after she was told that the disease was nonprogressive.

The patient's disease should also be differentiated with segmental optic nerve hypoplasia (tilted optic disc syndrome). The latter is also a congenital optic nerve hypoplasia in which the visual field impairment is usually found in the supratemporal quadrant, and one eye or both eyes are affected. But its fundus manifestations are a "D-shaped" or horizontal oval-shaped optic disc that tilts with the longitudinal axis accompanied by peripapillary atrophy and localized hypoplasia of the retina, choroid, or RPE [2, 3]. These characteristics can be used for differentiation.

Although the cause of visual function damage has been identified in this case, the diagnosis was only a descriptive one. The pathogenesis was still unclear and no relevant literature was found for review. The patient was still young, and there was no evidence showing local inflammatory, vascular, and oppressive lesions. Therefore, congenital dysplasia was considered to be highly possible. The outcome of the patient was worth following up via visual field monitoring.

References

1. Reynolds JD. Pediatric retina. Translated by Wang Yusheng. Xi'an: The Fourth Military Medical University Press; 2013.
2. Moschos MM, Triglianos A, Rotsos T, et al. Tilted disc syndrome: an OCT and mfERG study. Doc Ophthalmol. 2009;119(1):23–8.
3. Karna S. Atlas of neuro-ophthalmology. Translated by Zhao Jialiang. Beijing: Beijing Science and Technology Press; 2007.

Unusual "Narrow Anterior Chamber"

27

Ning Fan, Xuyang Liu, and Jiantao Wang

Two young females were observed with unusual bilateral shallow anterior chamber, narrow anterior chamber angle, short ocular axis, and symmetrical macular foci. One of them was even found with high intraocular pressure (IOP) and glaucomatous optic nerve damage. Did the shallow anterior chamber and glaucoma and the maculopathy belong to a single syndrome or two different diseases? Was there any inherent connection between the anatomical abnormality found in the anterior segment and the macular focus? If so, what's mechanism for the connection?

27.1 Case 1

27.1.1 Case Presentation

A 19-year-old female patient presented with gradual decrease of visual acuity in both eyes for over 3 years and swelling pain in the left eye for 1 month without any significant trigger. She had received trabeculectomy 2 years before due to high IOP in the right eye. IOP control after the operation was fine. Trabeculectomy had been performed again 4 months before due to high IOP in the left eye. Swelling pain in the left eye had started 1 month before.

Upon examination, the best corrected visual acuity (BCVA) was 20/100 OD and 20/40 OS. The IOP was 17 mmHg OD and 55 mmHg OS. Filtering bleb of the conjunctiva showed generalized mild elevation in the right eye and was flat in the left eye. The cornea was transparent in the right eye and suffered from mild fog-like epithelium edema in the left eye. The anterior chamber was shallow, and irregular peripheral anterior synechia of the iris could be observed in both eyes. The diameter of the pupil was 2.5 mm OD and 4 mm OS. The lens was transparent in both eyes. Fundus examination revealed that the C/D ratio was about 0.4 OD and about 0.7 OS. In both eyes, the yellowish flecks, which were denser in the macula, could be observed in the posterior pole, and local shallow macular detachment could also be found (Fig. 27.1). The axial length was 21.37 mm OD and 21.78 mm OS.

Visual field examination demonstrated a relative scotoma in the center of the right eye, light sensitivity reduction in superior quadrant of the left eye, and supranasal and central scotomas in the left eye (Fig. 27.2).

Ultrasound biomicroscopy (UBM) showed a shallow anterior chamber in both eyes. Anterior synechia was revealed in the four quadrants of

N. Fan · J. Wang (✉)
Shenzhen Eye Hospital, Shenzhen University, Shenzhen, China

X. Liu
Xiamen Eye Center of Xiamen University, Xiamen, China

Shenzhen Eye Hospital, Shenzhen University, Shenzhen, China

N. Wang et al. (eds.), *Optic Disorders and Visual Field*, Advances in Visual Science and Eye Diseases 2, https://doi.org/10.1007/978-981-13-2502-1_27

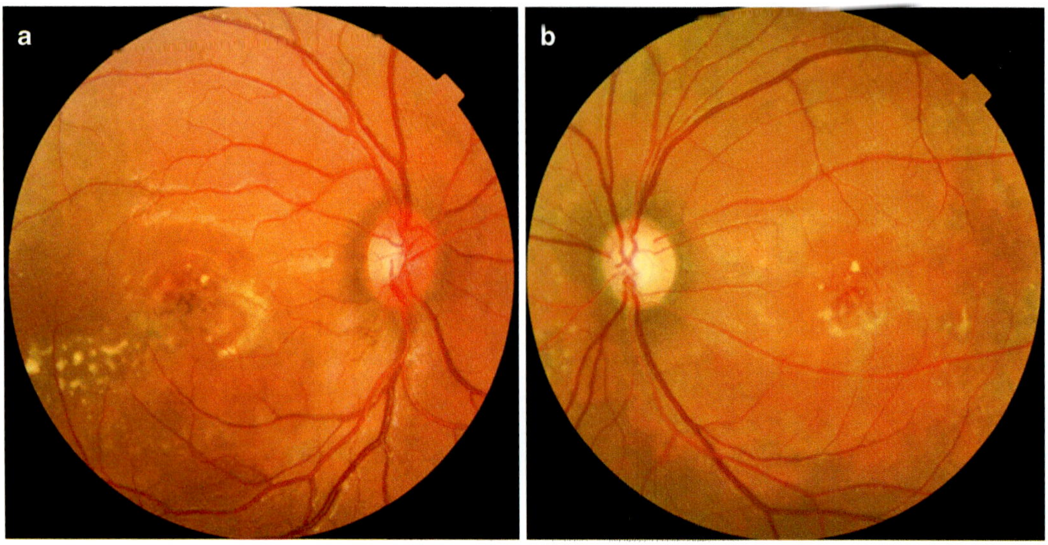

Fig. 27.1 Fundus photographs. Yellowish flecks foci, which were denser in the macula, could be observed in the posterior pole in both eyes, and local shallow detachment could also be seen. The C/D ratio was about 0.4 OD and about 0.7 OS. Panel a: Right eye. Panel b: Left eye

peripheral iris. The trabecular opening of the right eye could be seen vaguely with sparse filtering bleb and the iris peripheral anterior synechia. The trabecular incision in the left eye was unclear, and no significant filtering bleb formation was seen (Fig. 27.3).

27.1.2 Case Analysis

The patient was 19 years old with high IOP caused by angle closure and iris peripheral anterior synechia in both eyes. Glaucomatous visual field damage (supranasal scotoma) and optic disc change (neuroretinal rim thinning) were also found in the left eye. The clinical manifestations were similar with those of angle-closure glaucoma. Besides, the macular foci suggested that the scotomas found in the central visual fields of both eyes were originated from the maculopathy. These two conditions were very rarely found in young females. Then, what disease did the patient suffer from in the macula? Did the disease have any inner connection with the shallow anterior chambers and angle adhesion and closure in the anterior segment? To find the answers, we performed further examinations on the retina and macula.

Fundus fluorescein angiography (FFA) showed irregular speckled hyperfluorescence in the posterior pole and hive-like punctate hypofluorescence in the macula in both eyes at the early stage of angiography. No significant fluorescence leakage was shown at the late stage (Fig. 27.4).

Optical coherence tomography (OCT) of the macula revealed scattered high-reflection material depositions on the surface of the RPE accompanied by neurosensory retinal detachment in both eyes (Fig. 27.5).

Electrooculography (EOG) demonstrated that the light peak was decreased in both eyes and the Arden ratio (light peak potential/dark-trough potential) was 0.92 OD and 0.95 OS (Fig. 27.6).

The patient's fundus and EOG findings supported the diagnosis of Best disease. But was there any connection between the Best disease and her "angle-closure glaucoma?" Best disease is inherited in an autosomal dominant manner, so did the patient have a family history? Could the patient be diagnosed with Best vitelliform macular dystrophy (BVMD)?

A second inquiry on her medical history disclosed that the patient was an adopted orphan and

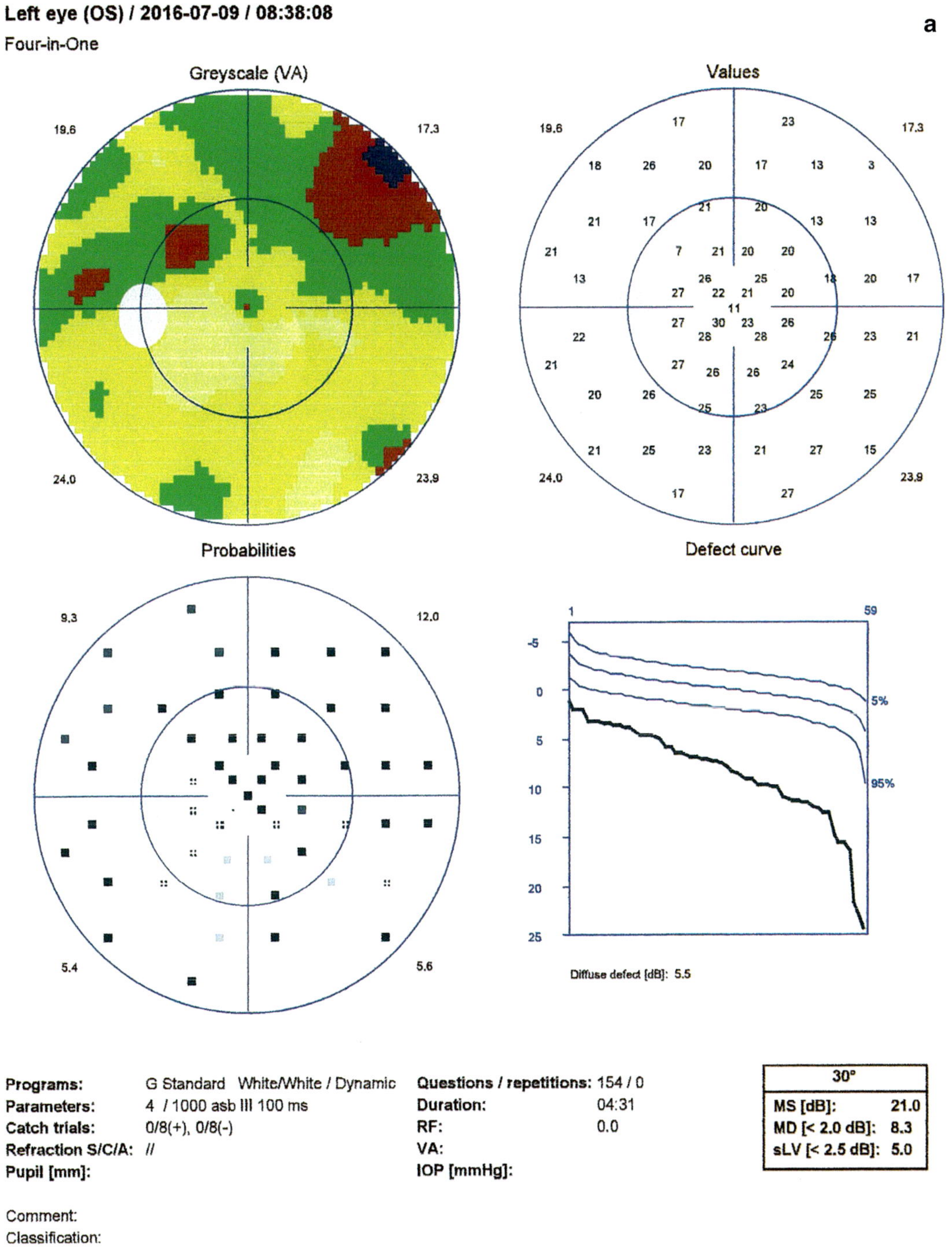

Fig. 27.2 Octopus visual field analysis printouts. Panel a: Light sensitivity reduction in superior quadrant and supra-nasal and central scotomas could be seen in the left eye. Panel b: A relative scotoma could be seen in the center of the right eye

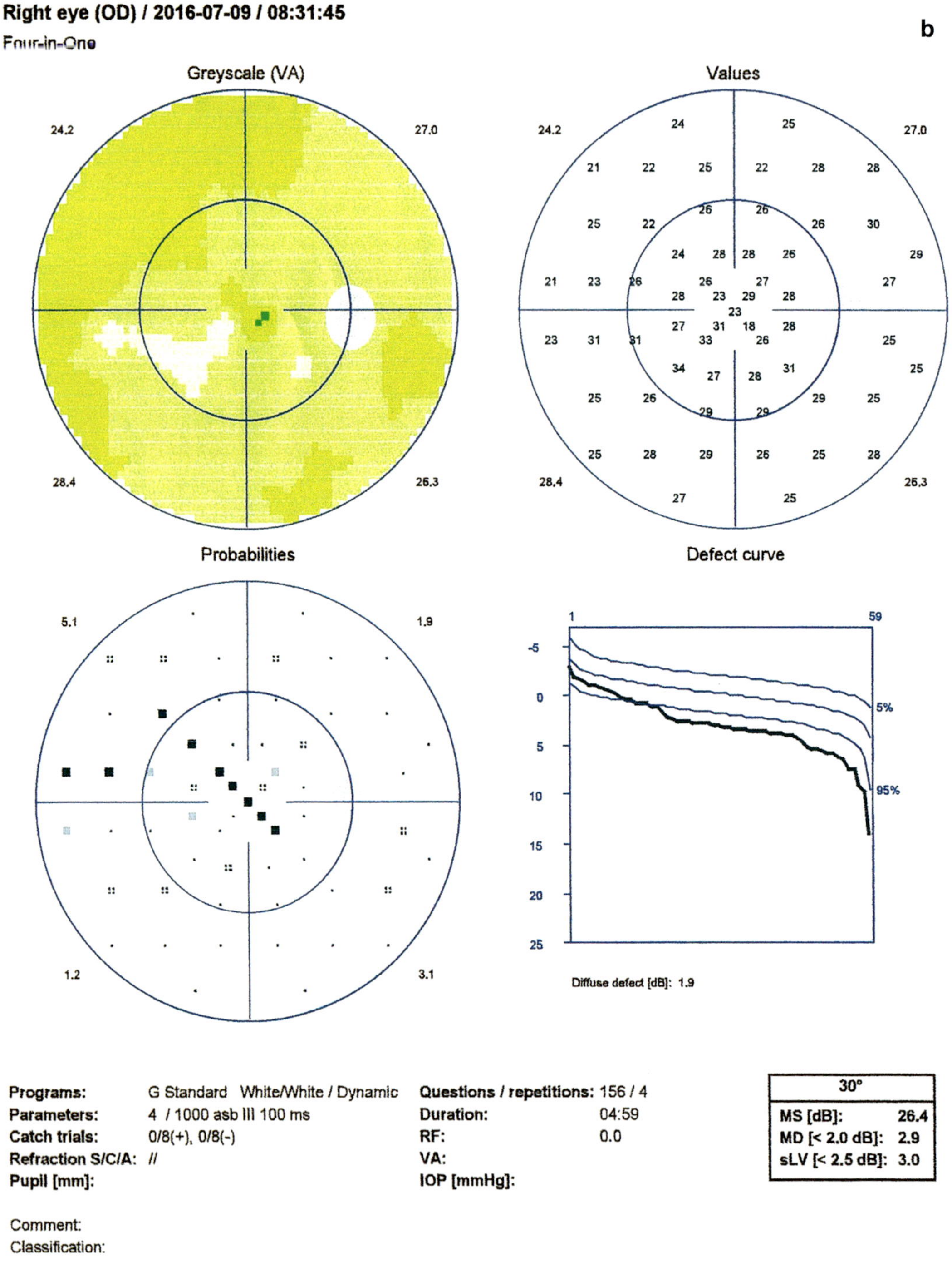

Fig. 27.2 (continued)

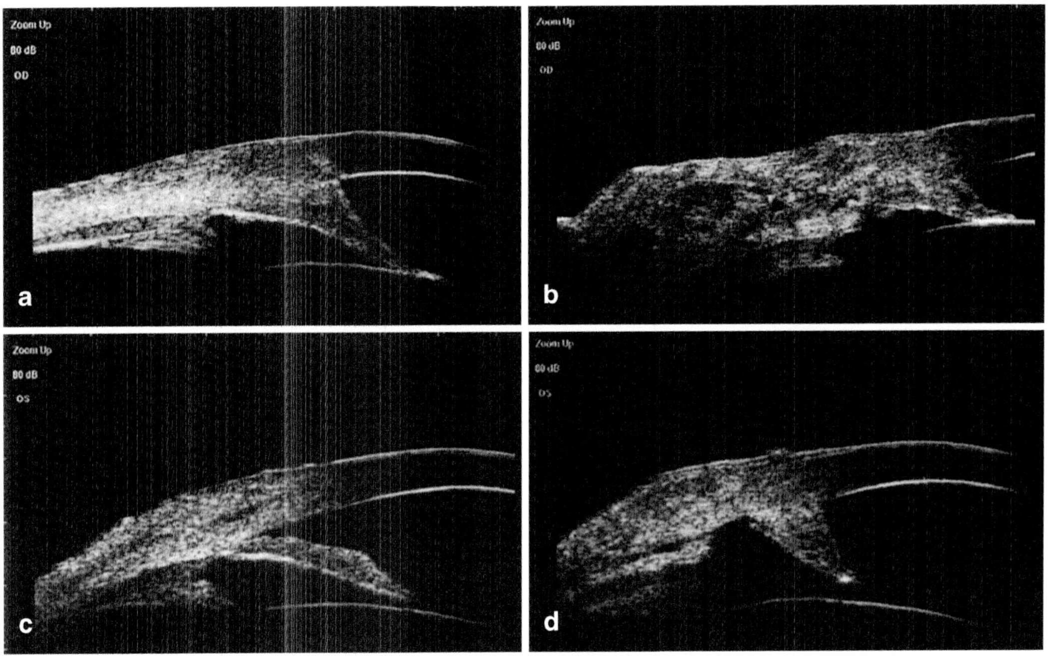

Fig. 27.3 UBM images of both eyes. UBM showed a shallow anterior chamber in both eyes. Anterior synechia was revealed in the four quadrants of peripheral iris. The trabecular opening of the right eye could be seen vaguely with sparse filtering bleb and the iris peripheral anterior synechia. The trabecular incision in the left eye was unclear, and no significant filtering bleb formation was seen; Panel a, b: Right eye. Panel c, d: Left eye

the health conditions of her biological parents were unknown.

Gene test revealed that BEST1 had a homozygous p. Arg255Gln (c.764G > A) mutation, i.e., G mutated into A at the position 764 and arginine into glutamine at the position 255.

BEST1 gene mutation was detected in the patient, which didn't conform to the pattern of autosomal dominant inheritance, and because the detection on her parents, brothers, and sisters could not be performed, it could not be ascertained that the inheritance pattern was autosomal recessive inheritance. However, the analyses on the genotype and phenotype of the patient suggested that what the patient had should be autosomal recessive bestrophinopathy (ARB), which is extremely similar to the BVMD and caused by BEST1 gene mutation. It is known that the BEST1 gene is connected with the anterior segment development of the eyes (refer to "discussion" for details). Therefore, the angle closure of her both eyes was actually relevant to the inborn dysplasia in the anterior segments. Hence, a more accurate description of her glaucoma should be developmental glaucoma.

27.1.3 Final Diagnosis

The final diagnosis was bilateral autosomal recessive bestrophinopathy (ARB) and bilateral developmental glaucoma.

27.2 Case 2

27.2.1 Case Presentation

A 32-year-old female patient presented with recurrent bilateral eye fullness and pain accompanied by ipsilateral headache for several months. The patient had been suffering from bilateral eye fullness and pain accompanied by ipsilateral headache after fatiguing work in previous several months. The symptoms could remit spontaneously after

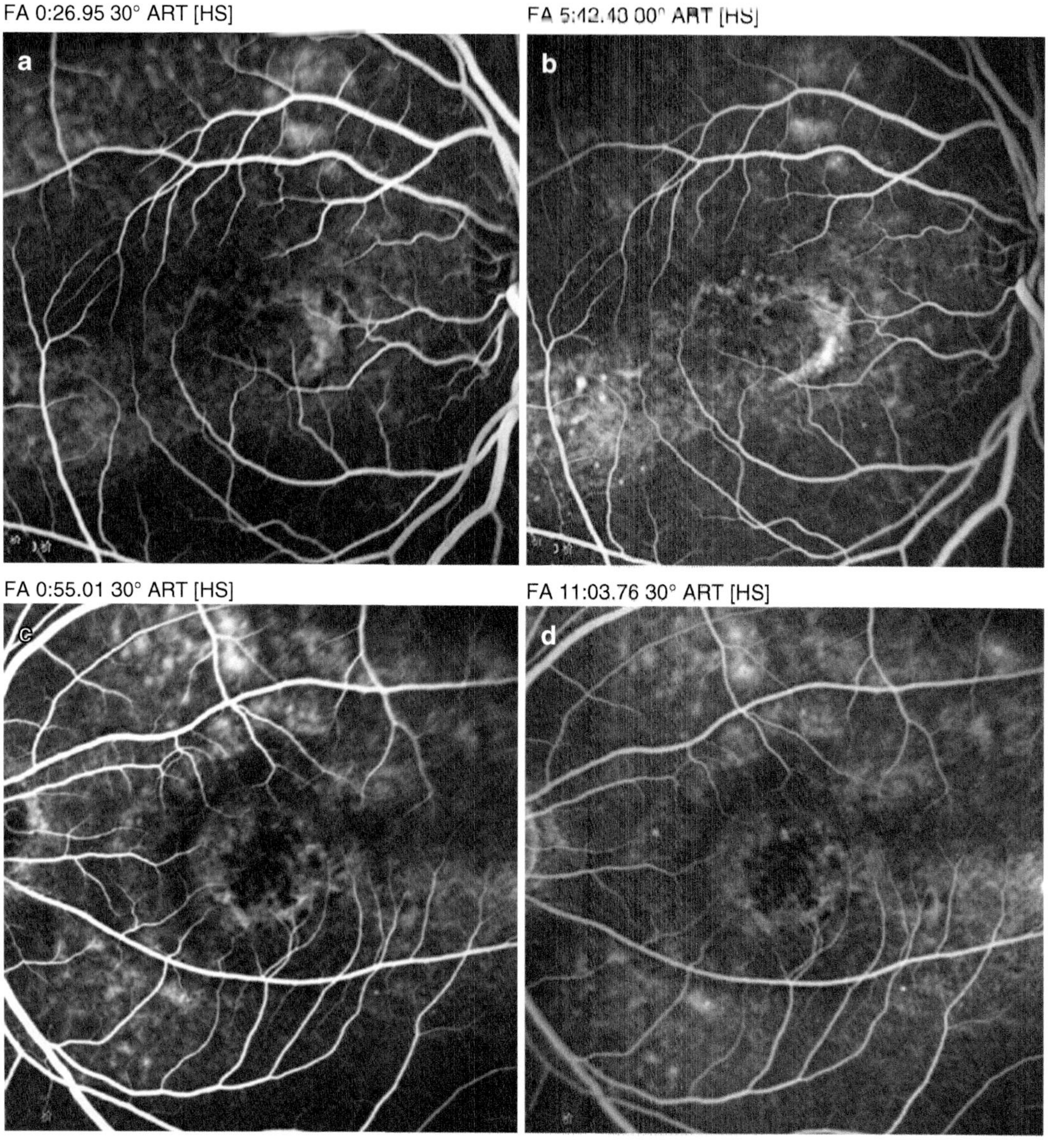

Fig. 27.4 FFA images of both eyes. FFA showed irregular speckled hyperfluorescence in the posterior pole and hive-like punctate hypofluorescence in the macula in both eyes at the early stage of angiography. No significant fluorescence leakage was shown at the late stage. Panel a: Early stage of angiography for the right eye. Panel b: Late stage of angiography for the right eye. Panel c: Early stage of angiography for the left eye. Panel d: Late stage of angiography for the left eye

rest. Bilateral acute painless vision decrease had been experienced by the patient when she was 8 years old, and she was diagnosed with maculopathy at another hospital. The visual acuity of both eyes improved gradually after drug treatment for several years, and no recurrence had been reported so far. Histories of trauma, operation, systemic diseases, and familial diseases were denied.

Upon examination, the BCVA of the right eye was 20/32 and the UCVA of the left eye was 20/20. The IOP measured with a noncontract tonometer was 19 mmHg OD and 20 mmHg OS. Slit-lamp examination of her anterior segments showed that, in both eyes, conjunctival congestion was absent, the cornea was transparent, the anterior chamber was shallow, peripheral

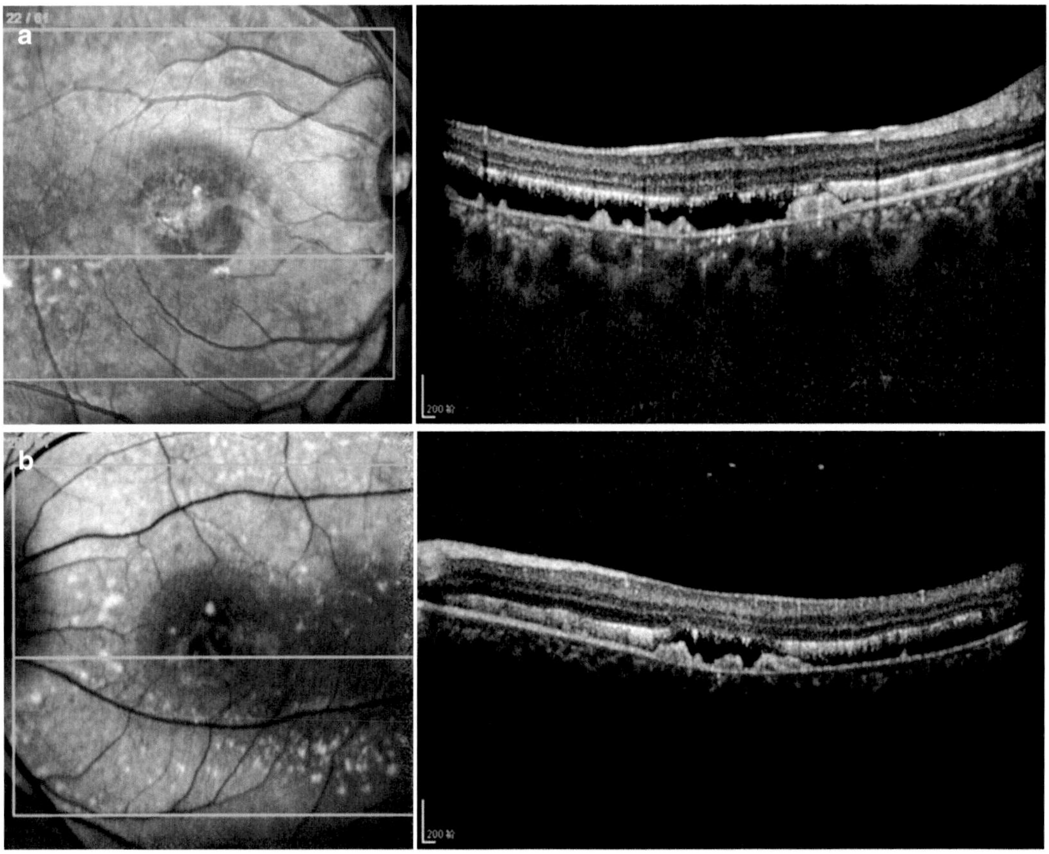

Fig. 27.5 OCT scanning of the macula. OCT revealed scattered high-reflection material depositions on the surface of the RPE accompanied by neurosensory retinal detachment in both eyes. Panel a: Right eye. Panel b: Left eye

anterior chamber was narrowed, the pupil was round with a diameter of 3 mm, and the lens was transparent. Fundus examination revealed that the C/D ratio was 0.2 OD and 0.3 OS, the optic disc was pink in color with a clear boundary in both eyes, and symmetrical white foci could be observed in the macula (Fig. 27.7). The axial length was 20.94 mm OD and 21.13 mm OS.

Visual field examination with the 10-2 test revealed a central relative scotoma in both eyes (Fig. 27.8).

UBM before laser iridotomy revealed the following findings: the central anterior chamber depth was about 1.82 mm in the right eye and 1.78 mm in the left eye; in both eyes, the anterior chamber angle narrowing, forward rotation of the ciliary body, and peripheral iris elevation could be observed in four quadrants (Figs. 27.9a and 27.10a). The reexamination after laser iridotomy showed the following results: the central anterior chamber depth was about 1.91 mm in the right eye and 1.85 mm in the left eye; in both eyes, the angle between the iris and the surface of trabecular meshwork became wider, and significant deepener was revealed in the peripheral anterior chamber, which suggested that the pupillary block was involved in the pathological process of angle closure (Figs. 27.9b and 27.10b).

OCT of the macula showed a fovea that lost its normal shape with only 82 μm in thickness and abnormal hyperreflectivities in the subretinal space in the right eye, and the abnormal hyperreflectivities in the subretinal space accompanied by neurosensory retinal detachment at the macula were seen in the left eye (Fig. 27.11).

FFA demonstrated round-speckled hyperfluorescence foci mixed with fluorescence blockage by pigment in the macula in both eyes. No

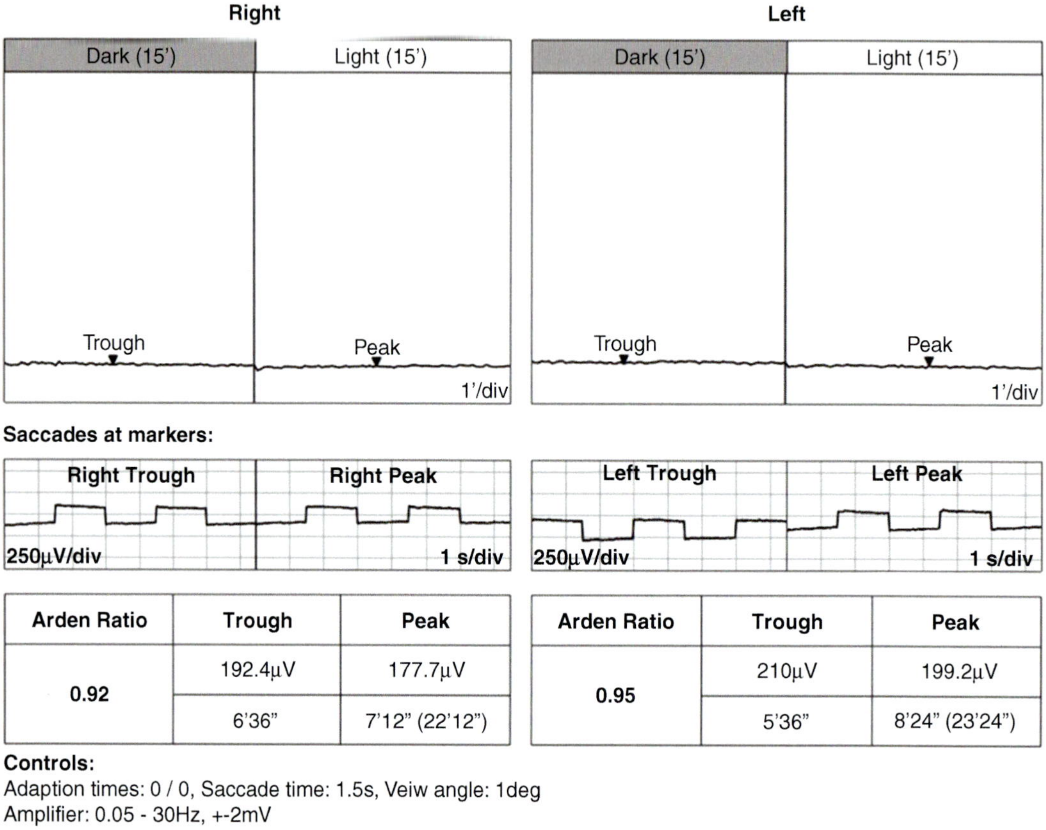

Fig. 27.6 Electrooculograms of both eyes. EOG demonstrated that the light peak was decreased in both eyes and the Arden ratio (light peak potential/dark-trough potential) was 0.92 OD and 0.95 OS

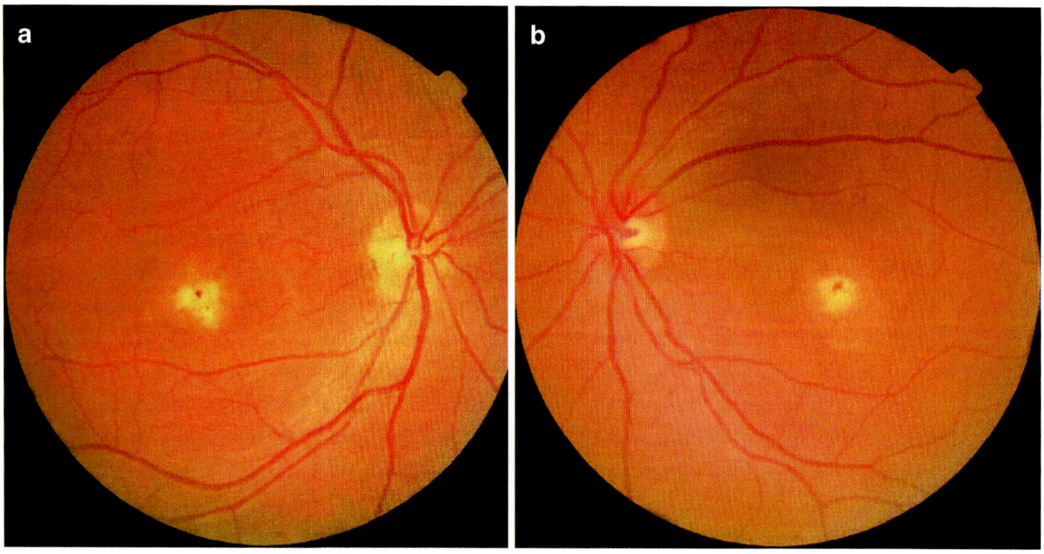

Fig. 27.7 Fundus photographs of both eyes. It could be seen that the optic disc was red with a clear boundary in both eyes, and symmetrical white foci were present in the macula. The C/D ratio was about 0.2 OD and about 0.3 OS. Panel a: Right eye. Panel b: Left eye

significant fluorescent leakage was shown at the late stage (Fig. 27.12).

Multifocal electroretinogram (mf-ERG) showed abnormal waveform and amplitude reduction in both eyes, and the central peak was not formed in the right eye (Fig. 27.13).

27.2.2 Case Analysis

Compared with the above case, no IOP increase but significant pupillary block could be found in this case. Outflow of aqueous humor from the posterior chamber was observed when the peripheral iris was

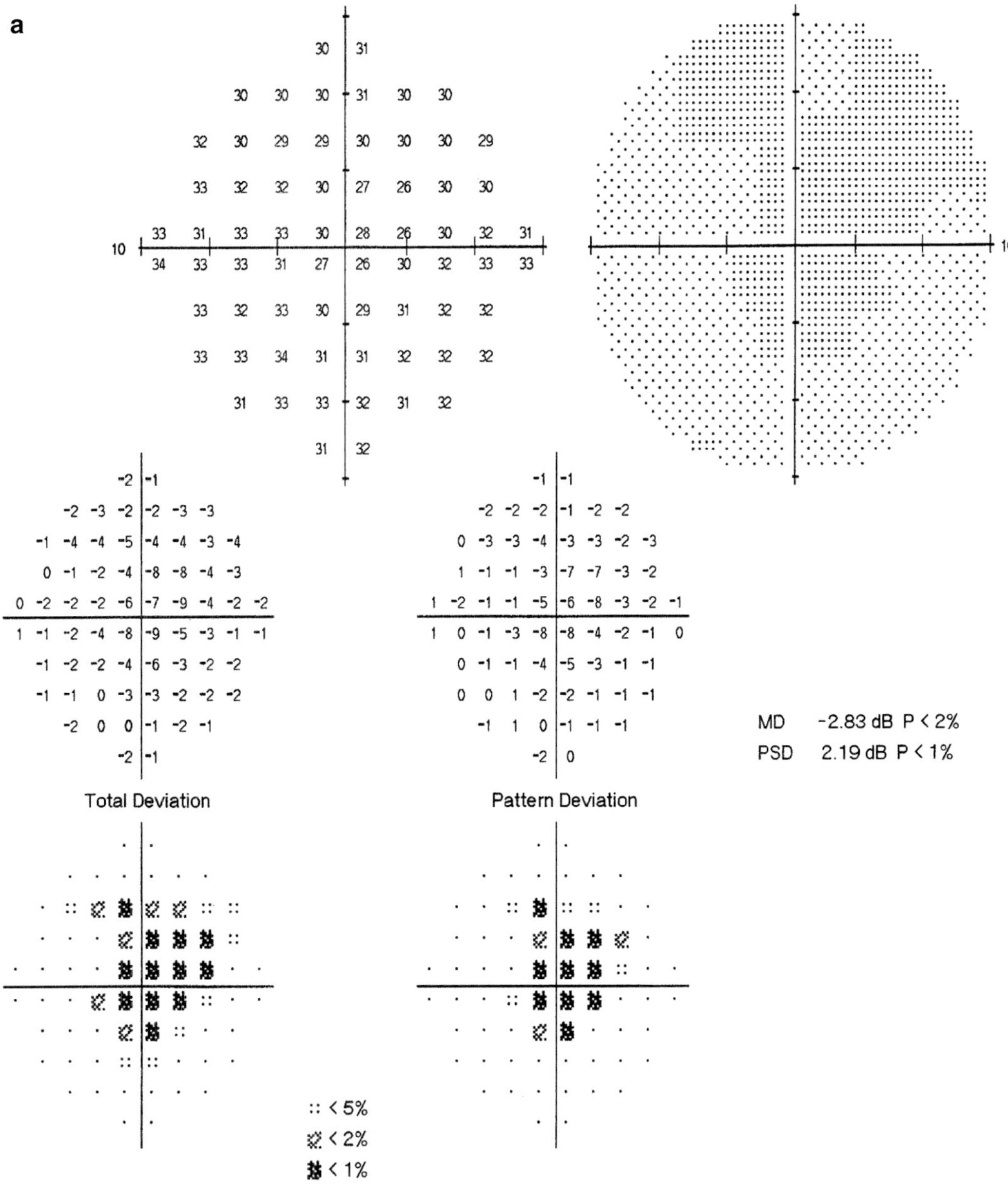

Fig. 27.8 Humphrey visual field analysis printouts. The examination with the 10-2 test revealed a central relative scotoma in both eyes

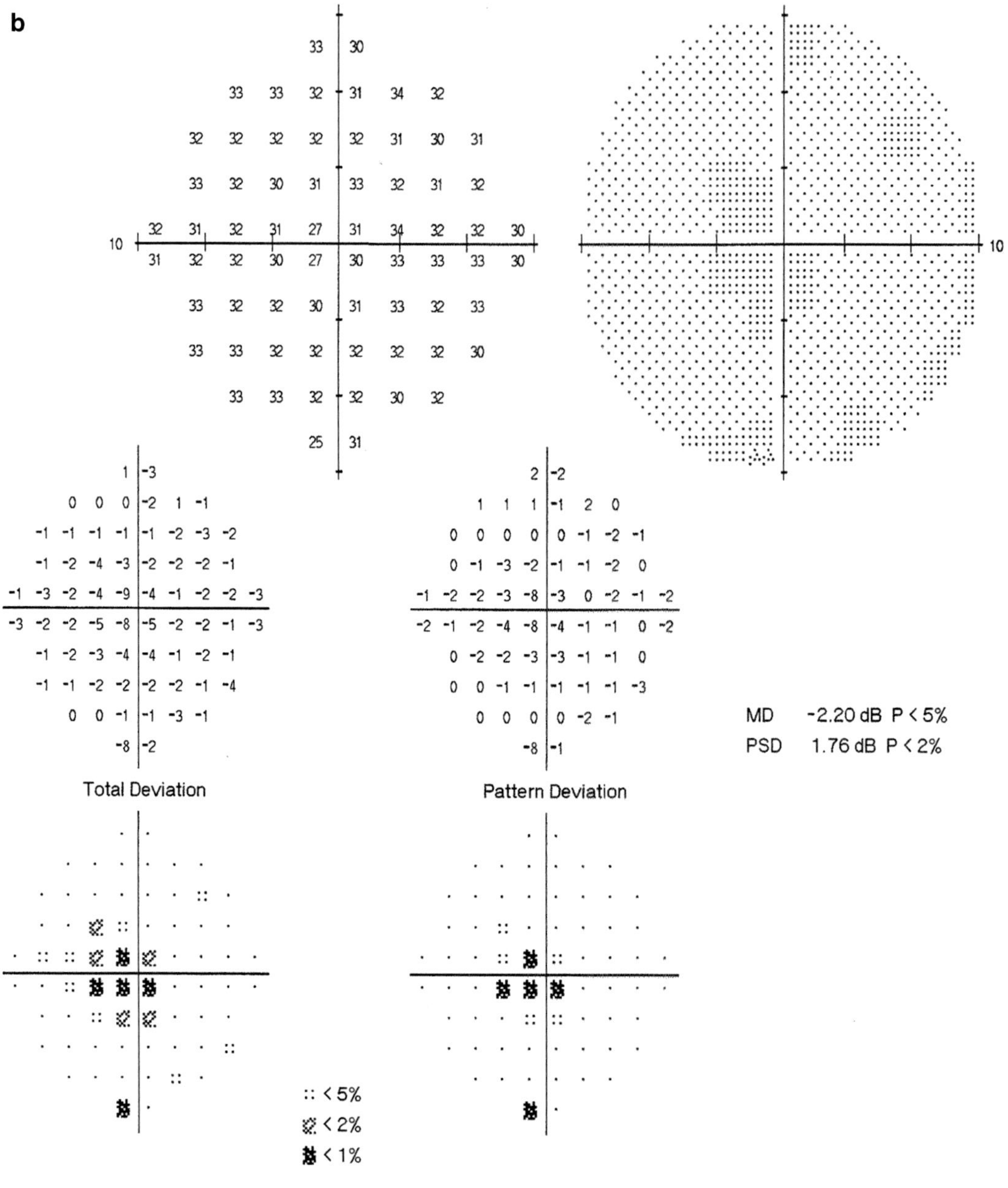

Fig. 27.8 (continued)

cut open by laser, and the peripheral anterior chamber became deeper immediately. The findings suggested that the patient had the anatomical basis of angle-closure glaucoma. Her fundus manifestations were also similar with those found in the above case, but the fundus disease duration was longer in this case, and scarring of the retinal foci was shown in the right eye. In order to get closer to the diagnosis, gene test was then performed.

BEST1 gene screening on the DNA of peripheral venous blood of the patient identified disease-related mutations.

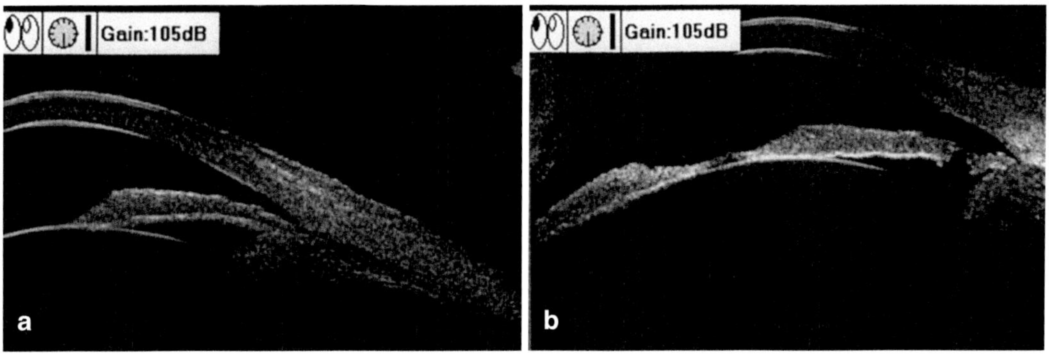

Fig. 27.9 UBM images of the right eye before and after laser iridotomy. Panel a: The 6 o'clock position UBM image taken before operation showed anterior chamber angle narrowing, forward rotation of ciliary body, and peripheral iris elevation. Panel b: The UBM image taken from the same site after operation showed the angle between the iris and the surface of trabecular meshwork became wide, and significant deepening was revealed in the peripheral anterior chamber

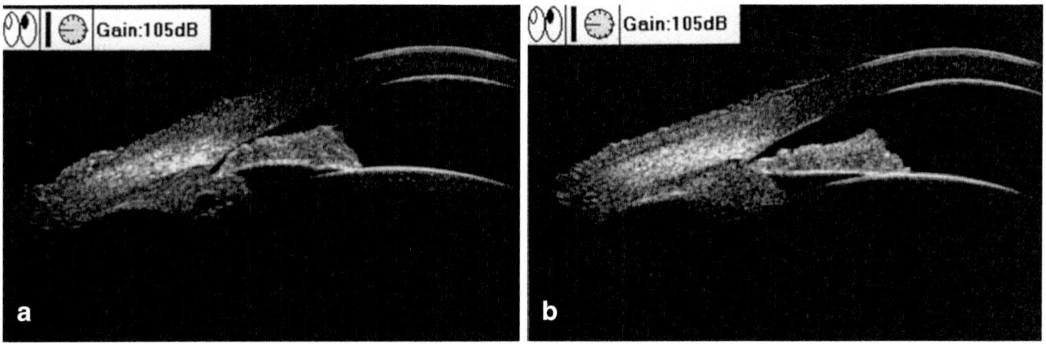

Fig. 27.10 UBM image of the left eye before and after laser iridotomy. Panel a: The 9 o'clock position UBM image taken before operation showed anterior chamber angle narrowing, forward rotation of the ciliary body, and peripheral iris elevation. Panel b: The UBM image taken from the same site after operation showed that the angle between the iris and the surface of trabecular meshwork became wide, and significant deepening was revealed in the peripheral anterior chamber

27.2.3 Final Diagnosis

The final diagnosis was bilateral autosomal recessive bestrophinopathy (ARB).

27.3 Discussion

BEST1 gene mutation can give rise to various clinical phenotypes. The most common one is BVMD, and the other phenotypes include adult-onset vitelliform macular dystrophy (AVMD), ARB, autosomal dominant vitreoretinochoroidopathy (ADVIRC), and MRCS syndrome (microcornea, rod-cone dystrophy, cataract, and posterior staphyloma) [1].

The clinical phenotypes of ARB and BVMD are similar. Their main difference is the inheritance pattern. The inheritance pattern of ARB is autosomal recessive inheritance while that of BVMD is autosomal dominant inheritance. Their clinical manifestations are also different. For instance, the typical yolk-like focus will not be shown in the macula in ARB. The main characteristics of ARB are vitelline material deposition, subretinal effusion, and macular edema, and it is usually distributed at the superior and inferior vascular arches outside the fovea. The EOG

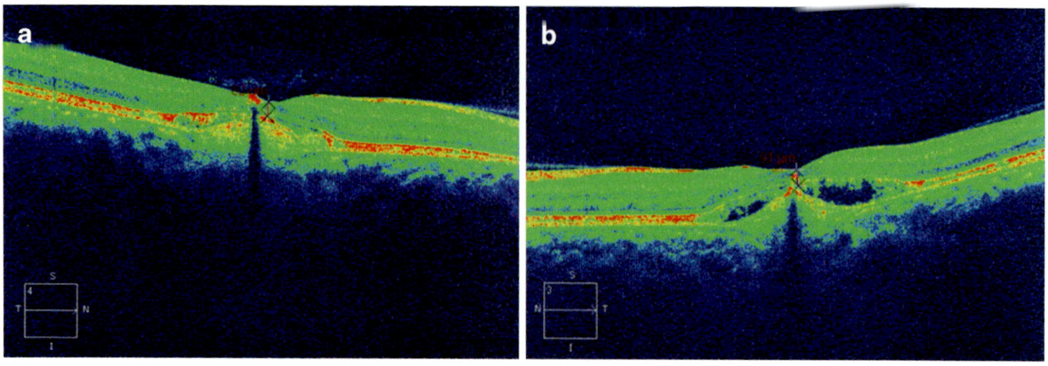

Fig. 27.11 Macular OCT images of both eyes. Panel a: A fovea that lost its normal shape with only 82 μm in thickness and abnormal hyperreflectivities in the subretinal space were seen in the right eye. Panel b: The abnormal hyperreflectivities in the subretinal space accompanied by neurosensory retinal detachment at the macula were seen in the left eye

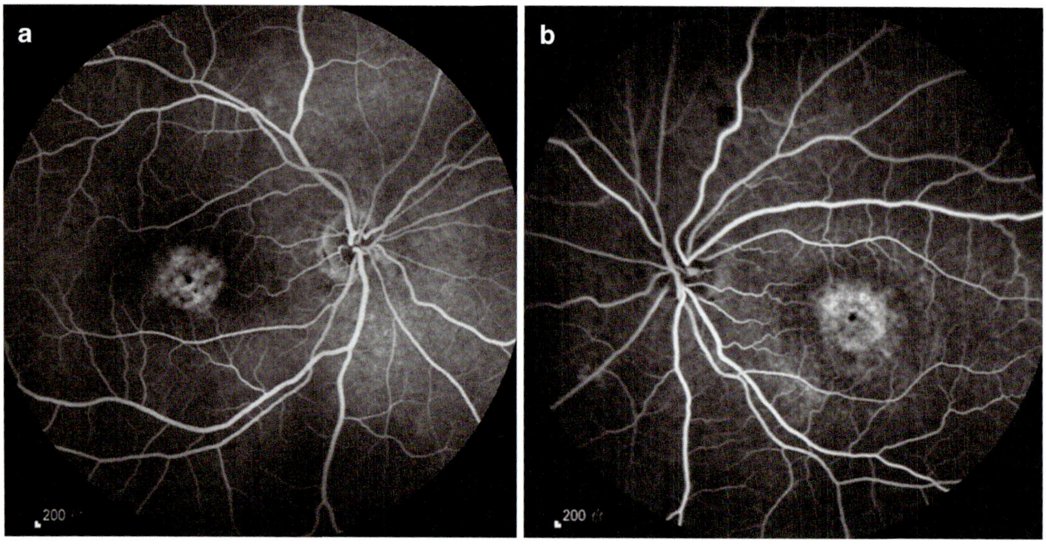

Fig. 27.12 FFA images of both eyes. Round-speckled hyperfluorescence foci mixed with fluorescence blockage by pigment could be found in the macula in both eyes. No significant fluorescent leakage was shown at the late stage. Panel a: Late stage of angiography for the right eye. Panel b: Late stage of angiography for the left eye

manifestations of ARB, which are significant decrease or disappearance of light adaptation and abnormal Arden ratio, are consistent with those found in BVMD. The ERG manifestations of ARB are decreases of both cone and rod responses [2]. The fundus manifestations and gene test results in the two cases mentioned in this section were both consistent with those of ARB. The fundus manifestations were multifocal yellowish material deposition accompanied by subretinal effusion. The gene tests revealed BEST 1 gene mutation. Therefore, the final diagnoses were both ARB. As a contrast, the fundus manifestations of the more common BVMD are yolk-like appearance formed by pale yellow lipofuscin deposition in the retinal pigment epithelium and/or below the retina (as shown in Fig. 27.14).

BEST1 gene encoding happens in the RPE bestrophin-1 protein. Bestrophin-1 protein is a multifunction protein and has functions including

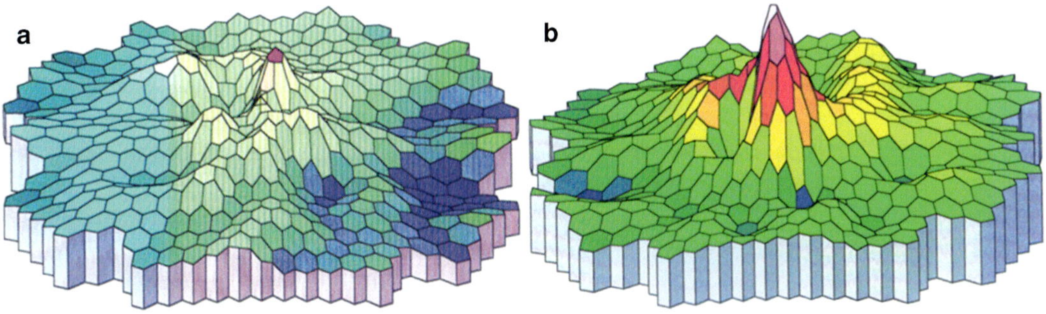

Fig. 27.13 mf-ERG images of both eyes. Abnormal waveform and amplitude reduction were revealed in both eyes. The central peak was not formed in the right eye. Panel a: Right eye. Panel b: Left eye

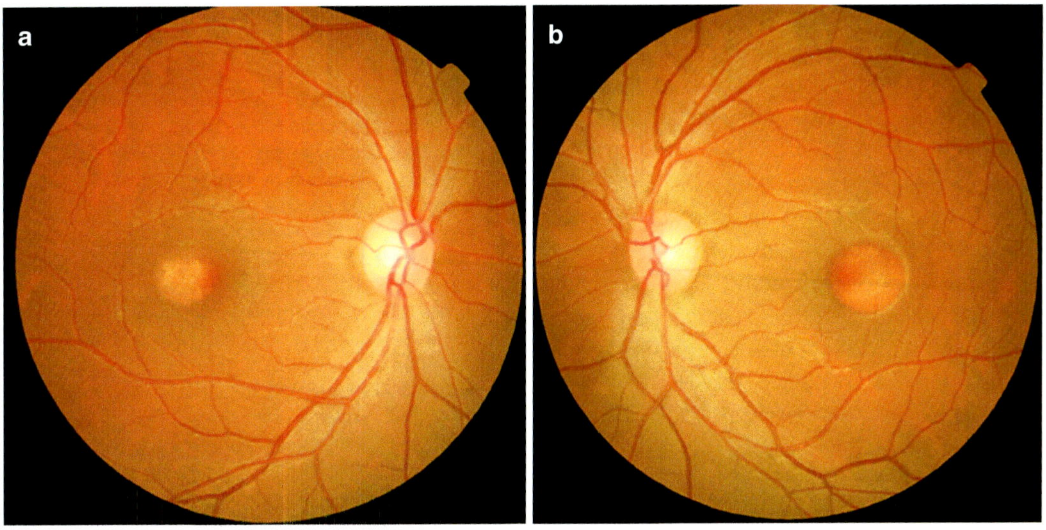

Fig. 27.14 Fundus photographs of both eyes. Fundus examination showed yolk-like appearance formed by pale yellow lipofuscin deposition in the macula. Panel a: Right eye. Panel b: Left eye

regulation of chloride and calcium channels, etc. BEST1 gene mutation will lead to the function disorder of bestrophin-1 protein and may cause channel function disorder. Consequently, abnormality of liquid and ion transport on RPE cell membrane, eyeball development defects, and retinal dystrophy can finally result [3, 4]. Moreover, some gene mutations may lead to haploinsufficiency or different abnormal phenotypes. For example, the manifestation of chloride channel function disorder is attenuated chloride ion current that is 10–40% that of the wild type [5].

The BEST1 gene is not only related to the function maintenance of RPE cells and photoreceptor cells but also related to eye development. Therefore, BEST1 gene mutation can produce simultaneously the anterior segment dysplasia, such as hypermetropic eye, short ocular axis, shallow anterior chamber, narrow anterior chamber angle, or even microphthalmia, etc. [2, 4], among which the incidence of glaucoma caused by angle closure related to anterior segment dysplasia (not primary angle-closure glaucoma technically but developmental glaucoma) is high. It has been reported in the literature that 50% of the ARB patients may also suffer from such kind of glaucoma [2]. Therefore, the manifestations of the fundus and anterior segment found in the patient could be explained by monism. This disease suggests that two or more types of seemingly irrelevant clinical phenotypes observed in one eye are likely to be interrelated in pathogenesis, and in-depth exploration on the molecular level is necessary. As far as this disease is concerned, the connection between maculopathy and shallow anterior chamber lies in the change of a base in a gene. This kind of connection between simple eye diseases is also true for the connection between an eye disease and a systemic disease.

Therefore, routine screening on the anterior segment should be carried out for patients with Best disease and vice versa, that is, for patients with unusual angle narrowing, especially young patients; screening for Best disease should also be performed. The mild decibel loss in the central visual field in these two situations shall be paid attention to, and macular or 10-2 perimetry will be more sensitive to such changes.

Furthermore, the theory and practice on molecular biology and gene treatment have been developing rapidly nowadays, and it's worth pointing out that elucidation of disease pathogenesis on the molecular level has very high significance. As far as this disease is concerned, the BEST1 gene is linked with the eye development. But how BEST1 gene mutation produces anterior segment dysplasia is still unknown. Therefore, it's still out of the question to consider treating anterior segment abnormalities from the prospective of the BEST1 gene. However, studies have made the correlation between the BEST1 gene and function maintenance of RPE cells and photoreceptor cells relatively clear [6]. The future gene treatment might be delivered via the following three routes: the first is to restore the structural contact and functional connection between the neuroepithelial cells and pigment epithelium cells; the second is to correct the RPE function abnormalities caused by mutant protein; and the third is to correct the function abnormalities of the chloride channel caused by haploinsufficiency resulting from gene mutation. It seems that the third route is more feasible for the moment because the correction requires only supplementation of bestrophin-1 protein, which could be a key to the precision treatment of this disease.

References

1. Boon CJ, Klevering BJ, Leroy BP, et al. The spectrum of ocular phenotypes caused by mutations in the BEST1 gene. Prog Retin Eye Res. 2009;28(3):187–205.
2. Crowley C, Paterson R, Lamey T, et al. Autosomal recessive bestrophinopathy associated with angle-closure glaucoma. Doc Ophthalmol. 2014; 129(1):57–63.
3. Hartzell HC, Qu Z, Yu K, et al. Molecular physiology of bestrophins: multifunctional membrane proteins linked to best disease and other retinopathies. Physiol Rev. 2008;88(2):639–72.
4. Yardley J, Leroy BHN, Lafaut BA, et al. Mutations of VMD2 splicing regulators cause nanophthalmos and autosomal dominant vitreoretinochoroidopathy (ADVIRC). Invest Ophthalmol Vis Sci. 2004;45(10):3683–9.
5. Yu K, Xiao Q, Cui G, et al. The best disease-linked Cl^- channel hBest1 regulates Ca V 1 (L-type) Ca2+ channels via src-homology-binding domains. J Neurosci. 2008;28(22):5660–70.
6. Jansson RW, Berland S, Bredrup C, et al. Biallelic mutations in the BEST1 gene: additional families with autosomal recessive bestrophinopathy. Ophthalmic Genet. 2016;37(2):183–93.

Part IV

Optic Nerve Disorders

NLP Due to Incomplete Development of ON

28

Xiaojing Pan, Ning Fan, and Xuyang Liu

A patient with unilateral no light perception (NLP) showed a small disc, which was the only positive sign, in the affected eye. In this section, we will analyze this case of unilateral blindness.

28.1 Case

28.1.1 Case Presentation

A 26-year-old female patient complained that her right eye had been blind since childhood. After the patient was born, her parents found that her right eye could neither see objects nor follow the light, while her left eye was as normal as that of the children of the same age. The patient was otherwise healthy and denied histories of other eye diseases, systemic diseases, trauma, and familial diseases.

On examination, her visual acuity was NLP (OD), and best corrected visual acuity (BCVA) was 20/20 with myopic correction (−4.50DS, OS). In both eyes, the intraocular pressures were within normal limits. Slit-lamp examination of her anterior segments was unremarkable except that the relative afferent pupillary defect (RAPD) was positive in the right eye. Fundus examination showed a small optic disc (about 1/4 of the left optic disc in size), surrounded by a yellow halo of hypopigmentation in her right eye, suggesting optic disc hypoplasia (incomplete development of the optic disc) characterized by a small optic disc with a larger concentric variably pigmented ring (the "double-ring" sign), and the ratio between the disc-to-macula distance (DM) and the disc diameter (DD) was obviously higher than that of the normal eye (Fig. 28.1). The left optic disc was pink in color with a sharp edge, and the size was within the normal limits. Figure 28.2 showed the disc of the left eye (the normal eye) and the right eye (optic nerve hypoplasia) and the outline of the "double ring." Figure 28.3 showed the relationship between DM and DD in the right eye. Her both eyes presented horizontal nystagmus and null point (stationary primary position). The position of the eye was checked by Hirschberg test (33 mm), which revealed fixation in her left eye and exotropia at a 15° angle in her right eye.

X. Pan
Shandong Eye Institute, Qingdao Eye Hospital, Qingdao, China

N. Fan
Shenzhen Eye Hospital, Shenzhen University, Shenzhen, China

X. Liu (✉)
Xiamen Eye Center of Xiamen University, Xiamen, China

Shenzhen Eye Hospital, Shenzhen University, Shenzhen, China

N. Wang et al. (eds.), *Optic Disorders and Visual Field*, Advances in Visual Science and Eye Diseases 2, https://doi.org/10.1007/978-981-13-2502-1_28

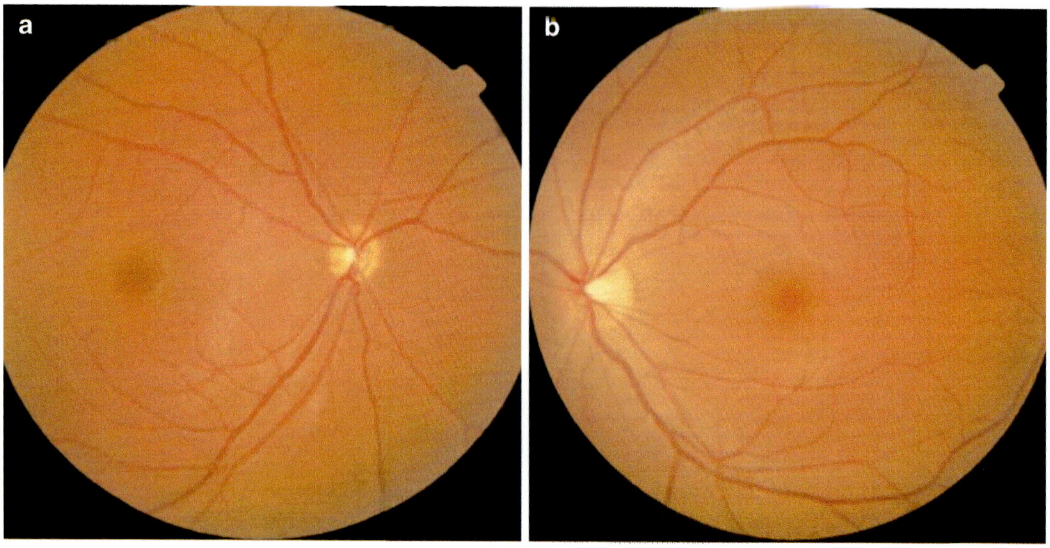

Fig. 28.1 Fundus photographs. Panel a: the right optic disc was small and surrounded by a yellow halo (i.e., the "double-ring" sign in which a small optic disc is surrounded by a larger concentric variably pigmented ring; see Fig. 28.2). The ratio between the disc-to-macula distance (DM) and the disc diameter (DD) was obviously higher than that of the normal eye; Panel b: the left optic disc was pink in color with a sharp edge, and the size was normal

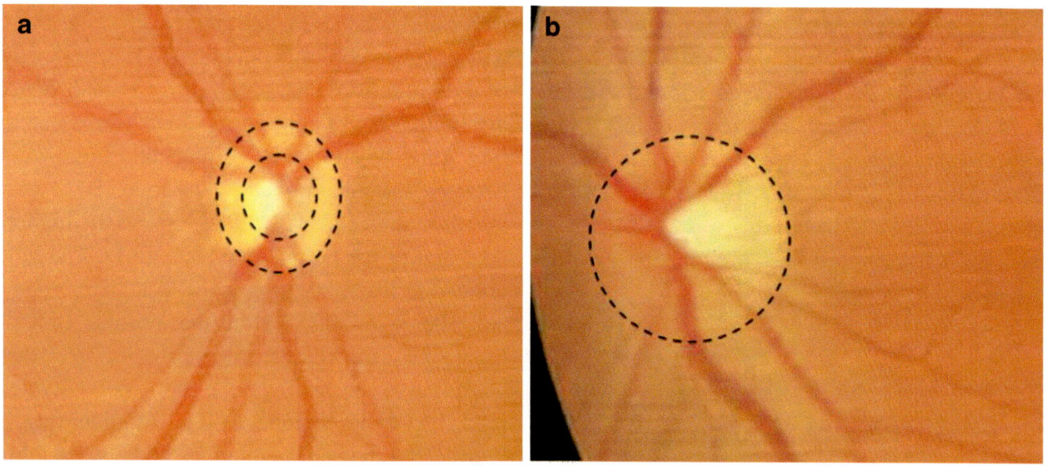

Fig. 28.2 The outlines of the optic disc. Panel a: the optic disc of the right eye which was obviously smaller and presented a "double-ring sign." Panel b: the normal optic disc of the left eye

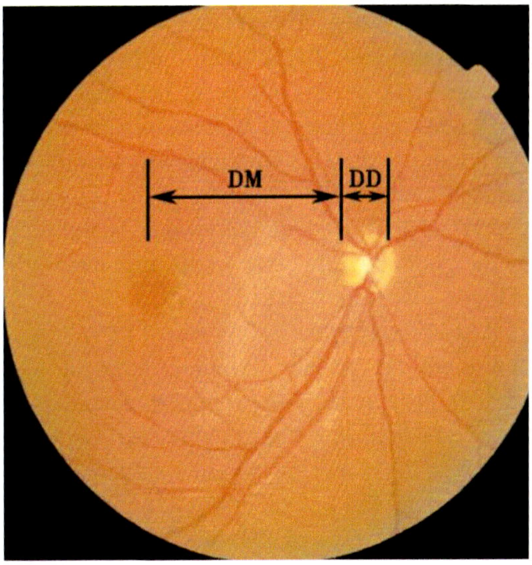

Fig. 28.3 Increased DM/DD ratio. *DM* the distance from the optic disc to the macula; *DD* optic disc diameter

Standardized automated perimetry revealed that the left eye was normal, while the right eye was totally blind.

The visual evoked potential (VEP) test showed no normal F-VEP waveform in the right eye, and normal latency and amplitude of P1 wave were revealed by F-VEP in the left eye (Fig. 28.4).

Cranial MRI indicated that the retrobulbar optic nerve of the right eye was significantly thinner than that of the left eye, and no other abnormalities were found.

28.1.2 Final Diagnosis

The final diagnosis was congenital optic nerve hypoplasia and sensory exotropia in the right eye and nystagmus in both eyes.

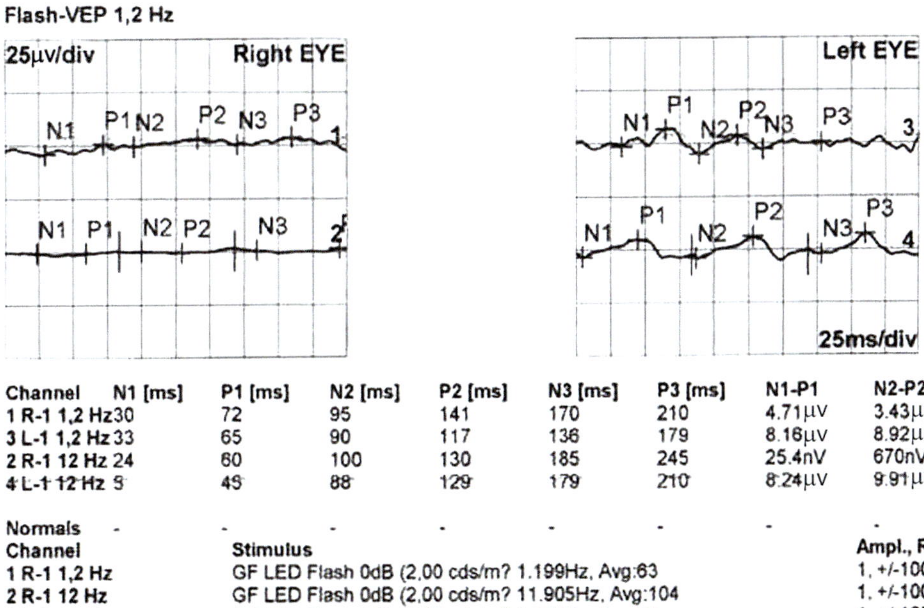

Channel	N1 [ms]	P1 [ms]	N2 [ms]	P2 [ms]	N3 [ms]	P3 [ms]	N1-P1	N2-P2	N3-P3
1 R-1 1,2 Hz	30	72	95	141	170	210	4.71µV	3.43µV	3.38µV
3 L-1 1,2 Hz	33	65	90	117	136	179	8.16µV	8.92µV	3.43µV
2 R-1 12 Hz	24	60	100	130	185	245	25.4nV	670nV	901nV
4 L-1 12 Hz	5	45	88	129	179	210	8.24µV	9.91µV	9.21µV
Normals	-	-	-	-	-	-	-	-	-

Channel	Stimulus	Ampl., Range, Filter
1 R-1 1,2 Hz	GF LED Flash 0dB (2,00 cds/m? 1.199Hz, Avg:63	1, +/-100µV 0.5-50Hz
2 R-1 12 Hz	GF LED Flash 0dB (2,00 cds/m? 11.905Hz, Avg:104	1, +/-100µV 0.5-50Hz
3 L-1 1,2 Hz	GF LED Flash 0dB (2,00 cds/m? 1.199Hz, Avg:63	1, +/-100µV 0.5-50Hz
4 L-1 12 Hz	GF LED Flash 0dB (2,00 cds/m? 11.905Hz, Avg:103	1, +/-100µV 0 5-50Hz

Fig. 28.4 F-VEP examination printouts. No normal F-VEP waveform was found in the right eye, but normal latency and amplitude of P1 wave were found in the left eye

28.2 Discussion

Congenital optic nerve hypoplasia (ONH) is a nonprogressive congenital anomaly. Histopathological studies have shown that the major pathological changes in the optic nerve include reduced axon number (only 1% of the normal quantity) [1], probably due to apoptotic pathological changes in the retinal nerve fiber layer (RNFL) or optic nerve during embryonic development, which is different from the delayed degenerative axonal loss in Leber's hereditary optic neuropathy (see Part IV, Chap. 34).

In the previous chapter, we have presented a case with partial optic nerve hypoplasia characterized by retinal nerve fiber defects. Furthermore, there is also another category of optic nerve hypoplasia as the result of developmental defects at the entrance to the optic nerve, which is characterized by a partially or completely defected optic disc and sometimes complicated by retinal and/or choroidal defects.

This patient was found to have unilateral visual acuity abnormality after birth (NLP) but had not been diagnosed. The optic disc of the affected eye demonstrated the characteristics of developmental defects—a small optic disc surrounded by a yellow halo in her right eye, suggesting optic disc hypoplasia (incomplete development of the optic disc) characterized by a small optic disc with a larger concentric variably pigmented ring ("double-ring" sign). The inner ring originated from the thickened retinal pigment epithelium and was connected with the hypoplastic optic nerve. The outer ring was derived from the junction of the lamina cribrosa and sclera, forming an ill-defined and irregular shiny ring around the optic disc, which was exposed sclera or hyperplastic fibrous tissues [2].

In this case, the NLP was directly related to the small optic disc, and fundus photography showed no reflection from the retinal nerve fiber layer in the right eye, indicating the number of axons of the optic nerve was significantly reduced when compared to those in the left eye, which was not only the anatomical basis of the small disc but also could fully explain the patient's profound vision loss. In addition, the photography also showed that the optic nerve hypoplasia was congenital or primary. If it was secondary, then even though she had no light perception, the reduced number of nerve fibers of the optic disc which had developed normally would be replaced by the glial tissue, in other words, the size of the optic disc would not change.

A dysplastic optic disc is off-white in color, and there are usually mottling halos in the parapapillary area with a hyperpigmented or hypopigmented ring (the "double-ring" sign). In histology, the inner ring is located in the junction of the sclera and lamina cribrosa, and the outer ring is the coverage of abnormally stretched retina and pigmented epithelium outside the lamina cribrosa. Furthermore, abnormalities such as retina thinning can also be found in the affected eye. What needs to be pointed out is that visual acuity can still be partially preserved, while visual field is being compromised in the case of optic nerve hypoplasia. But why did the patient in this case have no light perception? We believe that it was associated with the severity of optic nerve hypoplasia. The size of the patient's right optic disc (and the inner ring) was only 1/4 of that in the healthy contralateral eye. We speculated that her optic nerve was mainly composed of glial cells.

When such abnormalities occurred in both eyes of a patient, they are usually complicated by systemic endocrine and central nervous system abnormalities, including developmental retardation, short stature, cerebral agenesis, epilepsy, diabetes insipidus, forebrain anomalies, agenesis of corpus callosum or pellucid septum, etc. [3–5]. Therefore, early and correct diagnosis is very important because it can suggest that the patient needs endocrine and central nervous system disease screening.

And for the patients who are affected unilaterally, clinical signs include nystagmus, strabismus, uvea coloboma, microphthalmia, etc. [4, 5]. For instance, in this case, only nystagmus was observed, and there was no specific treatment method for it.

References

1. Kline LB, Foroozan R. Optic nerve disorders (Translated by Jun Xu, Qingsong Yang, Kai Ma). 2nd ed. Beijing: People's Medical Publishing House; 2014.
2. Liu Q, Fang Y. Optic disc diseases. Beijing: People's Medical Publishing House; 2015.
3. Hatsukawa Y, Fujio T, Nishikawa M, et al. Congenital optic tract hypoplasia. J AAPOS. 2015;19(4):383–5.
4. Pilat A, Sibley D, McLean RJ, et al. High-resolution imaging of the optic nerve and retina in optic nerve hypoplasia. Ophthalmology. 2015;122(7):1330–9.
5. Saadati HG, Hsu HY, Heller KB, et al. A histopathologic and morphometric differentiation of nerves in optic nerve hypoplasia and Leber's hereditary optic neuropathy. Arch Ophthalmol. 1998;116(7):911–6.

Changes in Visual Field Caused by Optic Disc Drusen

29

Xiaojing Pan, Ning Fan, and Xuyang Liu

Optic disc drusen is a clinically rare condition, and missed diagnosis of it can easily happen when the central vision is not affected. However, sometimes optic disc drusen can cause damage to the optic nerve and blood vessels. The standardized automated perimetry has important clinical value for the evaluation of its functional damage. Two cases will be presented below.

29.1 Case 1

29.1.1 Case Presentation

A 10-year-old female patient presented with the need of optometric review and fitting of spectacles. She had no ocular redness, eye pain, dark shadow, dizziness, paroxysmal blurred vision, or other discomforts. The patient had suffered from myopia for 2 years and denied histories of eye trauma, systemic diseases, or familial diseases.

On examination, the uncorrected visual acuity (UCVA) was 20/60 OD (−1.00DS) and 20/30 OS (−0.50DS), while the best corrected visual acuity (BCVA) was 20/20 OD and 20/20 OS. In both eyes, the refractive media was clear and the pupils were of equal sizes (3 mm in diameter), round, and reactive to direct light. Fundus examination showed the optic disc was elevated, but the area of elevation did not extend beyond the disc margin and was slightly pink in color with an unclear margin (Fig. 29.1).

Standardized automated perimetry revealed mild enlargement of the physiological blind spot in both eyes and a relative central scotoma in the left eye (Fig. 29.2).

The OCT results indicated that the nerve fiber layer was highly elevated in both eyes, and lump-produced signals with high reflection could be observed below it (Fig. 29.3).

B-Mode ultrasonography indicated a flat and solid hyperechogenic spot ahead of the optic disc in both eyes (Fig. 29.4).

29.1.2 Final Diagnosis

The final diagnosis was buried optic disc drusen in both eyes.

X. Pan
Shandong Eye Institute, Qingdao Eye Hospital, Qingdao, China

N. Fan
Shenzhen Eye Hospital, Shenzhen University, Shenzhen, China

X. Liu (✉)
Xiamen Eye Center of Xiamen University, Xiamen, China

Shenzhen Eye Hospital, Shenzhen University, Shenzhen, China

N. Wang et al. (eds.), *Optic Disorders and Visual Field*, Advances in Visual Science and Eye Diseases 2, https://doi.org/10.1007/978-981-13-2502-1_29

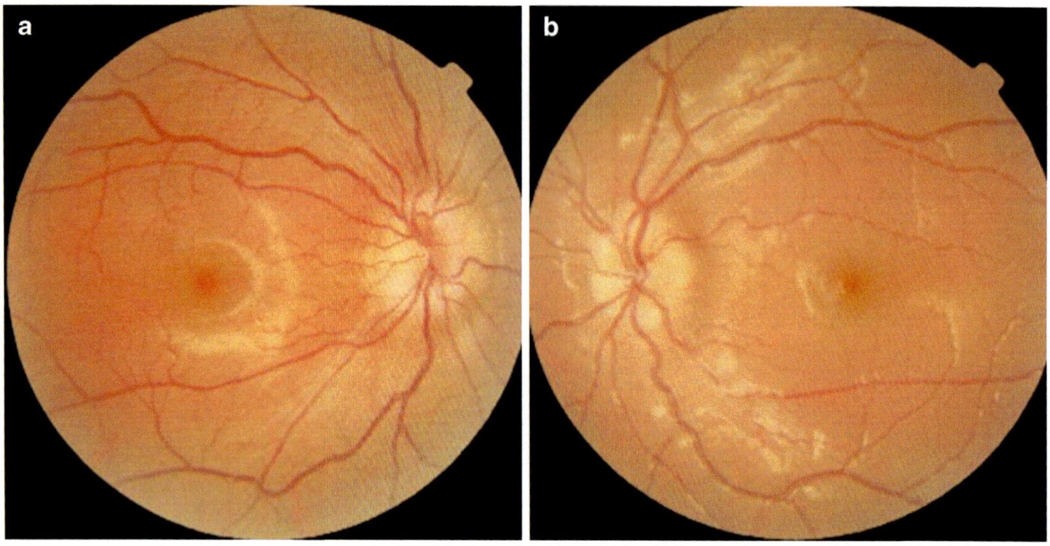

Fig. 29.1 Fundus photographs. The optic disc was elevated, but the area of elevation did not extend beyond the disc margin and was slightly pink in color with an unclear margin in both eyes. Panel a: right eye. Panel b: left eye

Fig. 29.2 Humphrey visual field assessment. The 24-2 test revealed mild enlargement of the physiological blind spot in both eyes and a pararelative central scotoma in the left eye. Panel a: grayscale map of the left eye. Panel b: grayscale map of the right eye. Panel c: pattern deviation probability map of the left eye. Panel d: pattern deviation probability map of the right eye

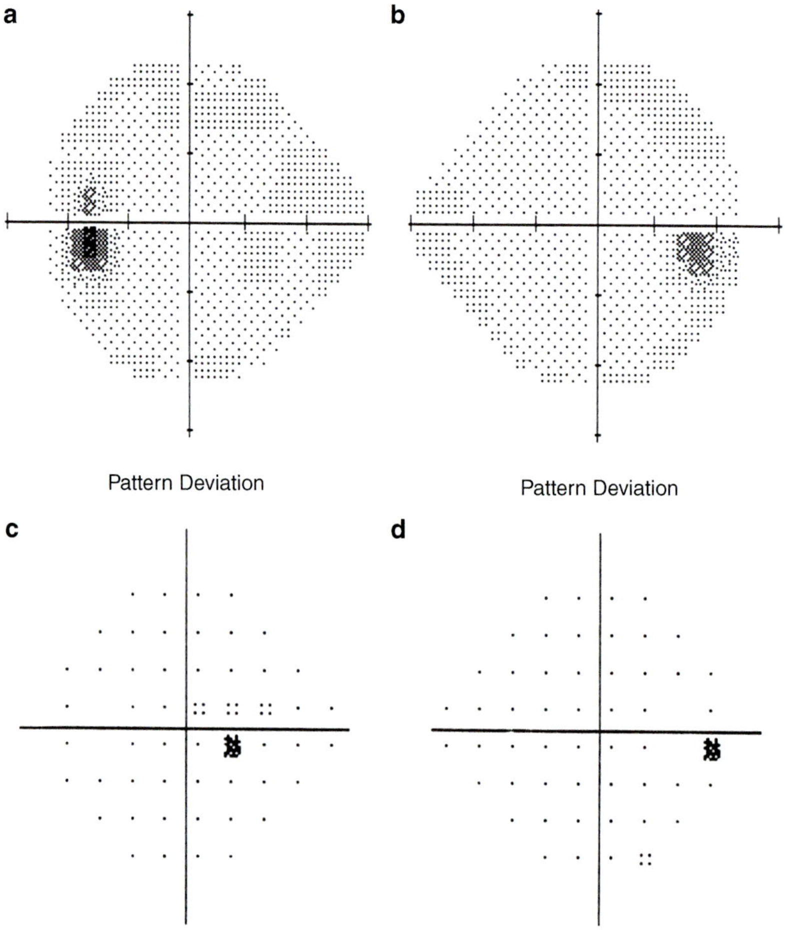

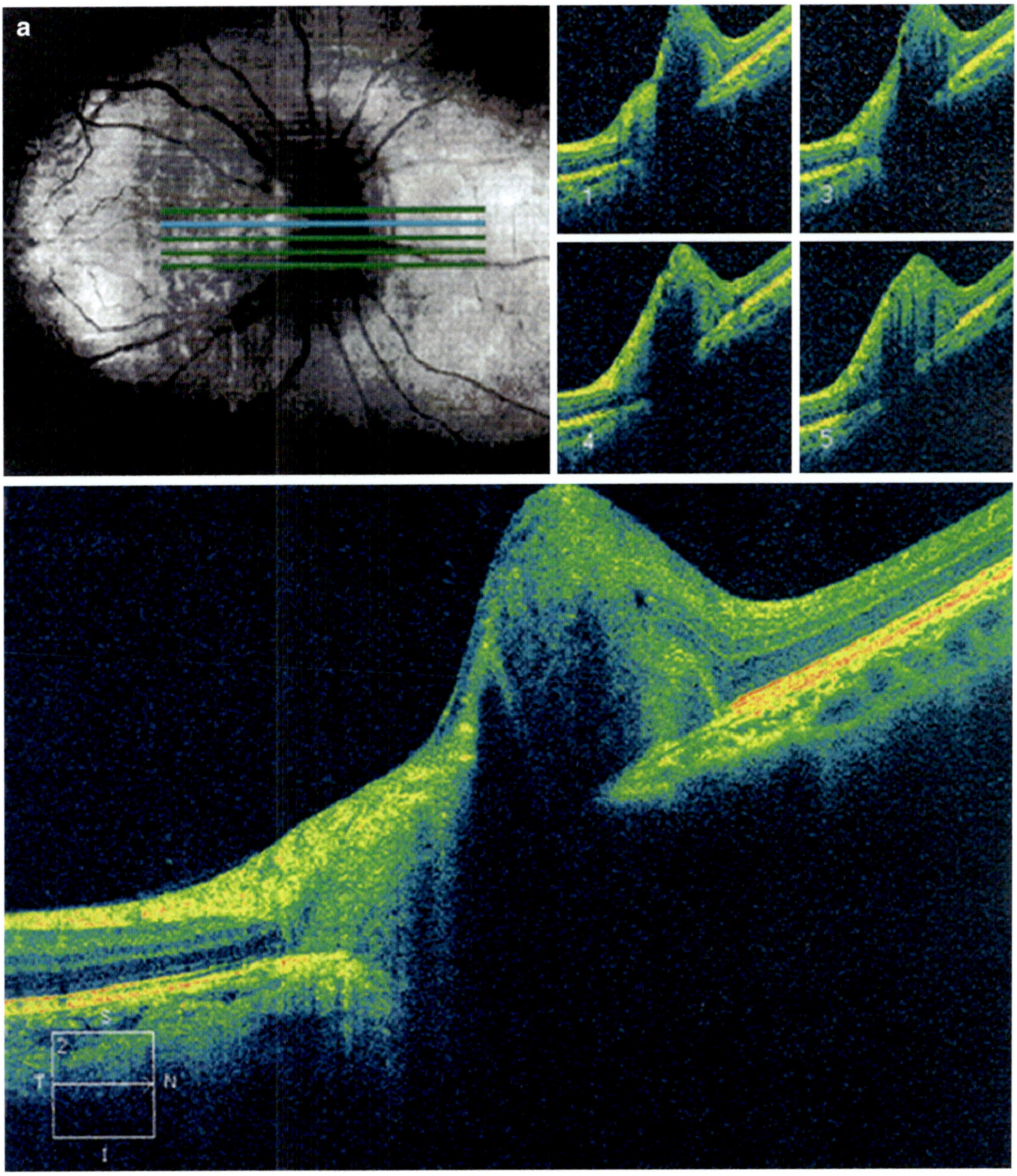

Fig. 29.3 OCT report of the optic disc. The nerve fiber layer was highly elevated in both eyes, and lump-produced signals with high reflection could be observed below it. Panel a: right eye. Panel b: left eye

29.1.3 Case Review

The patient was 10 years old and had no complaint of ocular discomfort. Buried optic disc drusen was observed in both eyes during the fundus examination before prescribing glasses, but no other abnormalities were found in the rest of the eye examination. The diagnosis was further confirmed by OCT, B-ultrasound, etc. An enlarged physiological blind spot was revealed

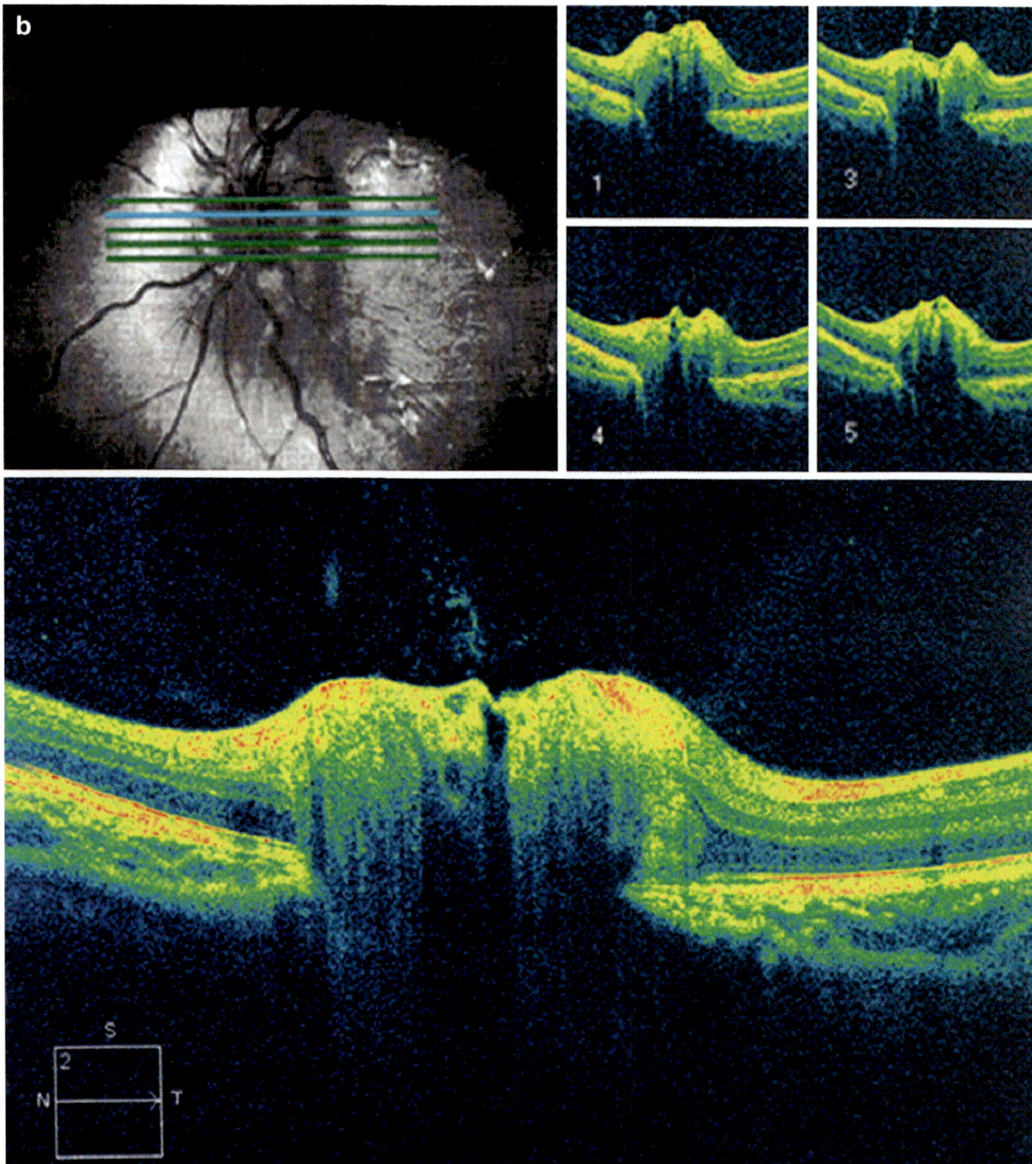

Fig. 29.3 (continued)

in both eyes with the visual field test, suggesting that the buried optic disc drusen might have been compressing the nerve fiber of the optic disc and caused damage. A relative central scotoma could still be observed in the left eye. Recheck and follow-up were required for visual field and fundus changes in both eyes. Complications might occur in buried optic disc drusen, such as optic disc hemorrhage, retinal vascular occlusion, anterior ischemic optic neuropathy, etc. Let's review the following case as an example.

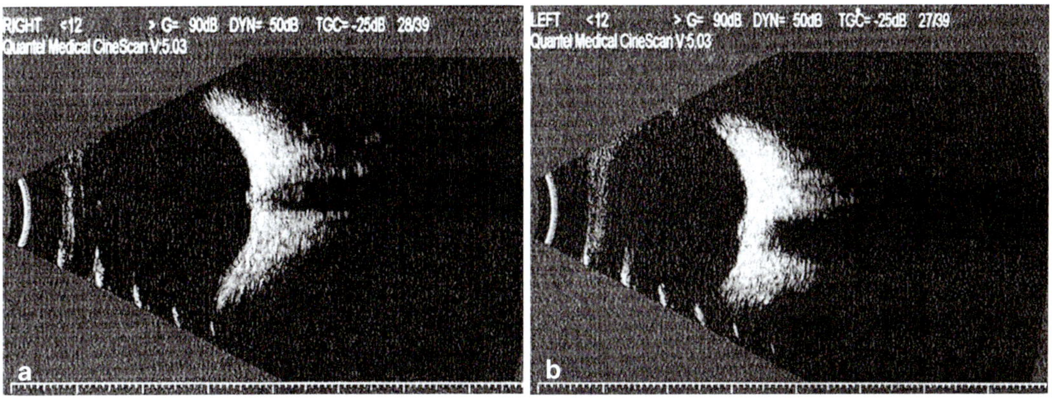

Fig. 29.4 B-ultrasound images. A hyperechogenic spot ahead of the optic disc in both eyes could be found. Panel a: right eye. Panel b: left eye

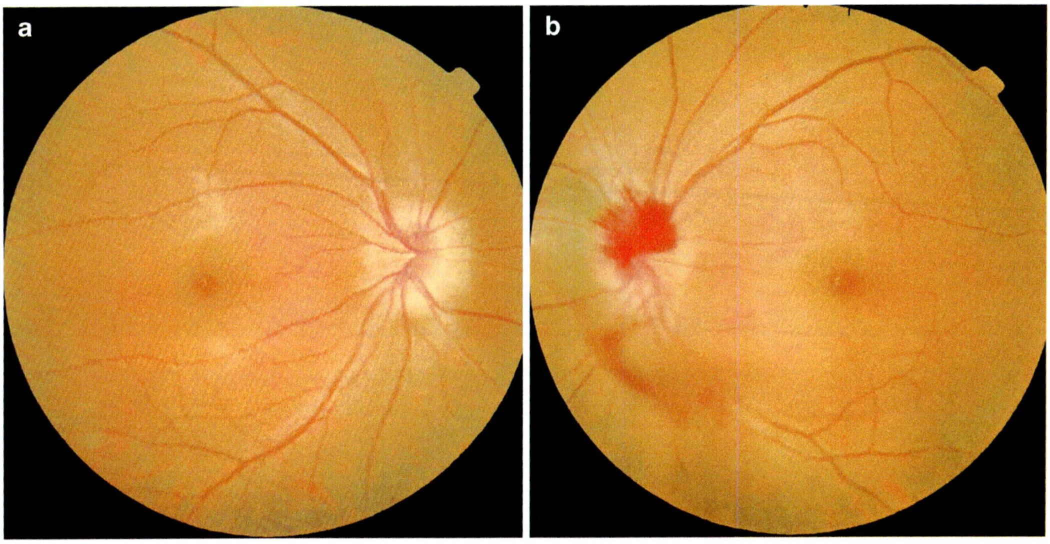

Fig. 29.5 Fundus photographs. In both eyes, the optic disc was elevated, but the area of elevation did not extend beyond the margin of the disc that had an unclear boundary. In the left eye, bright red hemorrhage foci in the superior optic disc were noted, and dark red subretinal hemorrhage foci and minor preretinal hemorrhage could be found in the nasal side. Panel a: right eye. Panel b: left eye

29.2 Case 2

29.2.1 Case Presentation

A 21-year-old female patient had noticed a black shadow floating in front of her left eye without identifiable causes 2 days before. No ocular discomforts, including eye redness, ophthalmalgia, decreased vision, etc., were presented. No history of dizziness or paroxysmal blurred vision was reported. Histories of trauma, systemic disease, and familial disease were also denied.

The UCVA was 20/20 OU. Intraocular pressure (IOP) was within normal limits OU. The refractive media was clear OU. The pupils were equal in size, round, and reactive to direct light. Fundus examination revealed that, in the right eye, the optic disc was elevated, but the area of elevation did not extend beyond the margin of the disc which was pink with an unclear boundary, while in the left eye, fresh hemorrhage foci in the superior optic disc and elevated inferior optic disc with an unclear boundary were seen, and dark red subretinal hemorrhage foci and minor preretinal hemorrhage were found in the nasal aspect (Fig. 29.5).

Throughout the process of fundus fluorescein angiography (FFA), small nodular fluorescence at the edge of the nasal optic disc without fluorescein leakage could be observed, and no abnormality was found in the retinal vessels in the right eye. The early-phase angiogram of the left eye showed a temporal cilioretinal artery, hemorrhage in the superior optic disc, subretinal and preretinal hemorrhage blocking fluorescence, and small nodular fluorescence at the edge of the inferior temporal optic disc without fluorescein leakage (Fig. 29.6).

The patient was treated with drugs to improve blood circulation. The recheck after 20 days

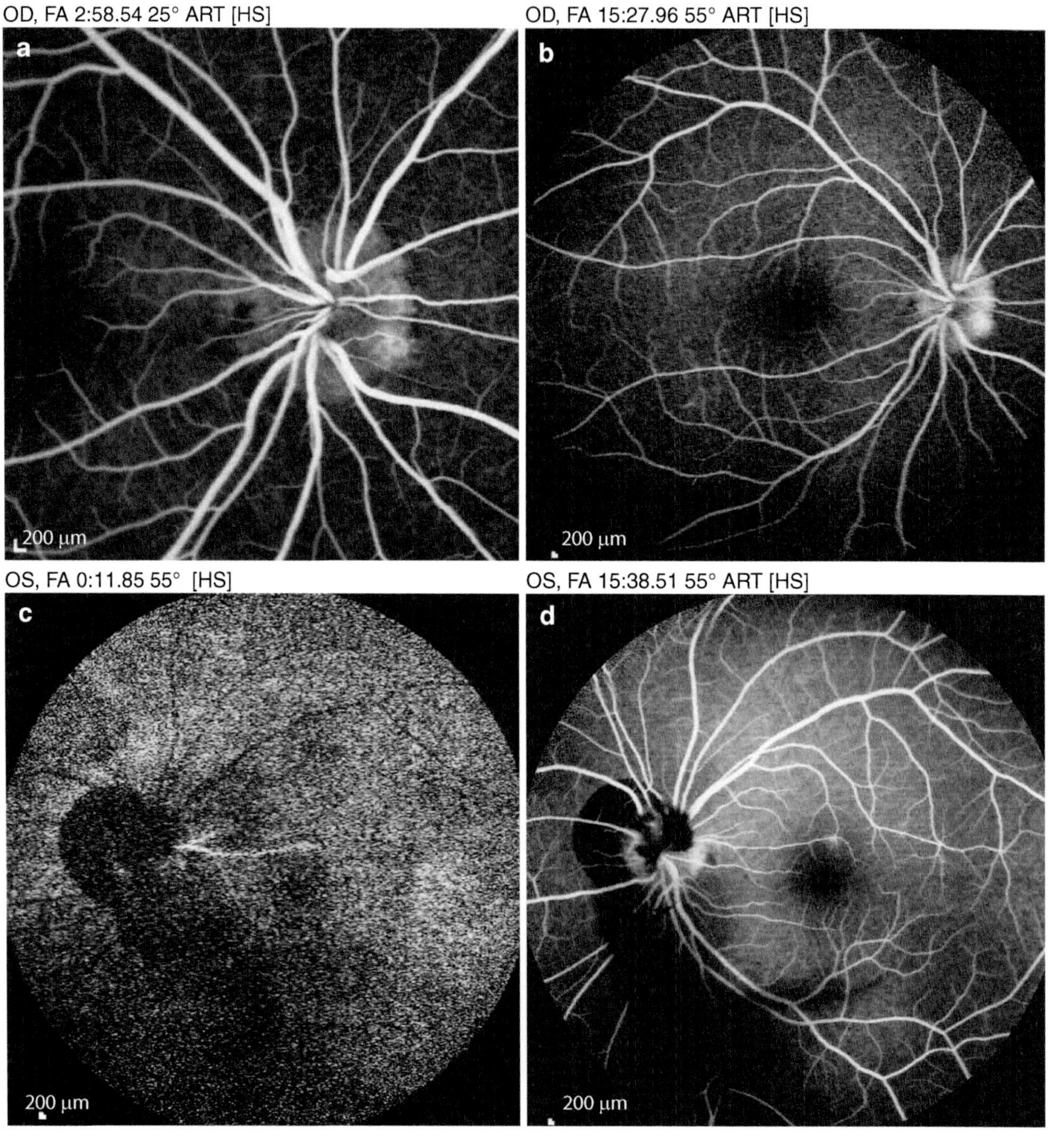

Fig. 29.6 FFA images of both eyes. Panels a, b: small nodular fluorescence at the edge of the nasal optic disc without fluorescein leakage could be observed, and the retinal vessels were free from leakage and staining in the right eye. Panel c: temporal cilioretinal artery could be seen in the early-phase angiogram of the left eye. Panel d: hemorrhage in the superior optic disc, subretinal and preretinal hemorrhage blocking fluorescence, and small nodular fluorescence at the edge of the inferior temporal optic disc without fluorescein leakage could be observed in the left eye

revealed that the retinal hemorrhage had been largely absorbed, and residual subretinal hard exudates could be observed in the nasal side of the optic disc which was elevated but without the area of elevation extending beyond its margin in the left eye (Fig. 29.7).

The recheck after 1 year demonstrated that the patient's vision was 20/20 OU. The fundus hemorrhage and exudates in the left eye had been absorbed. The optic disc in each eye was elevated with the area of elevation not extending beyond its margin and remained unchanged from that observed in the previous examination (Fig. 29.8).

Standardized automated perimetry showed an enlarged physiological blind spot in both eyes and a relative defect in the temporal side of the physiological blind spot in the left eye (Fig. 29.9).

B-Mode ultrasonography indicated flat and solid hyperechogenic spot ahead of the optic disc in both eyes (Fig. 29.10).

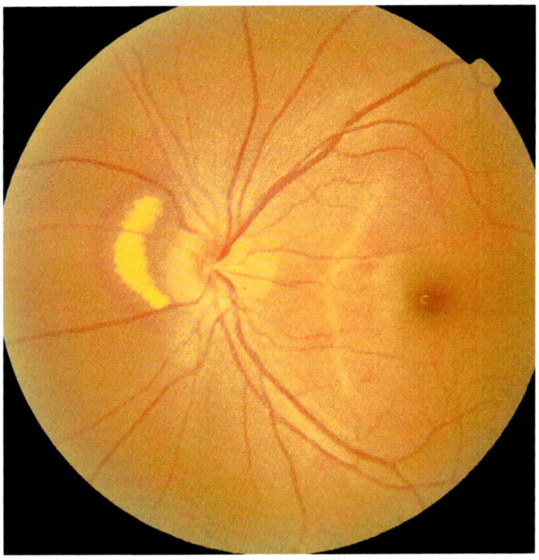

Fig. 29.7 Re-examination fundus photograph. The optic disc was elevated, but the area of elevation did not extend beyond the disc margin, and residual subretinal exudate foci in the nasal side of the optic disc could be observed in the left eye

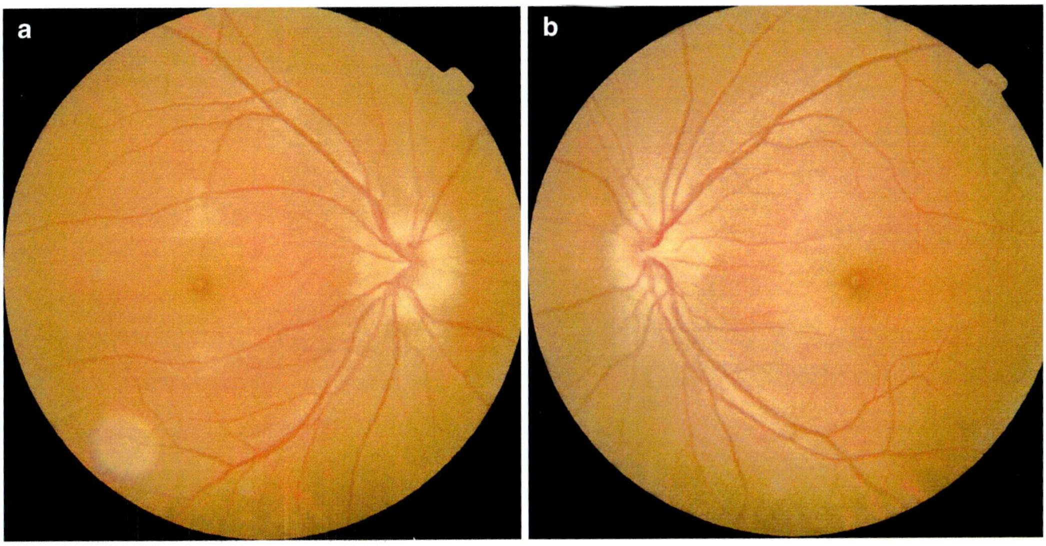

Fig. 29.8 Re-examination fundus photographs. The optic disc in each eye was elevated, but the area of elevation did not extend beyond the disc margin. Panel a: right eye. Panel b: left eye (Note: The spot-shaped shadow at the bottom left of Panel a was caused by lens contamination)

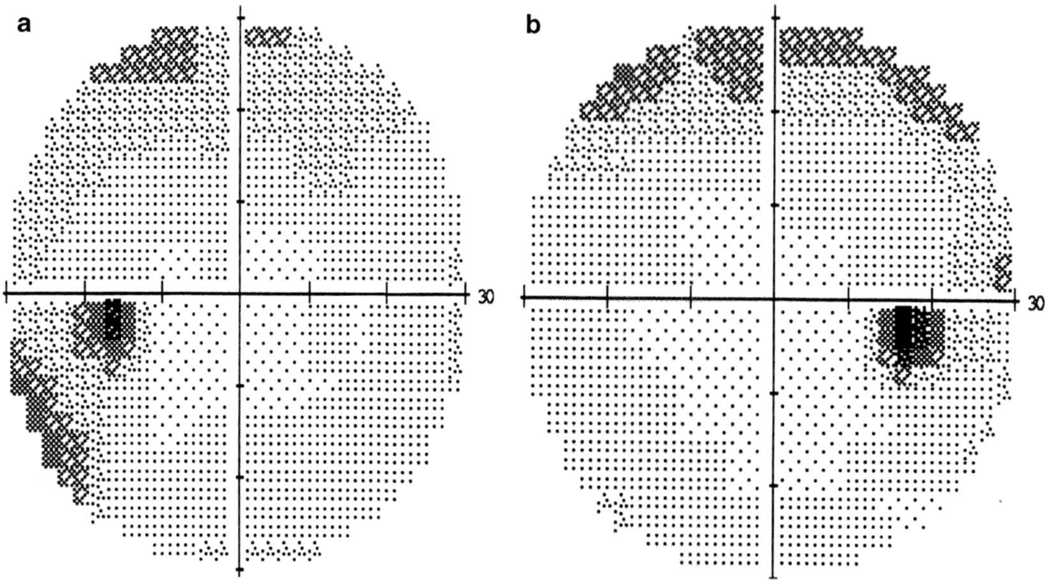

Fig. 29.9 Humphrey visual field grayscale maps. Enlargement of the physiological blind spot could be found in both eyes, and local light sensitivity reduction was observed in the temporal side of the physiological blind spot in the left eye. Panel a: left eye. Panel b: right eye

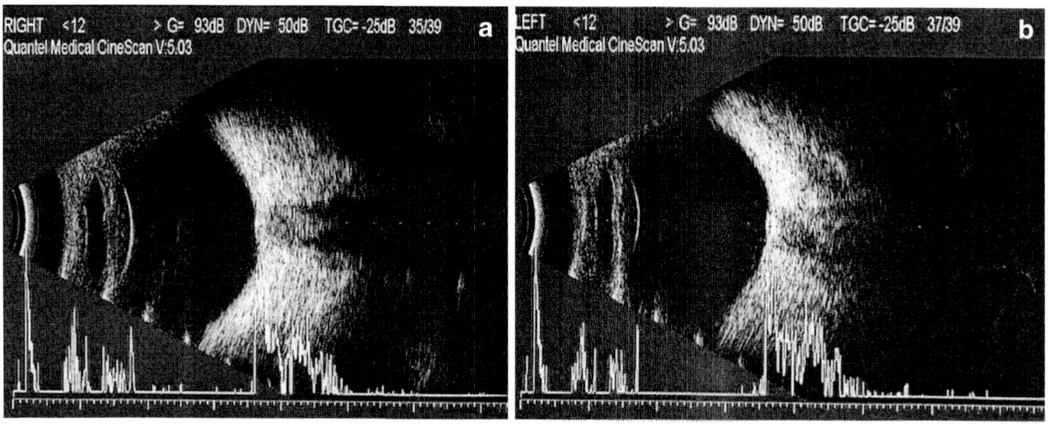

Fig. 29.10 B-Mode ultrasound images. A flat and solid hyperechogenic spot could be found in the spherical wall of the optic disc in both eyes. Panel a: right eye. Panel b: left eye

The OCT results indicated that lump-produced signals with high reflection could be observed below the nerve fiber layer of the optic disc in both eyes (Fig. 29.11).

29.2.2 Final Diagnosis

The final diagnosis was buried optic disc drusen in both eyes and optic disc hemorrhage in the left eye.

29.2.3 Case Review

A 21-year-old patient visited her doctor for the first time with the complaint of a black shadow floating in front of her left eye. The vision and intraocular pressure were normal. The fundus examination found that the optic disc was elevated but without the area of elevation extending beyond its margin in both eyes and revealed optic disc hemorrhage and subretinal and preretinal

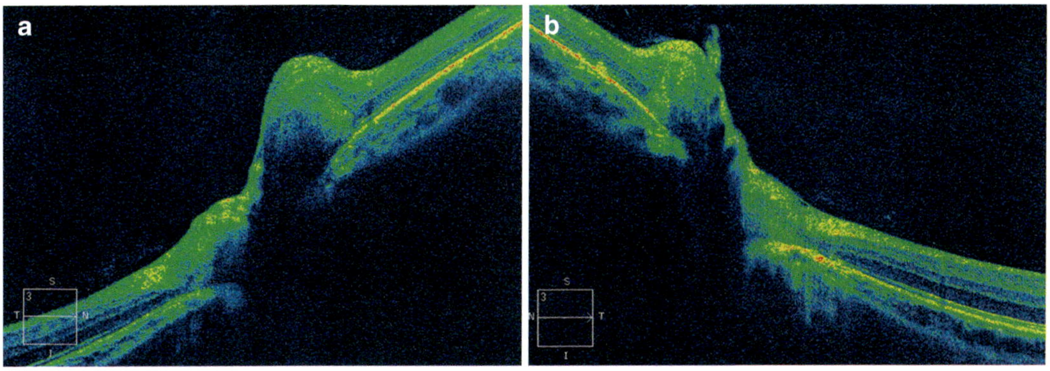

Fig. 29.11 OCT images of the optic disc. Lump-produced signals with high reflection could be observed below the nerve fiber layer of the optic disc in both eyes. Panel a: right eye. Panel b: left eye

hemorrhages in the left eye. The diagnosis of buried optic disc drusen in both eyes was further confirmed by 1-year follow-up. The optic disc and retinal hemorrhages in the left eye were considered to be caused by the damage to local vessels resulting from optic disc drusen. Fortunately, the visual field retest which was carried out after the blood was absorbed showed only an enlarged physiological blind spot and a relative scotoma in the temporal side of the physiological blind spot. Serious damage to the retinal nerve fiber and visual function was not identified.

In addition, a cilioretinal artery was seen in the patient's left eye. It was reported that the percentage of optic disc drusen patients with a cilioretinal artery (20–40%) was significantly higher than the prevalence of cilioretinal artery in the normal population.

29.3 Discussion

Optic disc drusen (ODD) are composed of hyaline-like calcific material within the optic disc. The morbidity of ODD in children is about 0.4%, and both eyes are usually affected [1]. The mechanism of ODD is not clear yet. It may be caused by hyperplasia and degeneration of immature optic neuroglia in the optic disc or disintegration and calcification of optic nerve fiber axoplasm or plasma protein sedimentation on the optic disc due to transmission barrier resulting from congenital vascular abnormality. There are some studies reporting that it is associated with genetic background.

Optic disc drusen can be divided into buried ODD and visible ODD according to the depth of the lesion [2]. The manifestations of the fundus in buried ODD include mild elevation of the optic disc with an unclear margin and sometimes pseudopapilledema. In general, a patient is usually free from subjective symptoms and sometimes has paroxysmal blurred vision probably due to the temporary ischemia as a result of drusen-induced vascular spasm. In this situation, the standardized automated perimetry usually reveals corresponding changes, such as an enlarged physiological blind spot, although the central vision has not been affected. Hemorrhage in the optic disc or surrounding areas can be caused by the compression or damage to the capillary vessels on or around the optic disc due to the drusen. Most patients do not see their doctor until a dark shadow appears after retinal hemorrhages. However, they are usually misdiagnosed as optic disc vasculitis, optic disc edema, or ischemic optic neuropathy through routine ophthalmologic examinations.

Currently, the main diagnostic methods include B-ultrasound, OCT, FFA, and CT. B-ultrasound is considered to be the most reliable method for diagnosis of ODD because the drusen contains calcium. As a result, hyperechogenic spot in front of the optic disc can still be observed even after gain reduction. High-resolution SD-OCT can display the characteristics of buried ODD more clearly [3]. The nerve fiber elevation of the optic disc and the lump-produced signals with high reflection below the optic disc can be observed. Localized intense fluorescence can be found at the edge of the optic disc at the early stage of FFA. Nodular fluorescence with clear border can be observed at the late stage, indicating the position and shape of ODD. There is usually no fluorescein leakage, which can be adopted for differentiation with optic disc vasculitis, papillitis, etc. For the ODD with calcification, CT examination can display dot-like hyperdense lesions clearly. For a patient with bilateral "optic disc edema," CT examination can be used to exclude intracranial space-occupying lesions, and it is helpful for differential diagnosis of the disease [4].

Although a lot of patients with buried ODD experienced missed diagnosis due to its asymptomatic manifestation, previous studies have reported that ODD can lead to progressive visual field defects. An enlarged physiological blind spot is a common type of visual field defect. A possible explanation is that some deeply buried and large drusen may directly compress the optic nerve fiber or block the blood supply so that visual field defects develop, and even the central vision is affected [5]. The acute decrease of vision found in a few patients may result from the vascular spasm or occlusion and refractive media opacity caused by vitreous hemorrhage.

Auw-Haedrich et al. stated that the patients with optic disc drusen are vulnerable to normal tension glaucoma (NTG)-like visual field impairment when compared with the normal population [2]. Therefore, for ODD patients with visual field impairment, IOP-lowering treatment shall be given even when intraocular pressure is normal, and no glaucomatous optic nerve damage is noted. Another case of ODD complicated by glaucoma will be discussed and analyzed in a later section (refer to Chap. 31 of Part IV for details).

In a word, standardized automated perimetry is an important method to identify and monitor optic disc drusen and has important clinical significance in the follow-up of this disease.

References

1. Zhang H. Atlas of ocular fundus diseases. Beijing: People's Medical Publishing House; 2007.
2. Auw-Haedrich C, Staubach F, Witschel H. Optic disk drusen. Surv Ophthalmol. 2002;47(6):515–32.
3. Merchant KY, Su D, Park SC, et al. Enhanced depth imaging optical coherence tomography of optic nerve head drusen. Ophthalmology. 2013;120(7):1409–14.
4. Sato T, Mrejen S, Spaide RF. Multimodal imaging of optic disc drusen. Am J Ophthalmol. 2013;156(2):275–82.
5. Wu Z, Guo M, Nie S, et al. Imageological diagnosis and analysis of buried optic disc drusen. Chin J Pract Ophthalmol. 2015;33(11):1272–4.

A Patient with Morning Glory Disc Anomaly in One Eye and Congenital Anophthalmia in the Contralateral Eye

30

Xiaojing Pan, Ning Fan, and Xuyang Liu

Congenital anophthalmia is a very rare and unilateral disease which is usually complicated by congenital abnormality in the contralateral eye. Below we will introduce a morning glory anomaly patient with congenital anophthalmia in the contralateral eye.

30.1 Case

30.1.1 Case Presentation

A 40-year-old female patient had a 3-year history of gradual decreased vision in her right eye. Congenital anophthalmia was found immediately after birth. No discomforts, including eye redness, eye pain, dark shadow, etc., were noticed. The photographs of both eyes were shown in Fig. 30.1. The patient was normally delivered full term. The patient denied that her mother had a history of any infectious disease or special drug treatment during pregnancy. The patient's body size was within normal limits. Her intelligence and language skills were normal. The histories of systemic diseases, trauma, and familial diseases were unremarkable.

The uncorrected visual acuity (UCVA) was 20/125, and no improvement was achieved with correction in the right eye. Intraocular pressure (IOP) was normal. Anterior segment showed no abnormalities. Fundus examination revealed significant enlargement of the optic disc and a funnel-shaped excavation filled with white glial tissue at the center of the disc. The blood vessels radiate out along the excavation edge and then extended in straight lines. The disc edge showed irregular circular ridge-like elevation with pigmentation on the surface. The optic disc was surrounded by a wide white chorioretinal atrophy, thus resembling a morning glory. Pigmentation anomalies, mild elevation, and cystoid edema were revealed in the macula. The peripheral retina showed no abnormalities (Fig. 30.2). Normal eyelid development, orbital collapse, and absence of eyeball were observed in the left eye.

Standardized automated perimetry indicated an enlarged physiological blind spot and a central defect in the right eye (Fig. 30.3).

The OCT results revealed a central funnel-shaped excavation through the linear scan on the optic disc in the right eye. Partial detach-

X. Pan
Shandong Eye Institute, Qingdao Eye Hospital, Qingdao, China

N. Fan
Shenzhen Eye Hospital, Shenzhen University, Shenzhen, China

X. Liu (✉)
Xiamen Eye Center of Xiamen University, Xiamen, China

Shenzhen Eye Hospital, Shenzhen University, Shenzhen, China

N. Wang et al. (eds.), *Optic Disorders and Visual Field*, Advances in Visual Science and Eye Diseases 2, https://doi.org/10.1007/978-981-13-2502-1_30

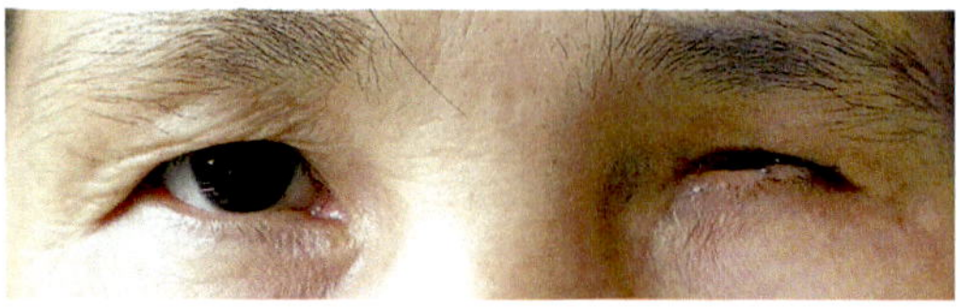

Fig. 30.1 Photos. Orbital collapse and absence of eyeball could be observed in the left eye

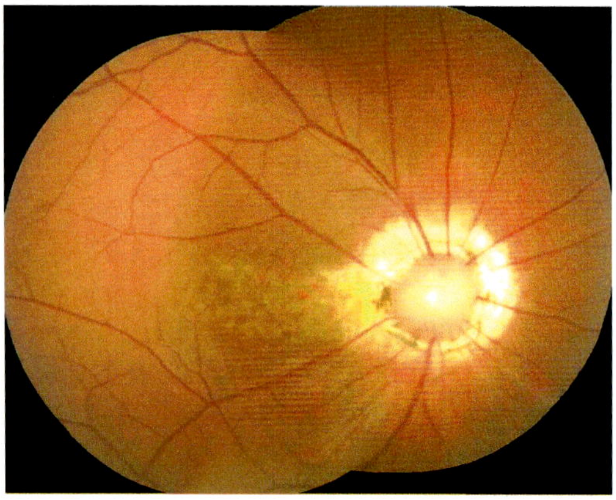

Fig. 30.2 Montage images of fundus photographs. Significant enlargement of the optic disc and a funnel-shaped excavation filled with white glial tissue in the central area were found. The blood vessels radiated out along the excavation edge and then extended in straight lines. The disc edge showed irregular circular ridge-like elevation with pigmentation on the surface. The peripheral optic disc was surrounded by a white chorioretinal atrophy. Pigmentation anomalies, mild elevation, and cystoid edema were revealed in the macula. The peripheral retina showed no abnormalities

ment accompanied by interlayer separation could be observed in the retinal neuroepithelium between the optic disc and the macula (Fig. 30.4). Refer to Fig. 30.5 for the 3D reconstruction image of the optic disc.

B-Mode ultrasonography showed deepening of the excavation in the optic disc of the right eye. Flocculent low-medium echoes could be found inside the vitreous cavity. The backward movement was positive. No eyeball echo was observed in the left eye (Fig. 30.6).

30.1.2 Final Diagnosis

The final diagnosis was morning glory disc anomaly with serous retinal detachment in the macula in the right eye and congenital anophthalmia in the left eye.

30.1.3 Case Review

Morning glory disc anomaly is usually unilateral onset. In this case, typical signs were shown in the right eye and were complicated by serous retinal detachment, leading to decreased vision. Her left eye was affected by congenital anophthalmia which was very rare. Our literature retrieval identified only one clinical report regarding an Indian child suffering from congenital anophthalmia in one eye and morning glory disc syndrome in the contralateral eye.

30.2 Discussion

Morning glory disc anomaly was firstly reported by Kindle in 1970. It was given the name because the optic disc looks like a bloom morning glory. The typical manifestations of the disease include optic disc excavation and enlargement, retinal vascular abnormality, pigmentation annulus surrounding the optic disc, and a characteristic central core of glial tissue [1]. The disease usually involves one eye, and bilateral involvement is rarely found. The prevalence rates in men and women are equal. The

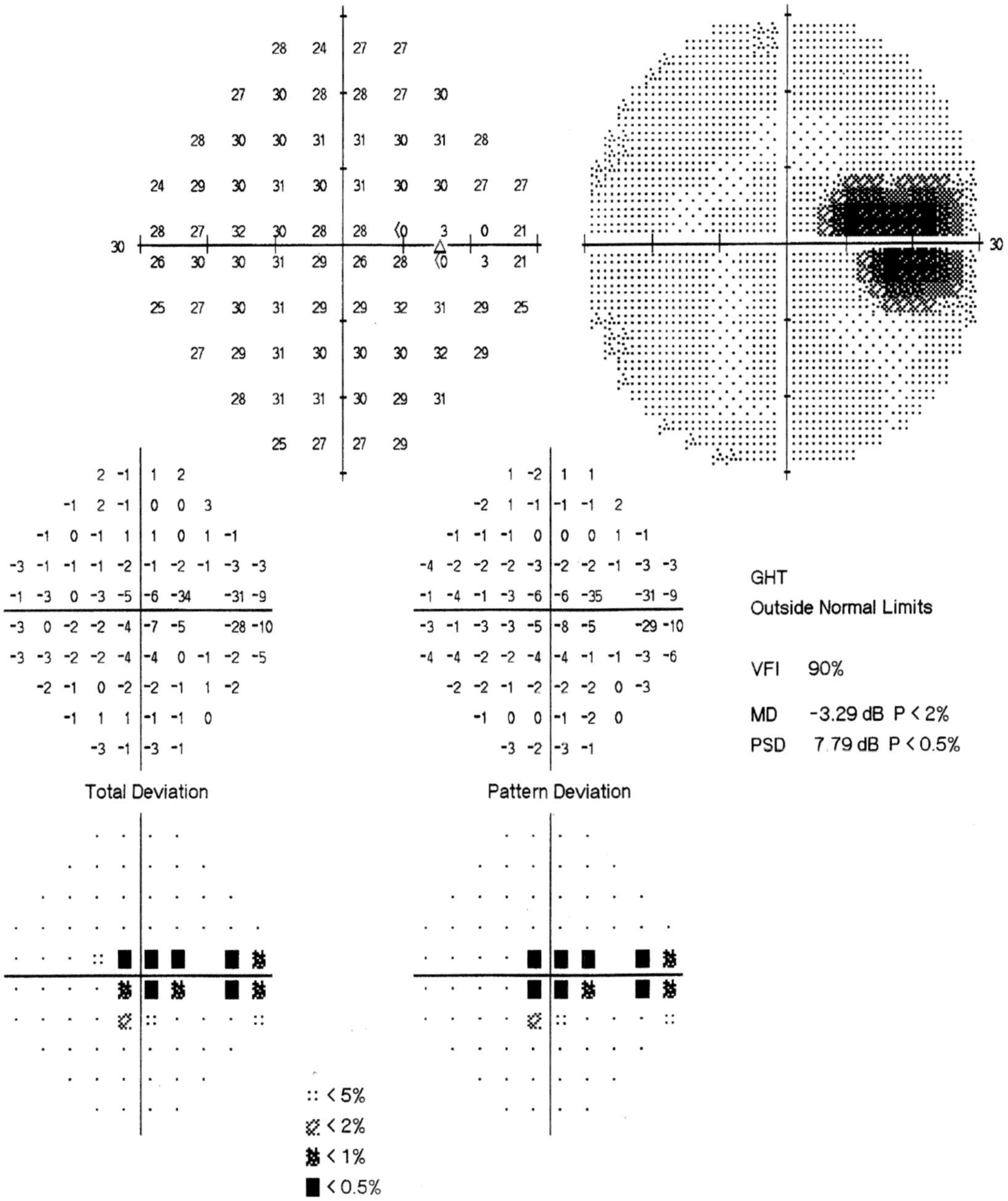

Fig. 30.3 Humphrey visual field analysis printout. The 30-2 test showed an enlarged physiological blind spot and a central defect

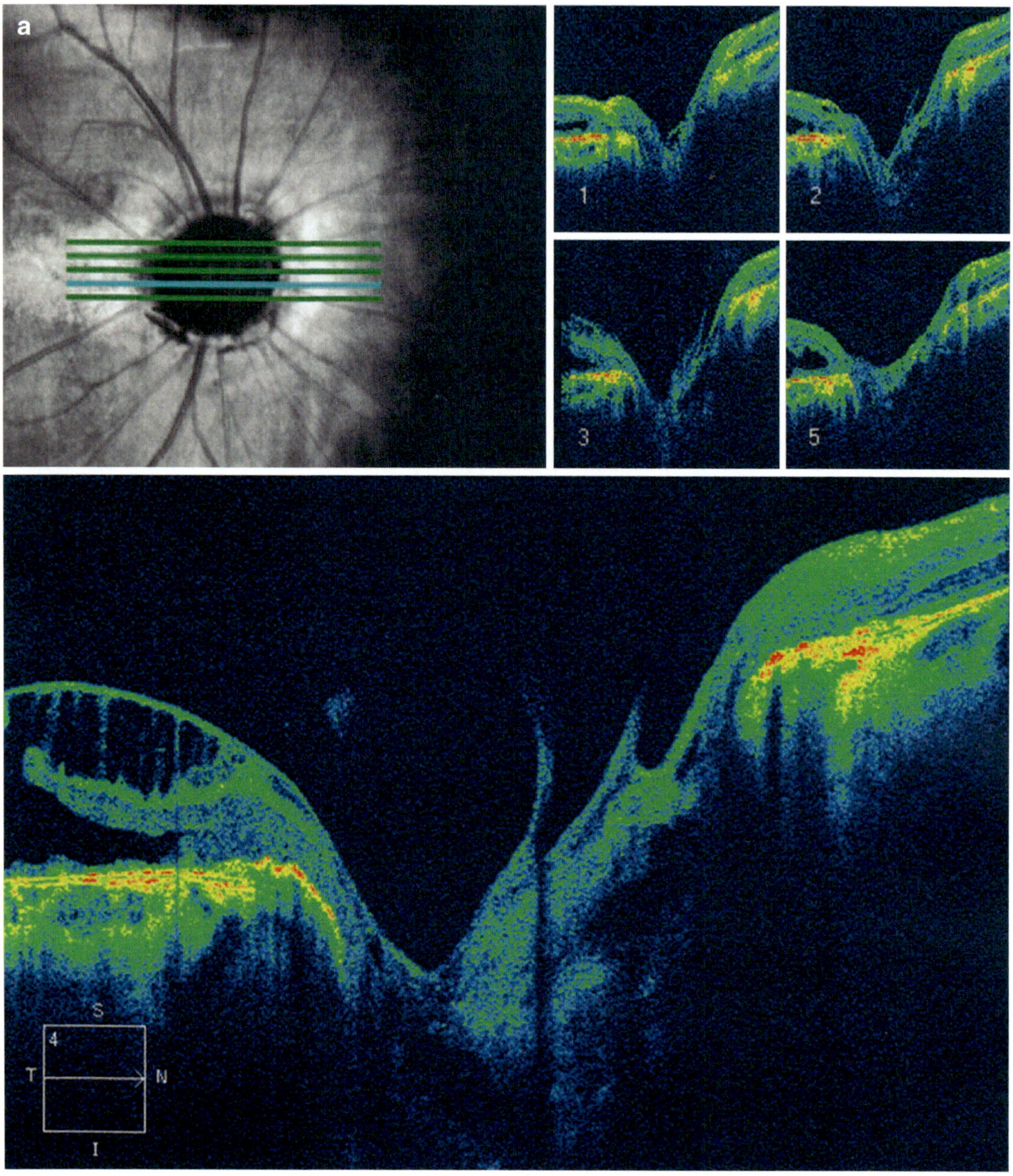

Fig. 30.4 OCT linear scanning of the optic disc and macula. A central funnel-like excavation was seen in the optic disc of the right eye. Partial detachment accompanied by interlayer separation could also be observed in the retinal neuroepithelium between the optic disc and the macula. Panel a: optic disc. Panel b: macula

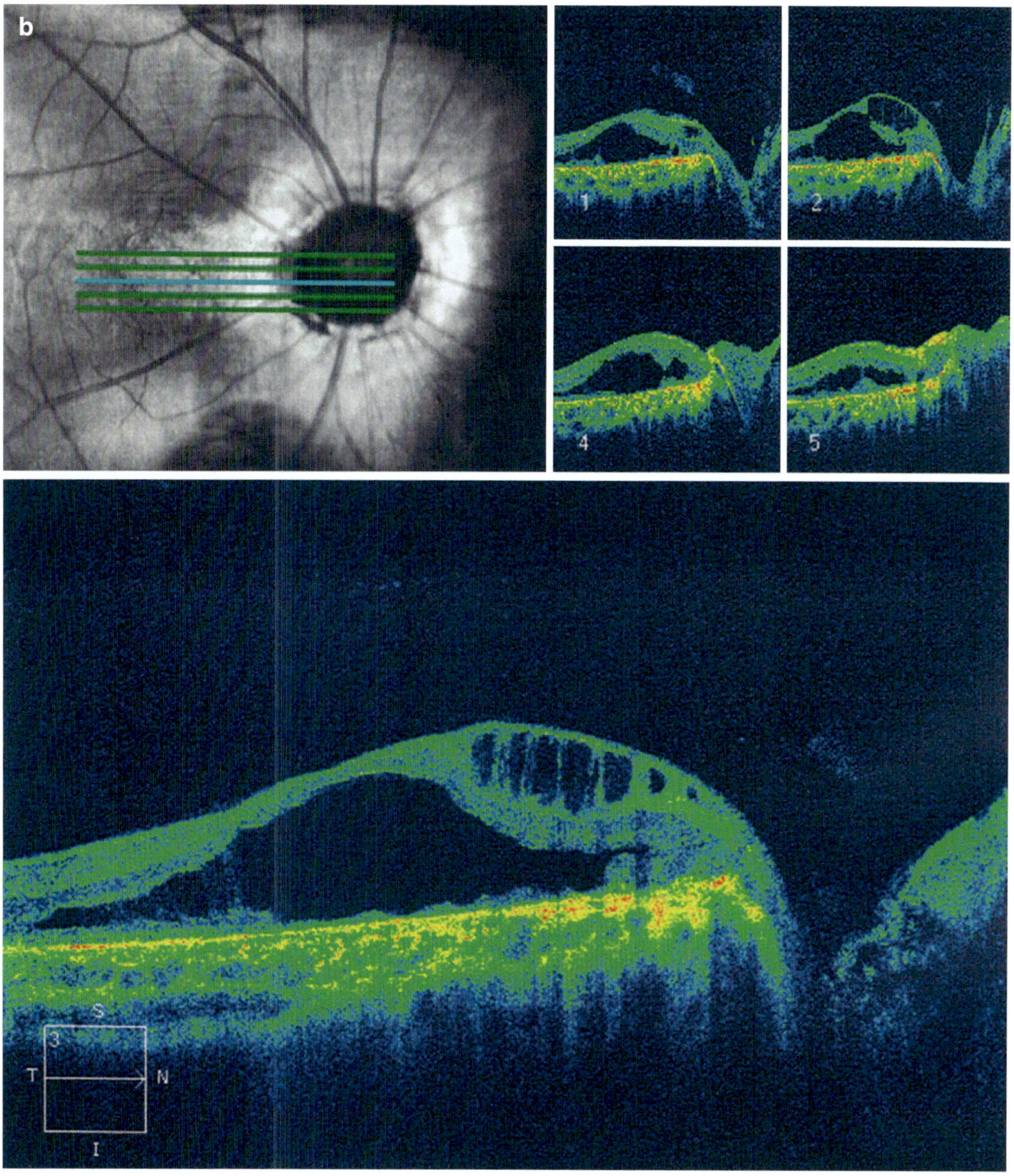

Fig. 30.4 (continued)

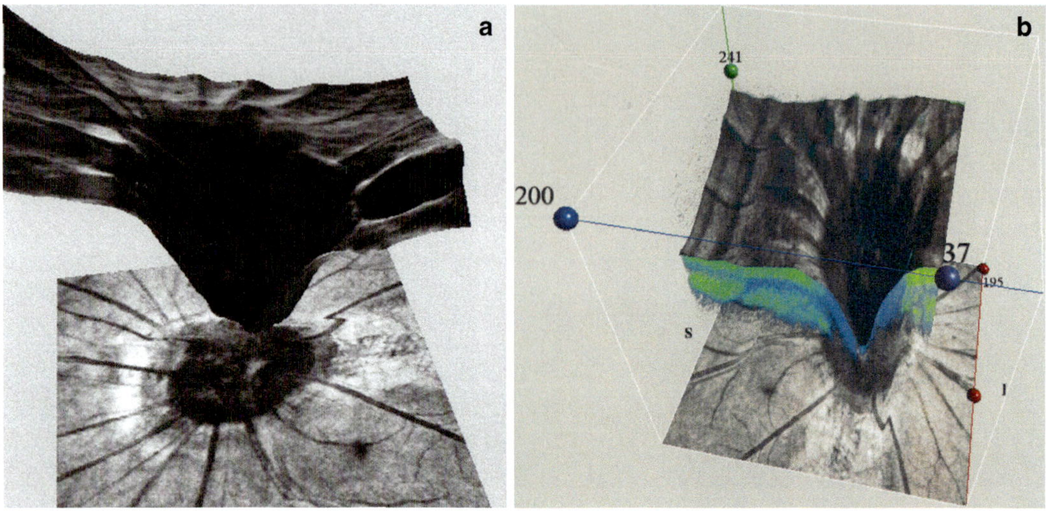

Fig. 30.5 3D reconstruction images of the optic disc. A funnel-like excavation could be found in the optic disc, and mild elevation was shown at the disc edge. Spoke-like climbing out and steep running could be found in the optic disc vessels

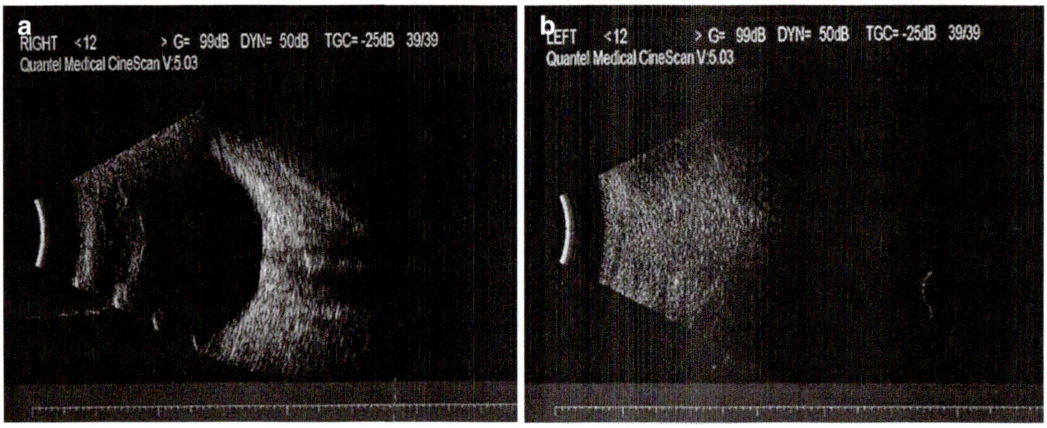

Fig. 30.6 B-ultrasound images. Panel a: deepening of the excavation was noted in the optic disc of the right eye. Flocculent low-medium-level echoes could be found inside the vitreous cavity. The backward movement was positive. Panel b: no eyeball echo was observed in the left eye

vision of patients with morning glory syndrome tends to be poor, and only about 30% of the patients have BCVA as well as 20/40 or better. Afferent pupillary defect and visual field defect are frequently observed. The main visual field change in morning glory syndrome is enlargement of the physiological blind spot. The other visual field defects could also be observed when corresponding retinal detachment develops simultaneously [2]. The manifestations in this patient included an enlarged physiological blind spot and a central visual field defect due to serous retinal detachment in the macula.

In addition, morning glory disc anomaly may be complicated by systemic congenital defects, including pituitary dwarfism and congenital abnormality of the internal carotid artery (e.g., moyamoya disease) [3, 4]. The pathogenesis has not been known yet. The patient had morning glory disc anomaly in one eye and congenital anophthalmia in the other, which suggested that there might be a common pathogenesis between the dysplasias in both eyes and which requires further studies in terms of molecular genetics. A literature review by us revealed that the relevant virulence gene of morning glory syndrome and congenital anophthalmia was PAX6 [4]. But a genetic sequencing analysis for such gene mutation was negative. Further studies should be done to understand the molecular biological mechanism of the disease.

About 38% of the patients with morning glory syndrome have complicating serous retinal detachment, which may be related to local dysplasia. The source of the serous fluid for retinal detachment may be the cerebrospinal fluid or the liquefied vitreous [2]. But it remains controversial.

There is still no effective and specific treatment for morning glory disc syndrome [3]. The possible complications should be ruled out by relevant examinations after the diagnosis of morning glory disc syndrome is confirmed. Standardized automated perimetry should be done for the diagnosis of the disease and complications.

References

1. Fei P, Zhang Q, Li J, et al. Clinical characteristics and treatment of 22 eyes of morning glory syndrome associated with persistent hyperplastic primary vitreous. Br J Ophthalmol. 2013;97(10):1262–7.
2. Chang S, Gregory-Roberts E, Chen R. Retinal detachment associated with optic disc colobomas and morning glory syndrome. Eye (Lond). 2012;26(4):494–500.
3. Cavazos-Adame H, Olvera-Barrios A, Martinez-Lopez-Portillo A, et al. Morning glory disc anomaly, a report of a successfully treated case of functional amblyopia. J Clin Diagn Res. 2015;9(10):ND01-03.
4. Magdalene D, Kalital DA, et al. Mild line craniofacial defects and morning glory disc anomaly with clinical anophthalmos-a distinct clinical entity. Orbit. 2010;29(1):57–9.

31 Glaucomatous Optic Neuropathy and Optic Disc Drusen

Xiaojing Pan, Ning Fan, and Xuyang Liu

Generally speaking, specific signs are critical to the diagnoses of some diseases. For example, bilateral papilledema is associated with intracranial hypertension. Enlargement of the optic disc cupping and neuroretinal rim thinning are important signs of primary open-angle glaucoma (POAG). However, we shall question the current diagnosis or go through the differential diagnoses when the typical signs that ought to be shown are not observed. The analysis process for a POAG case is presented as follows.

31.1 Case

31.1.1 Case Presentation

A 29-year-old male patient complained of blurred vision and pain in both eyes for over 1 year. But no headache, amaurosis, nausea, or vomiting was reported. The intraocular pressure in both eyes had been as high as 36 mmHg when examined at a local hospital, and latanoprost eye drops had been given to lower the intraocular pressure. No history of trauma or systemic diseases was found.

The uncorrected visual acuity (UCVA) was 20/200 OD and 20/65 OS, while the best corrected visual acuity (BCVA) was 20/20 OD and 20/20 OS. Intraocular pressure (IOP) by standard Goldmann applanation tonometry was measured as 28 mmHg OU. Slit-lamp examination of his anterior segments was unremarkable. Fundus examination showed mild elevation and an unclear boundary of the optic disc in both eyes. A wedge-shaped inferotemporal retinal nerve fiber layer (RNFL) defect (blue arrow) was present in the right eye. Reflection could be observed in the fovea (Fig. 31.1).

Standardized automated visual field test indicated that the central visual field in both eyes was normal (Fig. 31.2).

31.1.2 Case Analysis

Increased IOP in both eyes and a local RNFL defect in the right eye were observed in the patient. The diagnosis tended to be glaucoma. But why was optic disc elevation observed instead of optic disc excavation which is the

X. Pan
Shandong Eye Institute, Qingdao Eye Hospital, Qingdao, China

N. Fan
Shenzhen Eye Hospital, Shenzhen University, Shenzhen, China

X. Liu (✉)
Xiamen Eye Center of Xiamen University, Xiamen, China

Shenzhen Eye Hospital, Shenzhen University, Shenzhen, China

N. Wang et al. (eds.), *Optic Disorders and Visual Field*, Advances in Visual Science and Eye Diseases 2, https://doi.org/10.1007/978-981-13-2502-1_31

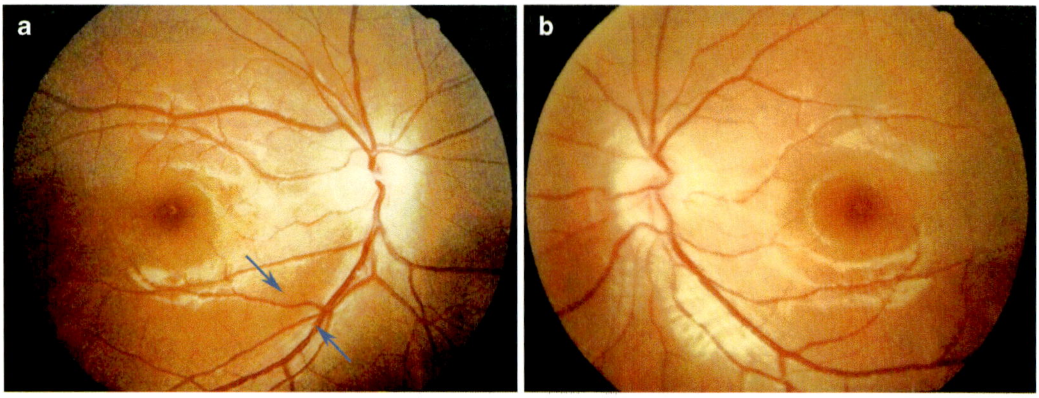

Fig. 31.1 Fundus photographs. Mild elevation and an unclear boundary were observed in the optic disc of both eyes. A wedge-shaped inferotemporal RNFL defect was found in the right eye (blue arrow). Panel a: right eye. Panel b: left eye

characteristic sign for glaucoma? What is the reason for the bilateral optic disc elevation?

1. Was it because the intracranial pressure increased? The lumbar puncture carried out at neurology department showed that the patient's intracranial pressure was 188 mmH_2O (13.8 mmHg), which was at the upper limit of normal intracranial pressures. No abnormality was found in the biochemistry and routine examinations of the cerebrospinal fluid.
2. Was it because of the intracranial hypertension caused by intracranial space-occupying lesions? No significant abnormality was revealed in the head MRI scan.

Based on the above examination results, the patient had no identifiable intracranial lesion. However, the intracranial pressure was at the upper limit of the normal range. Was this intracranial pressure high enough to cause bilateral optic disc elevation? The measured intracranial pressure of the patient was 13.8 mmHg. The intraocular pressure is 4–8 mmHg higher than the intracranial pressure under normal circumstances. The difference between the intraocular and intracranial pressures was 14.2 mmHg ($28 - 13.8 = 14.2$ mmHg), which suggested that it was significantly larger than normal range, and the optic disc should have been excavated. Therefore, the bilateral optic disc elevation found in the patient was not caused by the elevation of intracranial pressure. Other possible reasons needed to be identified.

We focused on the patient's eyes and optic disc again. Was it possible that the manifestation of the patient was in keeping with pseudopapilledema? Or was optic disc elevation caused by such factors as anatomic abnormality, inflammation, or ischemia? FFA, ICGA, and OCT were hence carried out.

Bilateral FFA + ICGA revealed no abnormality (Fig. 31.3).

Autofluorescence test of both fundi showed cluster-like autofluorescence inside the optic disc (Fig. 31.4).

The OCT results revealed lump-produced signals with high reflection inside the optic disc of both eyes. Thickness measurement of the RNFL around the optic disc showed inferotemporal RNFL thinning in the right eye and normal RNFL thickness in the left eye (Fig. 31.5).

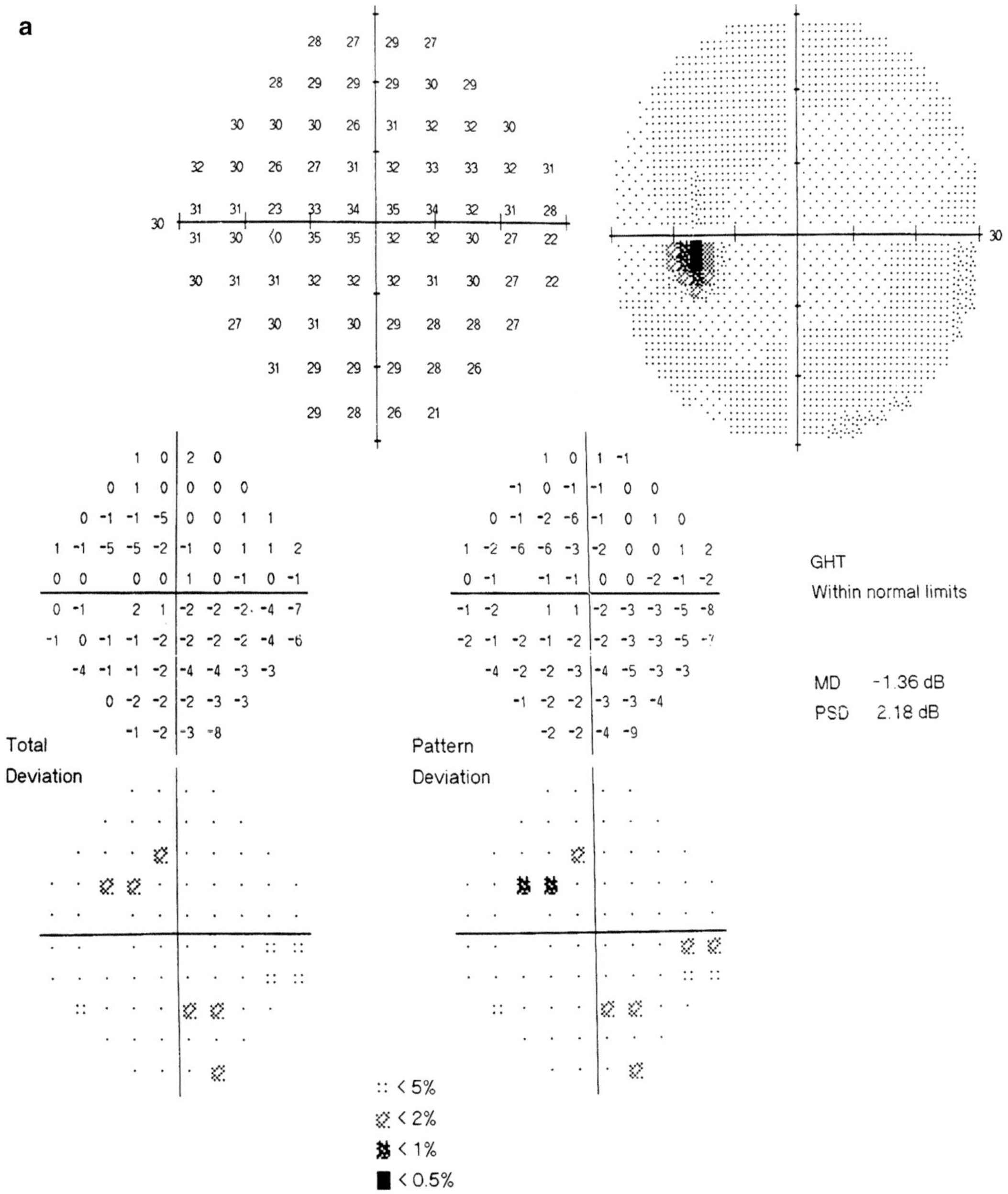

Fig. 31.2 Humphrey visual field analysis printouts. The 30-2 test revealed no significant abnormality in the visual field of both eyes. Panel a: left eye. Panel b: right eye

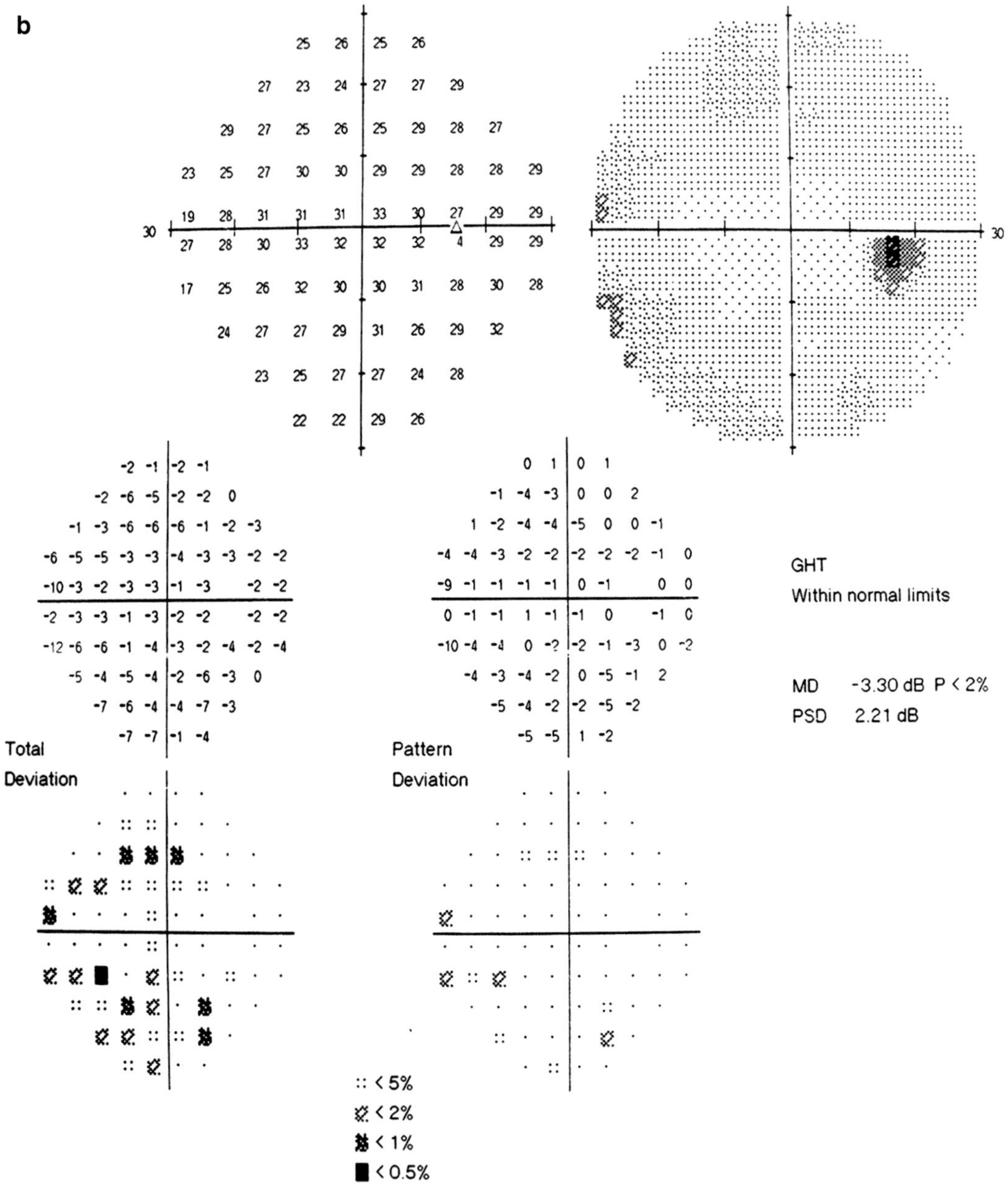

Fig. 31.2 (continued)

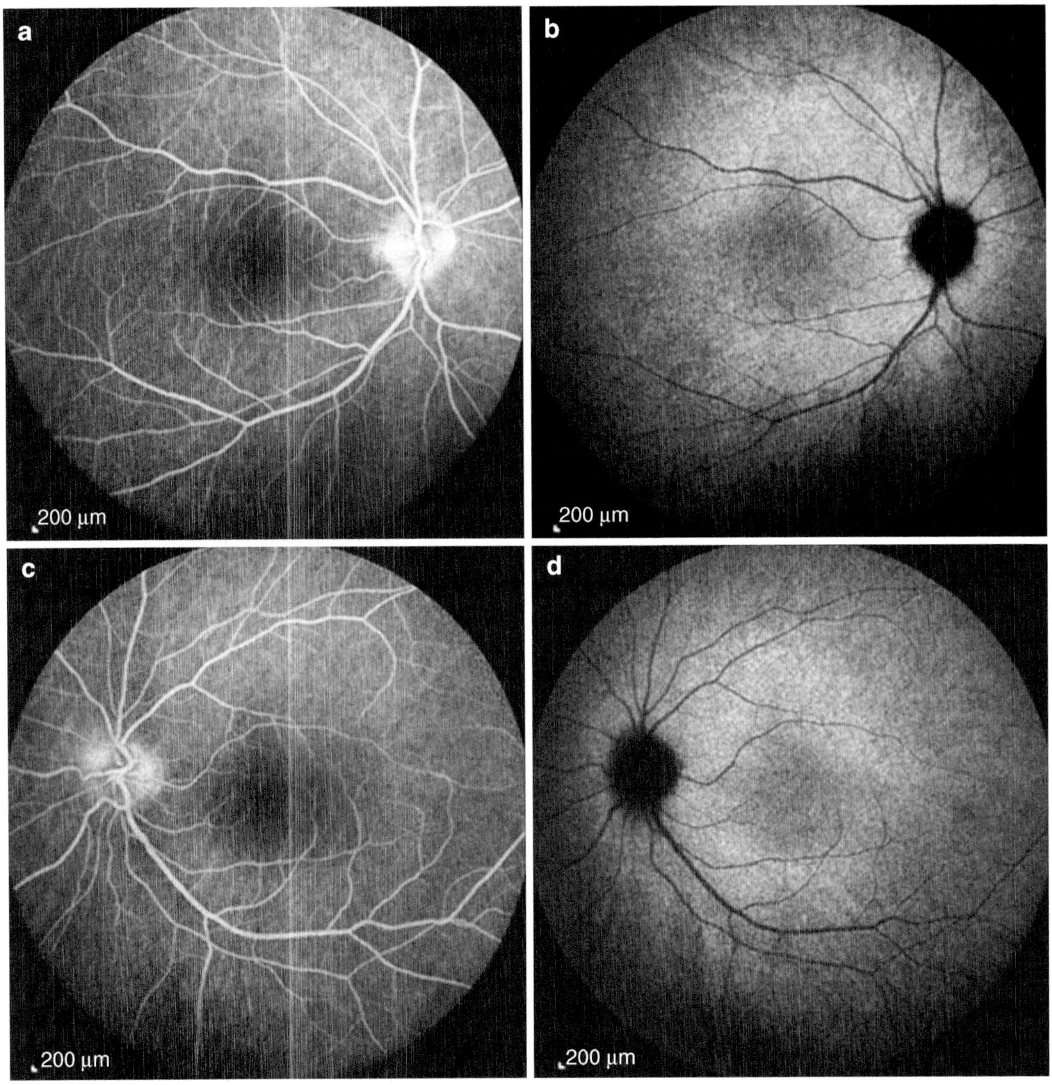

Fig. 31.3 FFA + ICGA images. Fluorescent staining could be observed in both optic discs at the late phase of the FFA. No fluorescein leakage was revealed. ICGA showed no abnormality in either eye. Panel a: FFA of right eye. Panel b: ICGA of the right eye. Panel c: FFA of the left eye. Panel d: ICGA of the left eye

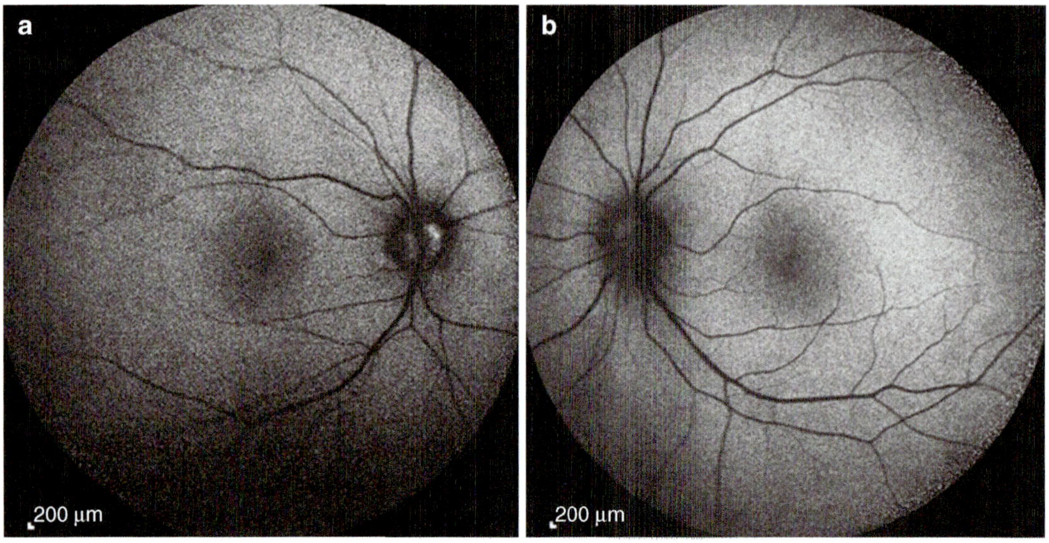

Fig. 31.4 Fundus autofluorescence images. Cluster-like autofluorescence was revealed inside the optic discs. Panel a: right eye. Panel b: left eye

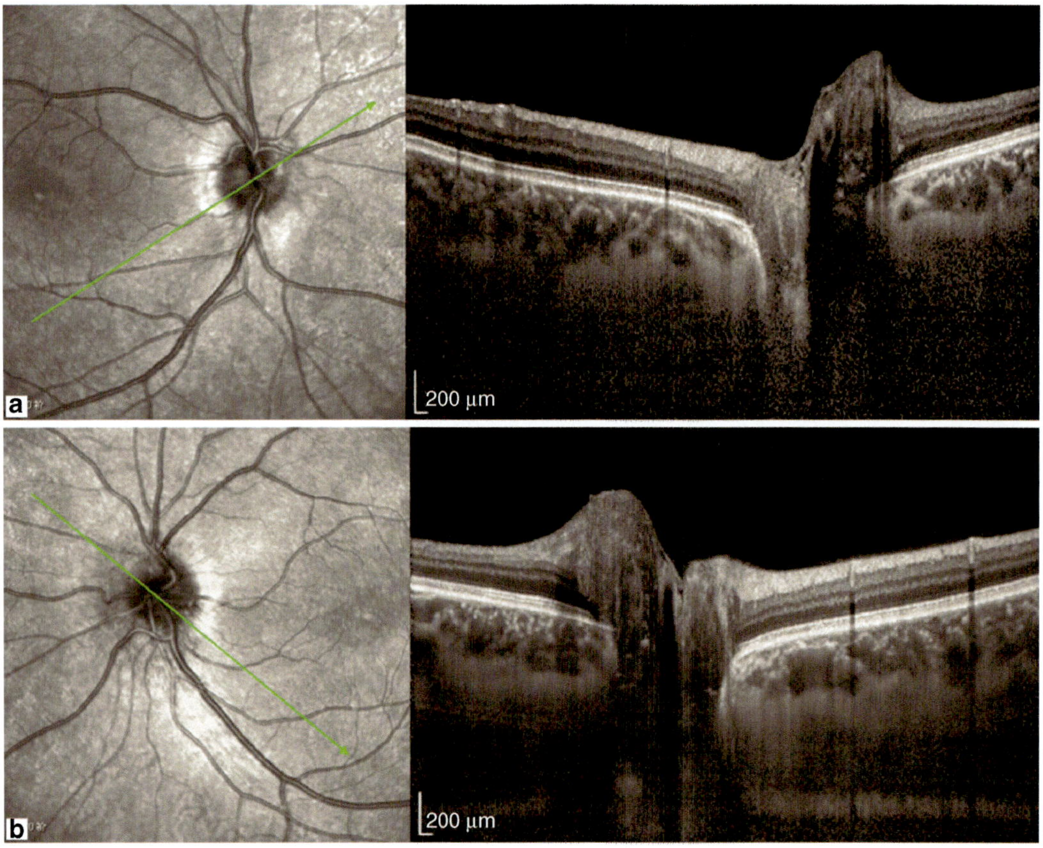

Fig. 31.5 OCT scanning of optic disc and RNFL thickness measurement. Lump-produced signals with high reflection could be observed inside the optic disc in both eyes. Panel a: right eye. Panel b: left eye. Panel c: the thickness measurement on RNFL around the optic disc showed inferotemporal RNFL thinning in the right eye (red arrow). Panel d: the RNFL thickness in the left eye was normal

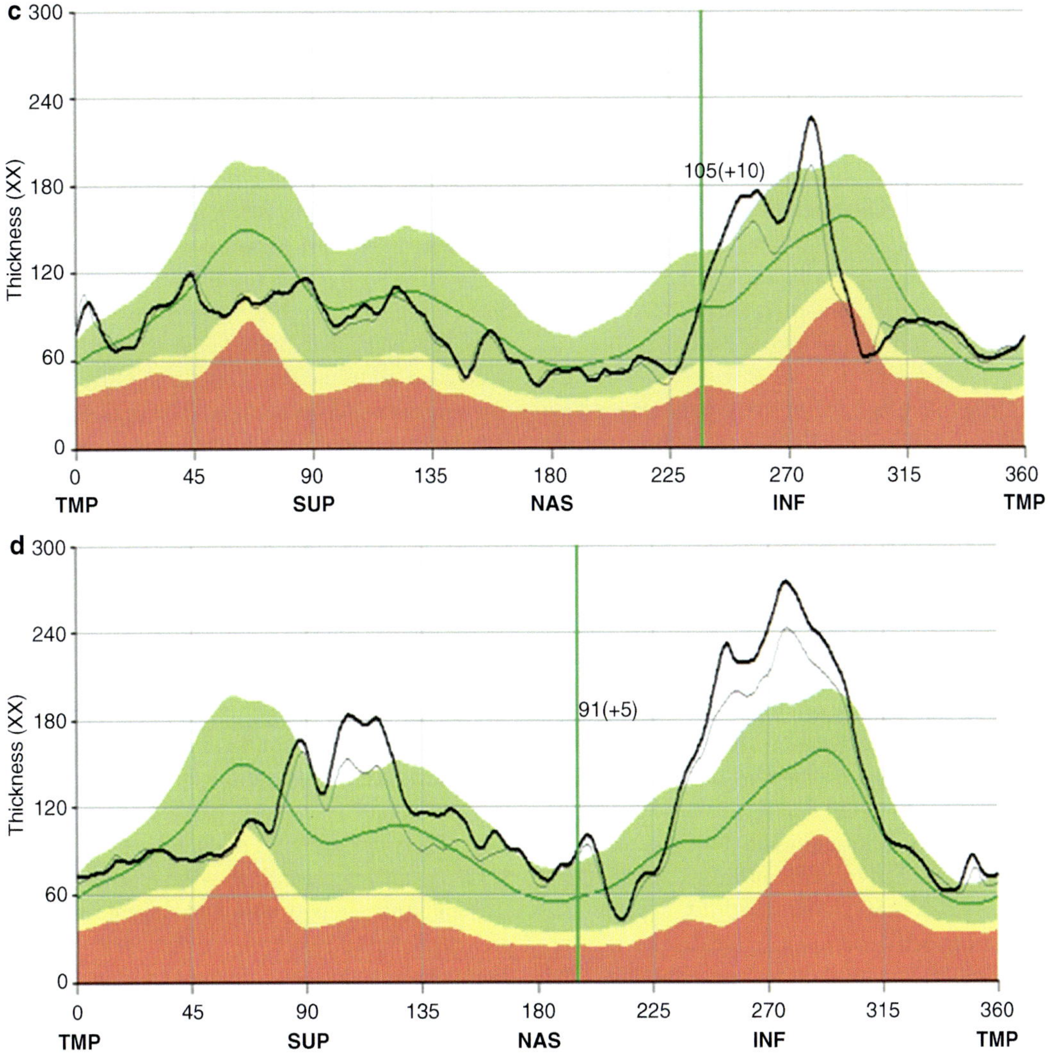

Fig. 31.5 (continued)

FFA revealed strong fluorescence in both optic discs, and no fluorescein leakage was observed. These findings did not conform to the FFA manifestations of papilledema. The autofluorescence in both optic discs and lump-produced signals with high reflection inside them shown by OCT scanning suggested the presence of buried optic disc drusen in both eyes.

With orbital CT, dot-like hyperdense lesions (calcification, Fig. 31.6) could be observed in the junction of the optic nerve and posterior wall of the eye ring in both eyes, which further confirmed the diagnosis of bilateral optic disc drusen.

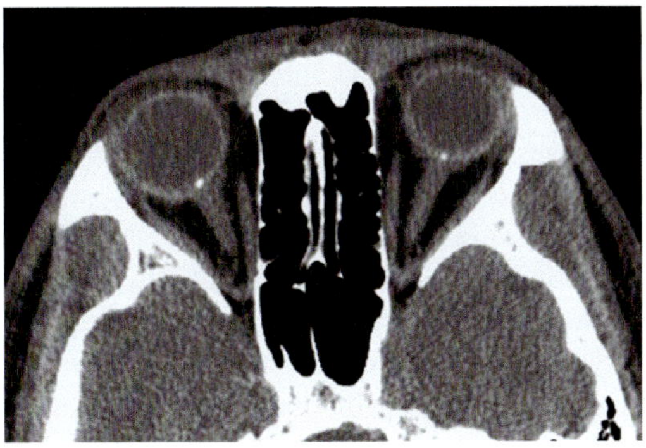

Fig. 31.6 Orbital CT image. Dot-like hyperdense lesions could be observed in the junction of the optic nerve and posterior wall of the eye ring in both eyes

The diagnosis of buried optic disc drusen in both eyes was confirmed based on the above findings, and the bilateral optic disc elevation could also be explained (pseudopapilledema).

31.1.3 Final Diagnosis

The final diagnosis was buried optic disc drusen in both eyes, pre-perimetric POAG in the right eye, and ocular hypertension in the left eye.

Drugs were prescribed to the patient to reduce intraocular pressures. Follow-up has been carried out for 3 years so far, and the disease condition has been stable. The defects of the visual fields and fundi showed no progression.

31.2 Discussion

Some specific signs are usually crucial for the diagnosis of some diseases clinically. For example, bilateral papilledema is associated with high intracranial pressure. Enlargement of the optic disc cupping and neuroretinal rim defects are usually indicative of primary open-angle glaucoma (POAG). We need to analyze the causes carefully and re-exam the diagnosis when the expected typical signs are missing. The patient in this section demonstrated typical glaucomatous RNFL defects and elevated IOPs. Although no visual field defect was identified, the patient could be diagnosed with POAG if corresponding enlargement of the optic disc cupping and neuroretinal rim damage existed. However, these expected changes did not manifest themselves. Instead, optic disc elevation and edema in both eyes were observed. Was the diagnosis of glaucoma correct? Or was it to be differentiated from other diseases?

During the differential analysis for the case, we wondered whether there was an association between optic disc elevation and high intracranial pressure. Based upon the analysis on the pressure gradient between the intraocular pressure and intracranial pressure, we found that the gradient was not sufficient to cause optic disc edema. Meanwhile, intracranial lesions were also ruled out by neuroimaging examination. Further investigation for the causes for optic disc elevation was carried out, and buried optic disc drusen in both eyes were confirmed.

With the presence of buried ODD, the patient did not demonstrate typical optic cupping and backward excavation because of the space-filling effect of the drusen body on the disc, even though the intraocular pressures were elevated, and only wedge-shaped defect was revealed in the RNFL without corresponding neuroretinal rim damage. The patient could still be diagnosed with POAG in the right eye even if there was no visual field impairment in this eye, because structural damage usually occurs prior to functional damage. And currently, only high intraocular pressure was found in the left eye, so the diagnosis was ocular hypertension.

Optic disc drusen usually involve both eyes, but visible optic disc drusen only develop in few affected eyes. It can be manifested as irregular pearl-like substances on the surface of the optic disc and is usually located in the nasal side of the optic disc. The cause of optic disc drusen is still unclear. It may be related to factors including hyperplasia and degeneration of premature optic neuroglia in the optic disc or disintegration and calcification of optic nerve fiber axoplasm, etc. The clinical manifestations of buried ODD include the following: (a) an elevated optic disc (but the area of elevation do not extend beyond the disc margin) and disappearance of the physiologic optic cup; (b) abnormal vascular changes in the optic disc, such as vascular branch abnormality, large vessels, increase in number or distortion of blood vessels, etc.; (c) multilayer hemorrhage in the superficial and peripheral areas; and (d) spontaneous retinal venous pulsation in some diseased eyes. B-ultrasound and CT have mainly been used in the diagnosis of optic disc drusen before. CT can display the calcified drusen clearly, but its sensitivity is lower than B-ultrasound. Currently, some new technologies, such as SD-OCT, fundus autofluorescence, FFA, etc., are also considered as the most valuable diagnostic tools for optic disc drusen [1, 2]. Two typical buried ODD cases have been introduced in Chap. 29 of this part, of which one case has been complicated by retinal hemorrhage. The discussion part in Chap. 29 has also elaborated the specific diagnostic methods for optic disc drusen.

There is no special treatment for optic disc drusen at present. For the patient in this case, the main treatment was to reduce intraocular pressure to prevent visual function damage. It is very important to monitor the potential progression of glaucoma and optic disc drusen with regular visual field follow-ups.

References

1. Merchant KY, Su D, Park SC, et al. Enhanced depth imaging optical coherence tomography of optic nerve head drusen. Ophthalmology. 2013;120(7):1409–14.
2. Sato T, Mrejen S, Spaide RF. Multimodal imaging of optic disc drusen. Am J Ophthalmol. 2013;156(2):275–82.

Congenital Optic Disc Pit

32

Xiaojing Pan, Ning Fan, and Xuyang Liu

Congenital optic disc pit is a type of developmental defect rarely found in the optic disc. There is a congenital nerve tissue defect at the pit. Most patients can be asymptomatic for life. However, abnormalities can usually be found in standardized automated perimetry which is helpful in determining the severity and possible complications of the disease.

32.1 Case 1

32.1.1 Case Presentation

A 72-year-old male patient who had undergone a cataract operation in the left eye at another hospital 1 month before presented for a recheck. His visual acuity recovered well after the operation. Discomforts such as distorted vision, dark shadow, etc. were denied. Histories of other ocular diseases, trauma, or familial diseases were denied.

X. Pan
Shandong Eye Institute, Qingdao Eye Hospital, Qingdao, China

N. Fan
Shenzhen Eye Hospital, Shenzhen University, Shenzhen, China

X. Liu (✉)
Xiamen Eye Center of Xiamen University, Xiamen, China

Shenzhen Eye Hospital, Shenzhen University, Shenzhen, China

The uncorrected visual acuity (UCVA) was 20/28 OD and 20/22 OS with no improvement with myopic correction. In both eyes, intraocular pressure (IOP) was normal, the cornea was transparent, the aqueous flare was negative, the pupil was 3 mm in diameter, and direct light reflex was sensitive. The intraocular lens was well positioned. In the left eye, the optic disc tilted to the inferotemporal area, and a deep pit with a clear boundary was observed in thc inferotemporal margin of the disc. Neuroretinal rim thinning accompanied by vascular crawling was revealed in the inferotemporal margin of the disc. The optic cup was relatively large, and the residual neuroretinal rim was pink in color. Reflection could be seen from the fovea (Fig. 32.1). The right fundus showed no abnormality.

Standardized automated perimetry showed that the physiological blind spot enlarged toward the temporal side in the left eye (Fig. 32.2).

OCT revealed a deep pit in the inferotemporal disc during both the vertical scan and 3D reconstruction of the optic disc. A nerve fiber tissue defect could be found in the pit area. Incomplete posterior detachment was found in the vitreous in front of the optic disc (Fig. 32.3).

32.1.2 Final Diagnosis

The final diagnosis was a congenital optic disc pit in the left eye.

N. Wang et al. (eds.), *Optic Disorders and Visual Field*, Advances in Visual Science and Eye Diseases 2, https://doi.org/10.1007/978-981-13-2502-1_32

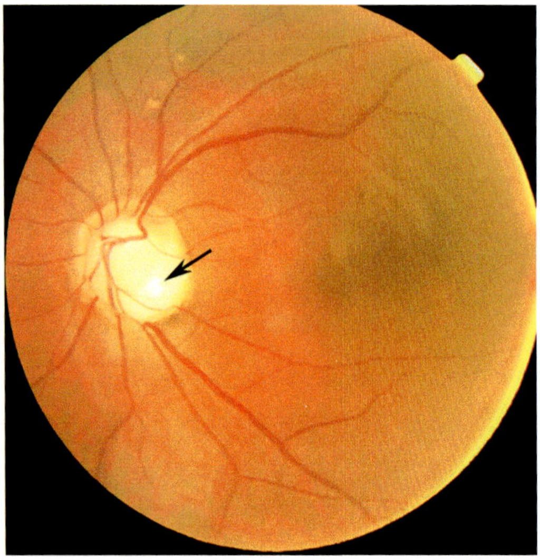

Fig. 32.1 Fundus photograph. A deep pit with a clear boundary could be seen in the inferotemporal margin of the optic disc. Vascular crawling and optic cup enlargement were revealed. The optic disc pit is indicated by the black arrow

32.1.3 Case Review

The patient in this case had a congenital optic disc pit and had been asymptomatic for a long time. A deep pit in the inferotemporal region of the optic disc was spotted during the fundus examination after the cataract operation. An enlarged physiological blind spot and a relative defect were identified in the visual field. The causes were mainly related to the nerve fiber tissue absence in the optic disc pit area. The relationship between the optic disc pit and tilted optic disc found in the patient was still unclear. A pit is a type of dysplasia, and it may compromise local physiological anatomy and barrier function. Therefore, a congenital optic disc pit may be complicated by other abnormalities and can lead to corresponding clinical symptoms and visual field changes. The following case is another example.

32.2 Case 2

32.2.1 Case Presentation

A 50-year-old female patient complained of gradual decrease in vision in her right eye without any identifiable cause for more than half a year, and no treatment was offered. One week before, the patient had felt that her symptoms got worse and micropsia had been noticed. Dysmorphopsia was denied. Histories of other ocular diseases, trauma, or familial diseases were denied.

The UCVA was 20/1000 OD with no improvement with myopic correction and 20/20 OS. Slit-lamp examination of her anterior segments was unremarkable. A pit in white color with a clear boundary was observed in the superior margin of the optic disc in the right eye. The optic disc was covered by glial tissue. Serous detachment and retinoschisis with a clear boundary were observed in the macula, and the superior and inferior archades were also involved. The peripheral retina was flat (Fig. 32.4). The left fundus showed no abnormality.

During the standardized automated perimetry, the 24-2 test revealed a defect in the inferior visual field and diffused reduction of light sensitivity in the superior visual field of the right eye (Fig. 32.5).

Eye B-Mode ultrasonography indicated localized retinal detachment in the temporal side of the right optic disc (Fig. 32.6).

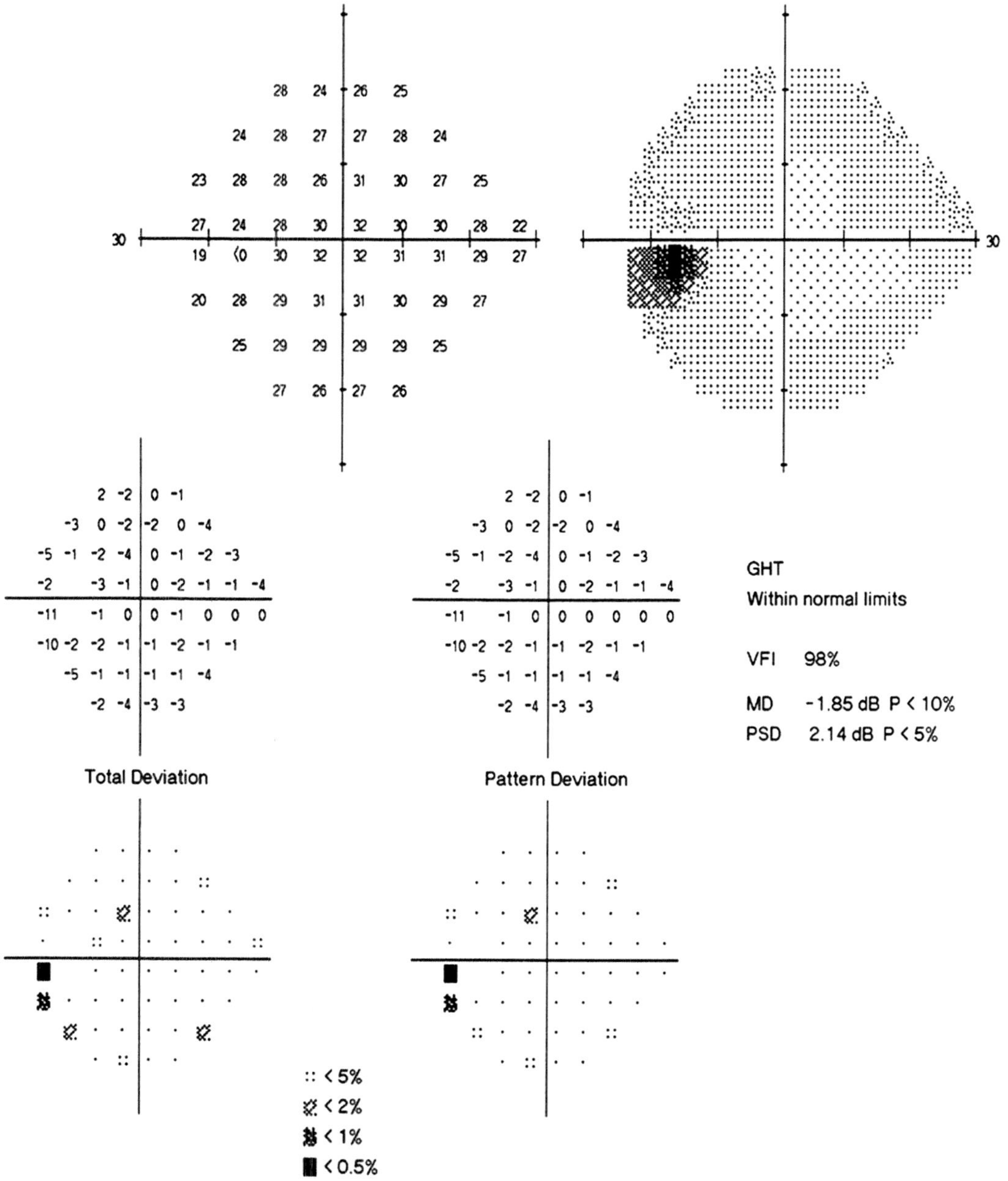

Fig. 32.2 Humphrey visual field analysis printout. The 24-2 test showed an enlarged physiological blind spot in the left eye

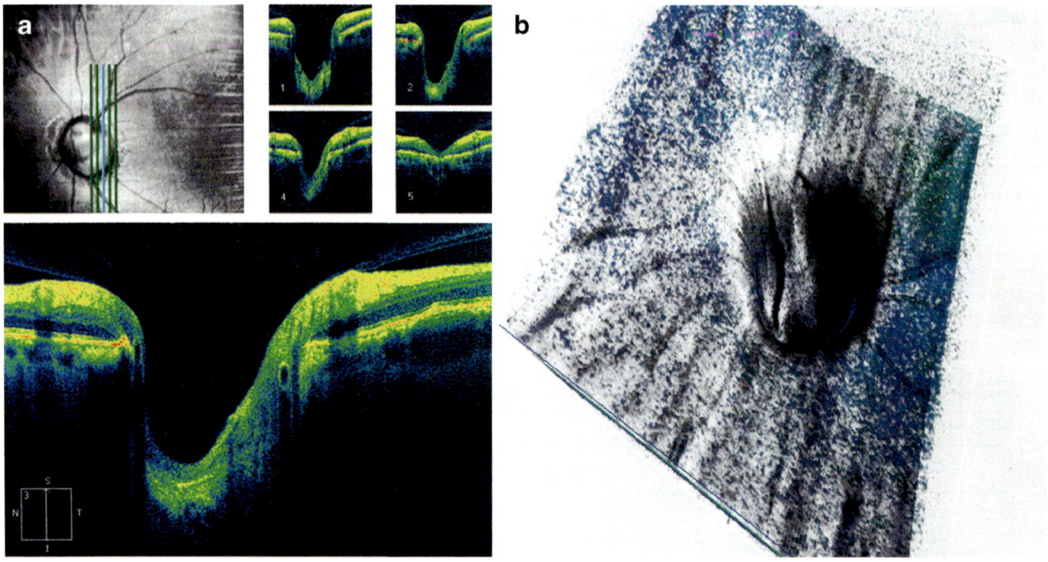

Fig. 32.3 OCT scanning and 3D reconstruction images of the optic disc. A deep pit in the inferotemporal area of the optic disc was observed, and no nerve fiber tissue was observed in the pit area. Panel a: vertical linear scan of the optic disc. Panel b: 3D reconstruction image of the optic disc

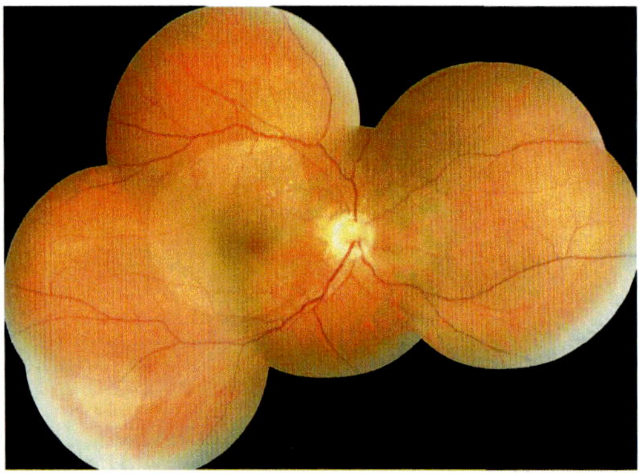

Fig. 32.4 Montage images of fundus photographs. A pit in white color with a clear boundary was observed in the superior margin of the optic disc. The optic disc was covered by glial tissue. Serous detachment and retinoschisis with a clear boundary were observed in the macula. The peripheral retina was flat

The OCT with horizontal linear scan showed the image of optic disc pit maculopathy, with cystoid spaces and schisis in multiple layers as well as subretinal fluid (Fig. 32.7).

During fundus fluorescein angiography (FFA), localized weak fluorescence at the early phase and significant enhanced fluorescence at the middle and late phases were observed in the superior optic disc of the right eye. Flaky transmitted fluorescence in the macula at the early phase and fluorescent staining between the macula and optic disc were seen at the middle and late phases (Fig. 32.8).

32.2.2 Final Diagnosis

The final diagnosis was a congenital optic disc pit and serous retinal detachment in the right eye.

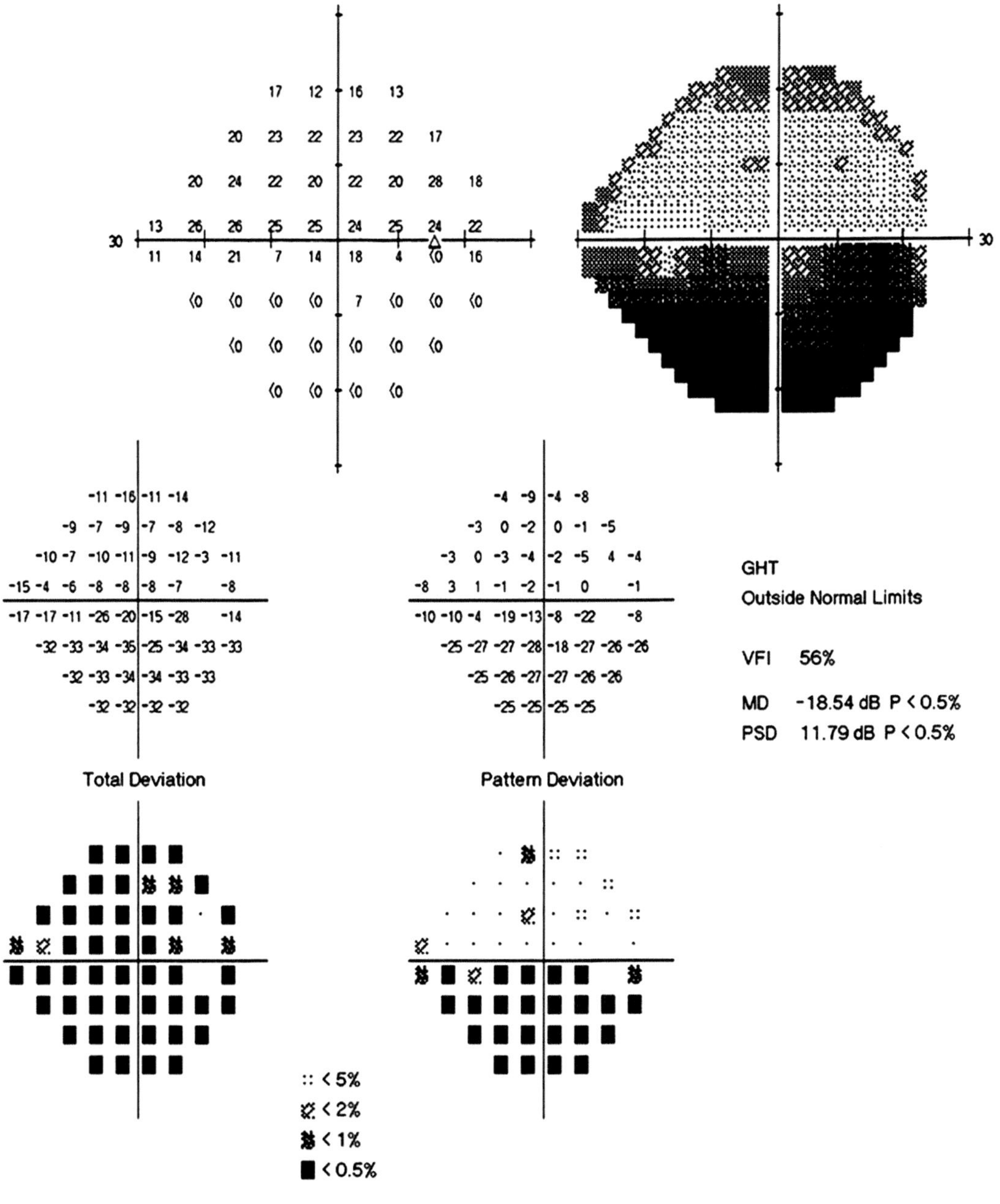

Fig. 32.5 Humphrey visual field analysis printout. The 24-2 test showed visual field defects in inferior region of the right eye

In consideration of the significant retinal detachment in the macula, vitrectomy was performed in combination with C3F8 gas tamponade. Local laser photocoagulation on the peripheral retina around the pit and retinal reattachment were achieved.

32.2.3 Case Review

The congenital optic disc pit can be accompanied by serous retinal detachment in 30–60% of all cases. The common complaint of such patients is central vision loss and the serous detachment of macular neuroepithelium in fundus [1]. The visual field defects, which can be manifested as absolute or relative central visual field defects, paracentral defects, or arcuate defects connecting to the physiological blind spot, are related to the range and degree of the neuroepithelium detachment. The visual field defects of this patient included diffused reduction of light sensitivity and an inferior defect which resulted from the facts that the optic disc pit was located in the superior region and maculopathy in the superior region was more severe.

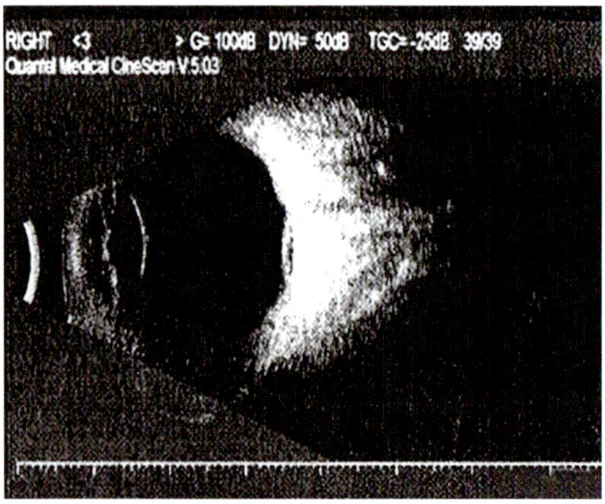

Fig. 32.6 B-ultrasound image. Localized retinal detachment in the temporal side of the optic disc was shown

Currently, different treatment schemes, including local laser treatment for the pit area, vitreous chamber gas tamponade, and vitrectomy combined with procedures, etc., are offered for the optic disc pit accompanied by serous retinal detachment according to the retinal detachment area and height and whether macular retinoschisis or holes are present or not.

32.3 Discussion

Optic disc pit is caused by the developmental defects of neuroectoderm, and it is connected with the poor embryonic fissure closure resulting from abnormal differentiation of primitive optic nerve head cells. Optic pits are usually unilateral onset, and approximately 15% of them are found to be bilateral. The morbidity is

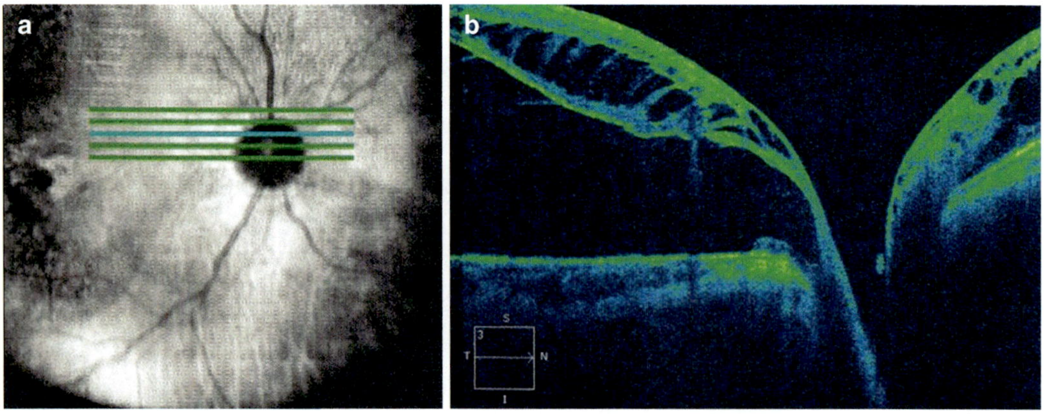

Fig. 32.7 OCT linear scanning of the macula and optic disc. The OCT linear scanning showed optic disc pit maculopathy, with cystoid spaces and schisis in multiple layers as well as subretinal fluid. Panel a: scanning position. Panel b: OCT image of the parapapillary retina

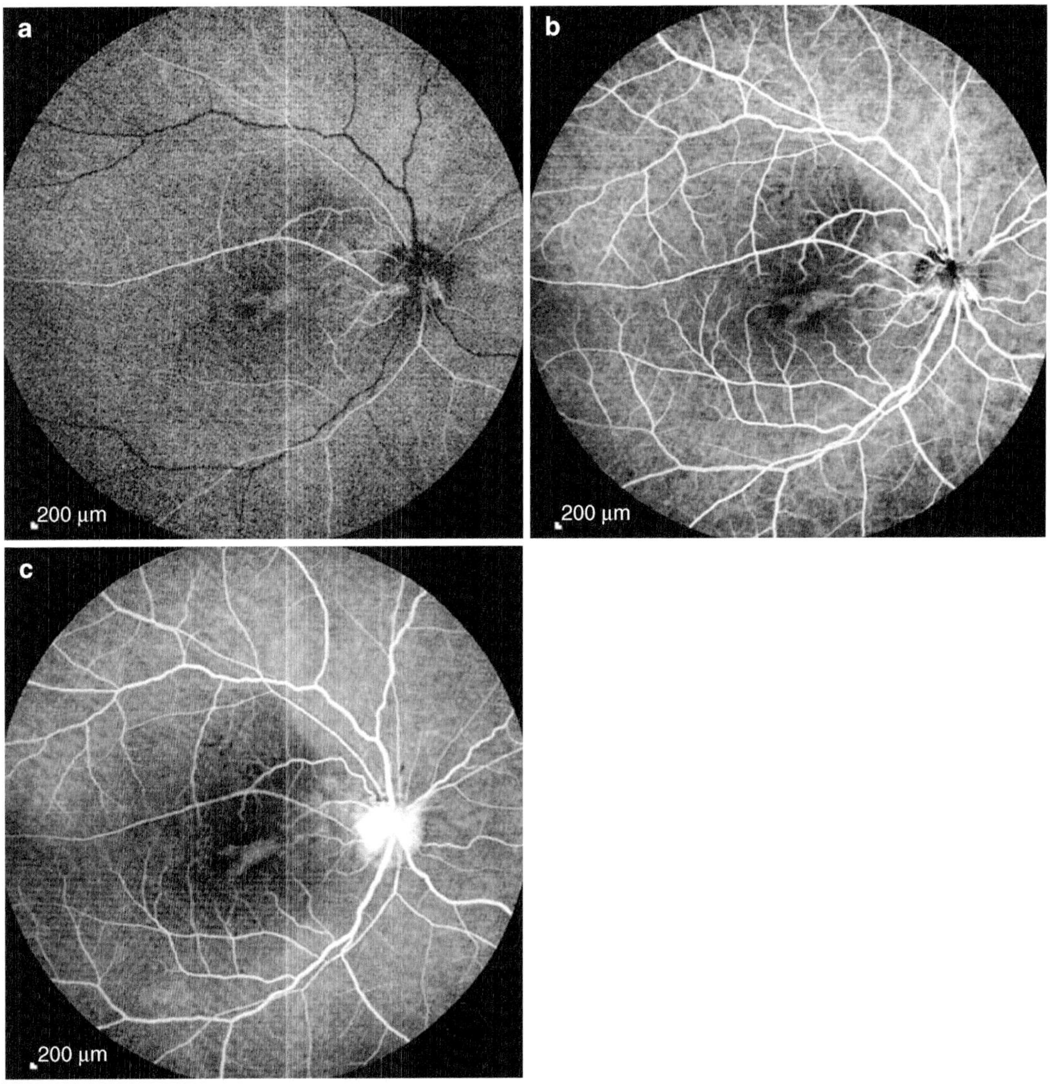

Fig. 32.8 FFA (fundus fluorescein angiography) images. Localized weak fluorescence at the early phase and significant enhanced fluorescence at the middle and late phases were observed in the superior optic disc of the right eye. Flaky transmitted fluorescence in macula at the early phase and fluorescent staining between macula and optic disc at the middle and late phases were revealed. Panel a: early-phase angiogram. Panel b: middle-phase angiogram. Panel c: late-phase angiogram

about 1:11,000. They had no obvious tendency of being hereditary [2]. The pit has already existed before the patient is born and is filled or covered by the residual tissues of the embryo in the early years. As the residues are gradually absorbed, the pit is exposed, which more often is found in young and middle-aged populations. It can also be accompanied by other congenital abnormalities, such as partial optic disc loss, prepapillary membrane, peripapillary atrophy, and residual vitreum artery. Macular diseases can be concomitant in 40% of eyes affected by optic disc pits, and it is usually found in the patients with a pit in the temporal side. These macular diseases include serous retinal detachment, retinoschisis, macular holes, and so on, and they can lead to serious damage to the central vision of the patient [3].

The common visual field defects in an optic disc pit include an enlarged physiological blind spot, paracentral defects, arcuate defects connecting to the physiological blind spot, etc. Visual field impairments get worse when complicated by retinal detachment, such as a quadrantic visual field defect, diffuse or localized light sensitivity loss, etc. The extent and severity of the damage are closely related to retinal diseases.

Both of the above cases are congenital optic disc pits. In one of them, the patient was a senior male without any symptom for a long time, and in the other, the patient was a middle-aged female with serious decrease in vision accompanied by macular changes. Why were different manifestations found in the same disease? What was the underlying mechanism for the occurrence of retinoschisis and retinal detachment? Where did the subretinal effusion originate from?

No clear answers to the above questions have been found based upon our literature review. It is speculated to be connected with the traction and liquefaction of the vitreous. In young and middle-aged patients with optic disc pits, the posterior vitreous detachment produces traction force on the optic disc and retina, and meanwhile, the liquefied vitreous is easier to pass through the optic disc pit and enter the area under the retinal neuroepithelium, which results in serous retinal detachment (the manifestations are similar to those of central serous chorioretinopathy, but their pathogeneses are different). Complications, including macular cleavage or holes, etc., are observed due to the occurrence of metabolic disorder and cystic degeneration, etc. found within the retina after detachment. And for senior patients with optic disc pits, posterior vitreous detachment has been complete, and the traction force on the optic disc and retina has been weakened or even resolved. Therefore, the possibility of occurrence of retinal detachment and macular cleavage is remote. Some people believe that the subretinal effusion is not only from the liquefied vitreous but also from the cerebrospinal fluid in the subarachnoid space and leakage of basal vessels in the pit.

Similar to the optic disc pit, morning glory syndrome is also a type of congenital dysplasia and can also be complicated by local serous retinal detachment (about 25%). Whether both of them have similar pathological mechanisms needs to be further investigated.

References

1. Türkçüoğlu P, Taskapan C. The origin of subretinal fluid in optic disc pit maculopathy. Ophthalmic Surg Lasers Imaging Retina. 2016;47(3):294–8.
2. Wang Y, Ren Q, Li L, et al. Two cases of congenital optic disc pit in one pedigree. Chin J Ocul Fundus Dis. 2006;22(6):421–2.
3. Wu Q, Zhang M, Zhang J. Characteristics of clinical and OCT scanning image of congenital optic disc pit with macular disease. Chin J Ocul Fundus Dis. 2015;31(4):385–7.

33 Melanocytoma of the Optic Disc

Xiaojing Pan, Ning Fan, and Xuyang Liu

Melanocytoma of the optic disc is a benign tumor originating from the optic disc, and it progresses slowly. If the tumor becomes larger, the visual acuity and visual field can be compromised. Attention should be paid to differentiating it from the malignant transformation of melanocytoma of the optic disc.

33.1 Case 1

33.1.1 Case Presentation

A 34-year-old female patient presented with fundus abnormalities observed during a physical examination. The patient had experienced no discomfort in either eye. She denied decreased vision, red and sore eyes, or persistent shadow in front of her eyes. Histories of other ocular diseases, systemic diseases, or familial diseases were denied.

X. Pan
Shandong Eye Institute, Qingdao Eye Hospital, Qingdao, China

N. Fan
Shenzhen Eye Hospital, Shenzhen University, Shenzhen, China

X. Liu (✉)
Xiamen Eye Center of Xiamen University, Xiamen, China

Shenzhen Eye Hospital, Shenzhen University, Shenzhen, China

In both eyes, the uncorrected visual acuity (UCVA) was 20/16, intraocular pressure (IOP) was normal, the refractive media was clear, and the pupils were of equal sizes (3 mm in diameter) and round with normal light reflex. A tumor in black color, mildly swelling, and with an unclear edge at the temporal optic disc was seen in the right eye, without bleeding and exudates (Fig. 33.1). There was no abnormality in the left eye.

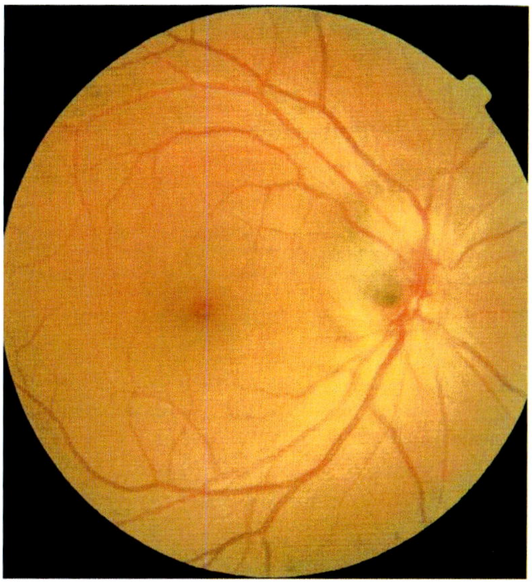

Fig. 33.1 Fundus photograph. A tumor in black color, mildly swelling, and with an unclear edge at the temporal optic disc was seen

N. Wang et al. (eds.), *Optic Disorders and Visual Field*, Advances in Visual Science and Eye Diseases 2, https://doi.org/10.1007/978-981-13-2502-1_33

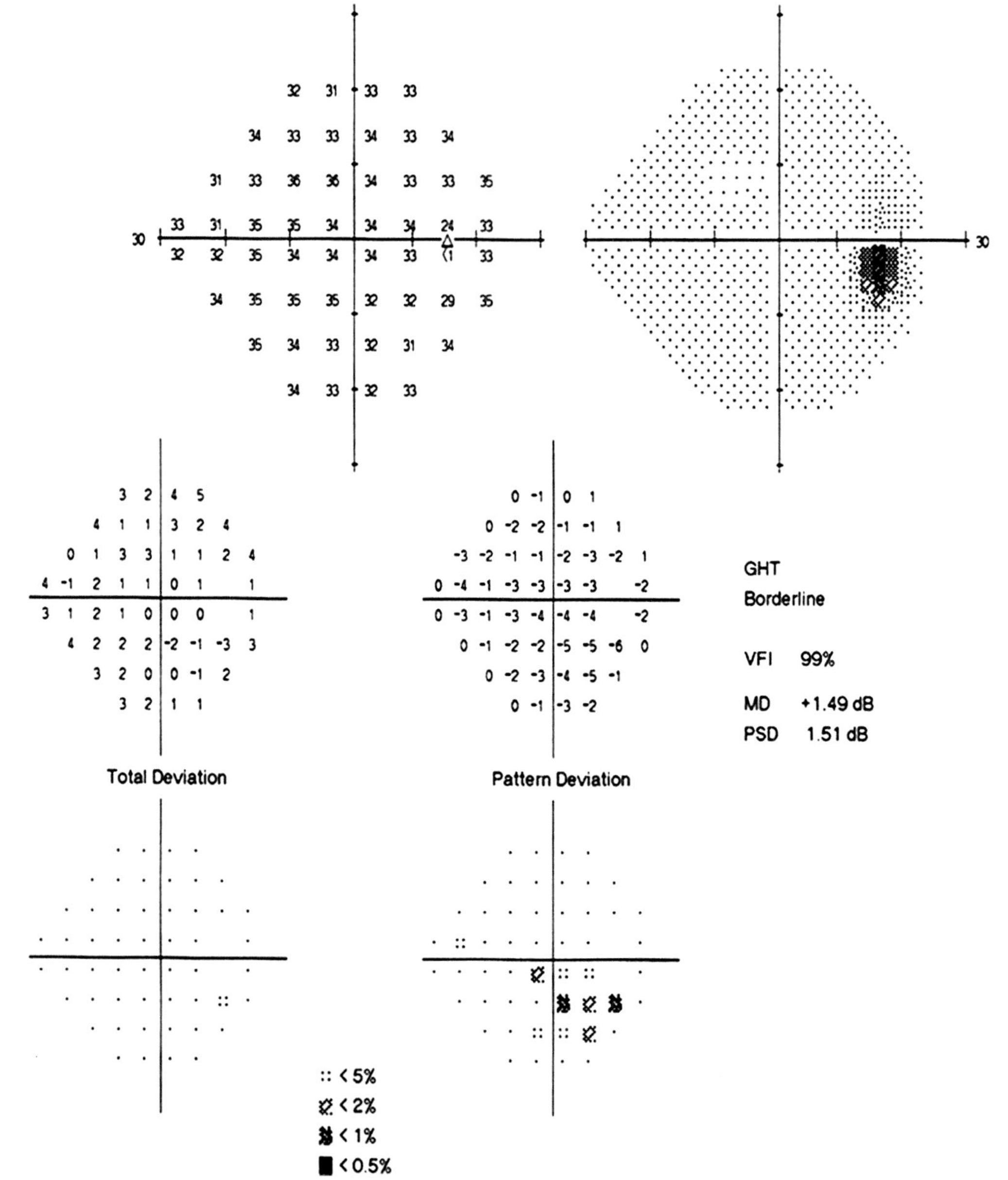

Fig. 33.2 Humphrey visual field analysis printout. An enlarged blind spot could be seen with the 24-2 test

Standardized automated perimetry with the 24-2 strategy showed an enlarged blind spot in the right eye (Fig. 33.2).

B-Mode ultrasonography showed a solid hyperechogenic spot on the optic disc surface of the right eye (Fig. 33.3).

The FFA examination showed weak fluorescence (melanin blocked the fluorescence) in the lesion at the early phase and no fluorescein leakage at the late phase (Fig. 33.4).

OCT revealed a high reflection signal lesion with local elevation in the optic disc, followed by a nonreflective black shadow (Fig. 33.5).

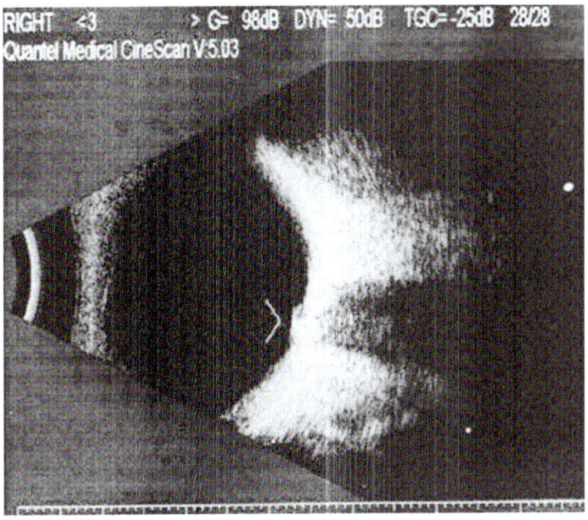

Fig. 33.3 B-ultrasound image. The B-Mode ultrasonography of the right eye showed a solid hyperechogenic spot on the optic disc surface

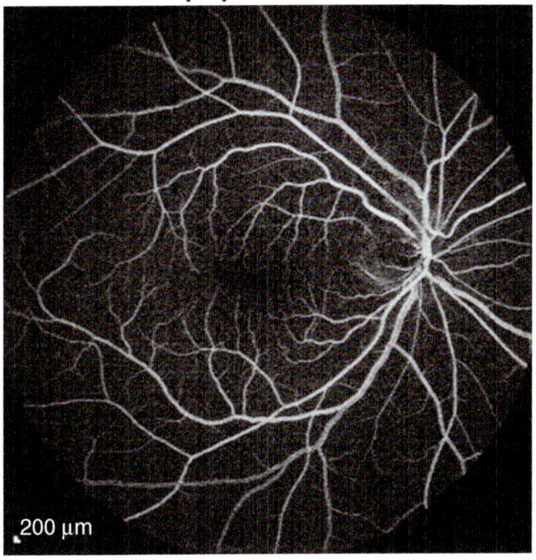

Fig. 33.4 FFA image. Weak fluorescence (melanin blocked the fluorescence) in the lesion could be seen at the early stage

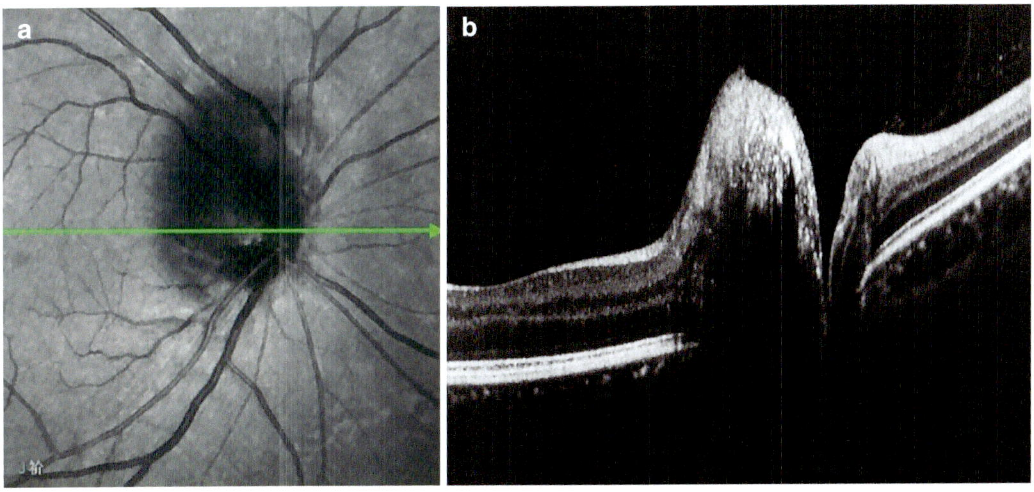

Fig. 33.5 OCT scanning of optic disc. The image showed a high reflection signal lesion with local elevation in the optic disc, followed by a nonreflective black shadow. Panel a: scan site. Panel b: OCT image

33.1.2 Final Diagnosis

The final diagnosis was melanocytoma of the optic disc of the right eye.

33.1.3 Case Review

The patient had melanoma in the optic disc of the right eye which had been asymptomatic for a long time and detected during a physical examination by accident. The boundary of the optic disc was unclear. A tumor in black color and mildly swelling could be seen. An enlarged blind spot was found, which could result from the following two reasons: either the tumor tissue infiltrated the retinal nerve fiber layer (RNFL) or the tumor tissue blocked the RNFL. The patient's visual acuity was 1.2, and the clinical recommendation was close monitoring.

When the melanocytoma compresses the tissue around the optic disc and results in retinal nerve fiber loss, edema or vascular occlusion, acute decrease of vision, and damage to the visual field would occur. Now let's take the patient in Case 2 as an example.

33.2 Case 2

33.2.1 Case Presentation

A 46-year-old male patient complained that his vision of the left eye had blurred 2 weeks before. He had no dysmorphopsia and denied the histories of other ocular diseases, trauma, or familial diseases.

In both eyes, the uncorrected visual acuities (UCVA) were 20/20 and IOP was normal. Slit-lamp examination of the anterior segment was unremarkable, and the vitreous was clear in each eye. The fundus examination of the left eye revealed that the superior margin of the optic disc was not clear with a red semi-translucent lump, and there was a superior RNFL defect (Fig. 33.6). No abnormality was found in the right eye.

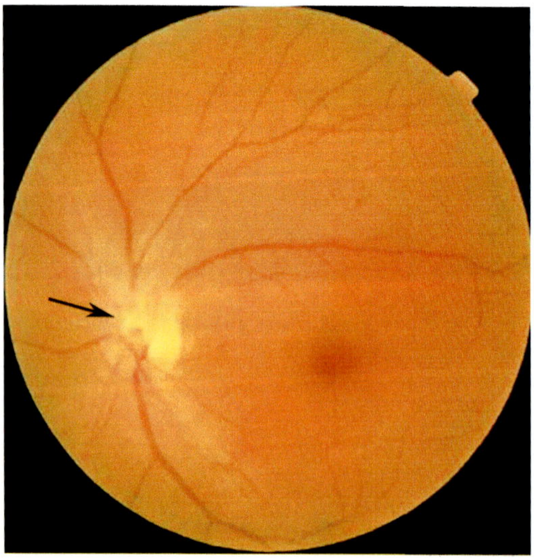

Fig. 33.6 Fundus photograph. The fundus examination of the left eye revealed that the superior optic disc had an unclear boundary, a mass was elevated slightly (black arrow), and there was a bundle defect in the superior RNFL

Standardized automated perimetry showed an inferior arcuate scotoma that extended from the physiological blind spot in the left eye (Fig. 33.7).

FFA showed weak fluorescence (tumor tissue blocked fluorescence) in the lesion at the early phase and enhanced fluorescence in the lesion at the late phase (Fig. 33.8).

OCT revealed a high reflection signal lesion with local elevation in the optic disc, followed by a nonreflective black shadow (Fig. 33.9).

33.2.2 Final Diagnosis

The final diagnosis was melanocytoma of the left optic disc.

33.2.3 Case Review

In this case, there was an arcuate scotoma extending from the blind point in the inferior visual field of the left eye, which resulted from the superior RNFL defect. The defect was caused by the expansion and erosion of tumor tissue toward the superior optic disc and superior retinal nerve fibers.

33.3 Discussion

Melanocytoma of the optic disc is a type of benign tumor, and it grows slowly, which is a variant form of nevi and originates from melanocytes in the uveal matrix. It may occur at any age, mostly in the optic disc and ciliary body. This disease is characterized as a rare, benign, unilateral, and slowly growing condition with little impact on visual acuity [1].

As the tumor enlarges slowly, the retinal nerve fibers and blood vessels around the optic disc are compressed, or blood supply is compromised by tissue necrosis within the tumor. Optic disc edema, retinal vessel occlusion, ischemic optic neuropathy, neovascular glaucoma, and other complications may occur, resulting in acute deterioration in visual acuity and damage to the visual field [2].

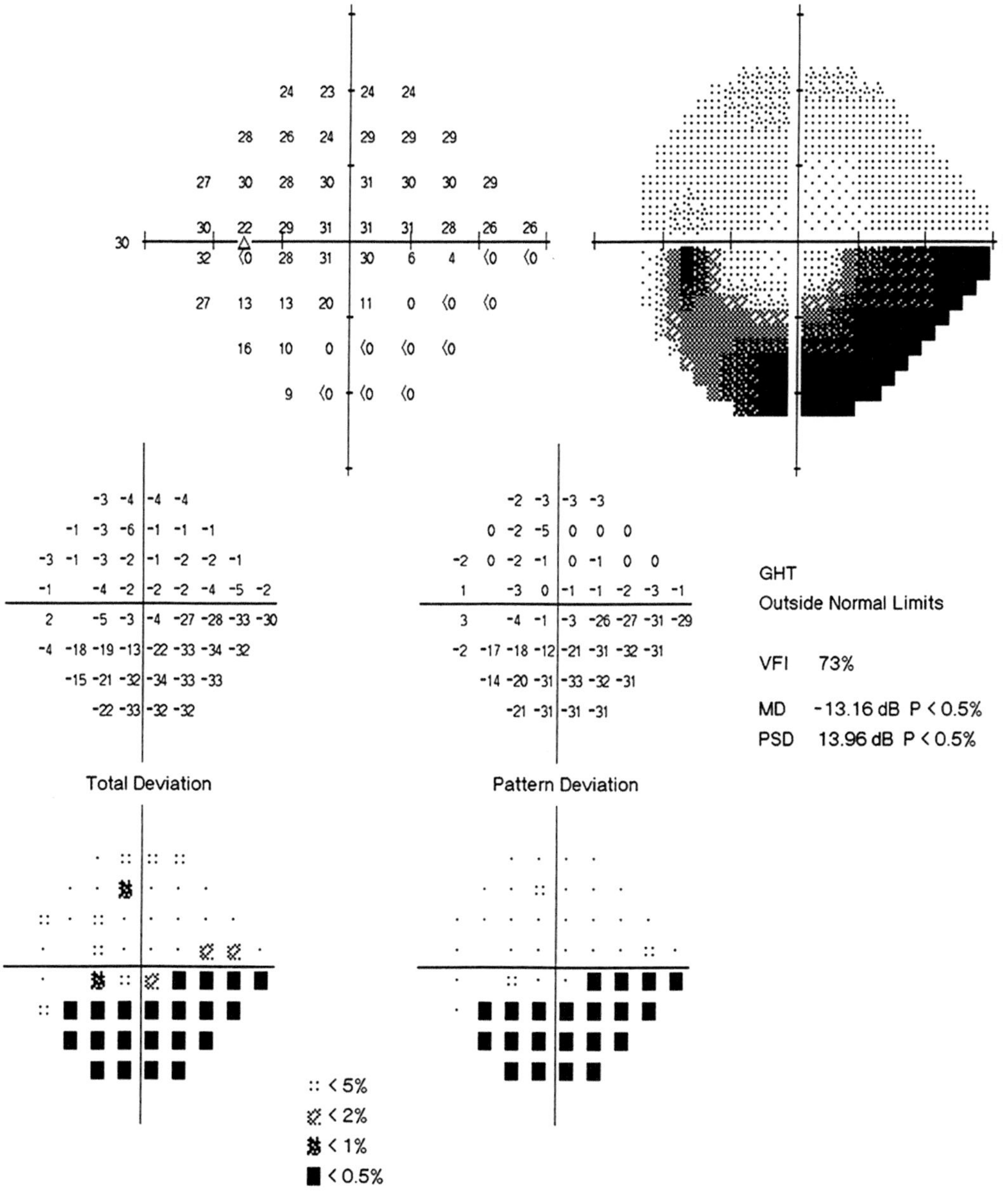

Fig. 33.7 Humphrey visual field analysis printout. The 24-2 test showed an inferior arcuate scotoma extending from the blind spot

The change of the visual field is related to the location and severity of the lesion. If the lesion develops beyond the margin of the optic disc, it can be characterized by an enlarged physiological blind spot. Subsequently, the tumor will compress the central retinal artery or infiltrate nerve fibers, and significant visual field damage will occur. The mechanism of visual field defects varies with the sizes and stages of the tumors. A small tumor at the early stage will cause changes to the visual field mainly due to the migration of pigment cells along retinal

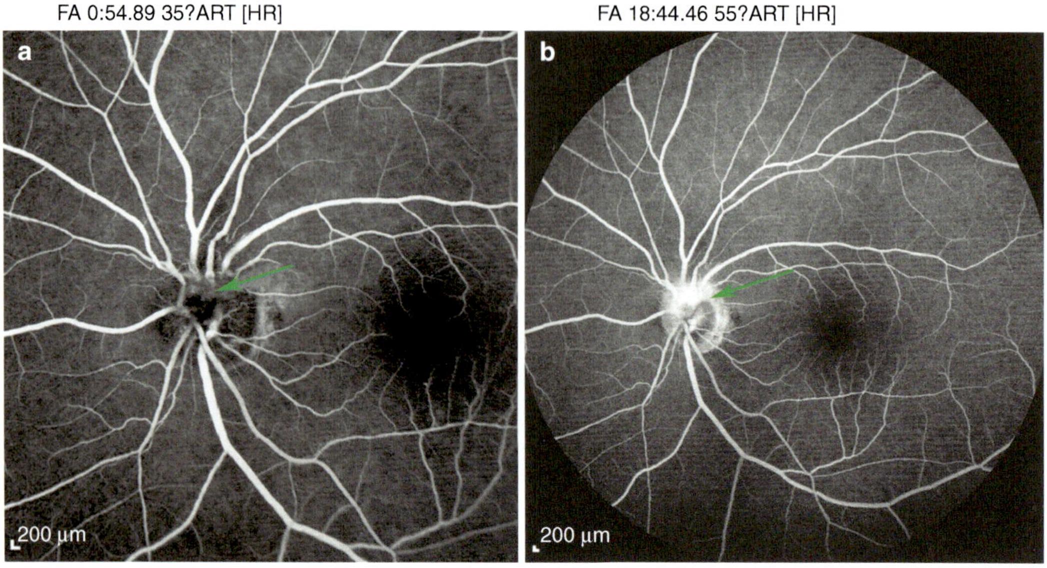

Fig. 33.8 FFA images of both eyes. Panel a: weak fluorescence (green arrow) in the lesion at the early phase. Panel b: enhanced fluorescence in the lesion at the late phase (green arrow)

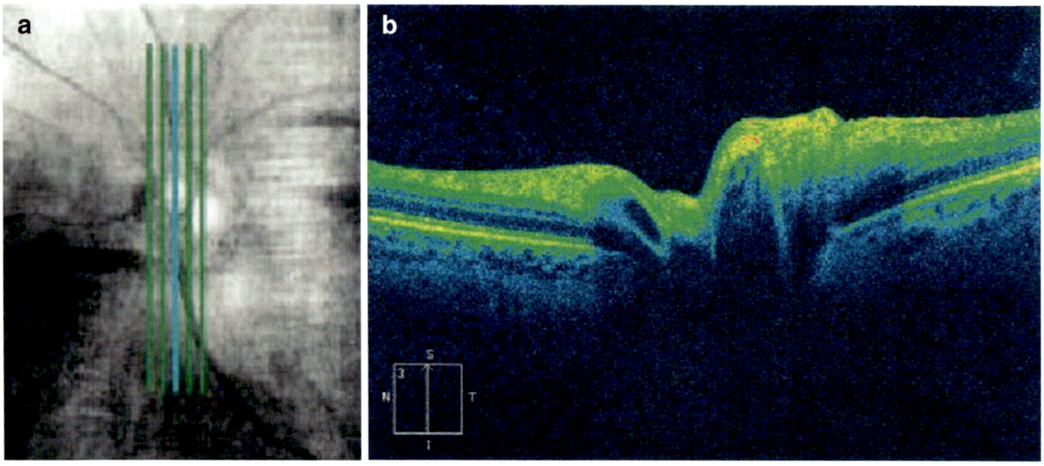

Fig. 33.9 OCT scan. The image showed a high reflection signal lesion with local elevation in the optic disc, followed by a nonreflective black shadow. Panel a: scan site. Panel b: OCT image

nerve fibers. A larger tumor at the middle and late stages will cause damage to the visual field due to the compression from the tumor.

In addition, melanocytoma of the optic disc needs to be followed up regularly. If the tumor is undergoing or accompanied by the following changes, such as enlargement to a certain volume, gradual color darkening, presence of satellite foci, significant vascularization in the tumor, bleeding, and significant deterioration of vision acuity and visual field, close monitoring should be carried out to determine whether it is malignant transformation of melanoma of the optic disc or not, which can be confirmed by needle biopsy.

References

1. Liu Q, Fang Y. Optic disc diseases. Beijing: People's Medical Publishing House; 2015.
2. Satya K. A therapy map of neuro-ophthalmology (Translated by Zhao Jialiang). Beijing: Beijing Science and Technology Press; 2011.

34 The Visual Field Defects of Leber's Disease

Xiaojing Pan, Ning Fan, and Xuyang Liu

Leber's hereditary optic neuropathy (LHON) is a maternal genetic disorder caused by point mutations of mitochondrial DNA (mtDNA). Visual field damage in LHON is mostly central defects of various sizes and shapes. In this section, several selected cases of the mutation of the same mtDNA are analyzed, and the pathogenesis of LHON is discussed at the molecular level.

34.1 Case 1

34.1.1 Case Presentation

A 16-year-old male patient complained of acute visual acuity decrease in both eyes for more than 20 days. He had mild pain on eye movement in both eyes but no eye redness and other discomforts. Histories of other ocular diseases, trauma, or systemic diseases were denied.

X. Pan
Shandong Eye Institute, Qingdao Eye Hospital, Qingdao, China

N. Fan
Shenzhen Eye Hospital, Shenzhen University, Shenzhen, China

X. Liu (✉)
Xiamen Eye Center of Xiamen University, Xiamen, China

Shenzhen Eye Hospital, Shenzhen University, Shenzhen, China

The uncorrected visual acuity (UCVA) was 20/400 OD (−1.00DS) and 20/665 OS, while best corrected visual acuity (BCVA) was 20/200 OD and no improvement OS. In both eyes, intraocular pressure (IOP) was normal, the refractive media was clear, the pupils were of equal sizes (3 mm in diameter) and round, and the direct light reflex was slightly slow. Fundus examination revealed slightly swollen optic discs with slight pallor at the temporal side (Fig. 34.1).

With a Humphrey perimeter, right superior homonymous quadrantanopia was shown (Fig. 34.2).

34.1.2 Case Analysis

The patient had right superior homonymous quadrantanopia. It is a classic visual field change with visual pathway damage, corresponding to the lesions around the left anterior temporal lobe and anterior horn of the lateral ventricle. The changes in the visual field are caused by the involvement of ventrally located fibers at the initial part of optic radiation (including the retinal nerve fibers from the inferonasal side in the right eye and the inferotemporal side in the left eye). The patient was a 16-year-old boy. He denied any history of trauma and had no discomfort. Therefore, we considered lesions of the visual pathway (left anterior temporal lobe lesions) first. The common causes, including arteriovenous

N. Wang et al. (eds.), *Optic Disorders and Visual Field*, Advances in Visual Science and Eye Diseases 2, https://doi.org/10.1007/978-981-13-2502-1_34

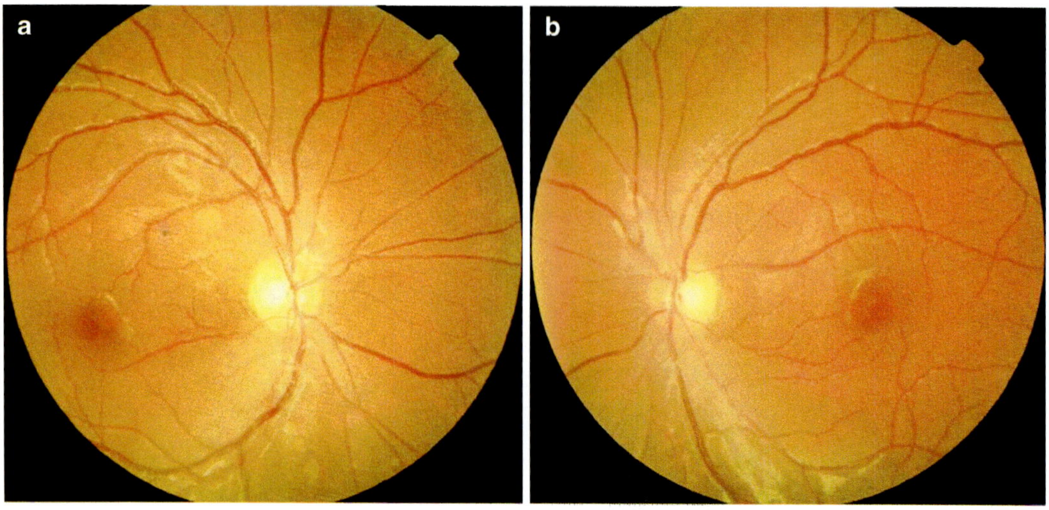

Fig. 34.1 Fundus photographs. Fundus examination revealed slightly swollen optic discs with slightly pale color at the temporal side. Panel a: right eye. Panel b: left eye

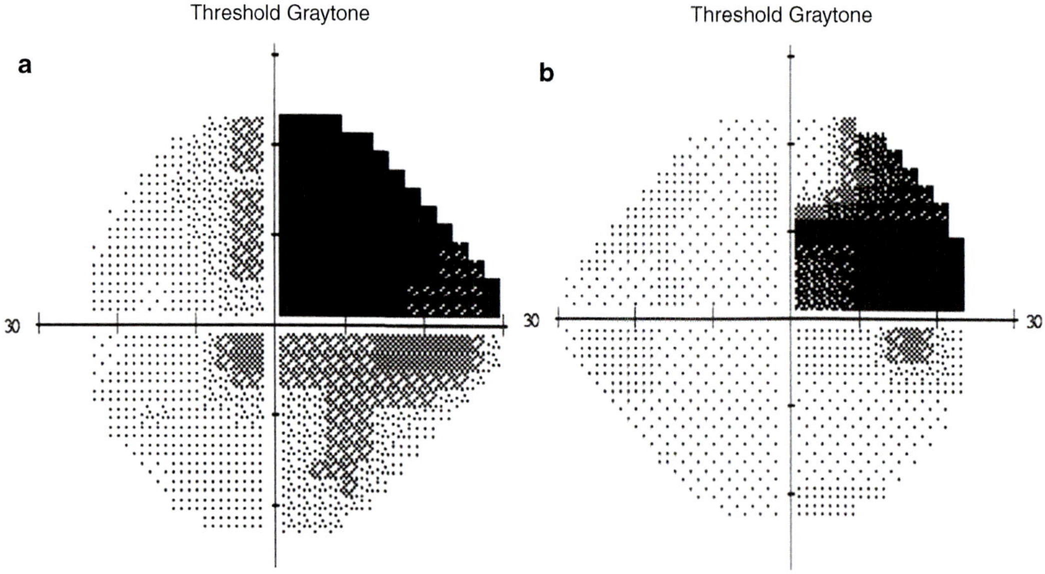

Fig. 34.2 The grayscale maps of Humphrey visual field assessment. The 24-2 test with a size V white visual target showed right superior homonymous quadrantanopia. Panel a: left eye. Panel b: right eye

malformations, trauma, or tumor, needed to be confirmed by cranial CT or MRI examination. However, after a series of consultations and imaging examinations in neurology and neurosurgery departments, the lesions of the visual pathway above the optic chiasma were ruled out. No demyelinating lesions of the nervous system including the optic nerve were found. After ruling out the lesions of the visual pathway at or above the optic chiasma, we had to reconsider the diagnosis and focus on the retina and optic nerve again.

FFA showed the fluorescence at the neuroretinal rim was slightly enhanced at the late phase in both eyes. No fluorescence leakage and no abnormal fluorescence in the macula were found (Fig. 34.3).

Fundus photography and FFA excluded retinopathy corresponding to the visual field defects

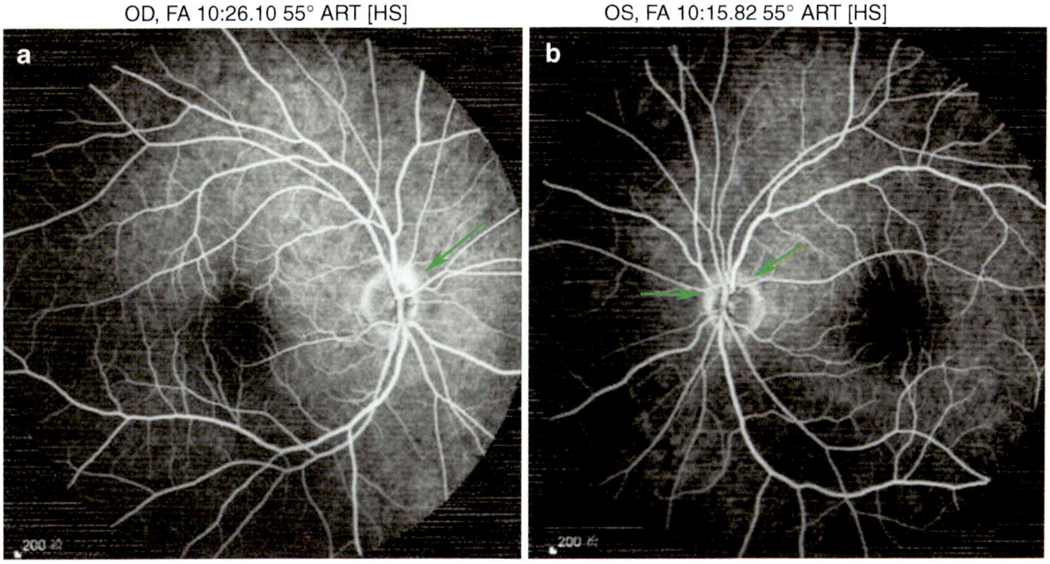

Fig. 34.3 The late-phase FFA images. The green arrow indicated local fluorescence enhancement of the optic disc. Panel a: right eye. Panel b: left eye

in the patient, but his direct light reflex of both pupils was slightly slow. While we focused on retrobulbar optic neuritis, posterior ischemic optic neuropathy, or even traumatic optic neuropathy and other considerations, one part of his family medical history was brought to our attention, i.e., one of his brothers who lived in another place also had poor eyesight. Is the disease familial? Did the Leber's hereditary optic neuropathy present as a typical visual field change due to lesions of the posterior visual pathway?

By mtDNA sequencing analysis on the peripheral blood of the patient, a nucleotide mutation that changed guanine nucleotide (G) into adenine nucleotide (A) was found at position 11778 (Fig. 34.4).

By mtDNA sequencing analysis of the patient's brother, nucleotide mutation was also found at position 11778. Visual field examination showed a central defect in both eyes of the brother (Fig. 34.5), consistent with the visual field changes in Leber's hereditary optic neuropathy. See Fig. 34.6 for the pedigree chart.

34.1.3 Final Diagnosis

The final diagnosis was Leber's hereditary optic neuropathy in both eyes.

The following cases of Leber's hereditary optic neuropathy are also associated with mtDNA G11778A, but the changes in the visual field are different.

34.2 Case 2

34.2.1 Case Presentation

A 14-year-old male patient complained of acute decrease in visual acuity for 1 year. He denied eye redness, eye pain, pain on eye movement, and other discomforts. Histories of ocular diseases, trauma, and systemic diseases were denied.

On examination, the UCVA was 20/200 OU with no improvement after refraction. IOP was normal OU. In both eyes, the refractive media was clear, the pupils were of equal sizes (3 mm in diameter) and round, and direct light reflex was slightly slow. Fundus examination showed that the optic disc had a clear boundary and was in pale color at the temporal neuroretinal rim in both eyes (Fig. 34.7).

Humphrey visual field testing showed a large central defect in the superior region of both eyes (Fig. 34.8).

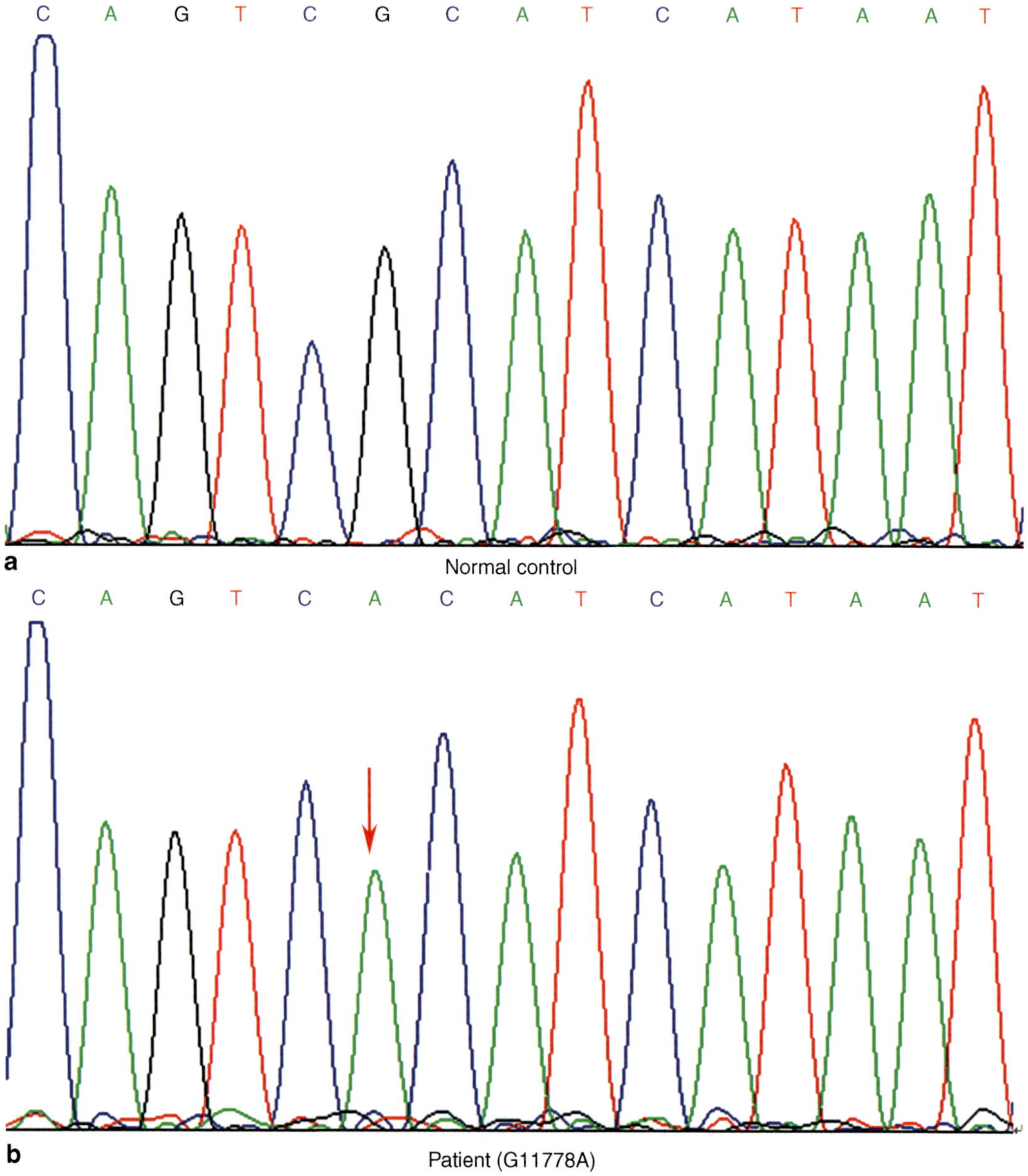

Fig. 34.4 mtDNA 11778 sequencing results. Panel a: mtDNA 11778 sequencing result of a normal control (arrow). Panel b: mutation at mtDNA G11778A in the patient (arrow)

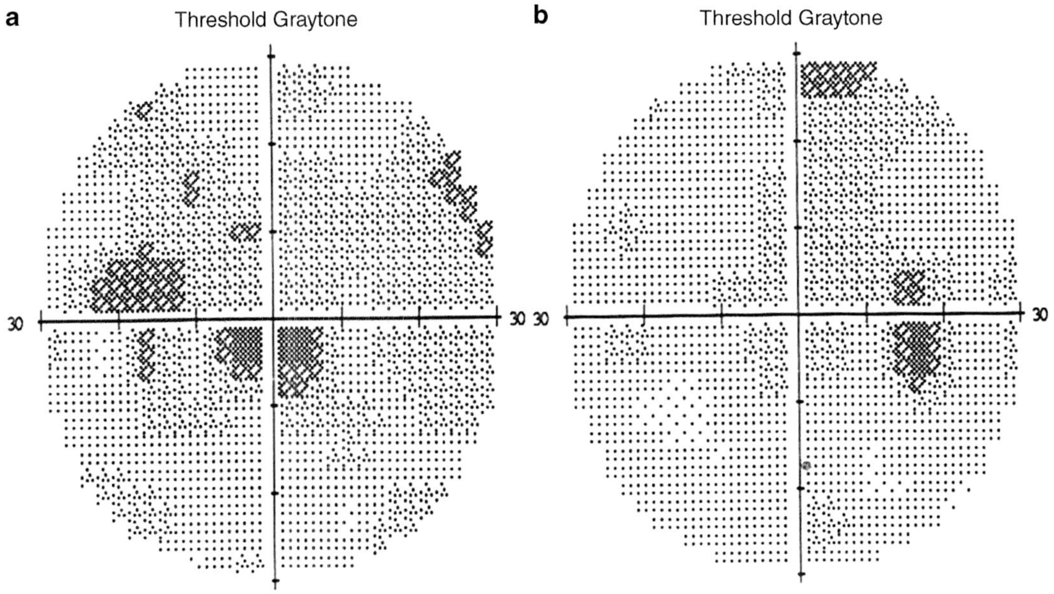

Fig. 34.5 The grayscale maps of Humphrey visual field assessment for the patient's brother. The 30-2 test showed a central defect in both eyes. Panel a: left eye. Panel b: right eye

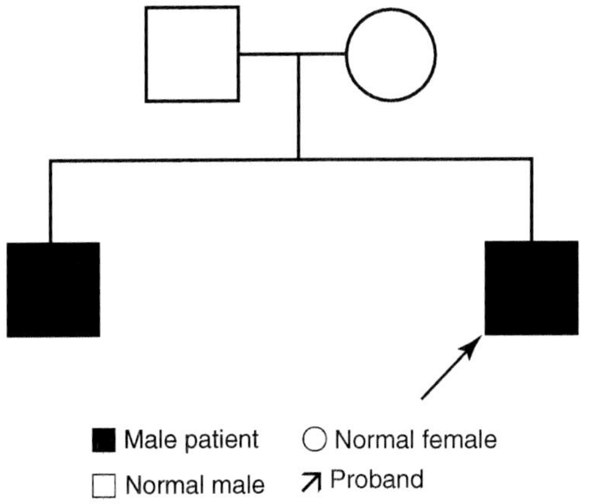

Fig. 34.6 Pedigree chart of Leber's hereditary optic neuropathy

By mtDNA sequencing analysis on the peripheral blood of the patient, a nucleotide mutation that changed guanine nucleotide (G) into adenine nucleotide (A) was found at position 11778.

34.2.2 Final Diagnosis

The final diagnosis was Leber's hereditary optic neuropathy in both eyes.

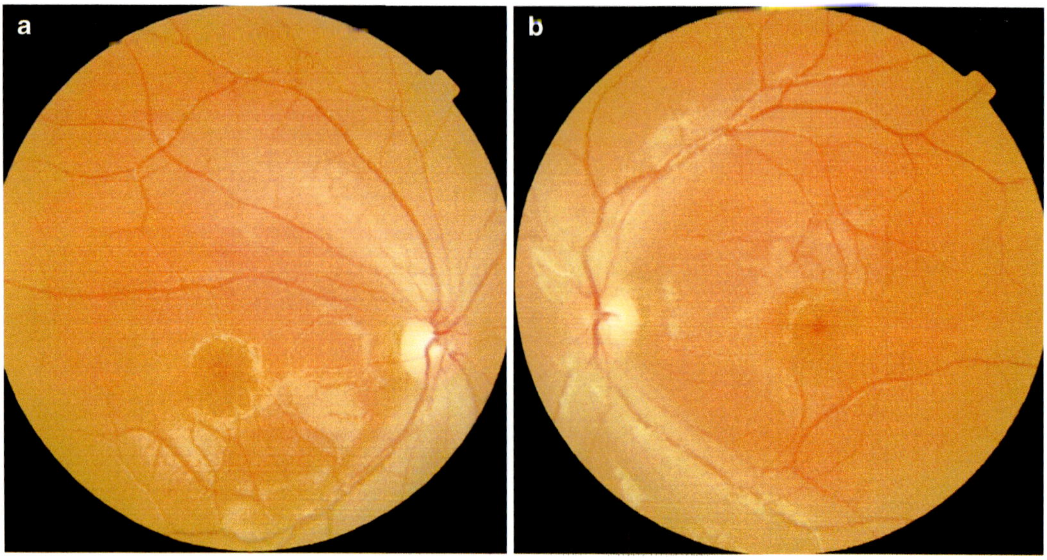

Fig. 34.7 Fundus photographs. The optic discs were with a clear boundary and in pale color at the temporal neuroretinal rim. Panel a: right eye. Panel b: left eye

34.3 Case 3

\

34.3.1 Case Presentation

A 9-year-old male patient complained of decreased visual acuity in both eyes for half a year. He denied any eye redness, eye pain, or other discomforts. There was no history of other ocular diseases, trauma, or systemic diseases.

On examination, the UCVA was 20/100 OD and 20/200 OS, with no improvement achieved with refraction. In both eyes, the IOP was normal, the refractive media was clear, the pupils were of equal sizes (3 mm in diameter) and round, and direct light reflex was slightly slow. Fundus examination showed an optic disc with a clear boundary and pale color in both eyes (Fig. 34.9).

Humphrey visual field testing showed an irregular and giant central defect in both eyes (Fig. 34.10).

By mtDNA sequencing analysis on the peripheral blood of the patient, a nucleotide mutation that changed guanine nucleotide (G) into adenine nucleotide (A) was found at position 11778.

34.3.2 Final Diagnosis

The final diagnosis was Leber's hereditary optic neuropathy in both eyes.

34.4 Case 4

34.4.1 Case Presentation

A 24-year-old male patient complained of acute decrease in visual acuity in the left eye for 2 months. He denied any eye redness, eye

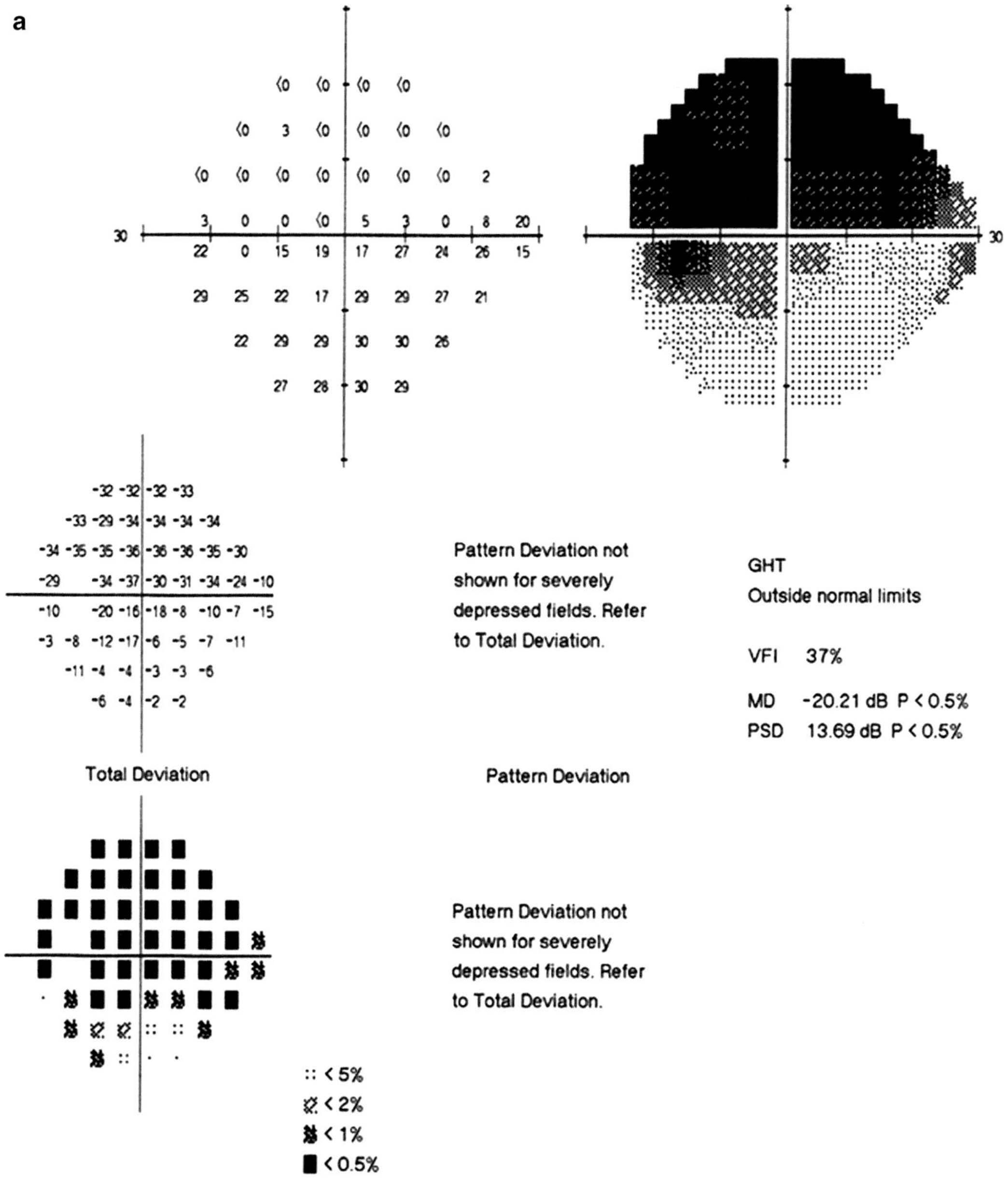

Fig. 34.8 Humphrey visual field analysis printouts. The 24-2 test showed a giant central defect in the superior region of both eyes. Panel a: left eye. Panel b: right eye

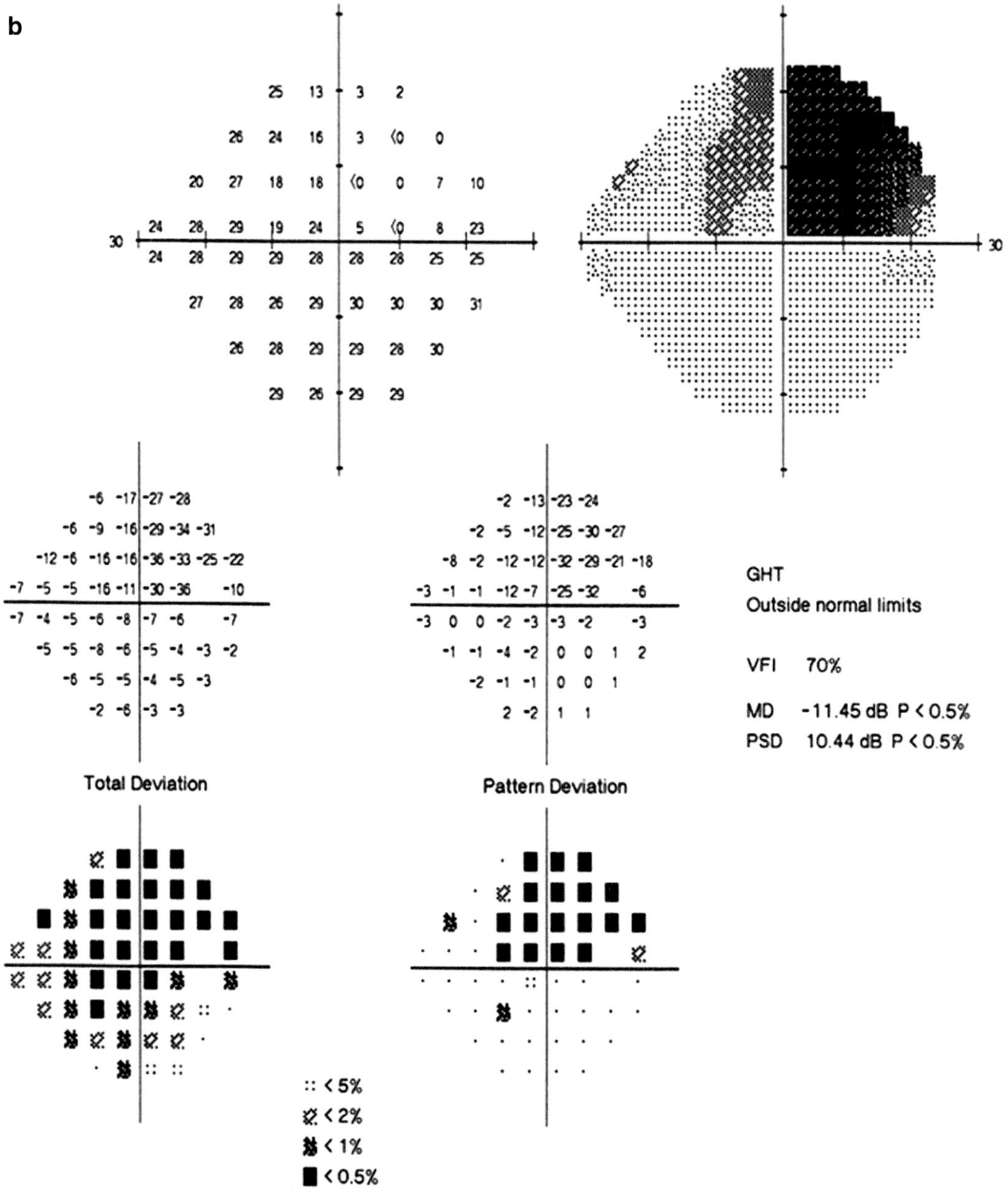

Fig. 34.8 (continued)

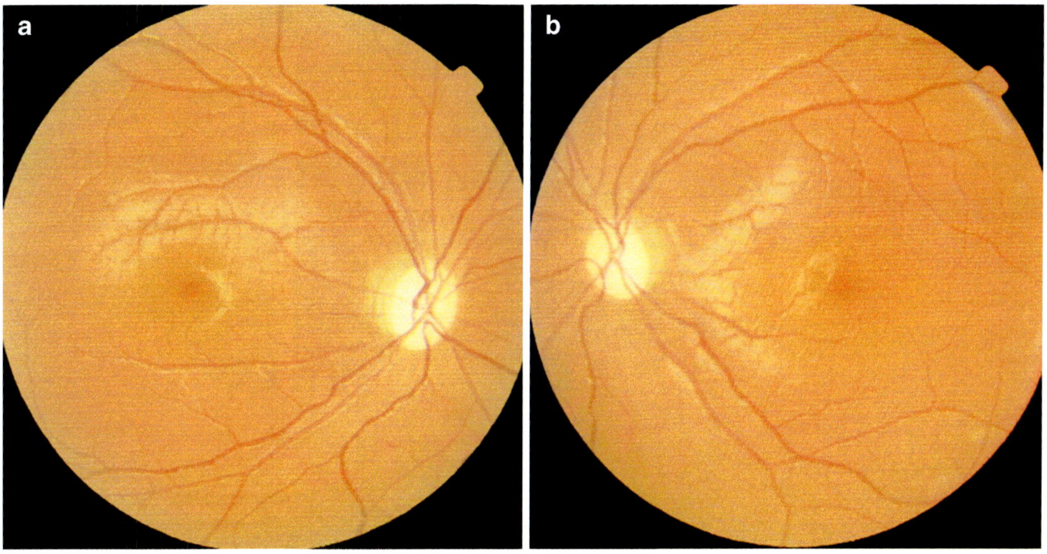

Fig. 34.9 Fundus photographs. In both of these photographs, we could see an optic disc with a clear boundary and pale color. Panel a: right eye. Panel b: left eye

pain, or other discomforts. There was no history of prior ocular diseases, trauma, and systemic diseases.

The UCVA was 20/20 OD and 20/200 OS (no improvement with refraction). In both eyes, IOP was normal, and the refractive media was clear. The pupils were of equal size (3 mm in diameter) and round. The relative afferent pupillary defect (RAPD) was positive in the left eye. Fundus examination revealed that the optic disc was hyperemic due to congestion, the boundary was clear, and the retinal veins were slightly tortuous and dilated in both eyes (Fig. 34.11).

Humphrey visual field testing showed an irregular central defect in the upper region of both eyes (Fig. 34.11).

By mtDNA sequencing analysis on the peripheral blood of the patient, a nucleotide mutation that changed guanine nucleotide (G) into adenine nucleotide (A) was found at position 11778.

34.4.2 Final Diagnosis

The final diagnosis was Leber's hereditary optic neuropathy in both eyes.

34.5 Case 5

34.5.1 Case Presentation

A 26-year-old male patient complained of decrease in the visual acuity of both eyes for half a year. He denied eye redness, sore eyes, headache, pain on eye movement, or other discomforts.

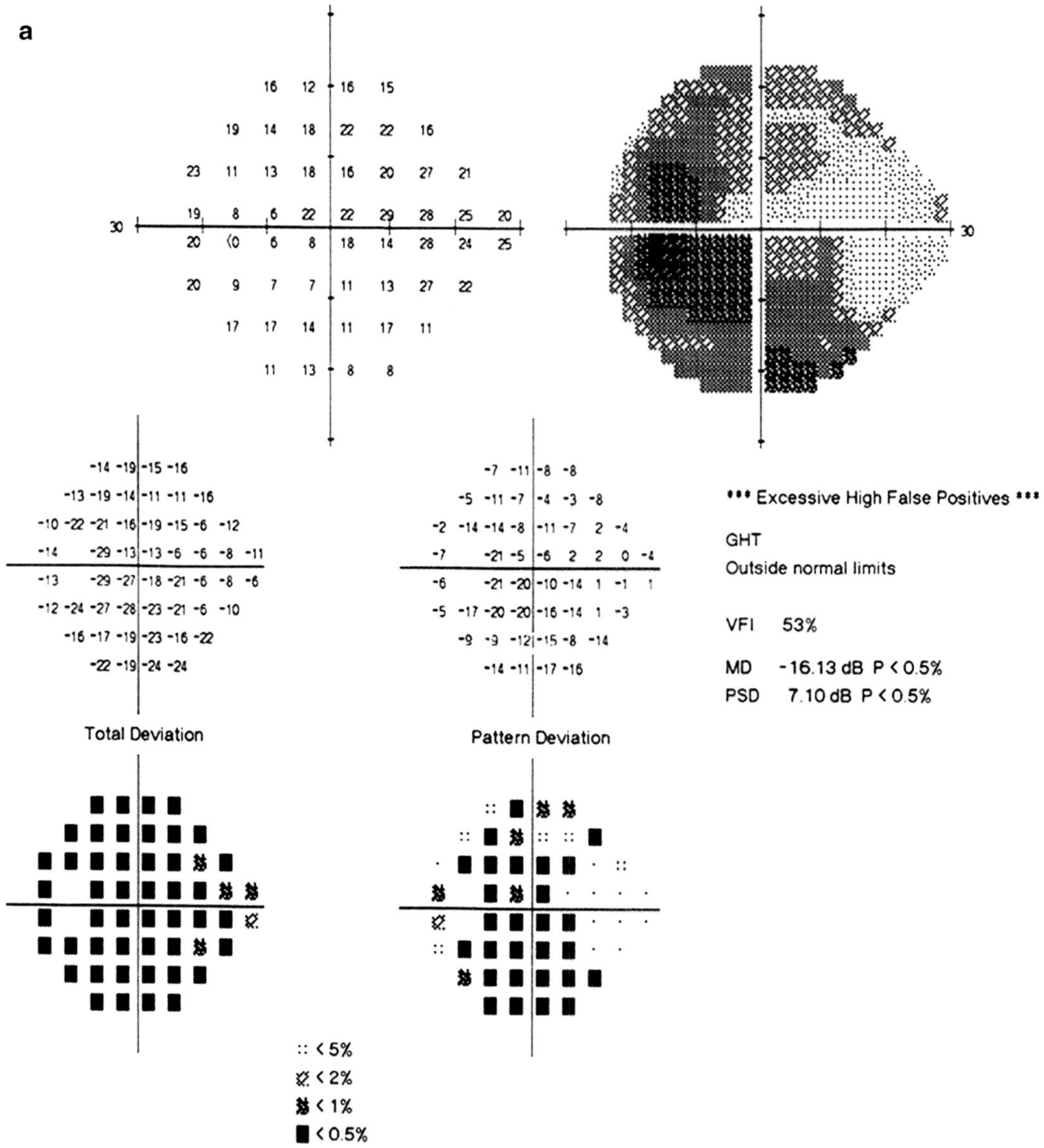

Fig. 34.10 Humphrey visual field analysis printouts. There was an irregular and giant central defect in each eye (24-2 test). Panel a: left eye. Panel b: right eye

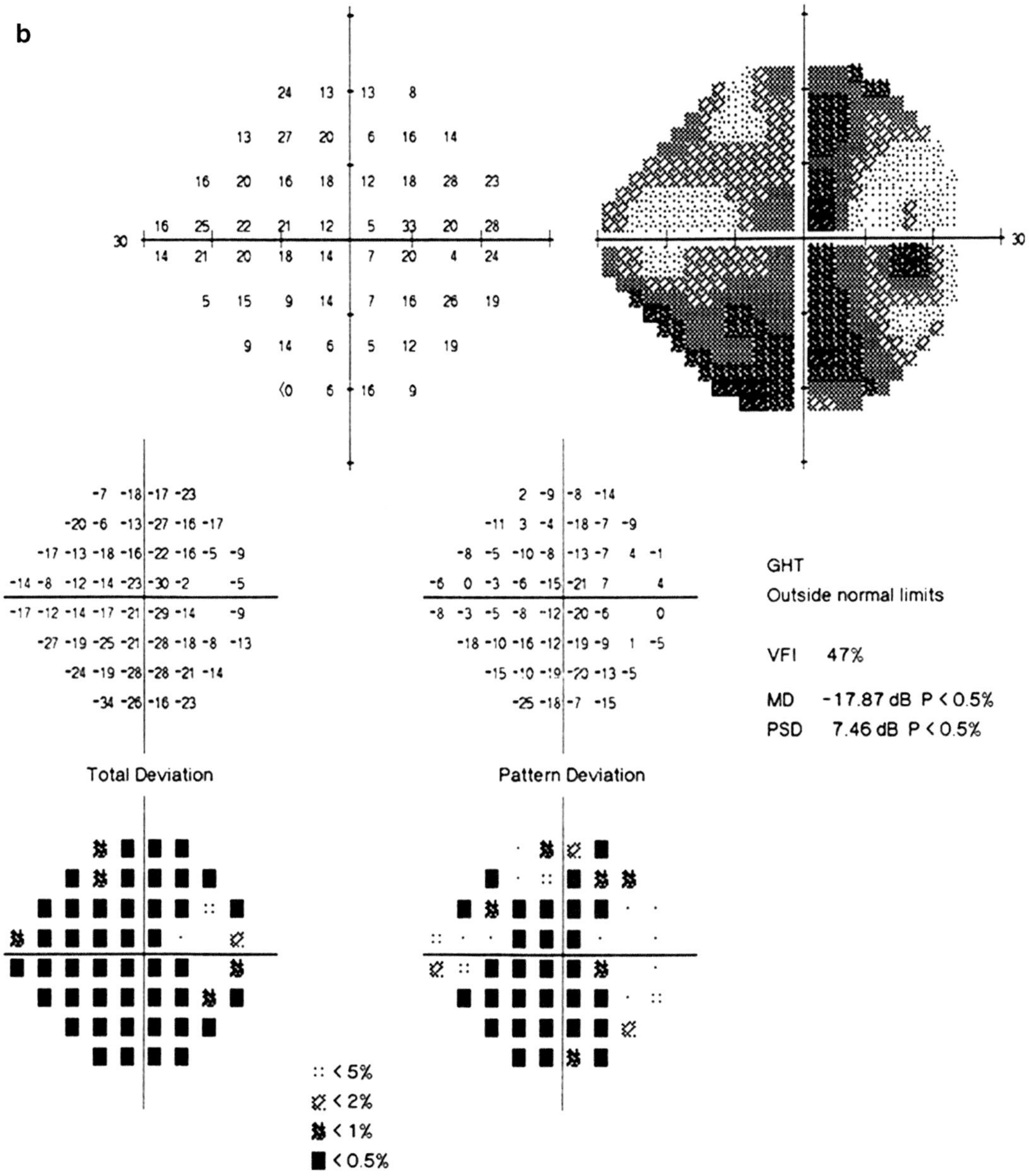

Fig. 34.10 (continued)

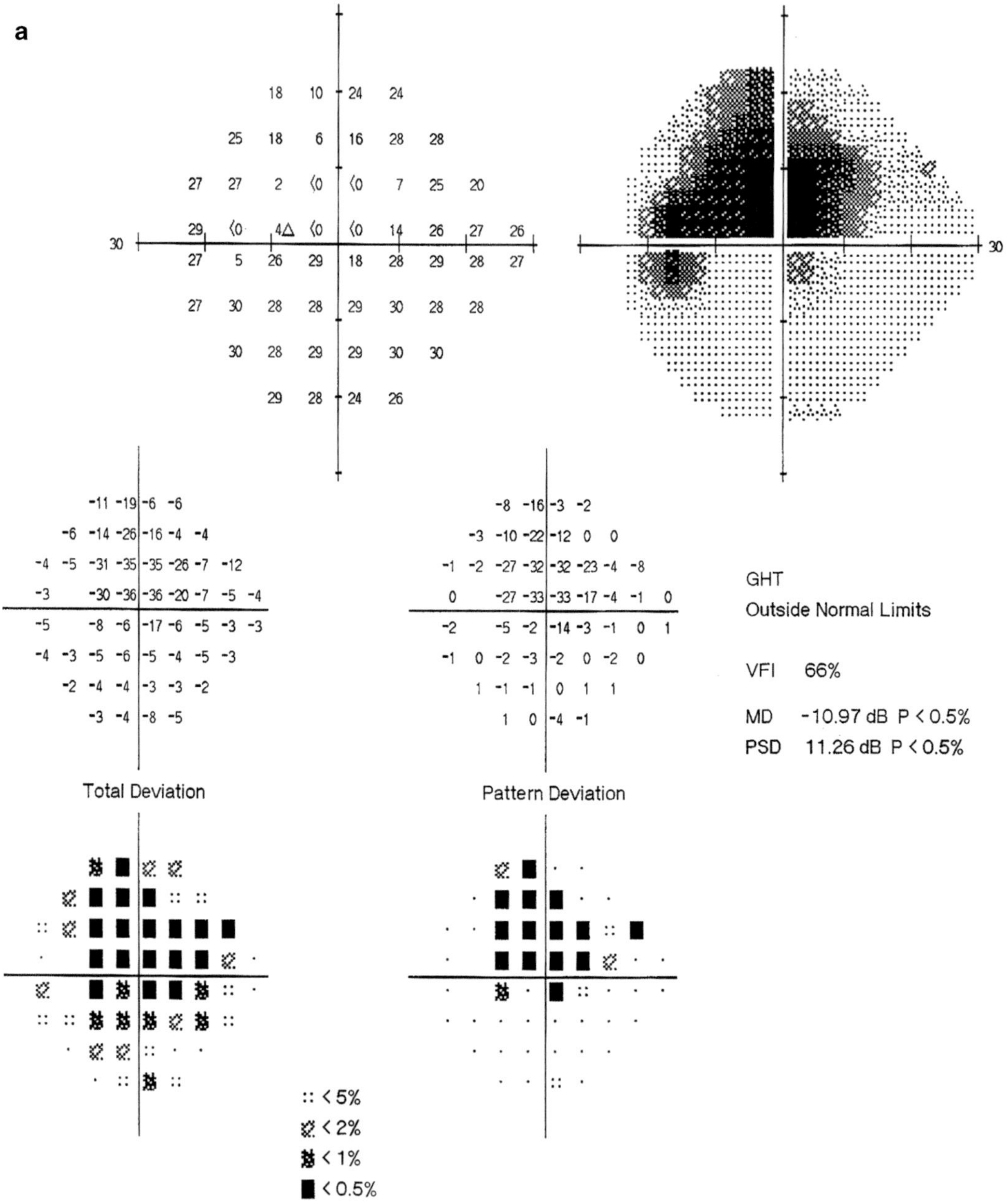

Fig. 34.11 Humphrey visual field analysis printouts. There was an irregular central defect in the superior region of both eyes. Panel a: left eye. Panel b: right eye

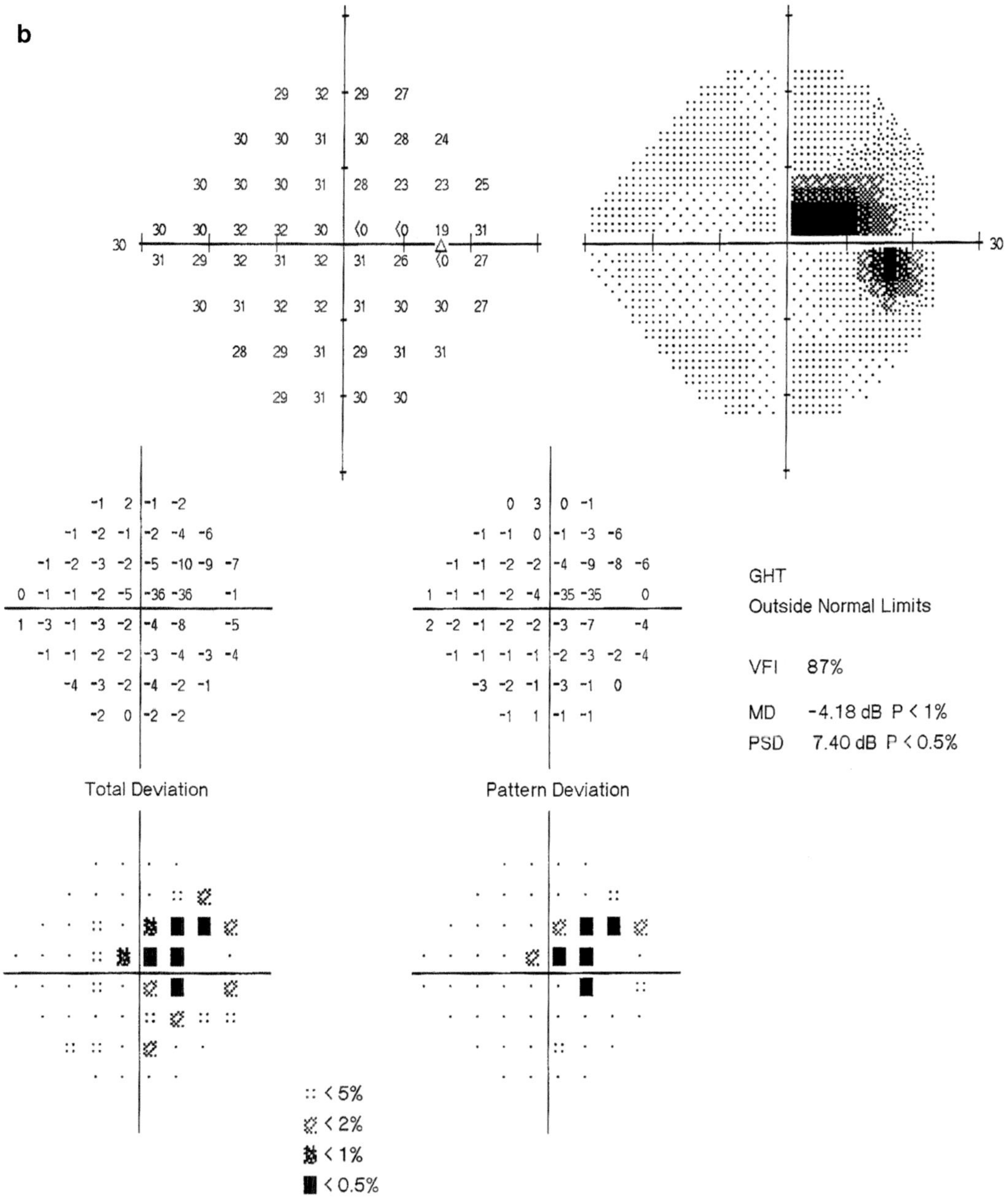

Fig. 34.11 (continued)

There had been no improvement in visual acuity with treatment in other hospitals. The histories of trauma, previous ocular diseases, and systemic diseases were denied. His maternal uncle had a similar medical history.

The BCVA had no improvement with refraction (20/28 OD and 20/25 OS). In both eyes, IOP was normal, slit-lamp examination of anterior segment was unremarkable, the pupil size was 3mm in diameter, and light reflex was sensitive. Fundus examination showed that the optic disc was slightly pale in color (particularly significant at the temporal rim) with a clear boundary, and the cup-to-disc (C/D) ratio was 0.8 in both eyes. The reflection of the inferior and temporal retinal nerve fibers was reduced in both eyes (Fig. 34.12).

Standardized automated perimetry showed a giant central defect extending from the blind spot in both eyes with the most severe damage in the superior region (Fig. 34.13).

OCT showed diffuse RNFL thinning in both eyes, which was more severe in the inferior and temporal quadrants (Fig. 34.14).

By mtDNA sequencing analysis on the peripheral blood of the patient, a nucleotide mutation that changed guanine nucleotide (G) into adenine nucleotide (A) was found at position 11778.

34.5.2 Final Diagnosis

The final diagnosis was Leber's hereditary optic neuropathy in both eyes.

34.6 Discussion

Leber's hereditary optic neuropathy is a maternal genetic disorder that was associated with mitochondrial DNA point mutations. Clinically, Leber's disease is characterized by painless, acute, or subacute loss of central vision simultaneously or sequentially in both eyes. The visual field usually presents a central defect in both eyes (e.g., Cases 2 and 3). At the early stage of the disease, the fundus exhibits dilated microangiopathy of capillaries around the optic disc, mild optic disc edema (pseudoedema), and no fluorescein leakage in the optic disc during FFA. At the late stage (6 months later), there is optic atrophy, mostly atrophy of the papillomacular bundle and temporal pale color of the optic disc. According to the histopathological observation, axon degeneration, a slight increase of astrocytes and fibroblasts counts, a reduction of optic nerve diameter, central axonal loss, and mild inflammatory changes were seen during the course of LHON.

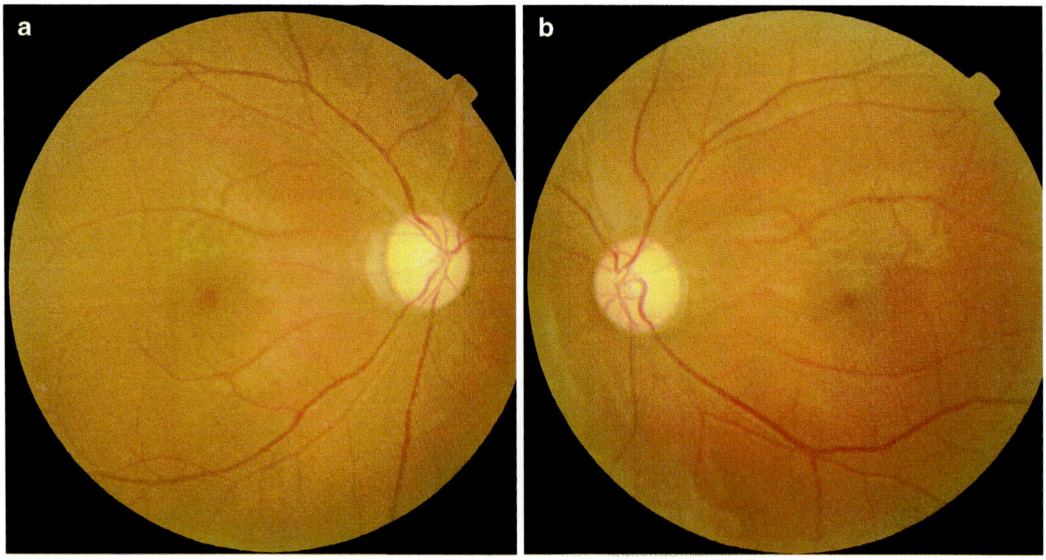

Fig. 34.12 Fundus photographs. In both eyes, the optic disc was pale in color (particularly obvious at the temporal rim) with a clear boundary, and the C/D ratio was 0.8. Panel a: right eye. Panel b: left eye

The features of mitochondrial DNA include semi-autonomy, maternal inheritance, threshold effect, and high mutation rates. Primary mtDNA mutation is a necessary condition rather than a sufficient condition for the occurrence of LHON. All maternal family members of a LHON patient carry the same mtDNA mutation, but most of them are asymptomatic carriers. The disease in 50% of the male mutation carriers and 10% of the female carriers will progress into optic neuropathy. LHON has obvious incomplete penetrance and gender bias, indicating that its development may be the result of synergistic effects of primary mutation with other factors.

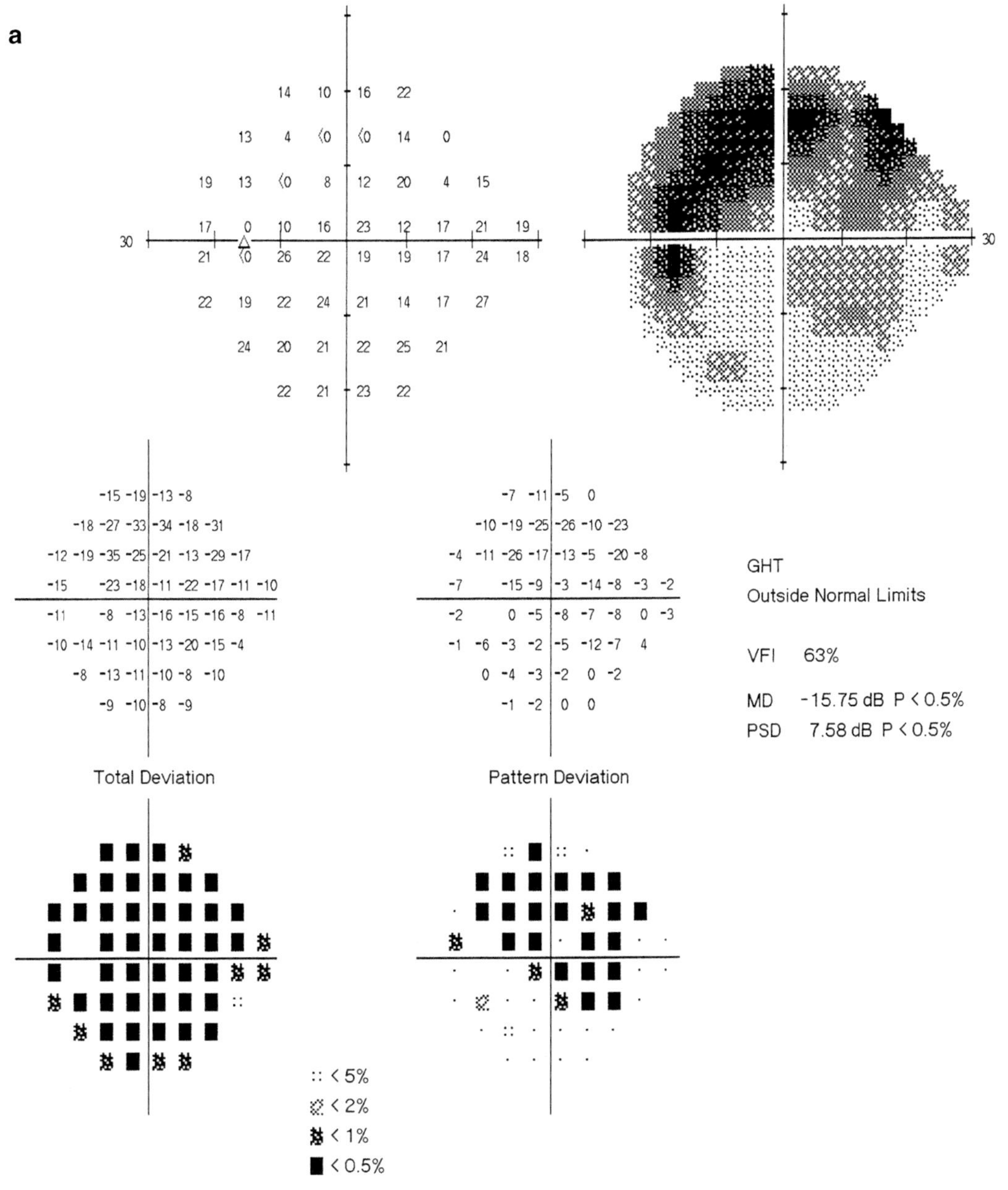

Fig. 34.13 Humphrey visual field analysis printouts. The 24-2 test showed a giant central defect extending from the blind spot in both eyes with the most severe damage in the superior region. Panel a: left eye. Panel b: right eye

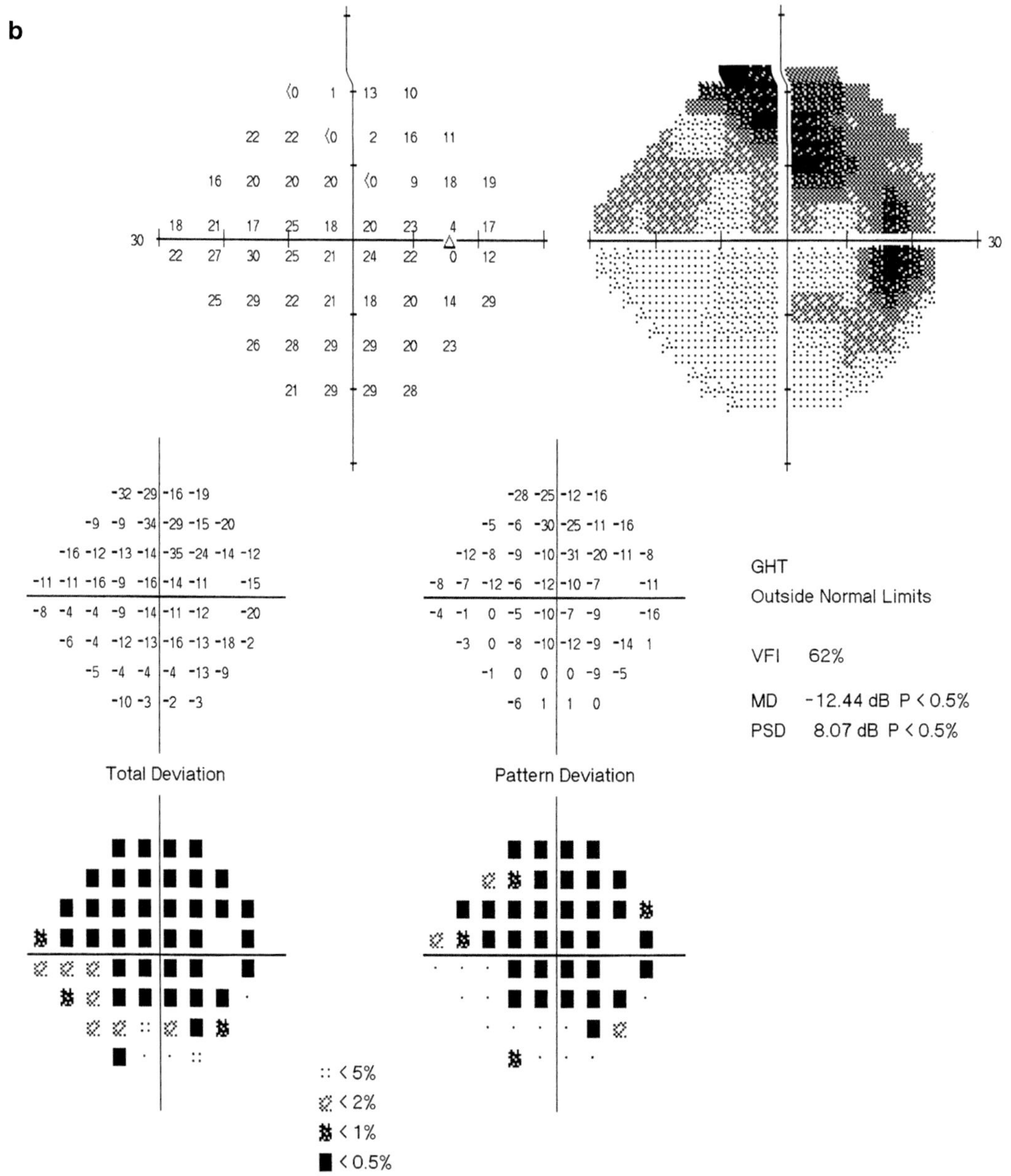

Fig. 34.13 (continued)

In Case 1 provided in this section, the nucleotide mutation was found at position 11778 in both the patient and his brother, but they experienced completely different forms of visual field damage. The elder brother showed a typical central defect in both eyes, while the other showed right superior homonymous quadrantanopia. It was speculated that the cause was mainly related to mtDNA mutation heteroplasmy [1]. In most of LHON patients and their family members, the pathogenic mtDNA mutation is homoplasmic. Only 14% of LHON patients carry wild-type-mutant hybrid mtDNA, a phenomenon known as heteroplasmy. It is found that the heteroplasmy level of primary mtDNA mutation is 75–80% in LHON. Once the number of copies of the mutant mtDNA at a site of the retina in both eyes is large enough to reach a certain degree, dysfunction

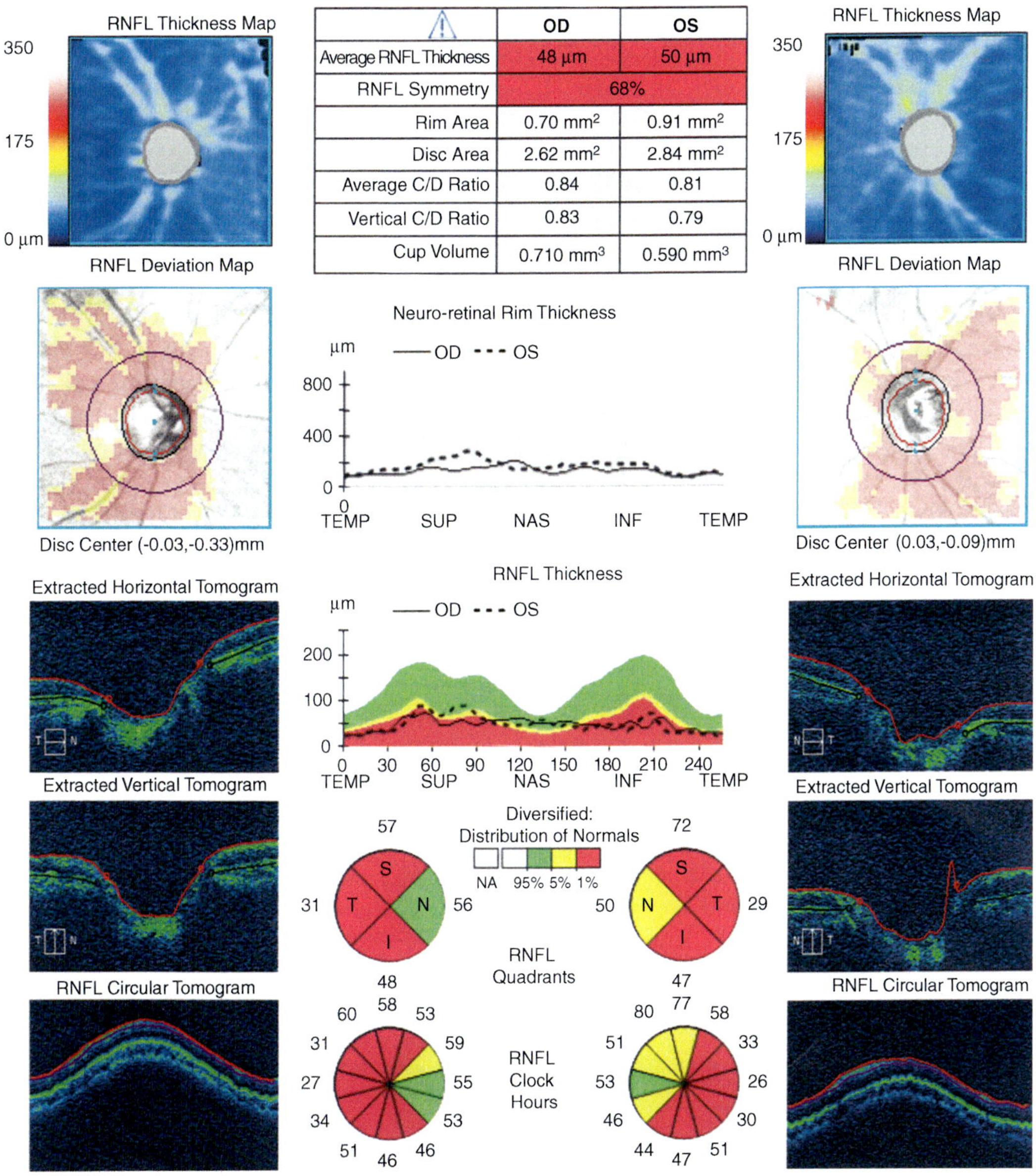

Fig. 34.14 OCT measurement printouts for the RNFL thickness. Diffuse RNFL thinning was noted in both eyes, which was more severe in the inferior and temporal quadrants

will appear, and thus there will be various kinds of visual field damage. The most common visual field damage is a diffuse giant central defect, but limited and bilateral symmetrical visual field damage is also possible. Different LHON patients, even from the same family, have significant differences in the heteroplasmy level of blood cell mitochondrial mutation load. This may be one of the reasons why family members have the same mutation but different visual field damage forms. The cases provided in this chapter remind us of the complexity of LHON and the diversity of its manifestations, and the molecular basis for its diversity is mainly the heteroplasmy of mtDNA mutation without "characteristics" or "regularity." In terms of visual field changes, they are also not "characteristic" and "regular." So, if there is a visual field change that is usually seen in typical visual pathway diseases (as in Case 1), this coincidence is not surprising.

In addition to the heteroplasmy, there are other potential genetic modifiers. Secondary point mutation; haploid; X-linked susceptibility gene; encoding nuclear gene; environmental factors including alcohol consumption, smoking, and other bad habits; and history of contact with toxic substances [2] will have a certain impact on the development and prognosis of LHON and result in different clinical phenotypes in LHON patients.

At present, there is no specific treatment for LHON. The current treatment methods mainly include mitochondria function improvement, support, and nutrition therapies. It is essential to avoid contact with harmful substances (cigarettes, alcohol, etc.) [2]. In recent years, idebenone, vitamin B12, vitamin C, cysteine sodium thiosulfate, coenzyme Q10, and ATP have been used for the treatment, but the effect is uncertain [3]. Previous studies have shown that the prognosis of LHON varies with mutation sites, which is directly related to the age of onset and the specific mtDNA mutation site. The three most common LHON mtDNA mutations are located at nucleotide positions 3460, 11778, and 14484. Among them, patients with 14484 point mutations have the best prognosis, followed by 3460, with 11778 being the worst, but clinically the mutation at position 11778 is the most common mutation type in Asia (50–70%).

It is encouraging that gene therapies for the disease have already been put into clinical application. For example, in a clinical trial performed in China, there were nine patients with LHON voluntarily receiving rAAV2-ND4 (recombinant adeno-associated virus vector expressing the ND4 gene) by intravitreal injection (the ND4 gene is a mitochondrial gene, the fourth subunit of the seven subunits encoding NADH dehydrogenase). The efficacy of the gene therapy was comprehensively evaluated by vision recovery, changes in VEP and OCT, changes in liver and kidney functions, and generation of AAV2 antibodies. Of the eight patients undergoing unilateral gene therapy, four had improvement of bilateral visual function, while the other four patients achieved visual function improvement in the opposite eye. No serious safety problem was observed in any receiver of the gene therapy during the 3 years of follow-up, and further investigation is still ongoing [4].

References

1. Ran R, Yang S, He H, et al. A retrospective analysis of characteristics of visual field damage in patients with Leber's hereditary optic neuropathy. Springerplus. 2016;5(1):843.
2. Giordano L, Deceglie S, d'Adamo P, et al. Cigarette toxicity triggers Leber's hereditary optic neuropathy by affecting mtDNA copy number, oxidative phosphorylation and ROS detoxification pathways. Cell Death Dis. 2015;6:e2021.
3. Saadati HG, Hsu HY, Heller KB, et al. A histopathologic and morphometric differentiation of nerves in optic nerve hypoplasia and Leber's hereditary optic neuropathy. Arch Ophthalmol. 1998;116(7):911–6.
4. Yang S, Ma SQ, Wan X, et al. Long-term outcomes of gene therapy for the treatment of Leber's hereditary optic neuropathy. EBioMedicine. 2016;10:258–68.

35 Optic Neuritis with Various Manifestations of Visual Field

Xiaojing Pan, Ning Fan, and Xuyang Liu

Optic neuritis is a clinically common disease which has various clinical manifestations. There is no pattern to find in its visual field damage. Several types and outcomes of visual field defects in optic neuritis are reviewed through several cases and literature review in this section.

35.1 Case 1

35.1.1 Case Presentation

A 36-year-old male patient complained of sudden decrease in visual acuity in his right eye for more than 10 days with pain upon eye movement. But there was no red or sore eyes, metamorphopsia, etc. He had experienced a cold and fever 1 week before the onset of the vision change, which had resolved. Histories of trauma, other ocular diseases, systemic diseases, or familial diseases were denied.

In the right eye, the uncorrected visual acuity (UCVA) was finger counting, and the best corrected visual acuity (BCVA) was 0.05 with refractive correction (−2.00DS − 0.75DC*180), the light projection was accurate, and red and green colors could be distinguished. In the left eye, the UCVA was 20/200, and the BCVA was 20/20 with refractive correction (−2.50DS−1.00DC*85). Intraocular pressure (IOP) was normal OU. Slit-lamp examination of the anterior segments was unremarkable except that the relative afferent pupillary defect (RAPD) was positive in the right eye. In the right eye, the optic disc exhibited an unclear margin, with congestion and edema. There was no abnormality in the left fundus (Fig. 35.1).

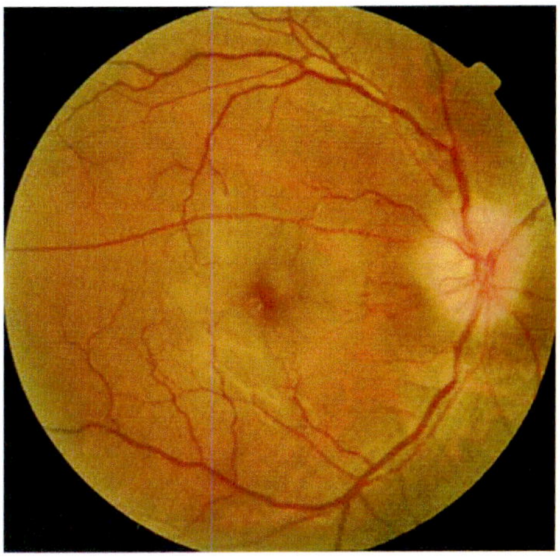

Fig. 35.1 Fundus photograph. The optic disc exhibited an unclear margin, with congestion and edema

X. Pan
Shandong Eye Institute, Qingdao Eye Hospital, Qingdao, China

N. Fan
Shenzhen Eye Hospital, Shenzhen University, Shenzhen, China

X. Liu (✉)
Xiamen Eye Center of Xiamen University, Xiamen, China

Shenzhen Eye Hospital, Shenzhen University, Shenzhen, China

N. Wang et al. (eds.), *Optic Disorders and Visual Field*, Advances in Visual Science and Eye Diseases 2, https://doi.org/10.1007/978-981-13-2502-1_35

Standardized automated perimetry showed a severe damage to the central visual field in the right eye with residual nasal visual field only (Fig. 35.2).

The F-VEP test showed abnormal waveform and decreased amplitude of the P2 wave under the stimulation at 1.2 Hz and normal waveform, normal latency, and decreased amplitude of the P2 wave under the stimulation at 12 Hz in the right eye, while there was no abnormality in the left eye (Fig. 35.3).

F-VEP showed abnormal waveform and decreased amplitude of the P2 wave under the stimulation at 1.2 Hz and normal waveform, normal latency, and decreased amplitude of the P2 wave under the stimulation at 12 Hz in the right

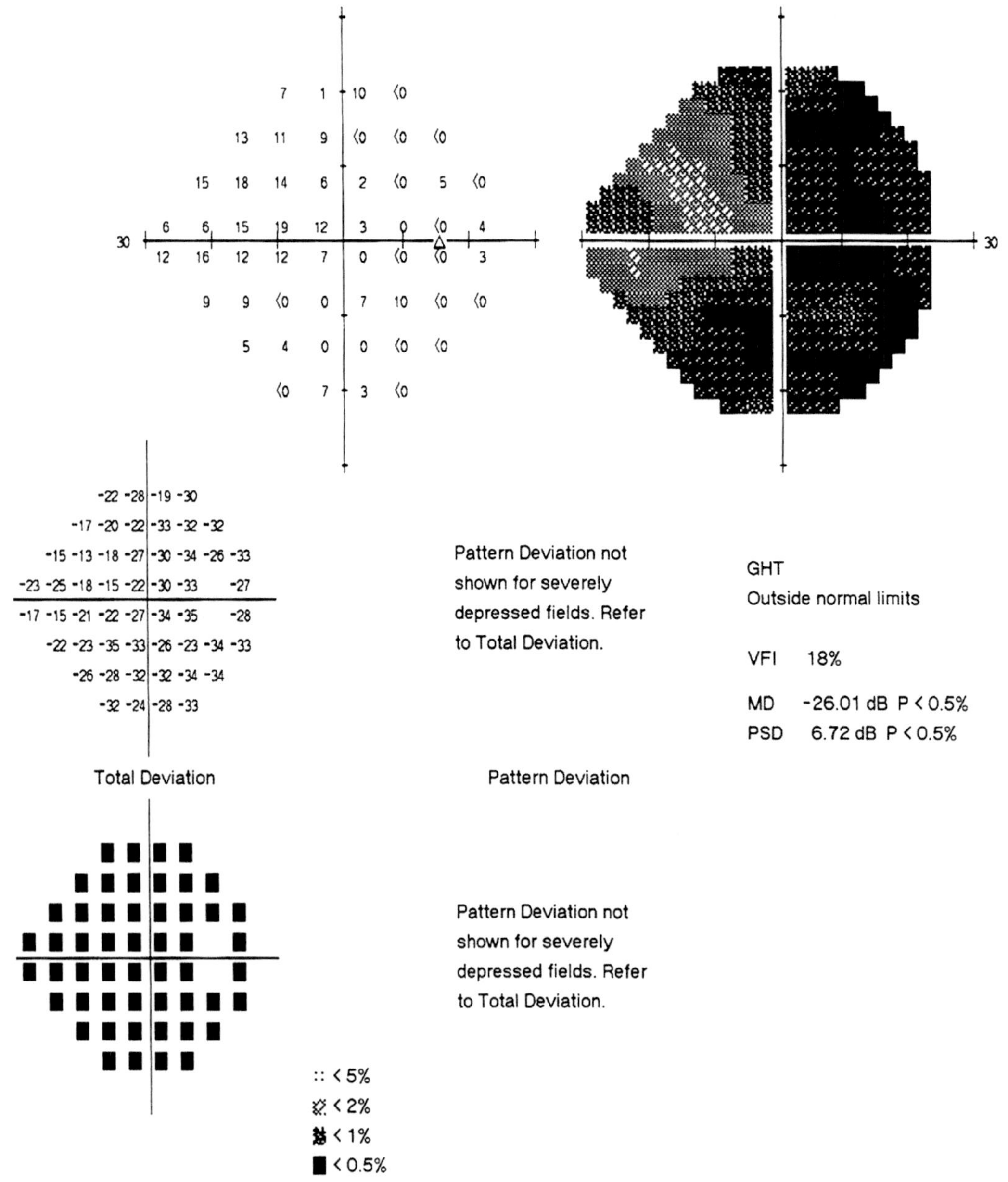

Fig. 35.2 Humphrey visual field analysis printout. The 24-2 test showed that there was only the nasal visual field remaining in the right eye, and the photosensitivity decreased diffusively and dramatically

Flash-VEP 1,2 Hz

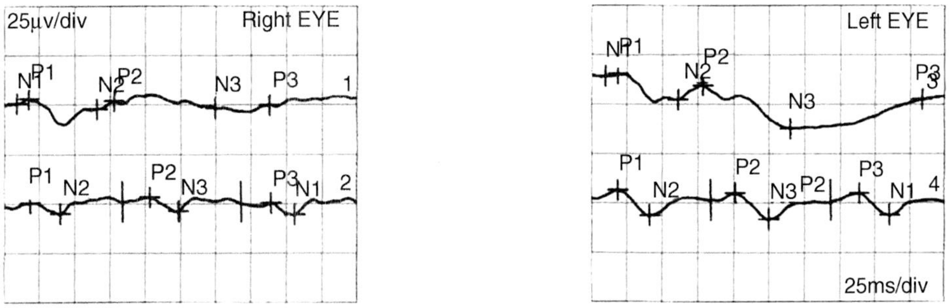

Channel	N1 [ms]	P1 [ms]	N2 [ms]	P2 [ms]	N3 [ms]	P3 [ms]	N1-P1	N2-P2	N3-P3
1 R-1 1,2 Hz	9	18	66	78	150	189	2.24μV	4.13μv	4.47μv
3 L-1 1,2 Hz	10	19	62	79	140	234	1.17μv	6.97μv	4.7μv
2 R-1 12 Hz	206	19	40	104	124	190	5.94μv	8.39μv	1.93μv
4 L-1 12 Hz	211	19	41	101	125	189	12.4μv	11.1μv	1.2μv
Normals	-	-	-	-	-	-	-	-	-

Channel	Stimulus	Ampl., Range, Filter
1 R-1 1,2 Hz	GF LED Flash OdB (2,00 cds/m? 1.199Hz, Avg:100	1, +/-100μv 0.5-50Hz
2 R-1 12 Hz	GF LED Flash OdB (2,00 cds/m? 11.905Hz, Avg:100	1, +/-100μv 0.5-50Hz
3 L-1 1,2 Hz	GF LED Flash OdB (2,00 cds/m? 1.199Hz, Avg:100	1, +/-100μv 0.5-50Hz
4 L-1 12 Hz	GF LED Flash OdB (2,00 cds/m? 11.905Hz, Avg:100	1, +/-100μv 0.5-50Hz

Fig. 35.3 F-VEP examination printouts

eye, while in the left eye, the waveform, latency, and amplitude were normal under the stimulation at both 1.2 and 12 Hz (Fig. 35.3).

FFA showed telangiectasia in the optic disc and in the top layer around the optic disc at the early phase, fluorescein leakage at the venous phase, and strong fluorescence in the optic disc at the late phase in the right eye (Fig. 35.4).

35.1.2 Final Diagnosis

The final diagnosis was papillitis in the right eye.

The patient was given methylprednisolone pulse therapy and oral hormones at sequentially reduced doses, which was supplemented with supportive therapies such as vitamin B and blood circulation improvement for 10 days. At the follow-up examination, the best corrected visual acuity (BCVA) was 1.2. RAPD was negative. The optic disc edema was resolved, and the standardized automated perimetry results were unremarkable in the right eye (Fig. 35.5). The F-VEP results showed that the waveform, latency, and amplitude of the P2 wave were all normal in the right eye. The cranial MRI revealed no abnormalities.

35.1.3 Case Review

Papillitis is an inflammatory disease that occurs in the optic papilla and its surrounding areas. It is a primary demyelinating optic neuritis and is closely related to central nervous system demyelinating diseases, such as multiple sclerosis or neuromyelitis optica. In most of the typical cases, the patients are unilaterally affected young adults, and the most common manifestation is visual field damage at the central 20°. VEP examination will show that the conduction velocity of nerve potential slows down due to the demyelination of nerve fibers, and then the latency is prolonged. When the axons of the nerve fibers are damaged, the conduction velocity may be normal, while the potential intensity is weakened, resulting in a decrease in amplitude. FFA will reveal capillary dilatation on the optic disc surface and fluorescein leakage on the vascular wall. In the late phase of radiography, the strong fluorescence of the whole optic disc and its surrounding tissues can be seen. The patient's visual field test, VEP, and FFA results matched the typical manifestations of optic nerve papillitis.

Currently, adrenal glucocorticoid is the main treatment for acute demyelinating optic neuritis. The optic neuritis treatment trial (ONTT) con-

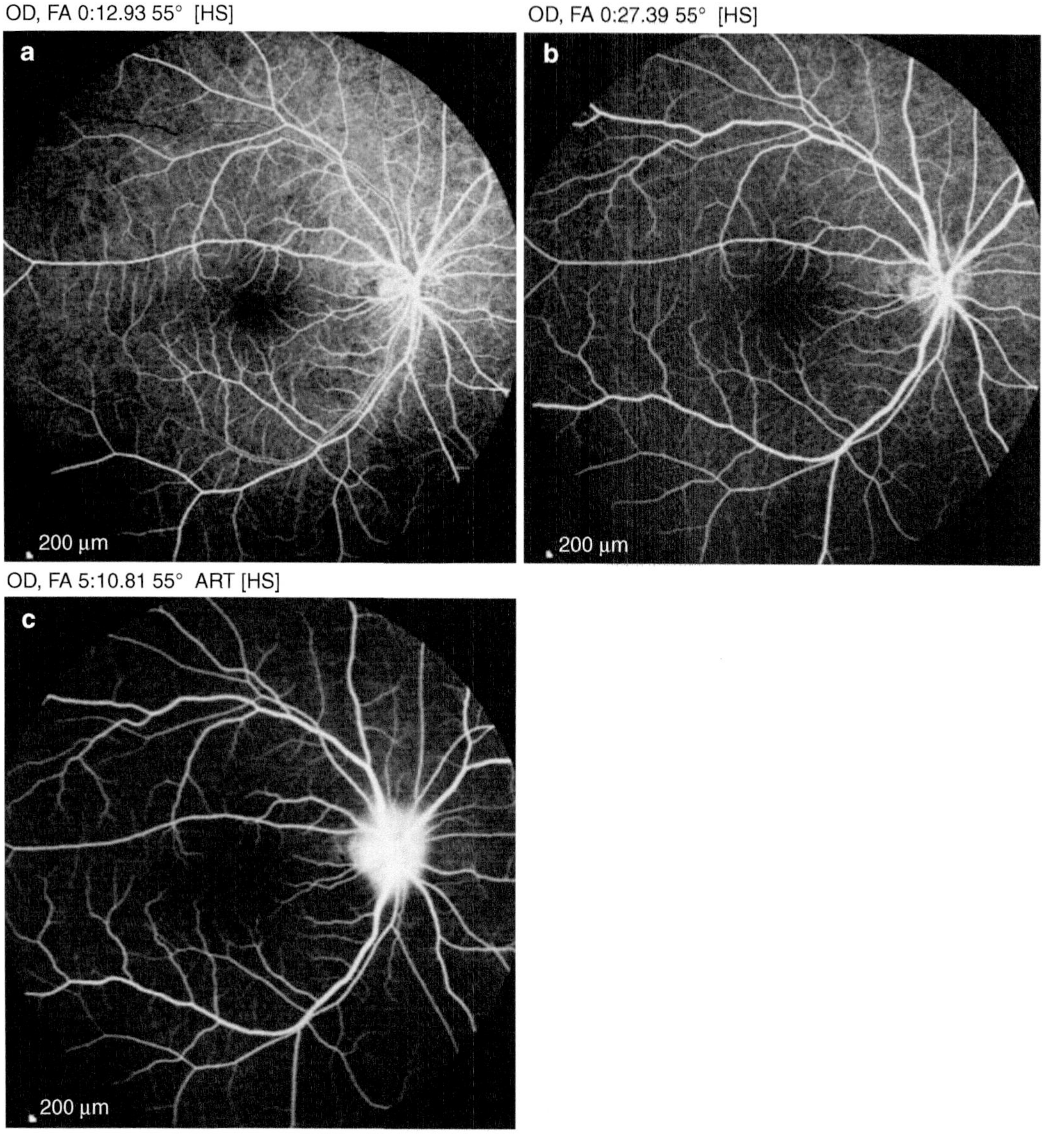

Fig. 35.4 FFA images. Panel a: telangiectasia in the optic disc and in the top layer around the optic disc at the early phase of angiography. Panel b: fluorescein leakage at the venous phase. Panel c: strong fluorescence of the optic disc at the late phase

firmed that pulse therapy with intravenous administration of high doses of methylprednisolone can obviously accelerate the recovery of visual function in these patients [1]. The patient in this case was treated according to the expert guidelines that were prepared by a neuro-ophthalmology group in China. After 10 days, the vision and visual field basically normalized without recurrence after reducing the dose of hormone sequentially.

For these patients, the cranial MRI examination is necessary, and clinical symptoms and necessary auxiliary examinations should also be considered to assist in determining whether there is any high-risk factor for progression into multiple sclerosis and neuromyelitis optica, especially in patients with recurrent papillitis and patients who are nonresponsive to hormone therapy.

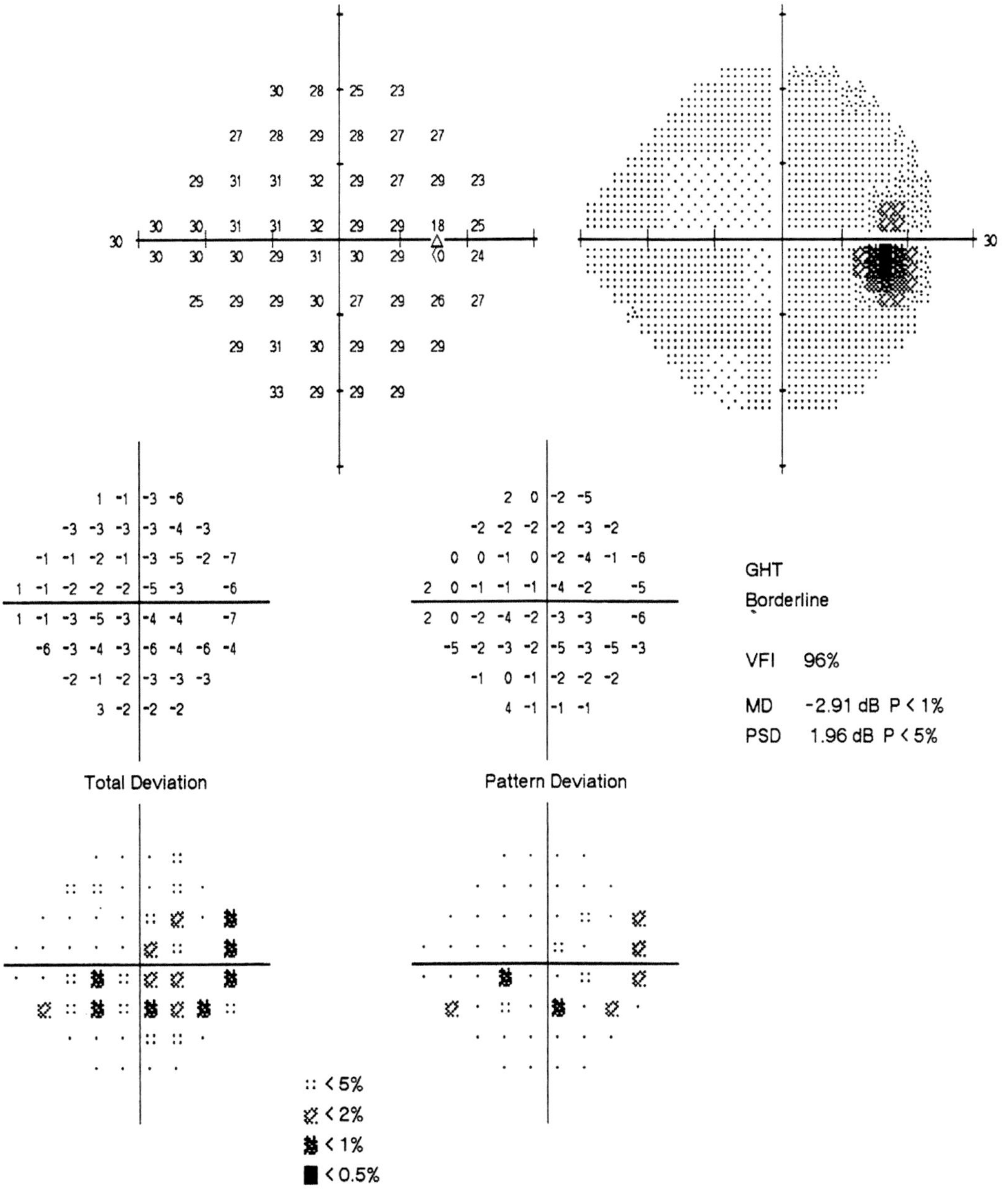

Fig. 35.5 Re-examination Humphrey visual field analysis printout obtained during the re-examination after treatment. The 24-2 test revealed a normal central field in the right eye

35.2 Case 2

35.2.1 Case Presentation

A 34-year-old male patient complained of feeling a shadow over the right eye accompanied by pain upon eye movement for 3 days. The patient did not feel any malaise. The patient did not have sore or red eyes, metamorphopsia, or other discomforts. There was no history of trauma, other ocular diseases, or systemic or familial diseases.

The UCVA was 1.2 OU. IOP was normal OU. Slit-lamp examination of his anterior segments was unremarkable. The RAPD was negative in the right eye. Fundus examination showed that the right optic disc was with an unclear boundary, congestion, and edema.

Standardized automated perimetry revealed nasal visual field defects in the right eye (Fig. 35.6).

The OCT results showed that the retinal nerve fiber layer (RNFL) thickness in the superior, inferior, and temporal quadrants increased significantly (Fig. 35.7).

FFA showed telangiectasia in the optic disc and the peripapillary surface layer at the early phase, fluorescein leakage at the venous phase, and obviously enhanced fluorescence of the optic

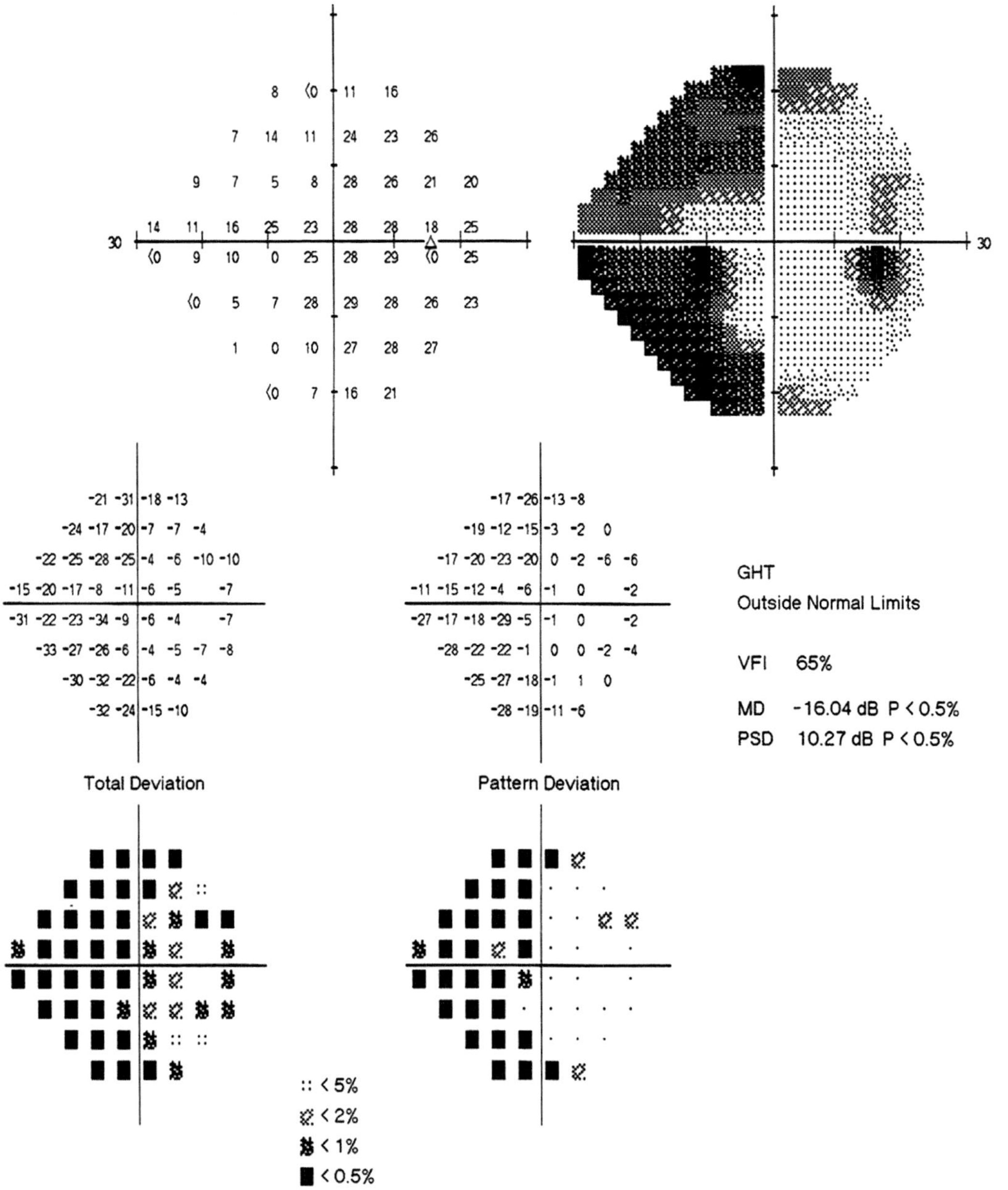

Fig. 35.6 Humphrey visual field analysis printout. The 24-2 test showed nasal visual field defects in the right eye

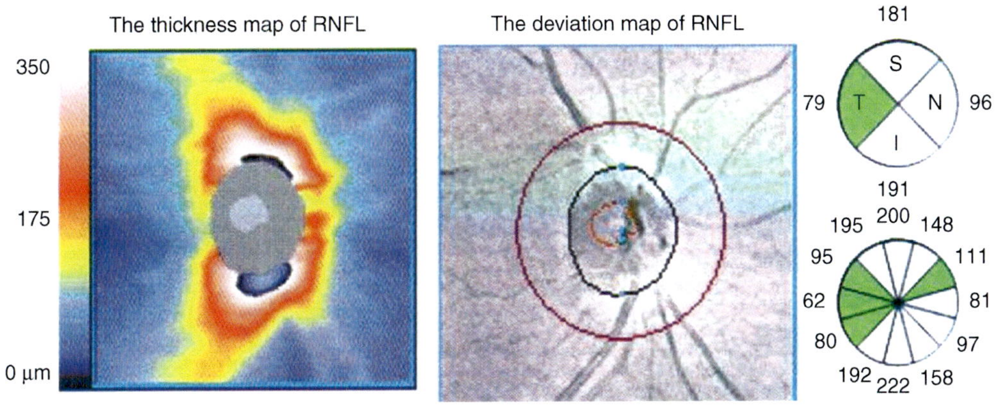

Fig. 35.7 OCT RNFL thickness analysis printout. The RNFL thickness in the superior, inferior, and temporal quadrants increased significantly

disc at the late phase in the right eye, but its disc boundary was still clear (Fig. 35.8).

The P-VEP results showed normal latency and a moderate decrease in the amplitude of the P100 wave in the right eye, and the P-VEP wave was normal in the left eye.

35.2.2 Final Diagnosis

The final diagnosis was papillitis in the right eye.

The patient was given methylprednisolone pulse therapy, oral hormones at sequentially reduced doses, and other supportive treatments including vitamin B and improvement of blood circulation. After 10 days, the follow-up examination showed a visual acuity of 20/20 OD, and the standardized automated perimetry revealed normal results (Fig. 35.9). No abnormalities were found during the head MRI examination.

35.2.3 Case Review

The patient was diagnosed with papillitis in the right eye. The visual field showed a nasal defect, which was consistent with the edematous RNFL areas (inferior, superior, and temporal quadrants) demonstrated by OCT. Considering the optic neuritis was localized around the optic disc, the local visual field damage was consistent, functionally and structurally, with the parapapillary RNFL thickness measured by OCT.

The amplitude of P-VEP in the right eye decreased significantly, and the latency was normal, suggesting that the lesion was mainly axonal injury of nerve fibers resulting in the reduction of the number of excitable axons. The normal latency indicated that the conduction function of myelin was normal, which suggested that demyelination was relatively mild.

35.3 Case 3

35.3.1 Case Presentation

A 25-year-old female patient complained recurrent vision loss in her left eye for more than 1 month. It had occurred without any obvious trigger. The patient had been treated with methylprednisolone, dexamethasone, prednisone, and other hormones in other hospitals. In the left eye, the visual acuity had been light perception at its worst, which was improved to 20/20 with refraction after treatment. However, the visual acuity in his left eye had decreased again 1 week before. He had no history of trauma, other ocular diseases, or systemic or familial diseases. His right eye was normal.

On examination, the UCVA was 20/20 OD and 20/28 OS, and there was no improvement with refraction. The IOP was normal. In both eyes, slit-lamp examination of anterior seg-

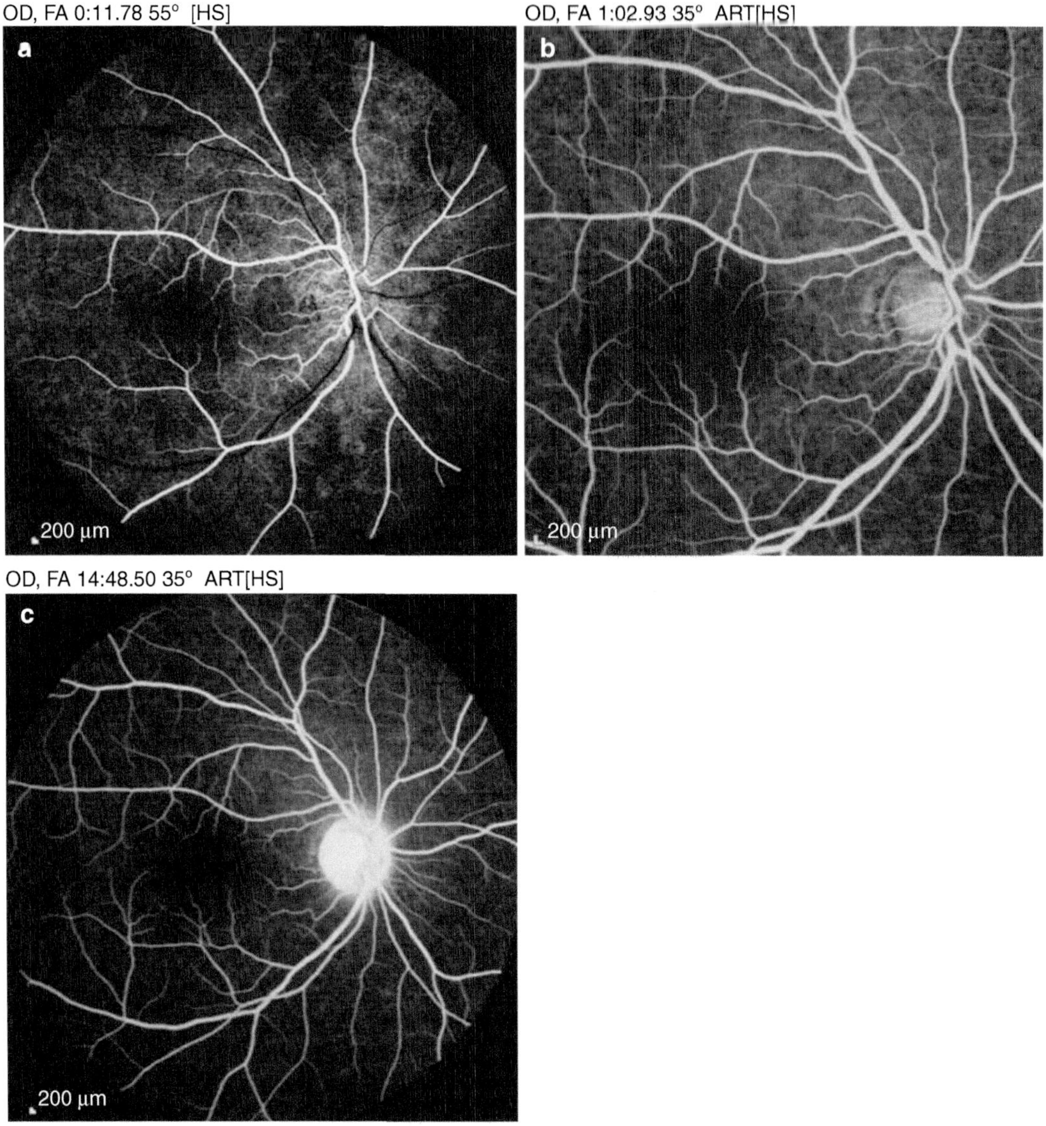

Fig. 35.8 FFA images. FFA showed telangiectasia in the optic disc and the peripapillary surface layer at the early phase, fluorescein leakage at the venous phase, and obviously enhanced fluorescence of the optic disc at the late phase in right eye, but its disc boundary was still clear. Panel a: the early-phase angiogram. Panel b: the venous-phase angiogram. Panel c: the late-phase angiogram

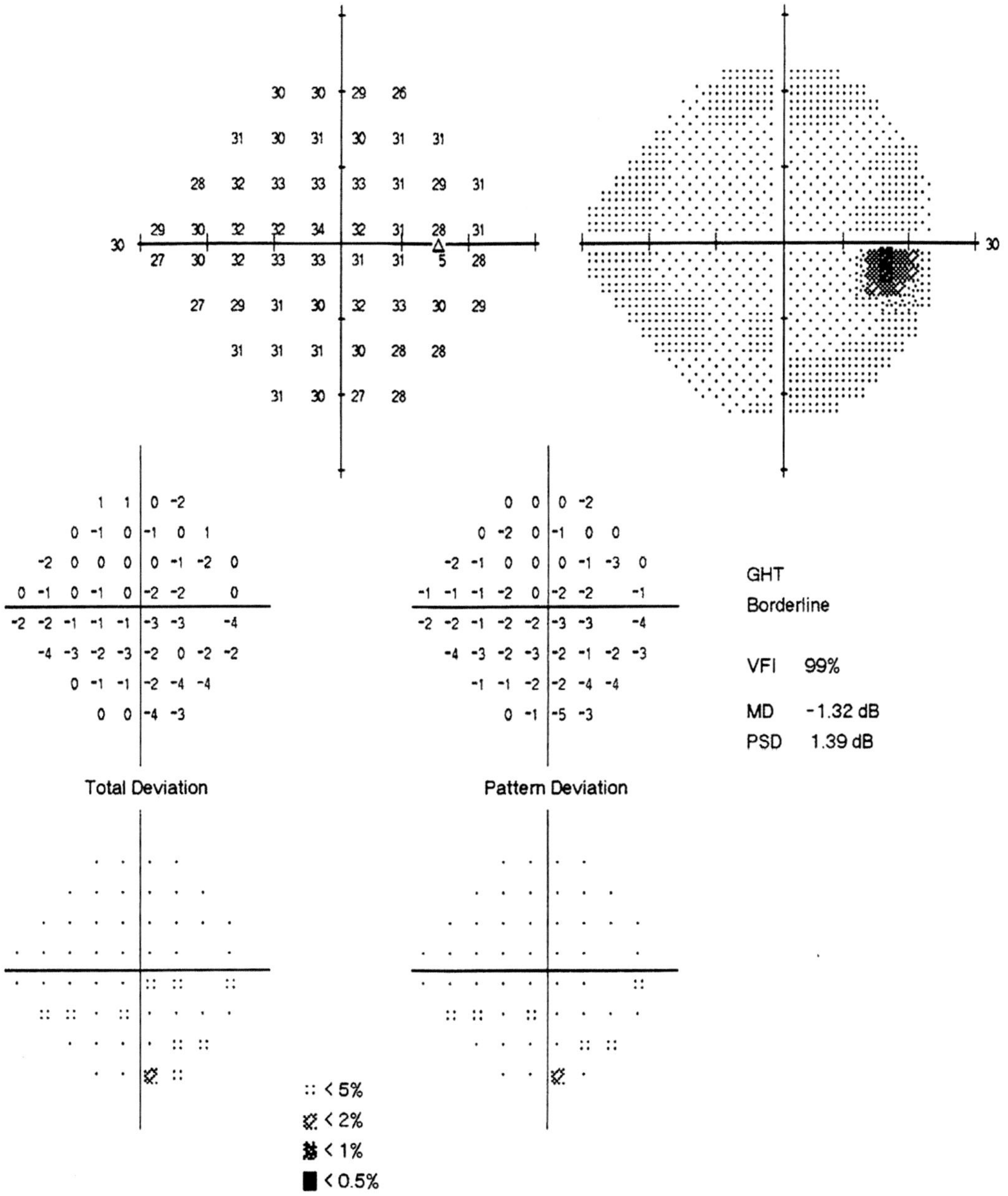

Fig. 35.9 Humphrey visual field analysis printout obtained during the re-examination after treatment. The 24-2 test showed normal results

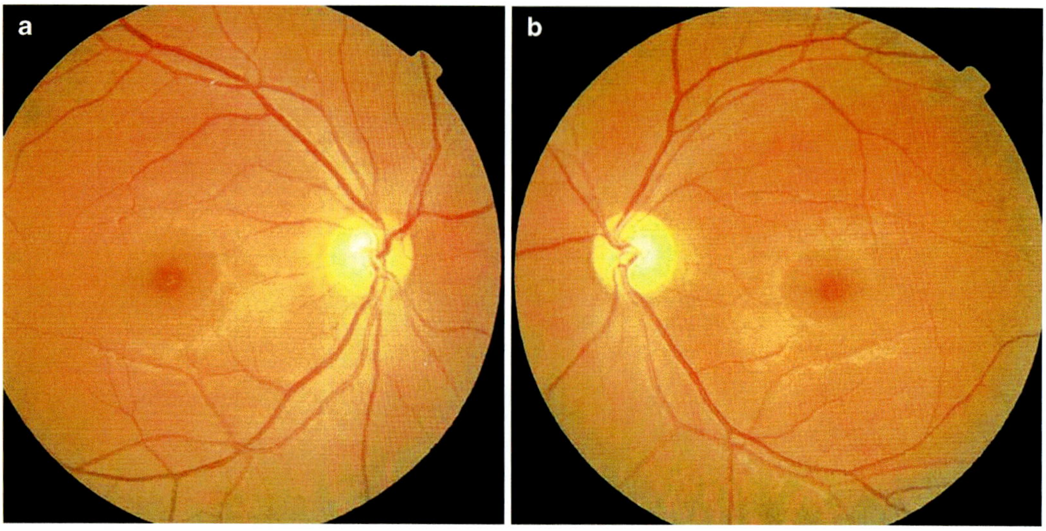

Fig. 35.10 Fundus photographs. Panel a: the right optic disc presented a clear boundary and a pink color, and the reflection of the RNFL was normal. Panel b: the left optic disc presented a clear boundary and a pale color, and the reflection of the RNFL was weakened

ments was unremarkable except that the RAPD was positive in the left eye. Fundus examination showed the left optic disc was pale in color with a clear boundary and a cup-to-disc (C/D) ratio of 0.5, and the reflection of RNFL was weakened. The right optic disc was pink in color with a clear boundary and a C/D ratio of 0.5, and the reflection of RNFL was normal (Fig. 35.10).

Standardized automated perimetry showed an irregular central defect in the left eye (Fig. 35.11).

The P-VEP results showed the waveform, latency, and amplitude of the P100 wave were severely abnormal in the left eye, while the P100 wave was normal in the right eye (Fig. 35.12).

FFA revealed normal findings in the left eye (Fig. 35.13).

35.3.2 Final Diagnosis

The final diagnosis was recurrent retrobulbar neuritis in the left eye.

35.3.3 Case Review

A central visual field defect is typical in optic neuritis, and it can appear in any phases of the course, such as the acute phase and recovery phase. At about 15 mm behind the eyeball or beyond, the core of the optic nerve is mainly macular fibers. Therefore, in case of retrobulbar neuritis, significant damage to macular fibers occurs first. As a result, a central defect appears in the visual field, similar to the visual field changes in patients with neuritis.

In this case, due to suboptimal hormone therapy after the onset, the condition recurred and deteriorated in a short period with thinning of retinal nerve fibers, suggesting optic atrophy. According to the natural course of idiopathic demyelinating optic neuritis, the visual function begins to recover 3–5 weeks after onset. When the visual acuity and visual symptoms improve at 4–6 weeks, the damaged nerve fibers begin to become thinner and the color of the optic disc paler.

35.4 Case 4

35.4.1 Case Presentation

A 34-year-old male patient complained of bulging pain for 1 week and decreased vision for 3 days in his right eye. The onset of disease had no

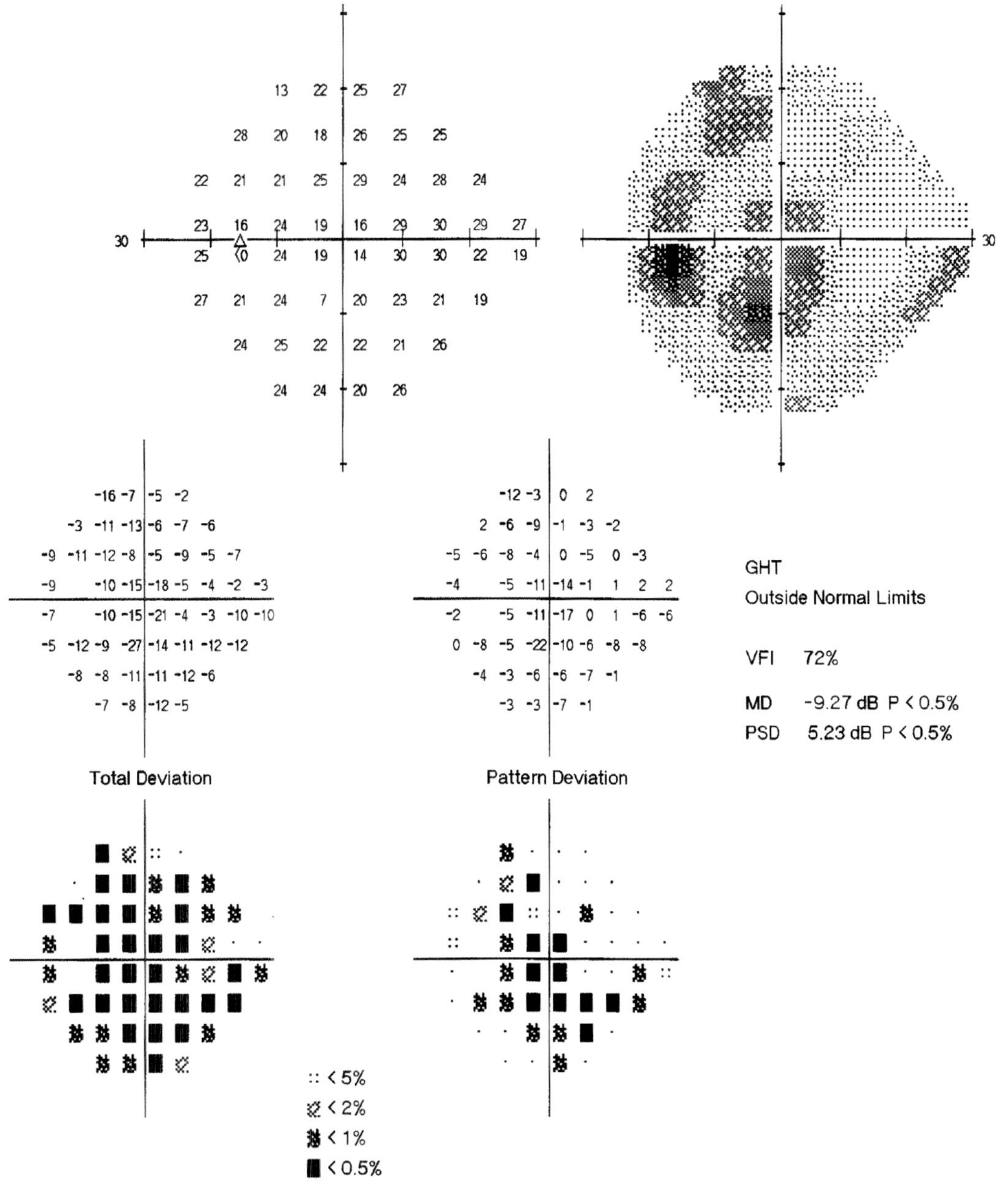

Fig. 35.11 Humphrey visual field analysis printout. The 24-2 test showed an irregular central defect in the left eye

obvious trigger. The patient denied any ocular discomfort. Histories of trauma, other ocular diseases, or systemic or familial diseases were denied.

The UCVA was 20/22 in the right eye, and it was not improved with manifest refraction. IOP was normal. Slit-lamp examination of his anterior segments was unremarkable except that the RAPD was positive in the right eye. Fundus examination revealed that the right optic disc had a clear boundary and was pale in color, with a C/D ratio of 0.6 (Fig. 35.14). No abnormality was found in the left eye.

Standardized automated perimetry showed quadrantanopia in the superior area of the right eye (Fig. 35.15).

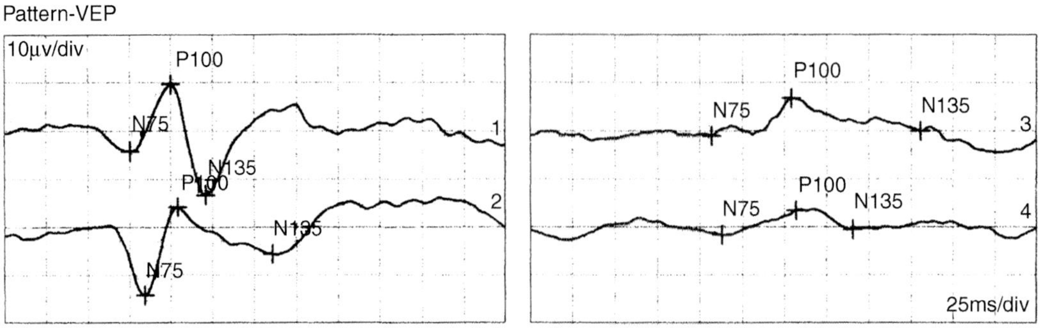

Channel	N75 [ms]	P100 [ms]	N135 [ms]	N75-P100	P100-N135
1 R-1 1,0	76	100	122	13.8µv	22.9µv
3 L-1 1,0	107	154 (!)	231	7.65µv	6.7µv
2 R-1 0,15	85	105	161	18.3µv	9.73µv
4 L-1 0,15	113	157 (!)	191	5.11µv	3.99µv
Normals	-	90-116-90-116	-	-	-

Channel	Stimulus	Ampl., Range, Filter
1 R-1 1,0	MON Patt. Rev. CB, 1?Full Field, Ctr:97% 1.5Hz, Avg:96	1, +/-100µv 1-50Hz
2 R-1 0,15	MON Patt. Rev. CB, 0?5' Full Field, Ctr:97% 1.5Hz, Avg:98	1, +/-100µv 1-50Hz
3 L-1 1,0	MON Patt. Rev. CB, 1?Full Field, Ctr:97% 1.5Hz, Avg:85	1, +/-100µv 1-50Hz
4 L-1 0,15	MON Patt. Rev. CB, 0?5' Full Field, Ctr:97% 1.5Hz, Avg:87	1, +/-100µv 1-50Hz

Fig. 35.12 P-VEP examination printouts. The waveform, latency, and amplitude of the P100 wave in the left eye were severely abnormal, and these are normal in the right eye

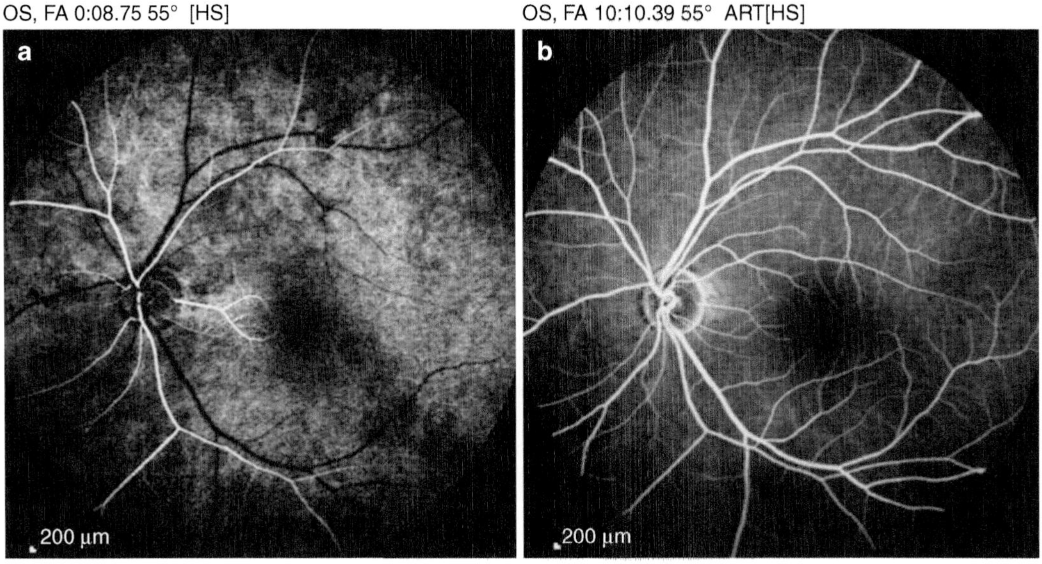

Fig. 35.13 FFA images. Panel a: FFA showed that the cilioretinal artery was filled with fluorescence at the early phase of angiography. Panel b: the FFA findings at the late phase of angiography were normal

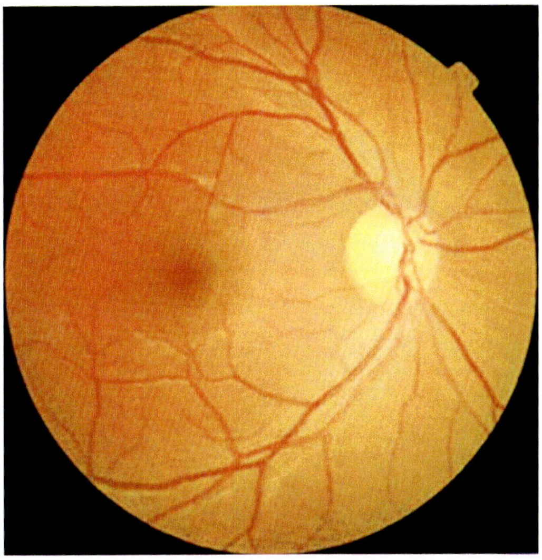

Fig. 35.14 Fundus photograph. The right fundus examination showed that the optic disc had a clear boundary and was pale in color with a C/D of 0.6

P-VEP showed that both the latency and amplitude of the P100 wave in the right eye were severely abnormal, and the P100 wave was normal in the left eye.

The FFA findings were normal in both eyes.

No abnormalities were found in the cranial MRI examination.

35.4.2 Final Diagnosis

The final diagnosis was retrobulbar neuritis in the right eye.

After 10 days of medical treatment, the follow-up examination showed that the visual acuity of the right eye was 20/20, and the visual field was normal (Fig. 35.16).

After 1 month of drug therapy, the patient was lost to follow-up and did not take medications as prescribed. The bulging pain and pain on eye movement in the right eye recurred after more than 2 months. The patient came back to the clinic 5 days later.

Eye examination showed the UCVA was 20/20 with no improvement with refraction in the right eye. IOP was normal. Slit-lamp examination of his anterior segments was unremarkable except that the RAPD was positive in the right eye. Fundus examination showed that the right optic disc had a clear boundary and was pale in color with a C/D ratio of 0.6. There was no abnormality in the macula. The findings in the left eye were normal.

Standardized automated perimetry showed an inferior arcuate scotoma in the right eye (Fig. 35.17).

P-VEP showed that both the latency and amplitude of the P100 wave were severely abnormal in the right eye, and the P100 wave was normal in the left eye.

FFA showed that no abnormalities were found in either eye.

35.4.3 Final Diagnosis

The final diagnosis was recurrent retrobulbar neuritis in the right eye.

The patient received medical treatment again. At the 10-day follow-up examination, a visual acuity of 20/20 and a recovering normal visual field were shown in the right eye (Fig. 35.18). The patient was discharged with medications and was asked to undergo regular examinations and take medicine as prescribed. During the 3-year follow-up, there was no recurrence of optic nerve disease.

35.4.4 Case Review

In this case, retrobulbar neuritis occurred two times within several months, which was mani-

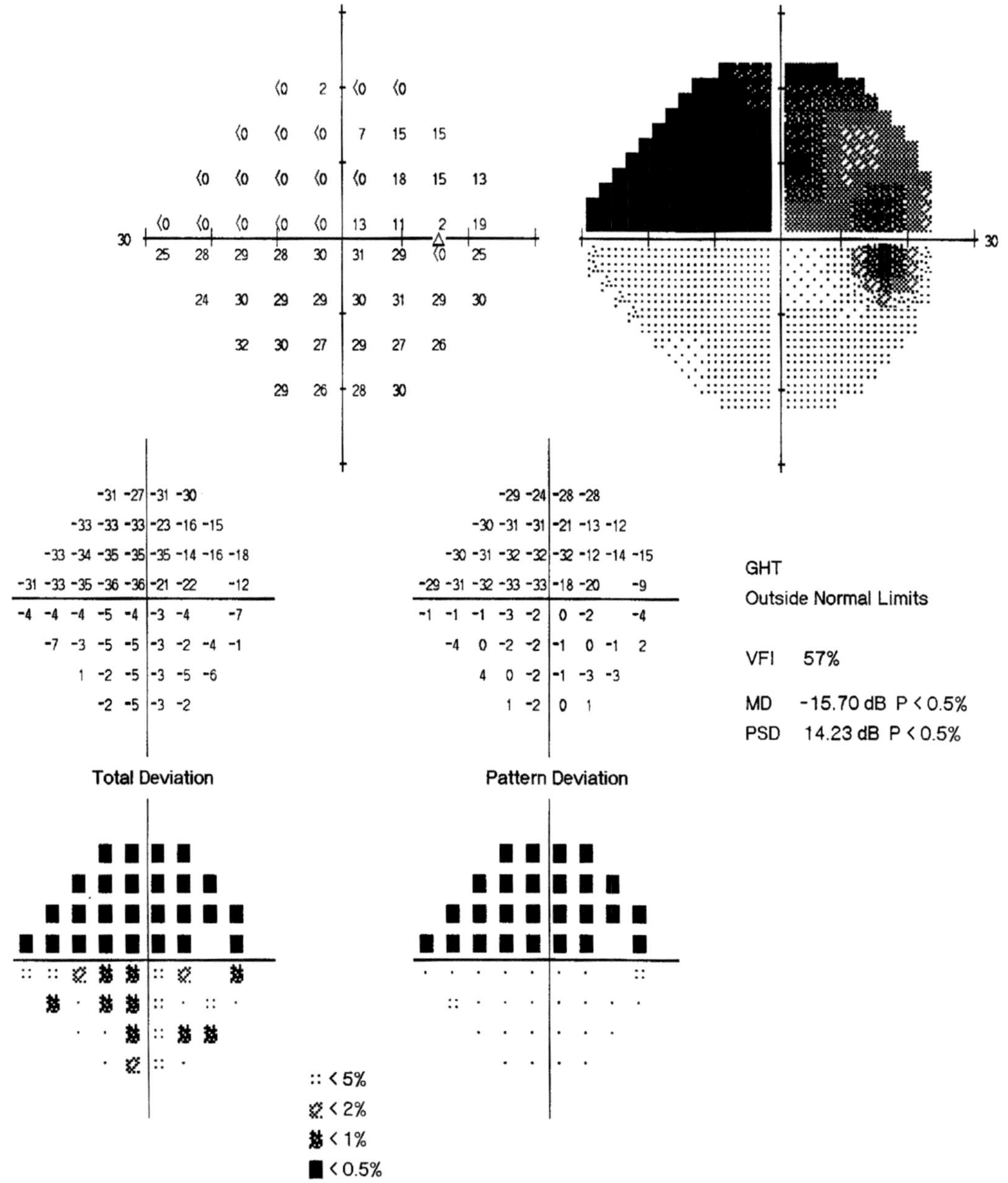

Fig. 35.15 Humphrey visual field analysis printout. The 24-2 test revealed quadrantanopia in the superior area

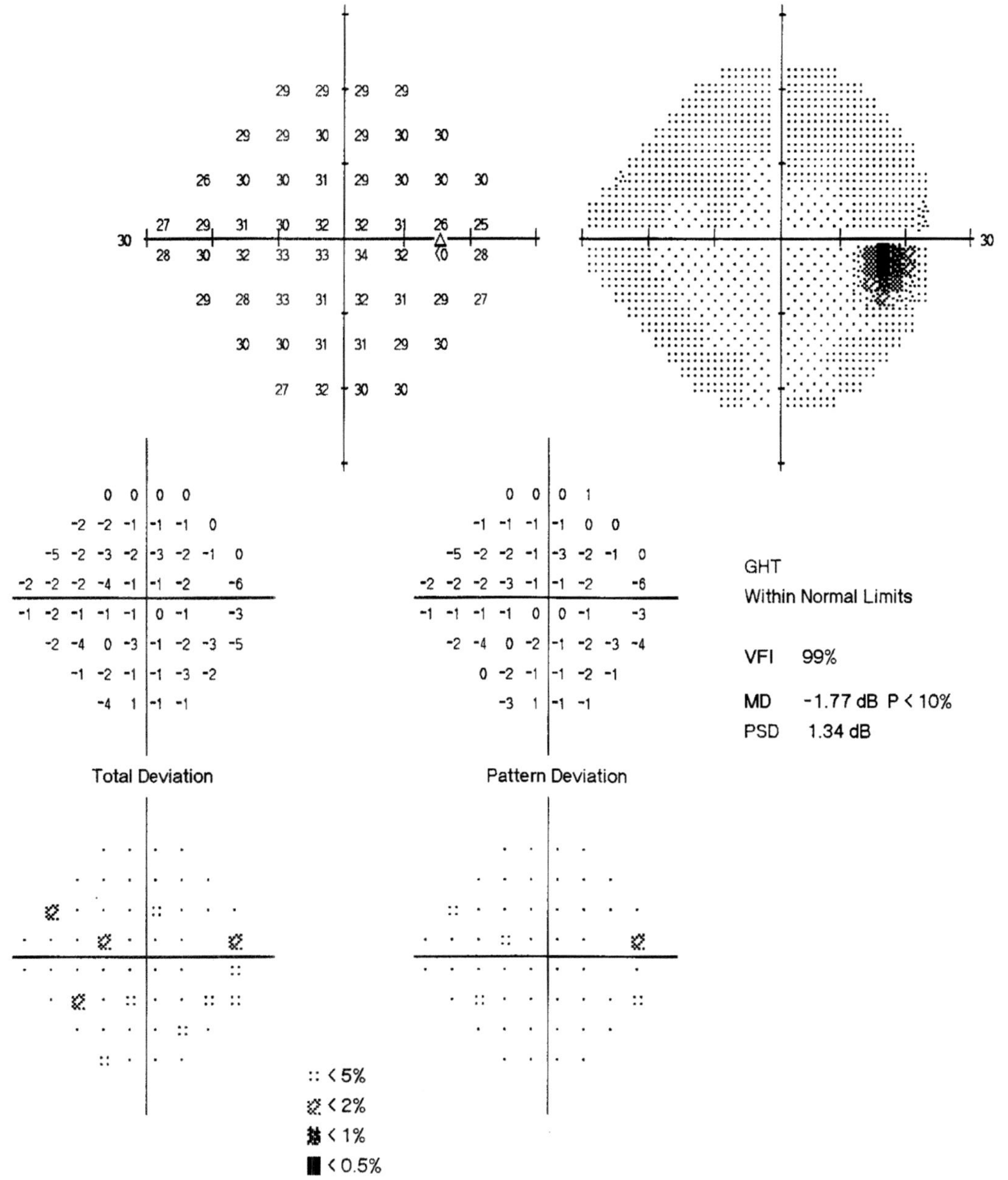

Fig. 35.16 Humphrey visual field analysis printout obtained during the re-examination after treatment. The 24-2 test showed normal results

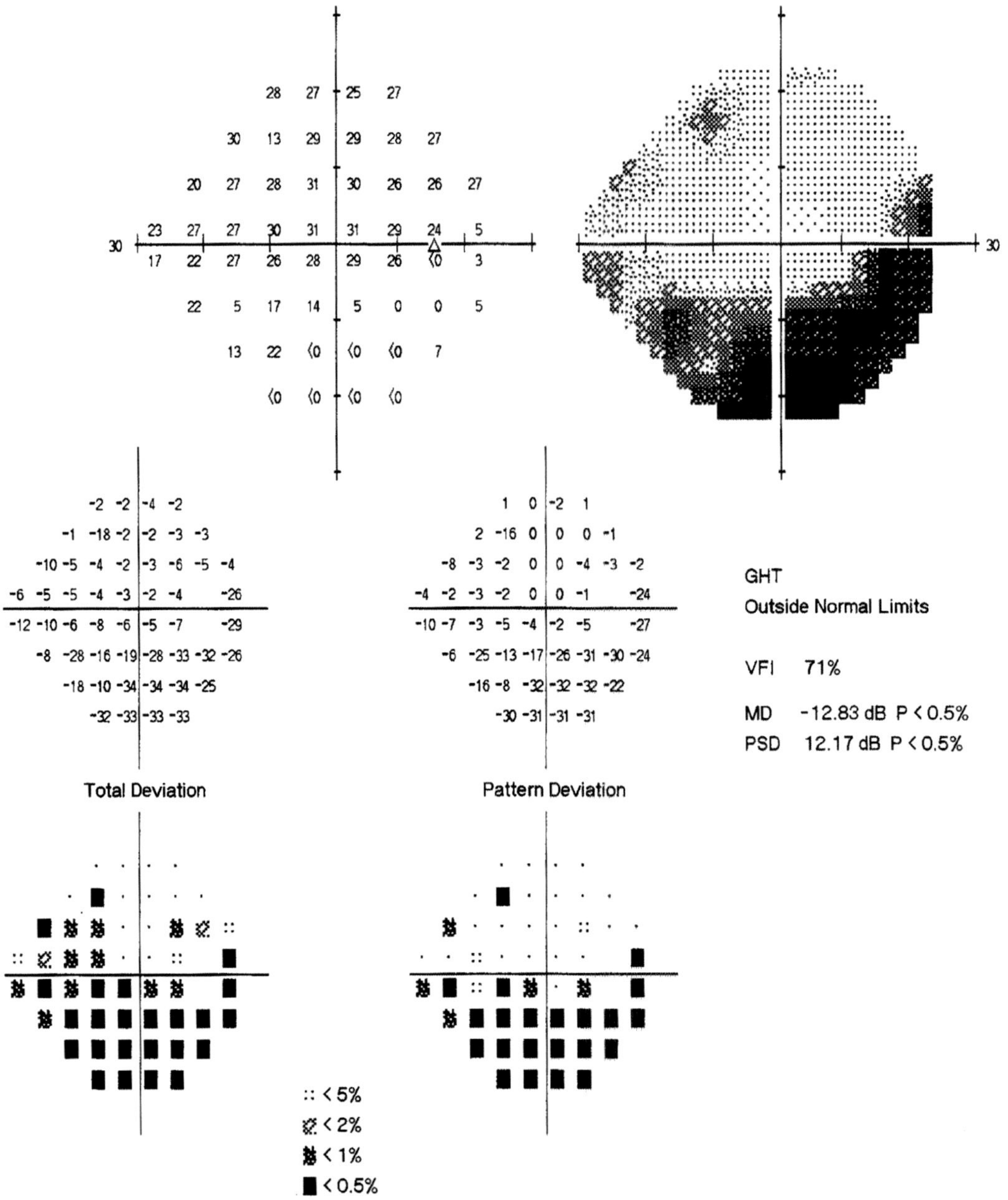

Fig. 35.17 Humphrey visual field analysis printout. The 24-2 test showed an inferior arcuate scotoma in the right eye

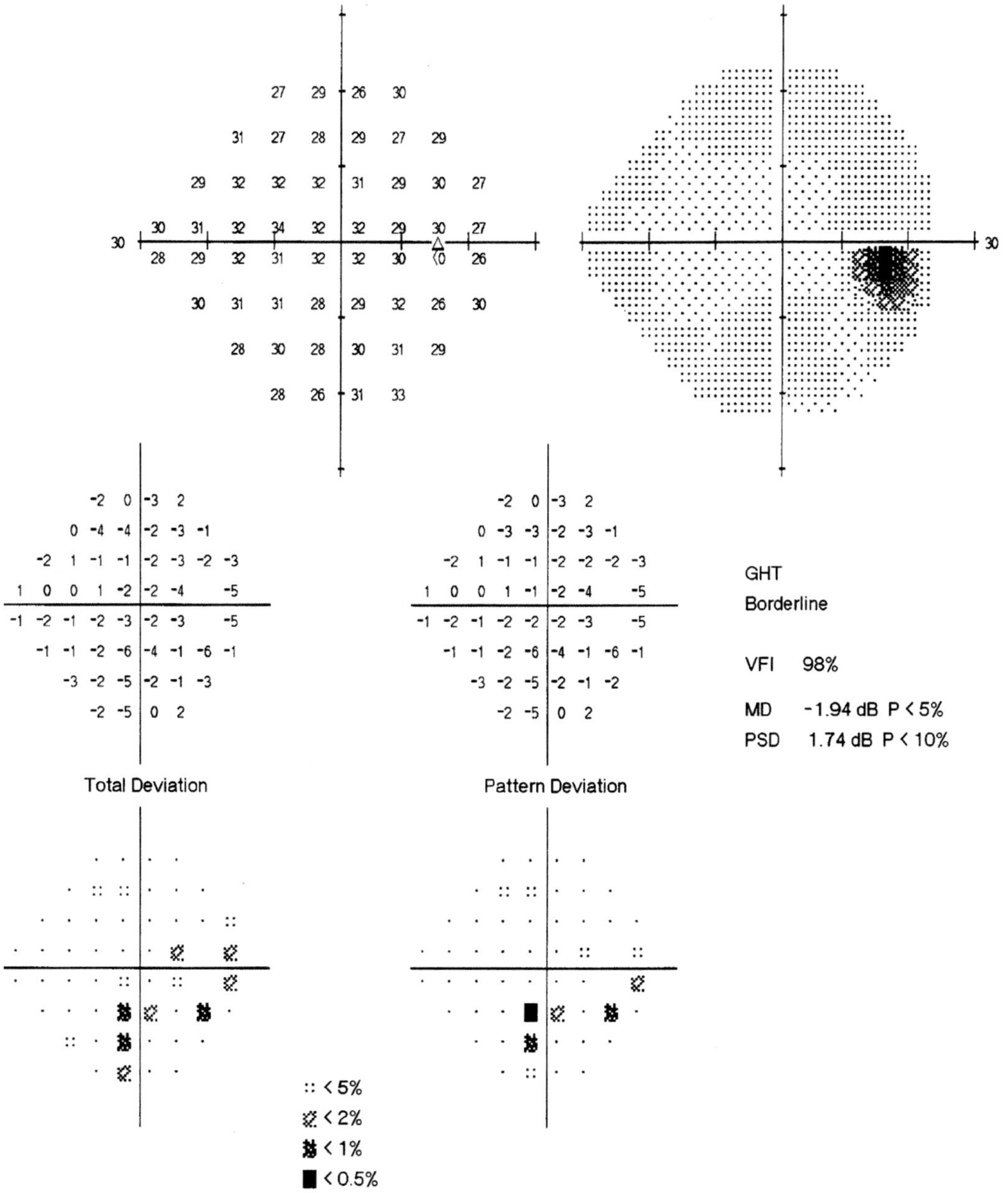

Fig. 35.18 Humphrey visual field analysis printout obtained during the re-examination after treatment. The 24-2 test showed a recovering normal result in the right eye

fested as a superior visual field defect and an inferior arcuate scotoma, respectively, further reflecting the variety of visual field changes in optic neuritis. In addition, it was recognized that standardized automated perimetry is not specific for diagnosing optic neuritis. In terms of morphology, the changes in the visual field in optic neuritis depend on the areas involved in inflammation and the composition of nerve fibers in these areas.

35.5 Discussion

The papillitis and retrobulbar neuritis discussed in this section are idiopathic demyelinating optic neuritis (IDON) that is the most common type of optic neuritis. This name is based on the previous knowledge that the disease is closely related to demyelinating diseases of the central nervous system, such as multiple sclerosis (MS) and neuromyelitis optica (NMO, also known as Devic disease). The clinical diagnosis is divided into papillitis, retrobulbar neuritis, optic perineuritis, and neuroretinitis according to the pathogenic site. Other types of optic nerve inflammation, including infectious optic neuritis, autoimmune optic neuropathy, and other optic neuropathy, like ischemic, genetic, compressing, nutritional and metabolic optic neuropathy, should be ruled out. According to the latest consensus on the diagnosis and treatment of optic neuritis, IDON may be MS-related optic neuritis. The latter is characterized by onset at multiple times and locations. The demyelination in NMO and its related optic neuritis is not exactly the same as that in MS, and the prognosis of NMO is also poorer [1, 2].

Of the 415 patients with defects at the central 30° of the visual field in the ONTT research, 48% were with diffusive defects, while 52% were with focal defects. In these patients with focal defects, 20% had nerve fiber bundle-induced focal visual field defects (including vertical, arcuate, and nasal step defects), only 8% had a central scotoma, and 5% had hemianopia [2].

The pattern of visual field damage in optic neuritis is rooted in the part of the retina corresponding to the nerve fibers involved. In the anterior optic nerve, because the central retinal arteries and veins occupy the center of the optic nerve, the fibers from the macula are squeezed in the lateral upper and lower position of the optic nerves, the retinal fibers from the superior and inferior nasal retina are located in the medial superior and inferior positions of the optic nerves, and the superior and inferior temporal fibers are located in the lateral superior and inferior positions of the optic nerves. In the optic nerve 15 mm behind the eyeballs or beyond, due to no passage of retinal vessels any more, macular fibers gradually shift to the axis part of the optic nerve, fibers from the temporal retina shift to the temporal part of the optic nerve, fibers from the nasal retina shift to the nasal part of the optic nerve, and a similar fashion applies to the fibers from the superior and inferior retina. Therefore, the location of the optic neuritis and the involved retinal nerve fibers determine the corresponding visual field changes. In the optic nerve 15 mm behind the eyeballs or beyond, macular fibers occupy about 1/4 of the core space, so the visual field damage with a central defect is relatively common, but other types of defect may also be found [3, 4].

References

1. The Neurophthalmology Group of Ophthalmology Branch in Chinese Medical Association. Expert consensus on the diagnosis and treatment of optic neuritis (2014). Chin J Ophthalmol. 2014;50(6):459–62.
2. Zhang X, Jing Y. A practical case analysis in Neurophthalmology Department of Beijing Tongren Hospital. Beijing: Science Press; 2010.
3. Heijl A, Patella VM. Principle for Humphrey perimetry and analysis (Translated by Yuan Yuansheng). Beijing: People's Medical Publishing House; 2005.
4. Heijl A. The essence of visual reading analysis: the introduction to Humphrey perimetry analysis (Translated by Yuan Yuansheng). Shanghai: Shanghai Popular Science Press; 2013.

36 A Visual Field Defect Extending from the Physiological Blind Spot: Ischemic Optic Neuropathy or Normal Tension Glaucoma?

Xiaojing Pan, Ning Fan, and Xuyang Liu

An arcuate visual field defect connecting to the blind spot indicates that the lesion results from the damage to the nerve fiber bundle extending from the optic disc. How can we determine whether this damage is the manifestation of the acute phase of ischemic optic neuropathy (ION) or normal tension glaucoma (NTG)? This section focuses on the similarities and differences between the two diseases in terms of pathogenesis, as well as the key points of clinical differentiation.

36.1 Case 1

36.1.1 Case Presentation

A 51-year-old male patient complained of blurred vision without any obvious cause in his right eye for half a year. He denied any acute vision loss, pain on eye movement, eye distention, headache, or other discomforts. The history of trauma as well as other ocular, systemic, or familial diseases was denied.

The uncorrected visual acuity (UCVA) was 20/28 OD and 20/40 OS, and the best corrected visual acuities (BCVA) were 20/18 OD (+0.50DC*165) and 20/20 OS (+0.50 DS). Intraocular pressure (IOP) by standard Goldmann applanation tonometry was measured as 15 mmHg OU. Slit-lamp examination of his anterior segments was unremarkable. The light reflex of the pupils was sensitive. In the right eye, the cup-to-disc (C/D) ratio was 0.5; the superior neuroretinal rim thinning and the reflection of the superior retina nerve fibers disappeared (Fig. 36.1). In the left eye, the C/D ratio was 0.4, and there was no abnormity in the retina. The central corneal thickness was 562 μm OD and 566 μm OS. The diurnal IOPs were 13–16 mmHg OD and 12–16 mmHg OS.

Standardized automated perimetry showed that an arcuate scotoma extended from the blind spot in the inferior visual field of the right eye (Fig. 36.2) and the visual field of the left eye was normal.

The OCT results showed the retinal nerve fiber layer (RNFL) thickness in the superior quadrant of the right eye was reduced, and the RNFL thickness in the left eye was within normal limits (Fig. 36.3).

X. Pan
Shandong Eye Institute, Qingdao Eye Hospital, Qingdao, China

N. Fan
Shenzhen Eye Hospital, Shenzhen University, Shenzhen, China

X. Liu (✉)
Xiamen Eye Center of Xiamen University, Xiamen, China

Shenzhen Eye Hospital, Shenzhen University, Shenzhen, China

N. Wang et al. (eds.), *Optic Disorders and Visual Field*, Advances in Visual Science and Eye Diseases 2, https://doi.org/10.1007/978-981-13-2502-1_36

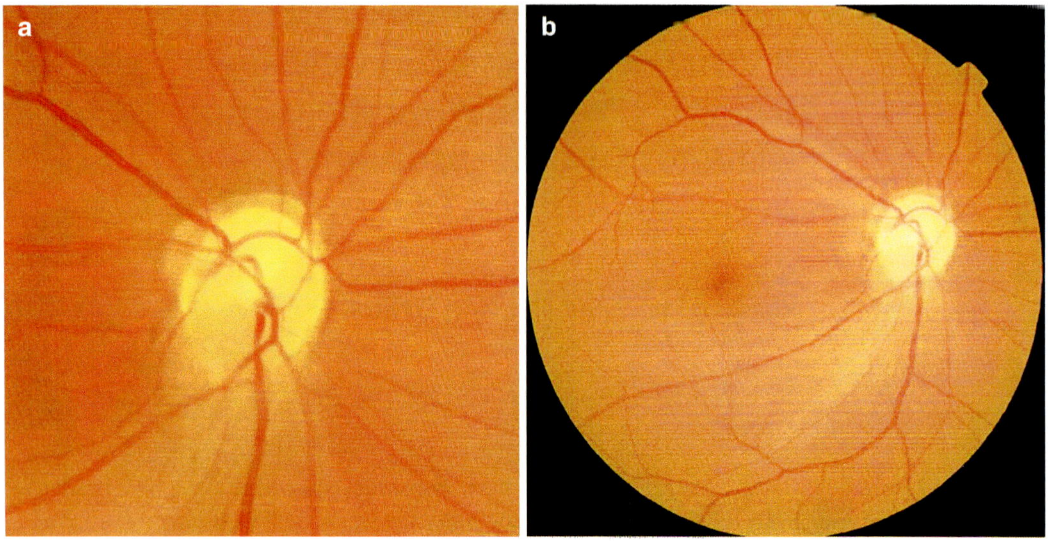

Fig. 36.1 Fundus photographs. Panel a: the C/D ratio was 0.5, and the superior neuroretinal rim was thinning. Panel b: the reflection of the superior retinal nerve fibers disappeared

The P-VEP results showed that the waveform of the P100 wave was normal in both eyes. In the right eye, under the stimulation at a low spatial frequency, the latency was normal, and the amplitude mildly decreased compared to that in the left eye; under the stimulation at a high spatial frequency, the latency was obviously delayed, and the amplitude slightly decreased compared to that in the left eye. In the left eye, the P100 wave was normal under the stimulation at both low and high spatial frequencies (Fig. 36.4).

The waveform of the P100 wave was normal in both eyes. In the right eye, under the stimulation at a low spatial frequency, the latency was normal, and the amplitude mildly decreased compared to that in the left eye; under the stimulation at a high spatial frequency, the latency was obviously delayed, and the amplitude slightly decreased compared to that in the left eye. In the left eye, the P100 wave was normal under the stimulation at both low and high spatial frequencies.

36.1.2 Final Diagnosis

The final diagnosis was ION (optic atrophy after the acute phase) or NTG in the right eye?

36.1.3 Case Review

The patient was a 51-year-old male with a complaint of decreased vision in the right eye for half a year, of which the onset had no obvious trigger and no definite time. There was no history of systemic diseases, such as abnormal blood pressure and diabetes. Examination showed normal intraocular pressure of the affected eye, decreased visual acuity, an arcuate scotoma which was connected to the physiological blind spot, and an enlarged and pale optic cupping. If we cannot figure out whether the patient had signs of the acute phase of ischemic optic neuropathy in the past, how could we make the diagnosis of NTG vs ION (optic atrophy after the acute phase)? In

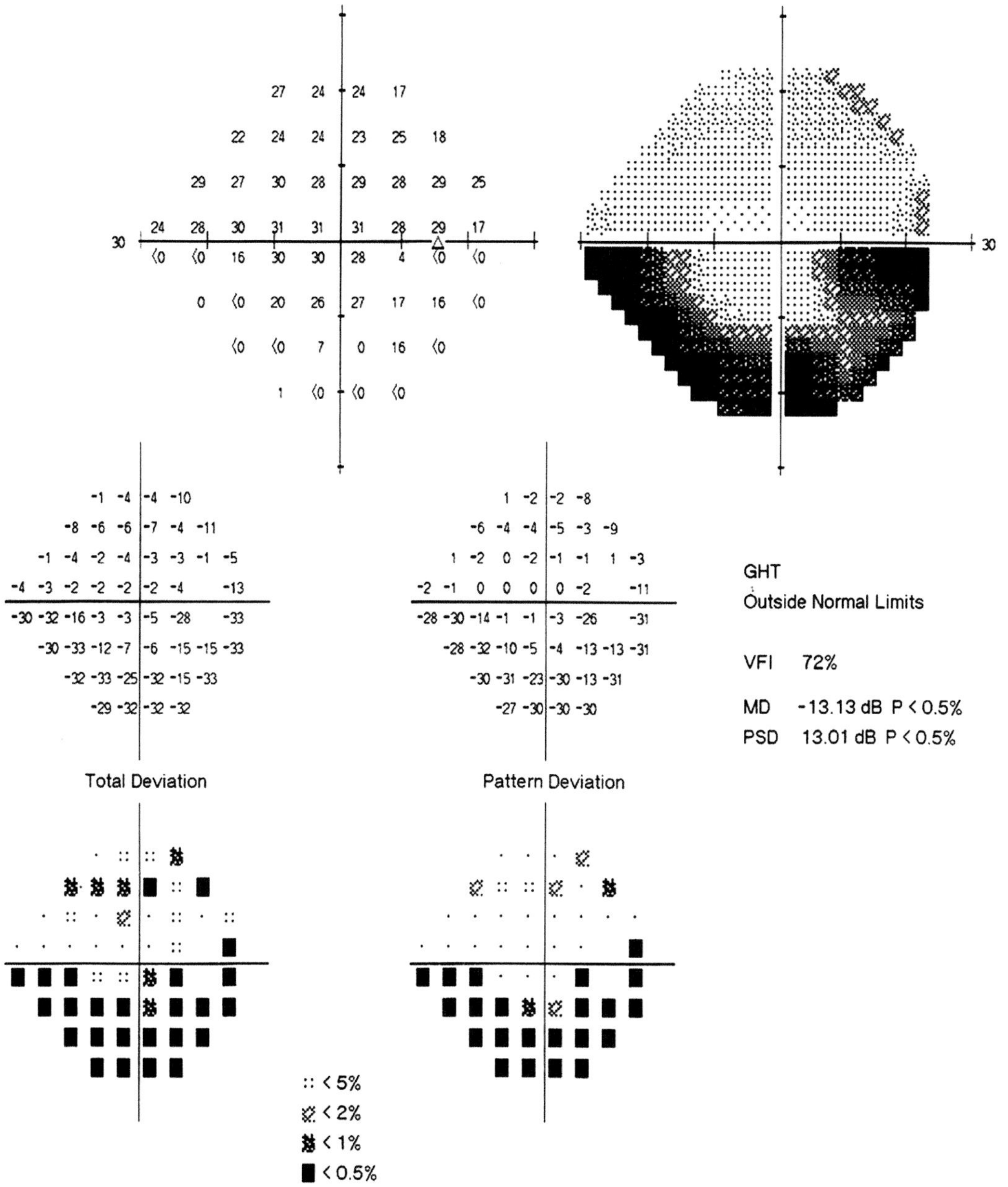

Fig. 36.2 Humphrey visual field analysis printout. The 24-2 test showed an inferior arcuate scotoma extending from the blind spot in the visual field of the right eye

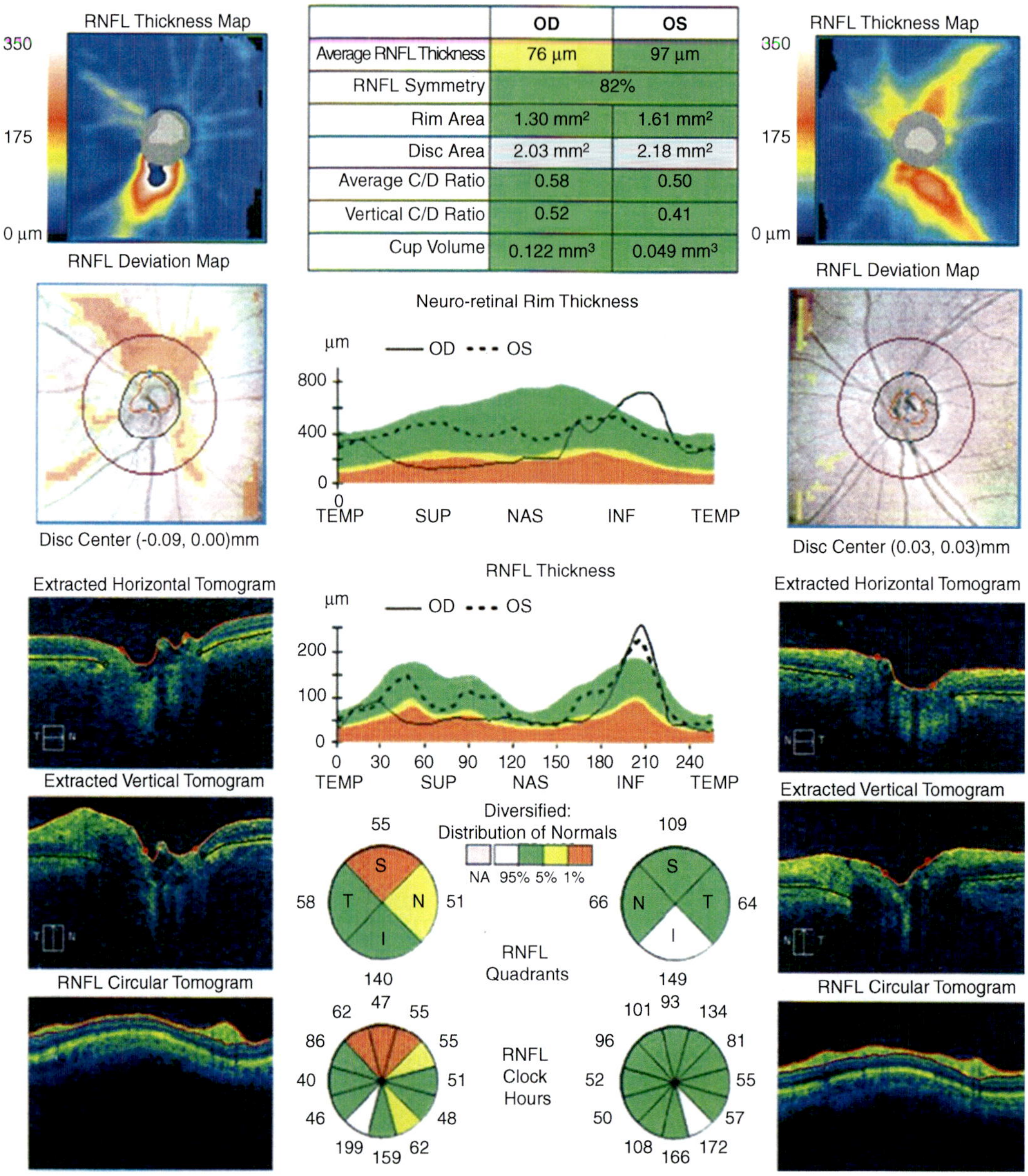

Fig. 36.3 OCT RNFL thickness analysis printouts. The RNFL thickness in the superior quadrant of the right eye was reduced, and in the left eye, it was within normal limits

this section, we will summarize the key points for the differential diagnosis of the two diseases (Table 36.1).

Based upon an in-depth review of this case, we found that there was evidence against NTG. Thus, our tentative diagnosis was ischemic optic neuropathy, and the reasons are as follows: (a) compared with that in typical glaucoma at moderate stage, the RNFL defect was relatively large in the affected eye; (b) the vision field showed an arcuate defect, without sparing the temporal side of the physiological blind spot; (c) the central corneal thickness (CCT) was not thinning; (d) the optic cup excavation was not deep, without vascular crawling and "bayonet-like" vessels; (e) there was a

Pattern-VEP

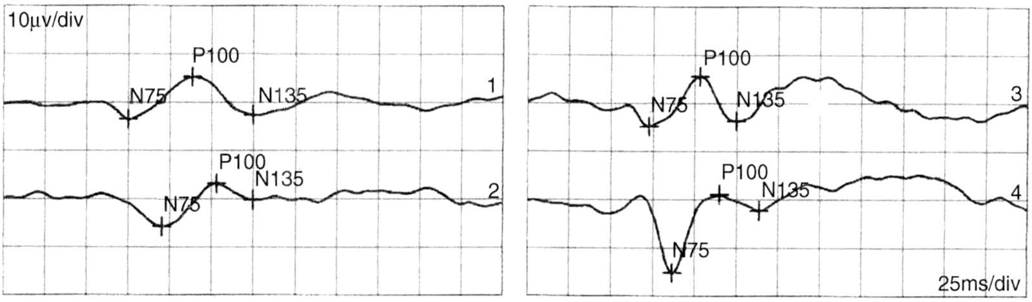

Channel	N75 [ms]	P100 [ms]	N135 [ms]	N75-P100	P100-N135
1 R-1 1,0	75	114	150	8.85µv	7.95µv
3 L-1 1,0	73	103	125	10.4µv	9.31µv
2 R-1 0,15	96	129 (!)	150	8.85µv	3.36µv
4 L-1 0,15	87	115	139	16.2µv	3.31µv
Normals	-	90-117-90-117	-	-	-

Channel	Stimulus	Ampl., Range, Filter
1 R-1 1,0	MON Patt. Rev. CB, 1?Full Field, Ctr:97% 1.5Hz, Avg:61	1, +/-100µv 1-50Hz
2 R-1 0,15	MON Patt. Rev. CB, 0?5' Full Field, Ctr:97% 1.5Hz, Avg:58	1, +/-100µv 1-50Hz
3 L-1 1,0	MON Patt. Rev. CB, 1?Full Field, Ctr:97% 1.5Hz, Avg:57	1, +/-100µv 1-50Hz
4 L-1 0,15	MON Patt. Rev. CB, 0?5' Full Field, Ctr:97% 1.5Hz, Avg:58	1, +/-100µv 1-50Hz

Fig. 36.4 P-VEP examination printouts

superior parapapillary atrophy; and (f) the patient was relatively old and with only one eye involved. However, there was no risk factor for anterior ischemic optic neuropathy (AION), i.e., a congested optic disc in the contralateral eye, and the pupil's response to light in the affected eye (the RAPD was negative) did not support the diagnosis, either. Therefore, we need to carry out FFA and, as necessary, cranial MRI, transcranial Doppler, and other neuroimaging examinations. Close follow-up of both eyes, even ruling out of Leber's disease, and nutritional therapy to improve circulation should all be considered, so as to make a correct differential diagnosis.

36.2 Case 2

36.2.1 Case Presentation

A 49-year-old male patient complained of feeling a shadow inferiorly over the right eye for several months. He denied pain on eye movement, eye distention, headache, or other discomforts. There was no history of trauma, other ocular diseases, or systemic or familial diseases.

In both eyes, the UCVA was 20/60. Best corrected visual acuities were 20/20 OU with refraction (−1.00 DS). IOP by standard Goldmann applanation tonometry was measured as 12 mmHg. Slit-lamp examination of his anterior segments was unremarkable. The direct light reflex was sensitive. In the right eye, the C/D ratio was 0.4, the color of the superior neuroretinal rim was pale, and the reflection of the superior RNFL was not observed (Fig. 36.5). In the left eye, the C/D ratio was 0.1, and there was no abnormity in the optic disc and the retina. The CCT was 520 µm OD and 522 µm OS.

Standardized automated perimetry showed an inferior arcuate scotoma connecting to the blind spot that was the most severe at the inferonasal quadrant in the right eye (Fig. 36.6).

36.2.2 Final Diagnosis

The right eye was AION in the right eye (optic atrophy after the acute phase).

The patient came back to the clinic 3 months later because of blurred vision in his left eye. The examination showed optic disc edema, noticeable pallor in the superior rim, and splin-

Table 36.1 Differentiation on the clinical manifestations and characteristics of NTG and ION

	Normal tension glaucoma NTG	Ischemic optic neuropathy ION
Onset characteristics	Mostly bilateral; with varying severities	Mostly unilateral; in 30–40% of cases, it might occur in two eyes; the bilateral visual field damage is relatively symmetrical
Visual acuity	The central vision is normal at the mild and moderate stages	Decreased central vision is usually observed
Visual field	Nasal step, paracentral scotoma, arcuate scotoma, annular scotoma, tube field, temporal island	Various types of visual field damage, with an arcuate scotoma connecting to the blind spot more often seen
Optic disc appearance	Vertical deepening and enlargement of the optic cupping could be seen; the residual neuroretinal rim is pink in color	The diseased part of the optic disc is pale (sometimes involved the temporal rim), and the cupping is relatively shallow; the pale area is bigger than the excavation area
RNFL	Slit-like or wedge-shaped RNFL defects which correspond to the rim notch and visual field damage sites are more often seen; diffuse defects can be observed at the advanced stage	The extent of RNFL atrophy is large, with a temporal atrophy being more common
FFA	Weak fluorescence in the optic disc can be found at the advanced stage	The fluorescence of the obstructed and non-obstructed areas in the disc is asymmetric
Contralateral eye	A large optic disc and a large optic cup are common	A small optic disc and a small optic cup ("crowded optic disc") can be observed
Refractive state	Myopia is common	Hyperopia or emmetropia is common
Pupils	Mostly normal	RAPD is positive when the unilateral visual function damage is serious
Intraocular pressure	Within normal range, sometimes with big fluctuations	Normal
CCT	Thinning is usually found	Normal
Family history	Family history of glaucoma	None
Systemic diseases	Hypotension, diabetes, migraine, or arteriosclerosis is often observed	Hypertension, diabetes, arteriosclerosis, massive bleeding, polycythemia, stenosis in carotid artery, or ophthalmic artery is commonly seen
Prognosis	Chronic progression can usually be found; central vision involvement or even blindness can be observed at the advanced stage	Decrease of the remaining central vision, optic atrophy, and visual field defects can be observed after acute stage; ipsilateral recurrence cases are rarely found

ter-shaped hemorrhage around the inferior rim of the left eye (Fig. 36.7). The infectious and immunological panels including erythrocyte sedimentation rate (ESR), C-reactive protein (CRP), antineutrophil cytoplasmic antibody (ANCA), and antinuclear antibody (ANA) were within normal limits. And syphilis, hepatitis B, and HIV infections were all excluded. The patient was diagnosed with non-arterial anterior ischemic optic neuropathy (NAION) in the left eye (acute phase).

36.2.3 Case Review

The first clinical findings in favor of NAION included superior neuroretinal rim being pale, reflection loss of the superior RNFL, an arcuate visual field defect connecting to the blind spot in the right eye, and smaller C/D ratio ("crowded optic disc") in the left eye. Though it is difficult to distinguish glaucoma from the sequela of AION by the visual field, the diagnosis of NAION can be confirmed for the patient based upon

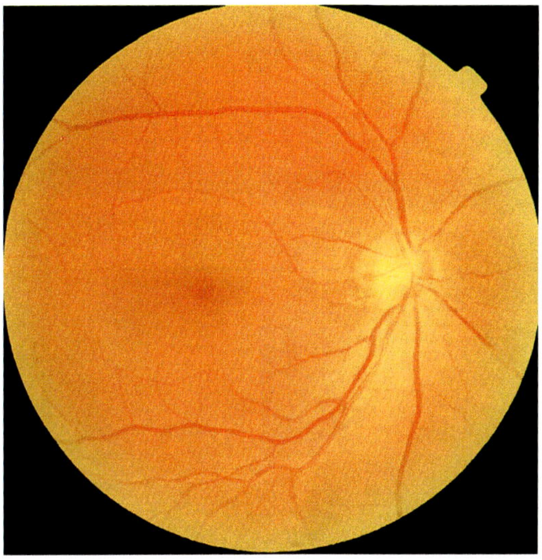

Fig. 36.5 Fundus photograph. The C/D ratio was 0.4, the color of the superior neuroretinal rim was pale, and the reflection of the superior RNFL disappeared

changes in the optic disc, neuroretinal rim, and RNFL. Acute onset of AION in the left eye 3 months later further confirmed the diagnosis. The patient developed AION in both eyes in a short period when he was only 49 years old. It is worth further exploration whether there are inflammatory factors involved in the onset of the disease and whether there are systemic underlying diseases.

36.3 Case 3

36.3.1 Case Presentation

A 43-year-old female patient complained that the visual acuity in her left eye had been decreasing for more than 1 month. She had no red and sore eyes, persistent shadow in front of eyes, metamorphopsia, or headache. The histories of trauma, other ocular diseases, and systemic or familial diseases were denied.

On examination, the UCVA was 20/40 OD and 20/60 OS. The BCVA was 20/20 OD (−5.00 DS) and 20/60 OS (plano). IOP by standard Goldmann applanation tonometry was 13 mmHg OU. Slit-lamp examination of her anterior segments was unremarkable except that the RAPD was positive in the left eye. In the right eye, the C/D ratio was 0.45, and wedge-shaped defects and loss of the reflection could be observed in the superior RNFL. In the left eye, the C/D ratio was 0.6, and the superior neuroretinal rim was slightly thinning with corresponding loss of reflection of the superior RNFL (Fig. 36.8). The CCT was 490 μm OD and 496 μm OS. Diurnal IOPs were measured as 12–15 mmHg OD and 11–14 mmHg OS.

Standardized automated perimetry showed an inferior paracentral scotoma in the visual field of the right eye and an inferior visual field defect in the left eye (Fig. 36.9).

36.3.2 Final Diagnosis

The final diagnosis was combined NTG and ION in the left eye and NTG in the right eye.

Bimatoprost ophthalmic solution was administered in both eyes, while compound anisodine hydrobromide, nimodipine, citicoline sodium, vitamin B, etc. were given to the left eye. The BCVA was then improved to 20/25 OS, and the visual field of the left eye showed significant improvement after 1 month of treatment (Fig. 36.10). The visual field of the right eye did not improve.

36.3.3 Case Review

Typical NTG was found in the patient's right eye. The visual field and optic disc shape conformed to the characteristics of glaucomatous damage. Meanwhile, the CCT was thin, and the IOP was not elevated. The visual field defect in the left eye involved the central area, and the vision acuity was compromised. The disease onset was sudden and its onset time was clearly identifiable. Also the treatment as for ischemic optic neuropathy was effective. Therefore, the diagnosis was combined AION and NTG. The coexistence of both diseases is very rare, and we will discuss the difference and association in pathogenesis between them later.

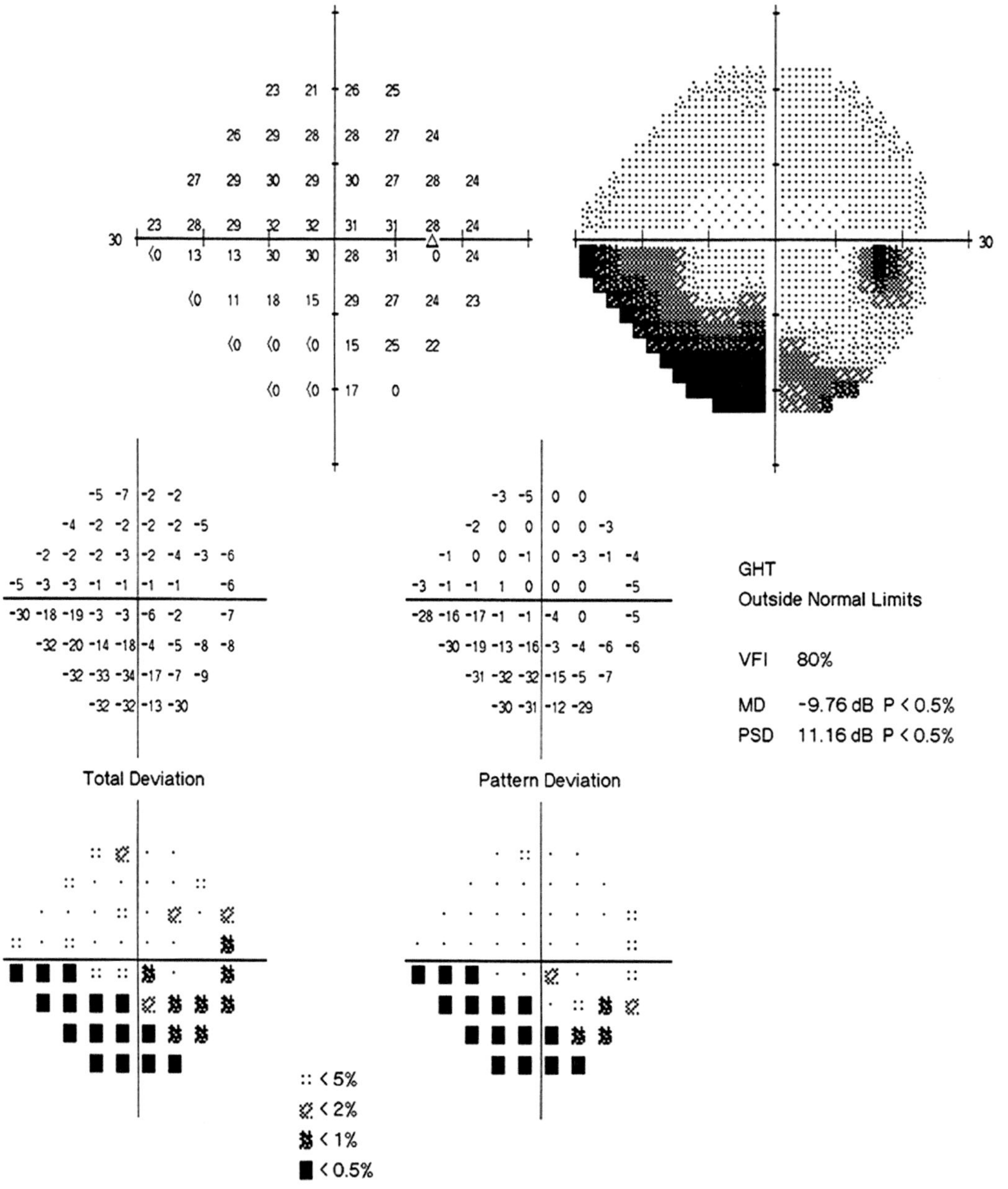

Fig. 36.6 Humphrey visual field analysis printout. The 24-2 test showed an inferior arcuate scotoma extending from the physiological blind spot that was the most severe at the inferonasal quadrant in the right eye

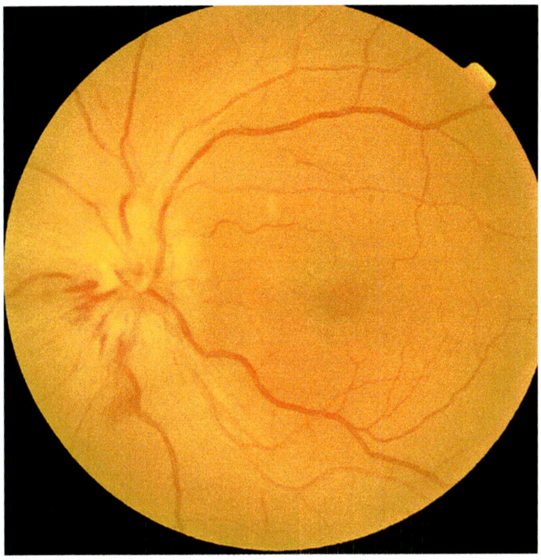

Fig. 36.7 Fundus photograph. Optic disc edema, pale color in the superior rim, and splinter-shaped hemorrhage around the inferior rim could be seen in the left eye

36.4 Case 4

36.4.1 Case Presentation

A 45-year-old male patient had suffered from glaucoma in both eyes for 6 months and had been treated with the medications for IOP lowering, but the compliance was not good. The patient felt that his eyes got tired easily, but no other discomfort was reported. He had a history of migraine for years and denied histories of trauma, other ocular diseases, and systemic or familial diseases.

On examination, the UCVA were 20/100 OU. Best corrected visual acuities were 20/20 OU with refraction (−4.50 DS). IOP by standard Goldmann applanation tonometry was 12 mmHg OU while being on medications. Slit-lamp examination of anterior segments was unremarkable.

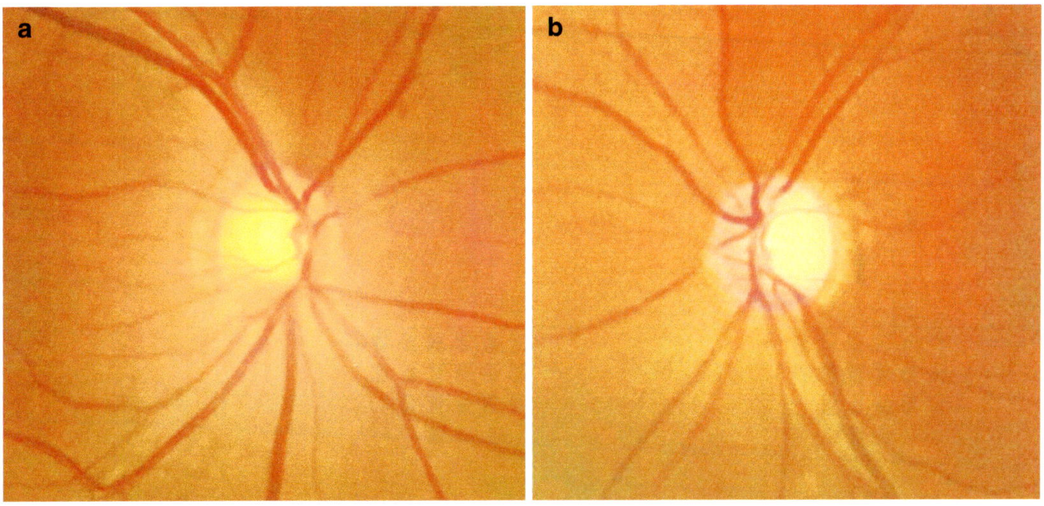

Fig. 36.8 Fundus photographs. Panel a: in the right eye, the C/D ratio was 0.45, and wedge-shaped defects and disappearance of the reflection were observed in the superior RNFL. Panel b: in the left eye, the C/D ratio was 0.6, and a thinning superior neuroretinal rim and disappearance of reflection of the superior RNFL were shown

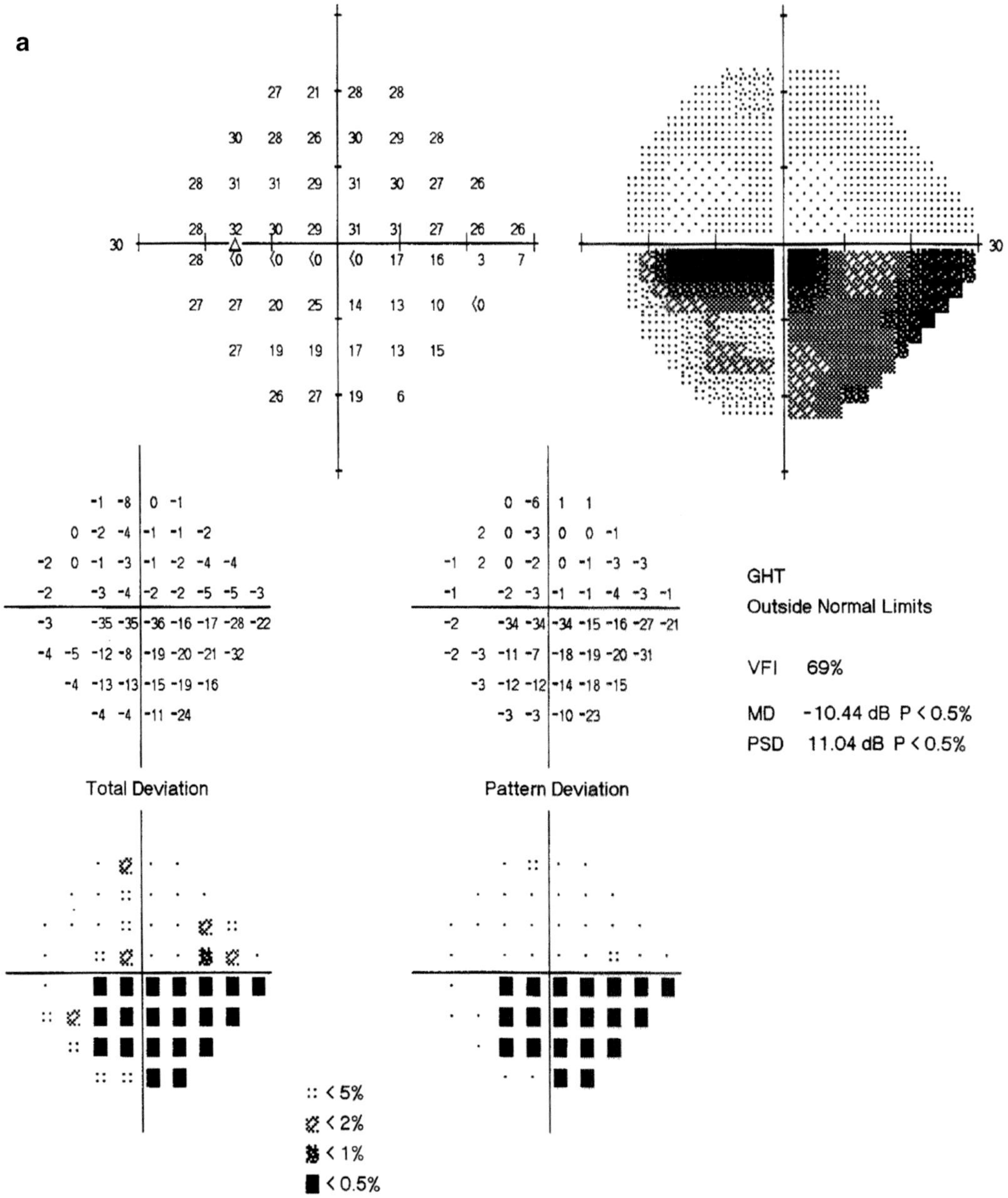

Fig. 36.9 Humphrey visual field analysis printouts. The 24-2 test revealed an inferior paracentral scotoma in the right eye and an inferior visual field defect in the left eye

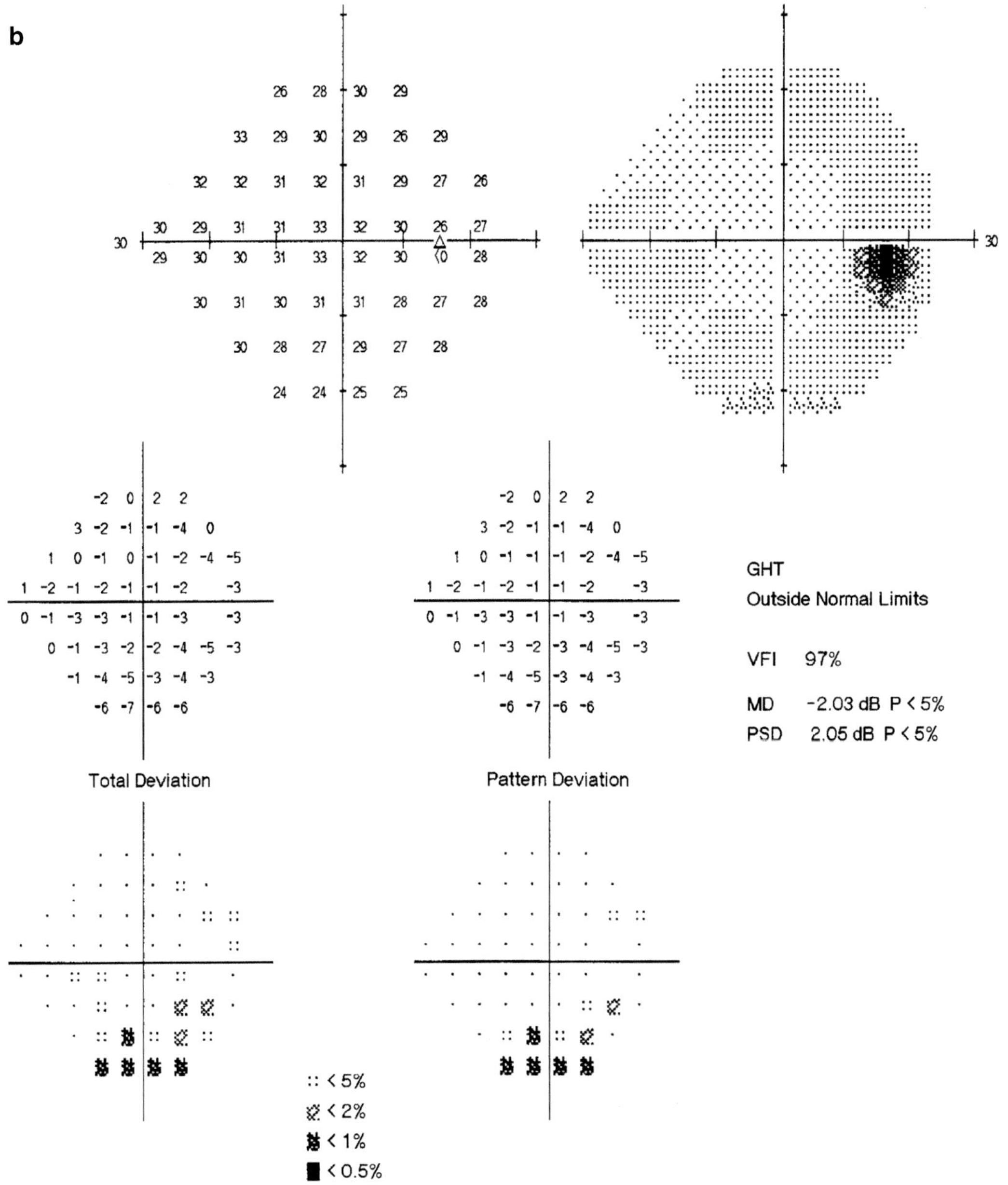

Fig. 36.9 (continued)

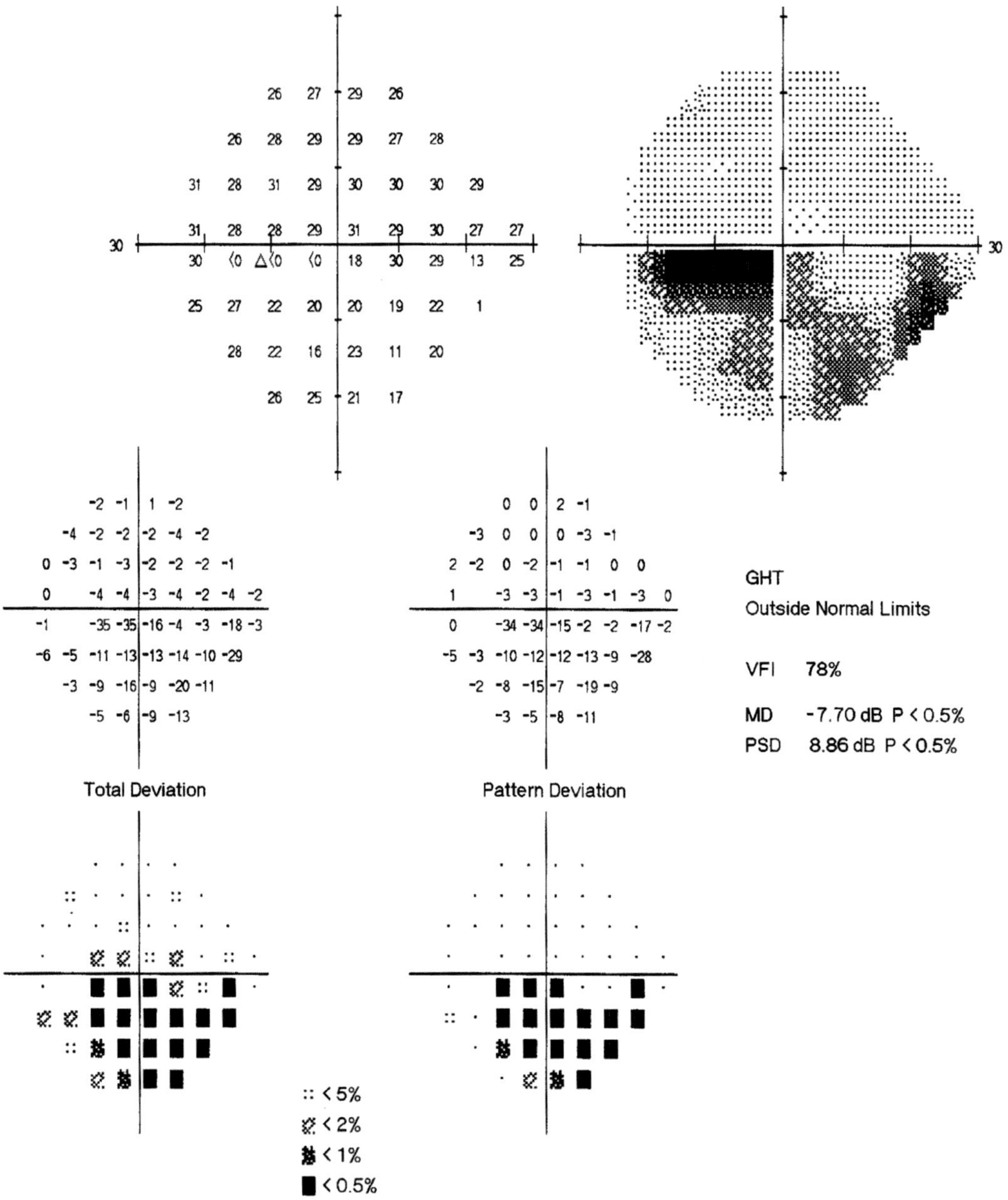

Fig. 36.10 Humphrey visual field analysis printout (re-examination after 1 month). The 24-2 test revealed an inferior visual field scotoma extending from the blind spot that showed improvement over the previous test result

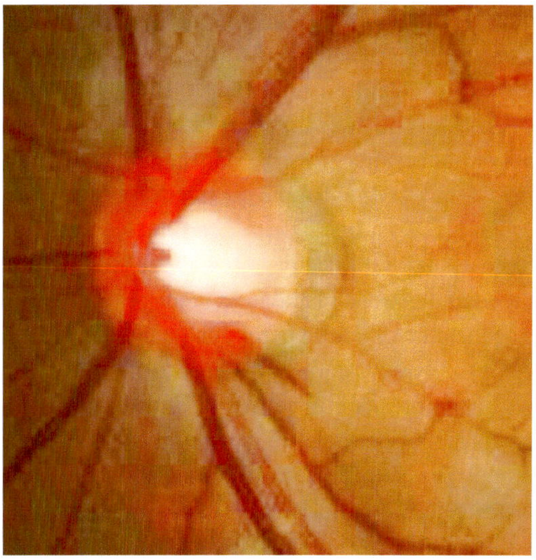

Fig. 36.11 Fundus photograph. The C/D ratio was 0.5 accompanied by splinter-shaped hemorrhage on the inferior rim and a slit-like RNFL defect in the left eye

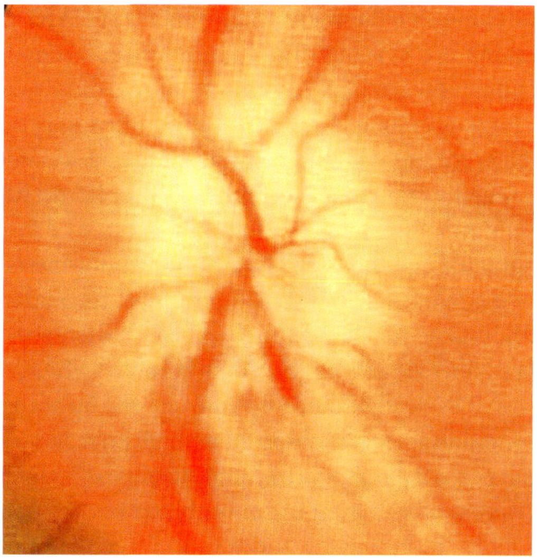

Fig. 36.12 Fundus photograph. Pale appearance, edema, inferior hemorrhage, venous tortuosity, and telangiectasis could be seen in the optic disc

In the right eye, the C/D ratio was 0.7, and wedge-shaped defects could be observed in the inferotemporal RNFL. In the left eye, the C/D ratio was 0.5 accompanied by splinter-shaped hemorrhage on the inferior rim and a slit-like RNFL defect (Fig. 36.11). The CCT was 496 μm OD and 501 μm OS.

36.4.2 Final Diagnosis

The final diagnosis was NTG in both eyes.

36.5 Case 5

36.5.1 Case Presentation

A 58-year-old male patient complained of sudden decreased vision in his left eye for 1 week. He had neither pain on eye movement nor a history of headache or cold. Histories of trauma and other ocular, systemic, or familial diseases were denied.

On examination, the UCVA was 20/200 OU, and it was not improved with refraction. IOP was normal OU. Slit-lamp examination of his anterior segments was unremarkable. In the right eye, the C/D ratio was 0.1, and the optic disc was pink in color with a clear boundary. In the left eye, pallor, edema, inferior hemorrhage, venous tortuosity, and telangiectasis could be observed in the optic disc (Fig. 36.12).

36.5.2 Final Diagnosis

The final diagnosis was NAION in the left eye (acute phase).

36.6 Discussion

The visual field changes in both NTG and ION after the acute phase can be manifested as an arcuate scotoma connecting to the physiological blind spot with a horizontal boundary. RNFL defects and/or a thinning neuroretinal rim at the corresponding site can also be found in both of them by fundus and OCT examinations [1]. It might be very difficult to make the differential diagnosis on both the diseases if we could not know whether the patient had acute manifestations of ischemic optic neuropathy or not, as in Case 1. Thus, we have summarized the following key points (Table 36.1).

Clinically, the coexistence of NTG and AION (as in Case 3) is rare. The former is usually found in the presence of myopia, a large optic disc, and a large optic cup. The latter is more often seen in the presence of hyperopia, a small optic disc, and a small optic cup. Dual factors of optic nerve ischemia and special anatomical structure of the optic disc are both involved in the pathogenesis of the two diseases. We will put emphasis on the discussion of the similarities and differences between the pathogeneses of NTG and ANION.

AION is an optic neuropathy caused by acute or serious ischemia observed in small branches of the posterior ciliary artery that supply the lamina cribrosa area or anterior area or blood vessels that supply the posterior optic nerves. Since the posterior ciliary artery is the terminal branch of the ophthalmic artery, it is very sensitive to the low perfusion caused by the blood pressure fluctuation. The sclerosis and stenosis of vascular walls, blood quality and volume abnormalities, etc. can all lead to ischemic optic neuropathy. The occurrence of AION has certain connection with a "disc at risk" [2]. Anatomical structure with a small optic disc diameter and C/D ratio ("crowded optic disc," usually seen in hyperopic eyes) will lead to crowding of the blood vessels and nerve fibers entering and exiting the lamina cribrosa and easy occurrence of ischemia in the small branches of the posterior ciliary artery. Each of the small branches of the posterior ciliary artery supplies a small part of nerve fibers in the optic disc, and a series of pathological changes caused by reduced blood supply, such as infarction, etc., can be found in the optic nerve fibers supplied by the branch if any branch or multiple branches develop ischemic optic neuropathy. The swollen optic nerve fibers have nowhere to go but squeeze each other because of the small optic disc and absence of an optic cup. Atrophy will finally be caused. In the obstructed area of the optic disc, color fading or pale appearance can be observed after the acute phase. The nerve fibers in the neuroretinal rim will reduce and be replaced by the glial tissues, resulting in excavation enlargement, but the area of paleness is significantly bigger than that of the excavation. The intensity of fluorescence revealed by FFA in the obstructed and non-obstructed areas is significantly asymmetric. The typical visual field change is an arcuate visual field defect connecting to the physiological blind spot, which proves that the disease is nerve fiber bundle damage starting from the optic disc. It can be free from a central defect since the disease rarely affects the papillomacular bundle. Such visual field change is easily confused with the glaucomatous visual field damage [3].

Systemic or ocular hemodynamic abnormality can usually be found in NTG patients [4]. Ocular perfusion pressure lowering will make the blood perfusion of the optic disc insufficient when the blood pressure and intraocular pressure are unbalanced or the blood viscosity increases, which will lead to ischemic damage to the small blood vessels in the optic disc and RNFL. The mechanism has been verified by FFA and hemorheological and hemodynamic studies. Hypotension, diabetes, migraine, and other cardiovascular diseases are also usually found in NTG patients clinically. However, compared with AION, NTG patients are younger when the disease occurs, and the mechanism of optic ischemia in it involves many non-systemic vascular factors. The anatomical structure of the optic disc in NTG patients may have certain defects, e.g., the connective tissue of the lamina cribrosa is thinner than that of the normal people, and the hole size in both upper and lower sides of the lamina cribrosa is big, which can more easily lead to collapse and backward excavation of the lamina cribrosa and distortion of the cribriform holes. The distorted cribriform holes will make the nerve fibers passing through them squeezed, and axoplasmic flow obstruction or compressive occlusion of the blood capillaries occurs, thus causing nutritional disturbance and finally atrophy in the optic nerves [5]. Studies have found that a longer ocular axis is often complicated by smaller wall hardness of eyeball and that a bigger excavation of the optic disc would more easily lead to glaucomatous excavation due to the impact of intraocular pressure. Therefore, clinically, NTG is usually found in the presence of myopia and a large optic cup.

With the progression of glaucoma, disturbances of axoplasmic flow and blood supply are observed in more and more nerve fibers. The lesion spreads upward along the neuraxon, and the nerve tissues in the neuroretinal rim reduce. More of the lamina cribrosa and distorted cribriform holes are exposed, and the optic disc excavation is further deepened and enlarged. The disease is characterized by chronic and progressive aggravation. Since the upper and lower connective tissues of the lamina cribrosa are the weakest, the upper and lower nerve fibers in the temporal optic disc are firstly damaged, and the undamaged nerve fibers are still shown as the neuroretinal rim in normal color. Therefore, glaucomatous optic cup enlargement is localized or diffused vertical enlargement, and the residual neuroretinal rim is in normal pink. This is exactly the important differentiation point for NTG and AION in terms of the optic cup enlargement caused by them.

Optic disc hemorrhage can be observed in different stages of both NTG and AION, as in Case 3 and Case 4, but the causes and clinical significances are different.

The optic disc hemorrhage in AION appears in the acute phase, and, due to the optic disc edema and flame-like hemorrhage in the shallow retinal blood capillaries beside the optic disc resulting from the acute or serious ischemia of the small branches of the posterior ciliary artery, it is usually connected with the ischemia severity. And infarction has usually been present in the nerve fibers corresponding to the hemorrhage focus. Optic disc hemorrhage in NTG is considered to be the risk factor of glaucoma progression, the occurrence rate of which increases gradually from the early stage to the middle stage and decreases gradually from the middle stage to the late stage. Optic disc hemorrhage is not observed in advanced glaucoma patients who are with no disc rim. Meanwhile, the recurrence rate of optic disc hemorrhage is relatively high in NTG, and the recurrence site may not be the original site as the recurrence tends to be distributed around the whole optic disc. Disc rim hemorrhage is indicative of vascular abnormalities and in a reciprocal causation relationship with glaucoma progression. Presumably, the optic disc hemorrhage in NTG is possibly caused by thrombosis, infarction, and rupture of microvessels. And then loss of corresponding nerve fibers and disc rim notch will appear, which is not completely identical with the ascending optic atrophy caused by POAG but similar to the mechanism of AION with the only differences being severity and acuteness. Therefore, NTG is different from the POAG in terms of pathogenesis and has similarities and common factors with AION. That is why some of the clinical manifestations of NTG and AION are easy to be confused and careful differentiation is required.

References

1. Cui H, Wang N. Ophthalmology. 2nd ed. Beijing: People's Medical Publishing House; 2014.
2. Zhang X, Jing Y. A practical case analysis in neurophthalmology. Beijing: Department of Beijing Tongren Hospital. Science Press; 2010.
3. Han S, Jung JJ, Kim US. Differences between nonarteritic anterior ischemic optic neuropathy and open angle glaucoma with altitudinal visual field defect. Korean J Ophthalmol. 2015;29(6):418–23.
4. Li M. Glaucoma. Beijing: People's Medical Publishing House; 2004.
5. Horowitz J, Fishelzon-Arev T, Rath EZ, et al. Comparison of optic nerve head topography findings in eyes with non-arteritic anterior ischemic optic neuropathy and eyes with glaucoma. Graefes Arch Clin Exp Ophthalmol. 2010;248(6):845–51.

37 Easily Ignored Signs of Non-arteritic Anterior Ischemic Optic Neuropathy: Secondary Serous Detachment in the Macula

Xiaojing Pan, Ning Fan, and Xuyang Liu

Non-arteritic anterior ischemic optic neuropathy (NAION) is a common optic nerve disease that is characterized by optic disc edema and visual field defects. Most of the previous treatments for and studies on NAION have been limited to the optic disc. With the widespread application of OCT in recent years, increased incidence of NAION complicated by serous detachment in the macula has been reported.

37.1 Case 1

37.1.1 Case Presentation

A 78-year-old male patient noticed sudden decreased vision in his right eye without any apparent cause for 2 weeks. He had no headache, eye pain, or red eyes. The visual acuity in the right eye was slightly improved after oral hormones were administrated at an unknown dose for 1 week in another hospital. He had been suffering from blurred vision in the left eye for more than 20 years due to optic atrophy. Histories of trauma, other ocular diseases, systemic diseases (including abnormalities of the blood pressure, blood sugar, blood lipid, etc.), and familial diseases were denied.

On examination, in the right eye, the uncorrected visual acuity (UCVA) was 20/400. Best corrected visual acuity (BCVA) was improved to 20/200 with refraction (+1.75DS). The light projection was accurate, and red and green colors could be distinguished. In the left eye, the UCVA was 20/400 without improvement with refraction, and the light projection was accurate. Intraocular pressure (IOP) was normal OU. Slit-lamp examination of his anterior segments was unremarkable except that the crystalline lens was not transparent. In the right eye, optic disc edema and hemorrhage were observed, without foveal reflex (Fig. 37.1). The optic disc was pale in color with a clear boundary in the left eye.

During the standardized automated perimetry, a diffuse depression was seen in the right eye (Fig. 37.2).

FFA showed significant delay in the filling of the central retinal artery at the early phase of the right eye. Weak fluorescence in the superior optic disc and telangiectasis in the optic disc could be seen at the middle phase. Strong fluorescence and significant fluorescein leakage were revealed in

X. Pan
Shandong Eye Institute, Qingdao Eye Hospital, Qingdao, China

N. Fan
Shenzhen Eye Hospital, Shenzhen University, Shenzhen, China

X. Liu (✉)
Xiamen Eye Center of Xiamen University, Xiamen, China

Shenzhen Eye Hospital, Shenzhen University, Shenzhen, China

N. Wang et al. (eds.), *Optic Disorders and Visual Field*, Advances in Visual Science and Eye Diseases 2, https://doi.org/10.1007/978-981-13-2502-1_37

the optic disc at the late phase. No fluorescein leakage point was observed in the macula during angiography (Fig. 37.3).

The F-VEP showed atypical F-VEP waveform, normal latency of the P1 wave, and significantly reduced amplitude of the P1 wave in both eyes (Fig. 37.4).

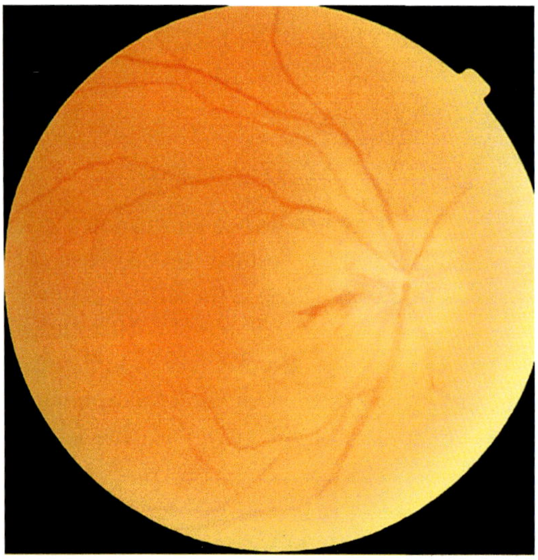

Fig. 37.1 Fundus photograph. Optic disc off-white edema and temporal linear hemorrhage were seen in the left eye. (Note: the image quality was slightly affected by phacoscotasmus)

The OCT of the macula revealed serous detachment of the sensory retina in the right eye. The subretinal fluid in the macula did not connect with the edematous optic disc (Fig. 37.5).

Blood sedimentation did not present any abnormality.

37.1.2 Final Diagnosis

The final diagnosis was NAION accompanied by secondary serous macular detachment of the neuroepithelium in the right eye.

37.1.3 Case Review

NAION is caused by local infarction in the supply area as a result of ischemia in small vascular branches of the posterior ciliary artery that supply the lamina cribrosa area or anterior area. It is clinically characterized by sudden decrease of vision, optic disc edema, and characteristic visual field defects (a fan-shaped defect connecting to the physiological blind spot). This patient was an elderly man who suffered acute decrease of unilateral vision and had a similar disease history in the contralat-

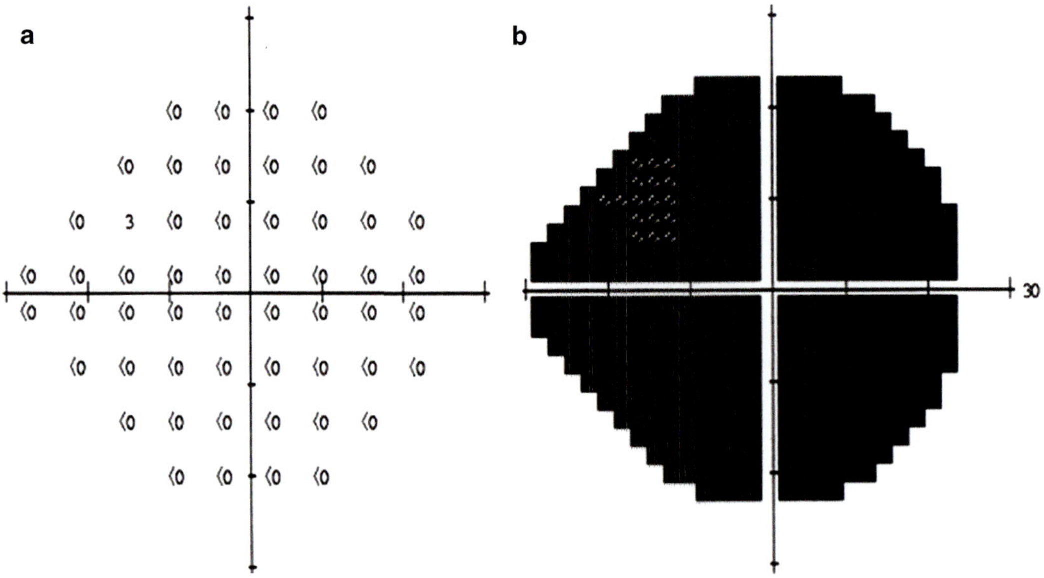

Fig. 37.2 The grayscale and threshold maps of Humphrey visual field assessment. The 24-2 test showed a diffuse depression of the visual field. Panel a: threshold map. Panel b: grayscale map

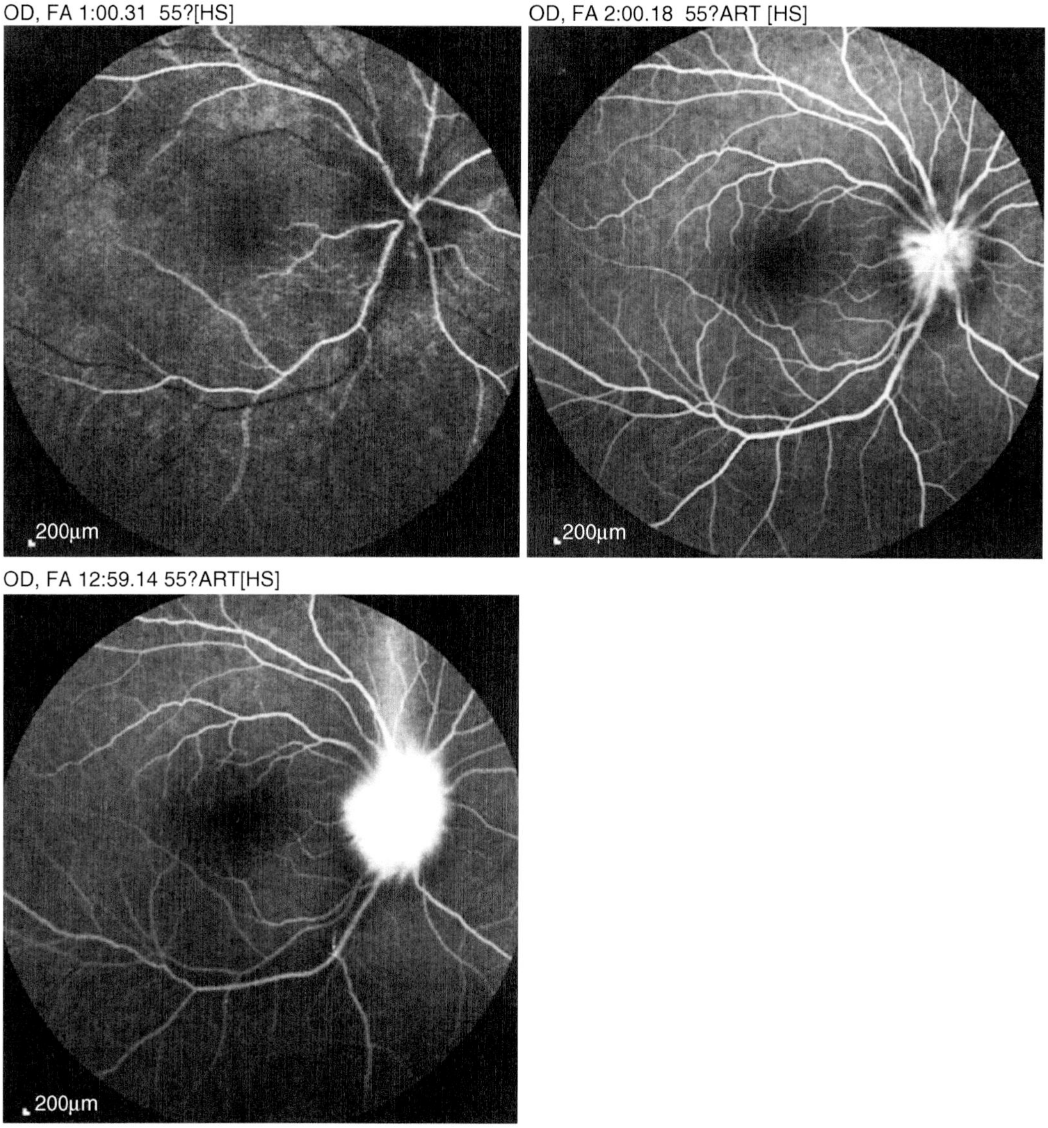

Fig. 37.3 FFA images. FFA showed significant filling time delay in the central retinal artery at the early phase of the right eye. Weak fluorescence in the superior optic disc and telangiectasis in the optic disc could be seen at the middle phase. Strong fluorescence and significant fluorescein leakage were revealed in the optic disc at the late phase. Panel a: the early-phase angiograph. Panel b: the middle-phase angiograph. Panel c: the late-phase angiograph

eral eye. He could be diagnosed with NAION according to the clinical manifestations. But he had some special characteristics, i.e., the vision, especially the visual field, showed serious diffuse damage; FFA indicated significant filling delay of the retinal artery at the early phase of angiography, but the central retinal artery occlusion could be excluded. OCT showed serous macular retinal detachment, but FFA revealed no fluorescein leakage point in the macular area.

The diffusive serious reduction of light sensitivity in the visual field of the patient's right eye suggested that the condition of NAION was serious. Significant filling delay in the retinal artery could be observed at the early phase of the

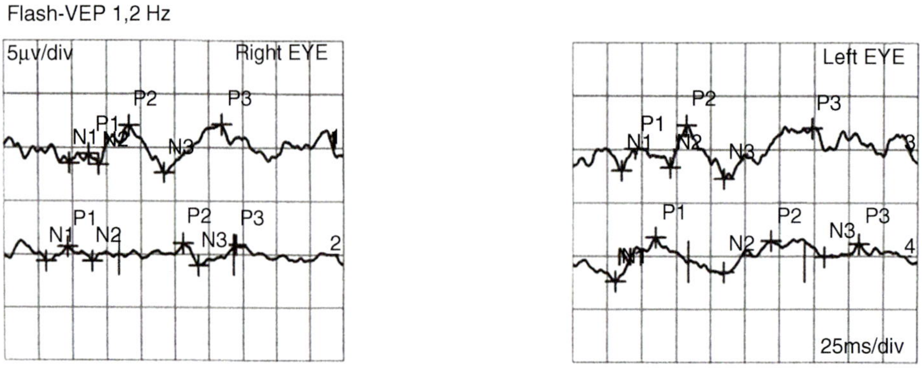

Channel	N1 [ms]	P1 [ms]	N2 [ms]	P2 [ms]	N3 [ms]	P3 [ms]	N1-P1	N2-P2	N3-P3
1 R-1 1,2 Hz	48	62	69	91	117	160	877nV	3.62µv	4.47µv
3 L-1 1,2 Hz	36	45	71	83	110	174	2.08µv	3.94µv	4.7µv
2 R-1 12 Hz	31	46	65	132	143	170	1.38µv	1.65µv	1.93µv
4 L-1 12 Hz	31	60	110	144	183	208	4.14µv	2.95µv	1.2µv
Normals	-	-	-	-	-	-	-	-	-

Channel	Stimulus	Ampl., Range, Filter
1 R-1 1,2 Hz	GF LED Flash 0dB (2,00 cds/m? 1.199Hz, Avg:34	1, +/-100µv 0.5-50Hz
2 R-1 12 Hz	GF LED Flash 0dB (2,00 cds/m? 11.905Hz, Avg:100	1, +/-100µv 0.5-50Hz
3 L-1 1,2 Hz	GF LED Flash 0dB (2,00 cds/m? 1.199Hz, Avg:35	1, +/-100µv 0.5-50Hz
4 L-1 12 Hz	GF LED Flash 0dB (2,00 cds/m? 11.905Hz, Avg:100	1, +/-100µv 0.5-50Hz

Fig. 37.4 F-VEP examination printouts. The F-VEP results showed atypical F-VEP waveform, normal latency of the P1 wave, and significantly reduced amplitude of the P1 wave in both eyes

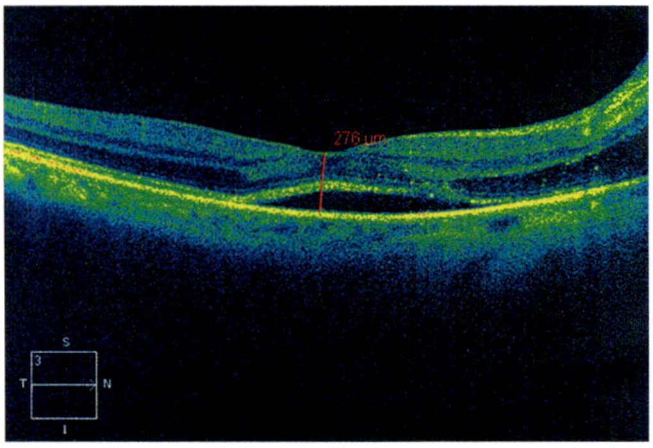

Fig. 37.5 Macular OCT images. Serous detachment of the sensory retina was seen in the macula. The subretinal fluid was not in contact with the edematous optic disc

FFA. The artery was completely filled at 1 min during angiography, but retinal arteries and veins could be completely filled at the middle and late phases without retinal leakage, indicating that there was serious low perfusion or obstruction in the ocular artery or internal carotid artery, which involved short posterior ciliary arteries supplying the superior and inferior anterior optic nerves and resulted in serious ischemic optic neuropathy. Therefore, the visual field was nearly total blindness. The cause of optic atrophy in the patient's contralateral eye was highly suspected to be NAION. The patient was advised to ask the internal medicine for consultation and undergo examinations including color ultrasonography of carotid artery, etc. to screen for severe atherosclerosis plaques in the internal carotid artery. The combined analysis of visual field and FFA was helpful for us to understand the NAION found in the patient.

37.2 Case 2

37.2.1 Case Presentation

A 61-year-old male patient complained of dim and blurred vision in the right eye for 3 days. He had no metamorphopsia or dark shadow in front of eyes and denied ocular diseases as well as histories of systemic diseases, trauma, or familial diseases.

On examination, the UCVA was 20/100 OD and 20/40 OS, and the BCVA was 20/20 OU. IOP was normal OU. Slit-lamp examination of his anterior segments was unremarkable except that the crystalline lens was slightly cloudy. Fundus examination revealed optic disc edema with an indistinctive boundary in the right eye and no foveal reflex; the optic disc of the left eye was pink in color with a distinctive boundary with a C/D ratio of 0.1 (Fig. 37.6).

Standardized automated perimetry revealed a relative scotoma extending from the blind spot that was the most severe at the inferonasal quadrant in the right eye (Fig. 37.7).

The OCT results showed optic disc swelling in the right eye. Serous neuroepithelium detachment was shown in the macula. The subretinal fluid was not in contact with the edematous optic disc (Fig. 37.8).

B-Mode ultrasonography indicated optic disc swelling in the right eye (Fig. 37.9).

Blood sedimentation did not show any abnormality.

37.2.2 Final Diagnosis

The final diagnosis was NAION accompanied by secondary serous macular detachment in the right eye.

37.2.3 Case Review

In this case, the onset was acute. The visual field defect was a relative scotoma connecting to the physiological blind spot. The optic disc edema was observed in the fundus. The findings conformed to the clinical characteristics of typical NAION. Local serous detachment was confirmed in the macular OCT scanning. The central vision was still 20/20, but the cause, mechanism, and clinical implications of the macular lesion deserved to be discussed.

37.3 Discussion

NAION is a clinically common optic nerve disease. It is usually found in middle-aged and senior patients over the age of 50. The disease onset can be unilateral or bilateral. The characteristics are sudden painless decrease of vision, localized or diffuse off-white edema in the optic disc, and arcuate and half- or multi-quadrant visual field defects.

The patients in both the above cases were middle-aged and aged males with acute unilateral onset and pale edema of the optic disc. Both of them could be diagnosed with NAION

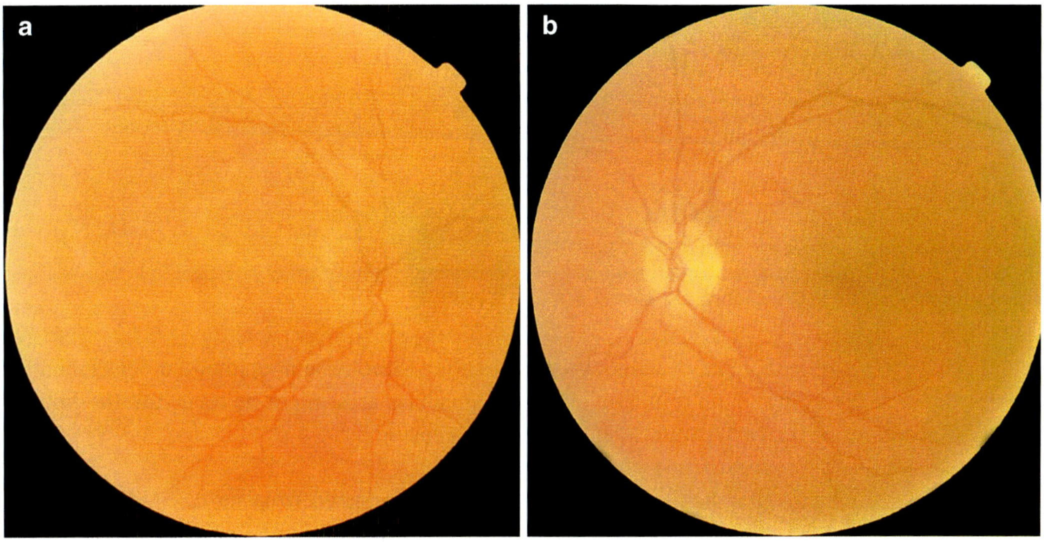

Fig. 37.6 Fundus photographs. Panel a: optic disc edema with an unclear boundary was noted in the right eye. Panel b: small optic cup was seen in the left eye (Note: the image quality was mildly affected by phacoscotasmus)

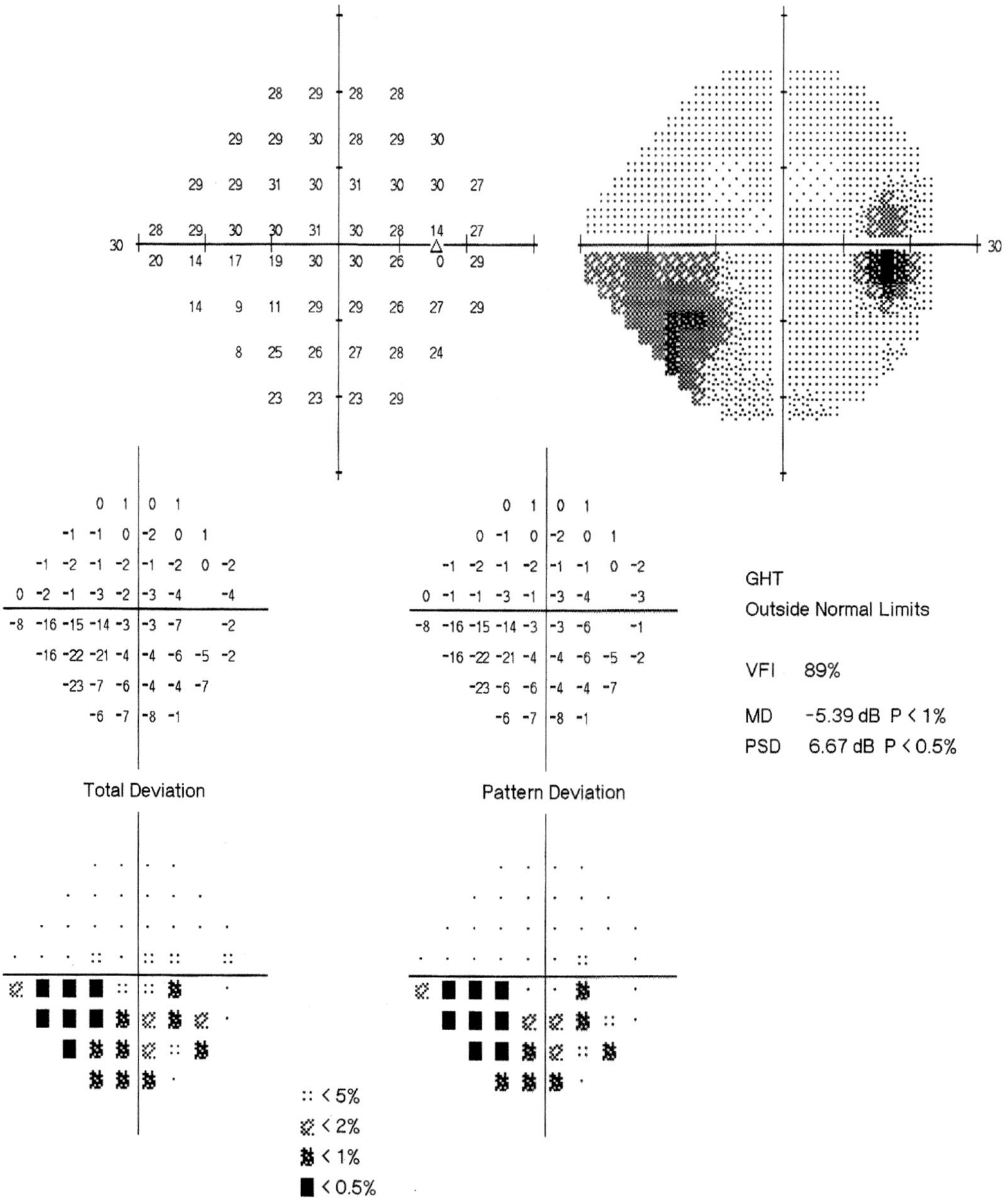

Fig. 37.7 Humphrey visual field analysis printout. The 24-2 test showed a relative defect extending from the blind spot that was the most severe in the inferonasal quadrant in the right eye

complicated by neuroepithelium detachment in the macular area according to the results of auxiliary examinations. The two patients showed different visions and prognoses due to different severities and extents of ischemia. However, both of them experienced serous neuroepithelium detachment in the macular area, which was relatively rare and had not received enough clinical attention. Serous neuroepithelium detachment in the macular area might be related to the following factors [1]:

(a) It is originated from the asymmetric edema of the optic disc: The asymmetric edemas in the upper and lower parts of the optic disc lead to an uneven stress on the optic disc.

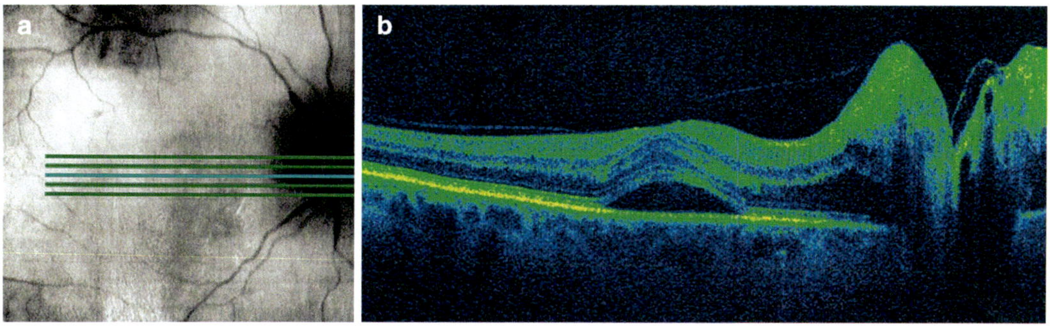

Fig. 37.8 OCT macula and optic disc scanning (9 mm linear scanning). Panel a: scanning site. Panel b: in the right eye, optic disc swelling, serous macular detachment, and subretinal fluid not in contact with the edematous optic disc were seen

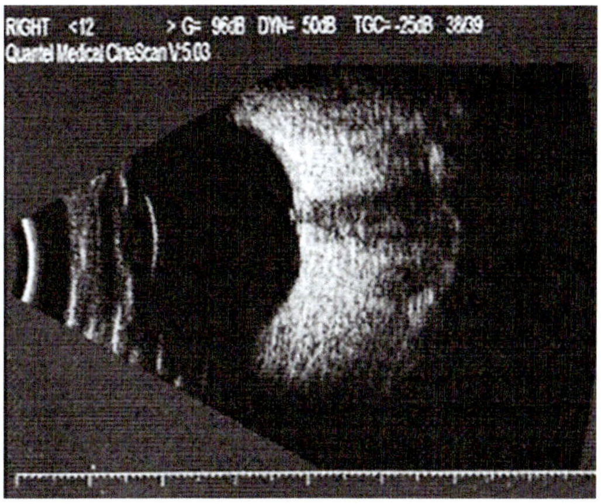

Fig. 37.9 B-ultrasound image. B-Mode ultrasonography indicated optic disc swelling in the right eye

When the edema was serious, the Kuhnt neuroglia tissues would be damaged, causing the fluid to flow between the retinal neuroepithelium and pigment epithelium and the optic disc fluid leakage to accumulate in the macular fovea.

(b) It is caused by the inflammation of the blood capillaries around the macula lutea: The inflammation causes abnormal permeability of the perifoveal retinal capillaries. The fluid leakage causes the neuroepithelium detachment at the fovea.

(c) It is caused by the leakage of the blood capillaries around the macula lutea: When optic disc edema was serious, the backflow of the venous blood was blocked, resulting in fluid leakage and accumulation in the neuroepithelium due to elevated internal pressure of the blood capillaries.

(d) It is caused by RPE barrier damage: The serous detachment of the sensory layer of the retina occurs due to "pump function" insufficiency and barrier function damage at the RPE level. The primary diseases of the choriocapillaris are also involved in the onset of this disease.

There are still no confirmed conclusions for the above deduction. The serous macular detachment will resolve with the resolution of optic disc edema, which suggests that the serous neuroepithelium detachment in the macula is closely related to optic disc edema. Since there is no leakage focus in the macula and FFA reveals no macular leakage point, the neuroepithelium detachment in the macula would usually be neglected [2]. The optic disc edema found in such patients is usually serious. Appropriate hormone therapy to alleviate the tissue edema at the early stage is essential for the recovery of neuroepithelium detachment in the macula and the improvement of vision. The pathological mechanism and clinical implication of neuroepithelium detachment in the macular area still need to be further studied.

It is worth pointing out that NAION complicated by neuroepithelium detachment in the macular area shall be distinguished from central serous chorioretinopathy (CSCR) which would occur when NAION is treated with glucocorticoids [3]. CSCR is a side effect of hormone application, which would cause macular serous retinal detachment and characteristic RPE lesions.

References

1. Xiaojun Z, Yun J. A practical case analysis in Neurophthalmology Department of Beijing Tongren Hospital. Beijing: Science Press; 2010.
2. Hedges TR, Vuong LN, Gonzalez-Garcia AO, et al. Subretinal fluid from anterior ischemic optic neuropathy demonstrated by optic coherence tomography. Arch Ophthalmol. 2008;126(6):812–5.
3. Alkin Z, Yilmaz I, Ozkaya A, et al. Steroid-induced central serous chorioretinopathy in a patient with non-arteritic anterior ischemic optic neuropathy. Saudi J Ophthalmol. 2015;29(3):232–4.

38 Optic Disc Vasculitis with Inconsistent Visual Field and Fundus Changes

Xiaojing Pan, Ning Fan, and Xuyang Liu

The signs of optic disc vasculitis usually include hyperemia and edema of the optic disc, tortuosity and dilation of retinal veins, and exudative hemorrhages of the optic disc and retina, while the damage to the visual field in impaired eyes was clinically insignificant. Therefore, clinical signs in the visual field and visual acuity are important for the differential diagnosis of it from other diseases with similar clinical presentations. Optic disc vasculitis is not uncommon in clinic. A selected case is presented as follows.

38.1 Case

38.1.1 Case Presentation

A 27-year-old female patient complained of dim vision in the right eye that had occurred without any obvious cause 2 months before. She had no red and sore eyes, metamorphopsia, shadow in the vision, or other discomforts. Histories of trauma and other ocular, systemic, or familial diseases were denied.

On examination, the uncorrected visual acuity (UCVA) was 20/200 OU, and the best corrected visual acuity (BCVA) was 20/20 OU. Light projection was accurate. Red and green colors could be distinguished. Intraocular pressure (IOP) was normal OU. Slit-lamp examination of her anterior segments was unremarkable. The relative afferent pupillary defect (RAPD) was negative. The right fundus showed optic disc hyperemia and edema, peripapillary telangiectasias, hemorrhages and exudates, and significantly tortuous superior temporal branch retinal vein (Fig. 38.1), while the left fundus was unremarkable.

FFA showed telangiectasia and microangioma of the optic disc at the arteriovenous phase. At the late phase, fluorescent staining and fluorescein leakage could be seen in the optic disc vessels (Fig. 38.2).

Standardized automated perimetry showed an enlarged physiological blind spot and paracentral defect at the inferonasal side of the right eye (Fig. 38.3).

The P-VEP results showed the waveform, latency, and amplitude of the P100 wave were normal in both eyes (Fig. 38.4).

X. Pan
Shandong Eye Institute, Qingdao Eye Hospital, Qingdao, China

N. Fan
Shenzhen Eye Hospital, Shenzhen University, Shenzhen, China

X. Liu (✉)
Xiamen Eye Center of Xiamen University, Xiamen, China

Shenzhen Eye Hospital, Shenzhen University, Shenzhen, China

N. Wang et al. (eds.), *Optic Disorders and Visual Field*, Advances in Visual Science and Eye Diseases 2, https://doi.org/10.1007/978-981-13-2502-1_38

38.1.2 Final Diagnosis

The diagnosis was Type I optic disc vasculitis in the right eye.

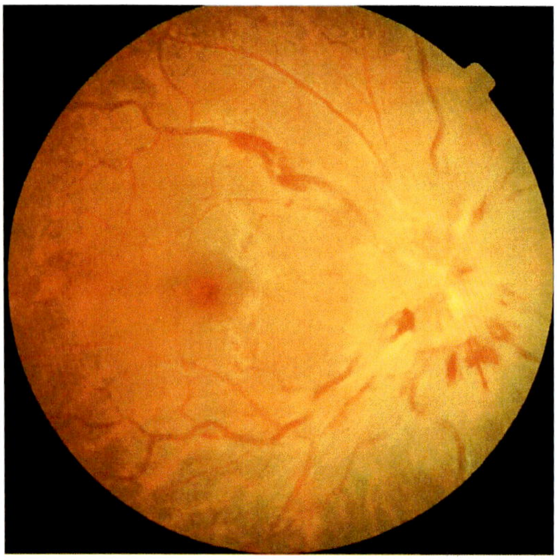

Fig. 38.1 Fundus photograph. The right fundus photograph indicated optic disc congestion and edema, peripapillary telangiectasias, hemorrhage and leakage, and obviously tortuous superior temporal branch retinal vein

38.2 Discussion

Optic disc vasculitis is a kind of inflammation which is limited to the vessels inside the papilla of the optic nerve, occurring usually in the vein of the optic disc [1]. The disease can be found in both men and women, mostly in young adults, and usually affects one eye. Optic disc vasculitis is divided into two types according to the clinical features, one of which is optic disc edema caused by inflammation of subbranches of ciliary vessels inside the optic nerve, called Type I optic disc vasculitis, while the other is central retinal vein occlusion caused by inflammation of the central retinal vein and its branches inside the optic disc, called Type II optic disc vasculitis [2].

The patient was diagnosed with Type I optic disc vasculitis. It is manifested clinically as edema and hemorrhage of the optic disc, retinal vein engorgement and tortuosity, formation of microaneurysm on the optic disc and high-degree capillary dilatation seen by FFA, and no obvious change in the artery. Optic disc vasculitis occurs in the anterior area of the optic disc, and it causes the permeability of the vascular wall increases, and the exudates accumulate in the loose tissue of

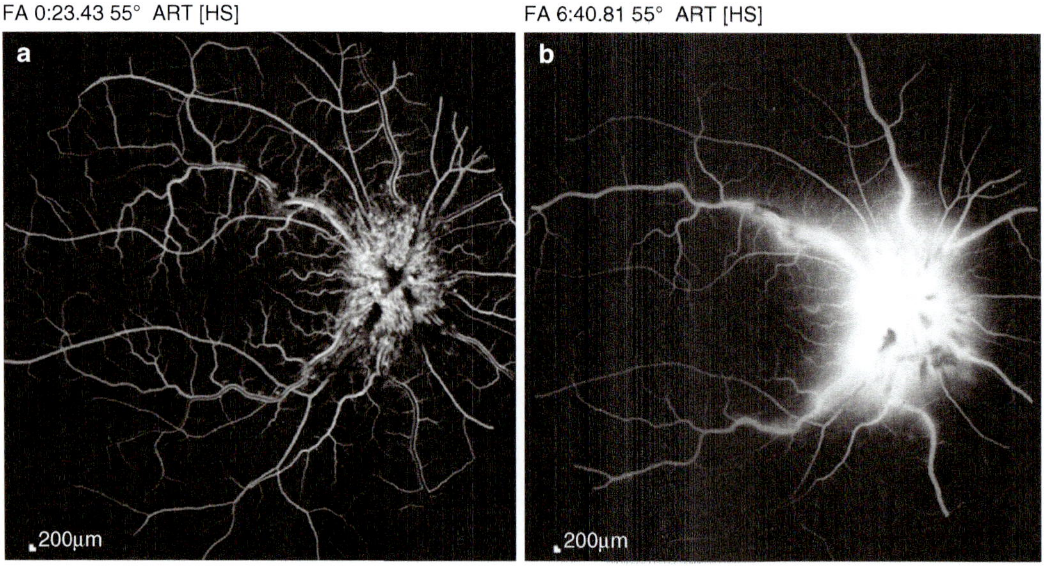

Fig. 38.2 FFA images. Panel a: telangiectasia and microangioma of the optic disc were seen at the arteriovenous phase. Panel b: staining and fluorescein leakage of the optic disc vessels were seen at the late phase

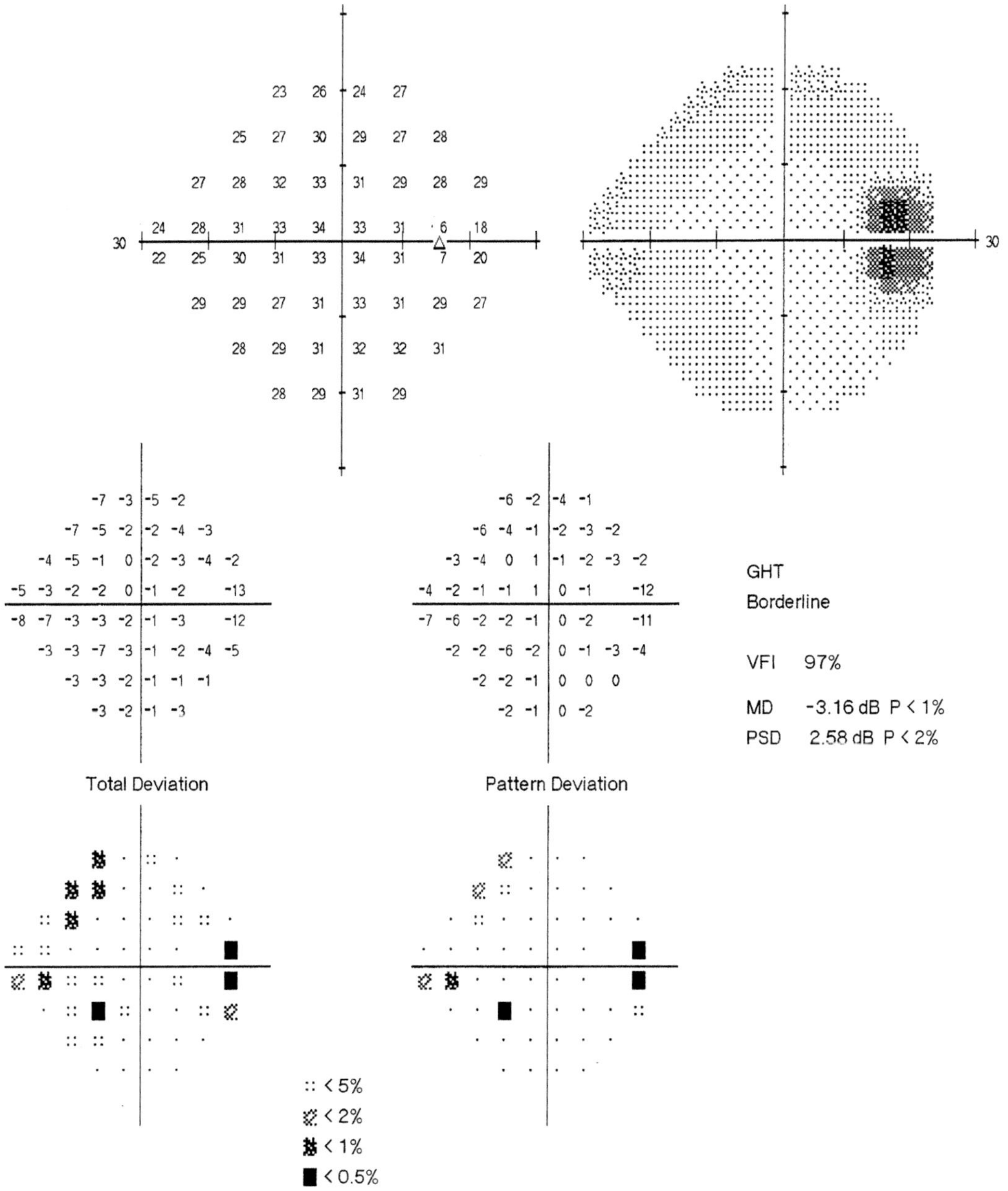

Fig. 38.3 Humphrey visual field analysis printout. The 24-2 test showed an enlarged physiological blind spot and paracentral defect at the inferonasal side of the right eye

anterior lamina cribrosa; these lead to aggravation of optic disc edema, significant blockage of blood flow, and increased fluorescence leakage through vascular wall [3]. But since the inflammation does not involve the central retinal artery and posterior ciliary artery, there is no significant influence on the artery blood supply to the retina, choroid, and posterior optic nerve, nor is there obvious effect on the macular area. So the impairment of visual acuity and visual field is relatively mild, presenting a seeming inconformity between visual field and fundus lesions.

Optic disc vasculitis has typical clinical manifestations, characterized by inconspicuous visual

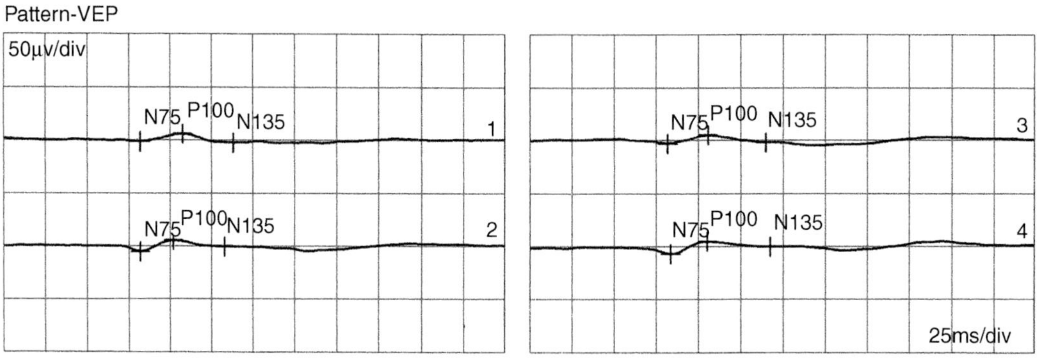

Channel	N75 [ms]	P100 [ms]	N135 [ms]	N75-P100	P100-N135
1 R-1 1,0	82	108	139	7.8µv	8.64µv
3 L-1 1,0	82	106	140	8.27µv	7.28µv
2 R-1 0,15	82	102	133	10.8µv	6.09µv
4 L-1 0,15	84	106	143	11.7µv	4.9µv
Normals	-	90-116-90-116	-	-	-

Channel	Stimulus	Ampl., Range, Filter
1 R-1 1,0	MON Patt. Rev. CB, 1?Full Field, Ctr:97% 1.5Hz, Avg:34	1, +/-100µv 1-50Hz
2 R-1 0,15	MON Patt. Rev. CB, 0?5' Full Field, Ctr:97% 1.5Hz, Avg:41	1, +/-100µv 1-50Hz
3 L-1 1,0	MON Patt. Rev. CB, 1?Full Field, Ctr:97% 1.5Hz, Avg:34	1, +/-100µv 1-50Hz
4 L-1 0,15	MON Patt. Rev. CB, 0?5' Full Field, Ctr:97% 1.5Hz, Avg:37	1, +/-100µv 1-50Hz

Fig. 38.4 P-VEP examination printouts. The waveform, latency, and amplitude of the P100 wave were normal in both eyes

function damage; thereby a differentiation from optic disc neuritis, retinal vein occlusion, retinal optic neuritis and ischemic optic neuropathy, and other diseases, which usually have an obvious damage to visual function, can be made. The damage to the vision field and visual acuity is an important basis for the differential diagnosis of this disease.

References

1. Zhang H. Atlas of ocular fundus diseases. Beijing: People's Medical Publishing House; 2007.
2. Liu Q, Fang Y. Optic disc diseases. Beijing: People's Medical Publishing House; 2015.
3. Oh KT, Oh DM, Hayreh SS. Optic disc vasculitis. Graefes Arch Clin Exp Ophthalmol. 2000;238(8): 647–58.

39 Diagnosis of Non-glaucomatous Optic Nerve Cupping Using Visual Field

Xiaojing Pan, Ning Fan, and Xuyang Liu

Non-glaucomatous optic nerve cupping is not uncommon clinically, and it is sometimes challenging to differentiate it from glaucomatous optic nerve cupping. In addition to structural assessment of the optic disc, optic cup, and neuroretinal rim, the visual field is also important for the differentiation between non-glaucomatous and glaucomatous optic nerve cupping. This section illustrates this from the perspective of the visual field.

39.1 Case 1

39.1.1 Case Presentation

A 60-year-old male patient complained of decreased vision in his right eye for many years. The patient had been diagnosed with "normal tension glaucoma" in another hospital, but he did not regularly take medications. The patient had no red and sore eyes, headache, and pain on eye movement or other discomforts in the right eye and denied a history of suddenly decreased vision in his right eye. Systemic disease histories and familial disease histories were also denied.

On examination, the uncorrected visual acuity (UCVA) was 20/200 OS with no improvement with refraction. UCVA was 20/25, and best corrected visual acuity (BCVA) was 20/20 OD with refraction (+1.25DS). Intraocular pressure (IOP) by standard Goldmann applanation tonometry was 12 mmHg OD and 13 mmHg OS. In both eyes, slit-lamp examination of his anterior segments was unremarkable, and the pupil size was 3 mm in diameter. Relative afferent pupillary defect (RAPD) was positive in the right eye. Fundus examination showed that the C/D ratio was 0.9 OD and 0.8 OS (Fig. 39.1).

39.1.2 Case Analysis

The patient was an elderly male. He presented with large optic cups in both eyes, yet the intraocular pressure was normal. Was the cupping physiologic or pathologic? Was it glaucomatous or non-glaucomatous? Was it from normal tension glaucoma? Were the eyes suffering from the same disease? Morphologically, the patient had a significantly enlarged optic cup and deep excavation in both eyes; his right eye showed deeper excavation, rim pallor, and absence of reflection of retinal nerve fibers; in the left eye, the color of the neuroretinal rim was

X. Pan
Shandong Eye Institute, Qingdao Eye Hospital, Qingdao, China

N. Fan
Shenzhen Eye Hospital, Shenzhen University, Shenzhen, China

X. Liu (✉)
Xiamen Eye Center of Xiamen University, Xiamen, China

Shenzhen Eye Hospital, Shenzhen University, Shenzhen, China

N. Wang et al. (eds.), *Optic Disorders and Visual Field*, Advances in Visual Science and Eye Diseases 2, https://doi.org/10.1007/978-981-13-2502-1_39

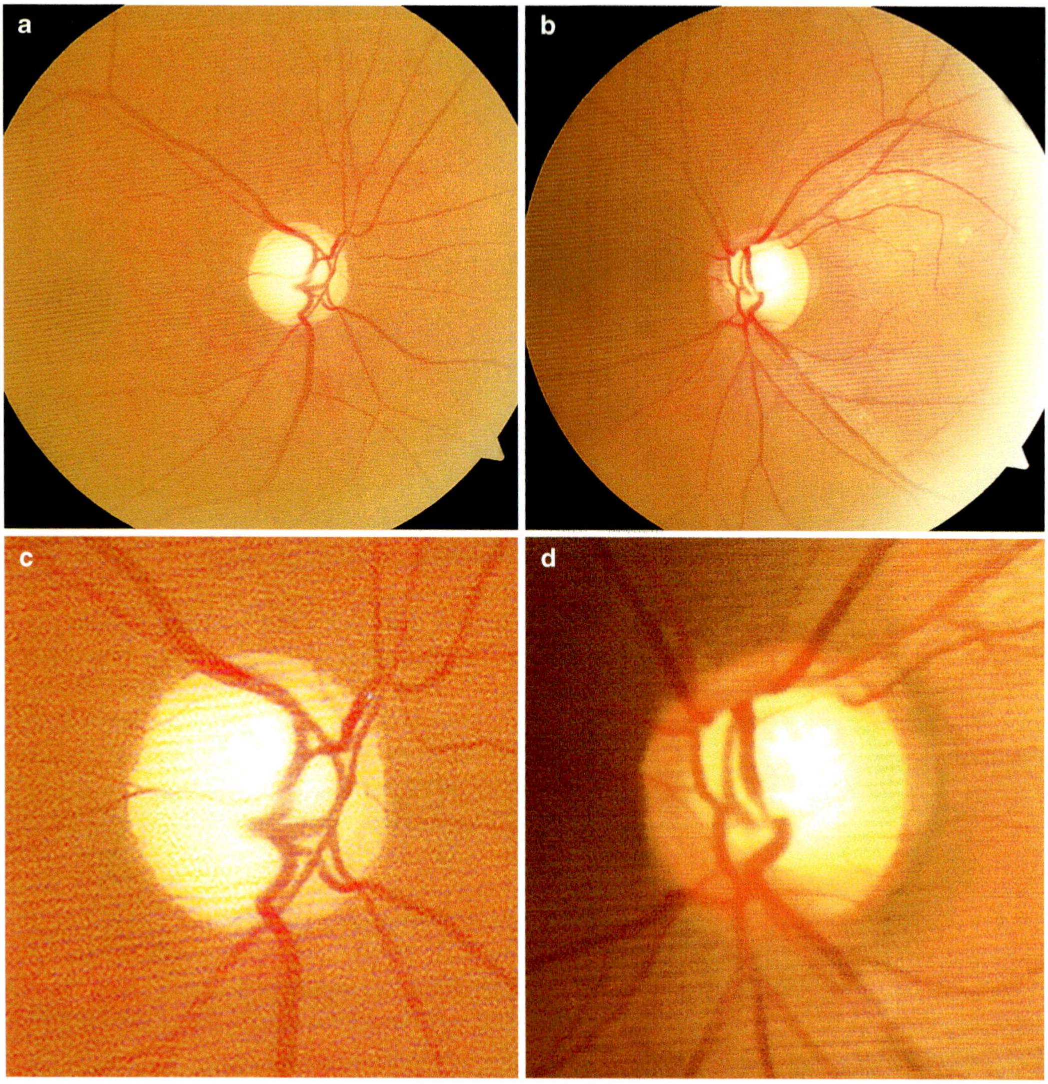

Fig. 39.1 Fundus photographs. The C/D ratio was 0.9 OD and 0.8 OS. Panels a, c: right eye. Panels b, d: left eye

unremarkable, and reflection of retinal nerve fiber was still observed, yet the significant excavation led to the fact that the upper neuroretinal rim and nasal disc seemed not to have followed the ISNT rules.

Non-glaucomatous optic nerve cupping includes physiologic large optic cups and various pathological large optic cups not caused by glaucoma. Common causes include retinopathy, optic neuropathy, compressive optic pathway diseases, etc. Then we quantitatively measured the retinal nerve fiber layer (RNFL) thickness. Central corneal thickness was also measured for intraocular pressure adjustment.

The OCT results showed that the RNFL thickness reduced, especially at the supratemporal and inferotemporal quadrants, and the RNFL thickness in the left eye was normal (Fig. 39.2).

The central corneal thickness was 493 μm in the right eye and 497 μm in the left eye.

The thin RNFL in the right eye was basically consistent with the characteristics of glaucoma, and the RNFL thickness in the left eye was normal. Was the condition in the right eye normal tension glaucoma? What about the left eye? We needed to assess visual function using standardized automated perimetry to confirm the diagnosis.

Standardized automated perimetry showed the visual field defect surrounding the physiological blind spot in the inferior quadrant and temporal

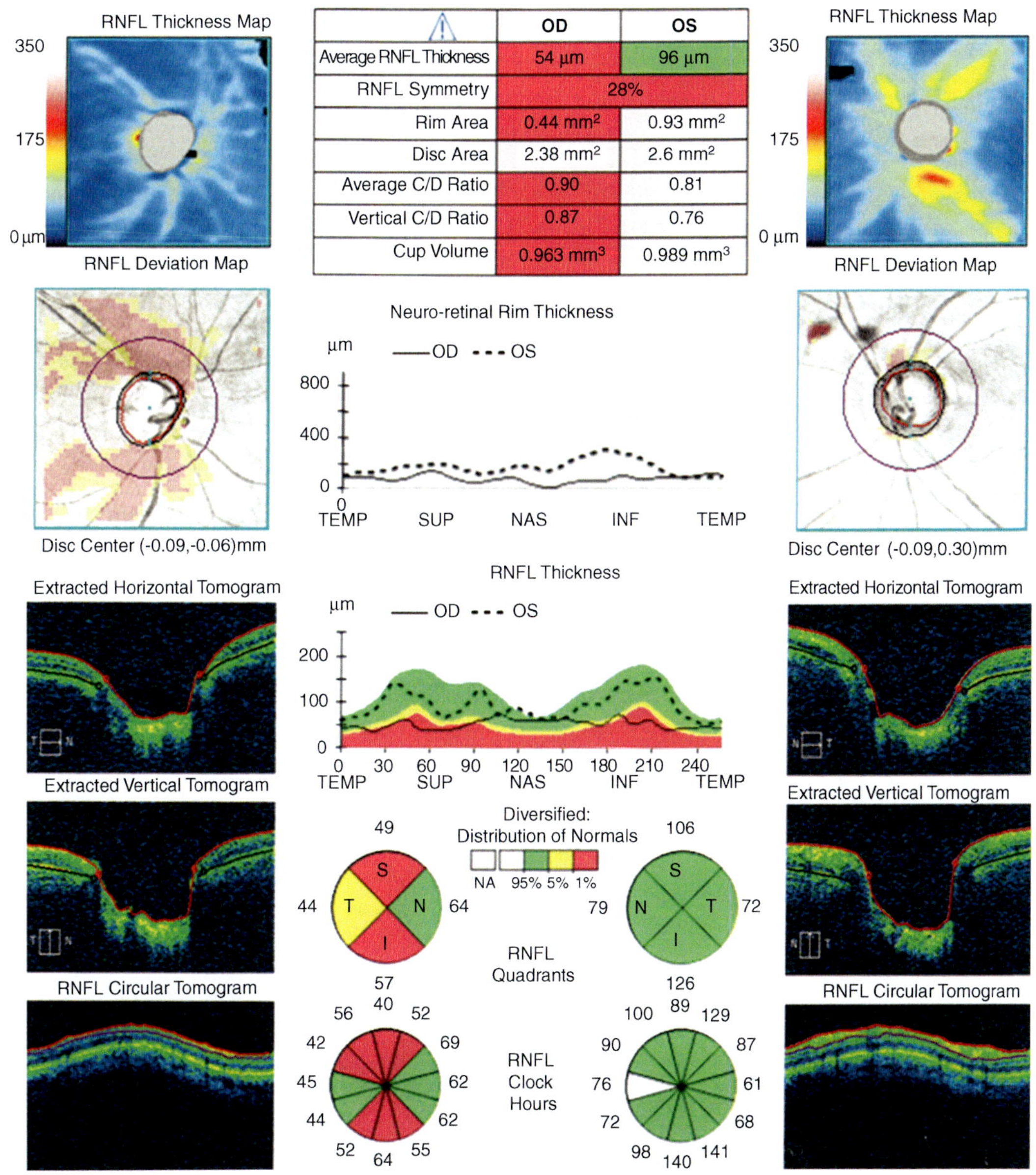

Fig. 39.2 OCT RNFL thickness analysis printout. The RNFL thickness reduced in the right eye, especially at the supratemporal and inferotemporal sides, and the RNFL thickness in the left eye was normal

quadrant of the left eye, and the central fixation was also involved; the visual field in the left eye was normal (Fig. 39.3).

The central vision in the right eye was poor, and the damage to the temporal visual field was serious, which was not consistent with the characteristics of visual function changes caused by glaucoma; based on the normal visual field and RNFL thickness in the left eye, the diagnosis of physiologic large optic cups was considered. Why did the right eye have unilateral optic atrophy?

Careful examination revealed linear scars on the skin of the right superciliary arch. The patient fell off from a bicycle more than 20 years ago. His right face touched the ground, and his right superciliary arch got injured. The visual function of the right eye was not examined, and no treatment was sought.

a

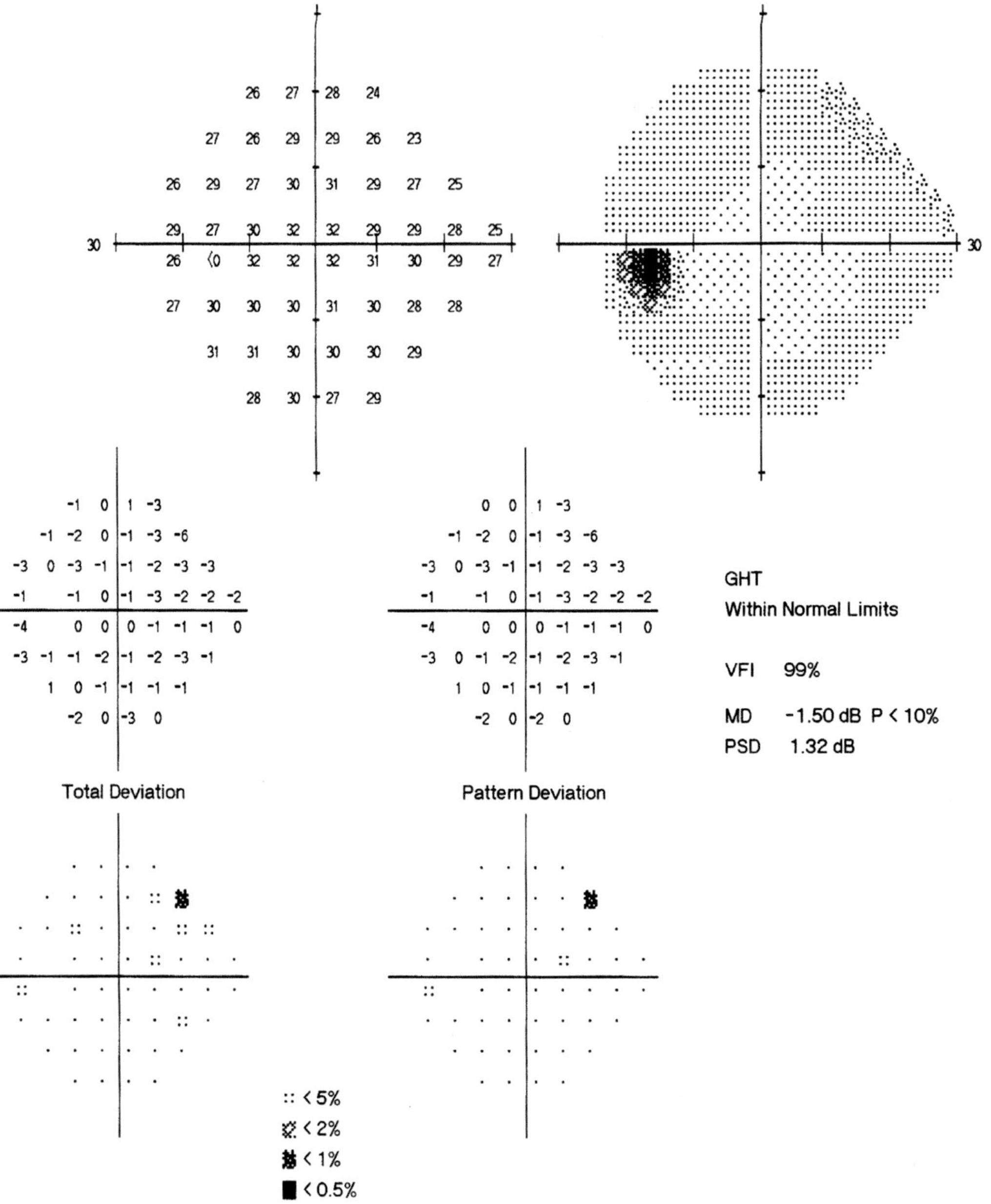

Fig. 39.3 Humphrey visual field analysis printouts. Panel a: normal left eye. Panel b: a visual field defect surrounding the physiological blind spot in the inferior quadrant and temporal quadrant of the right eye with the central fixation involved

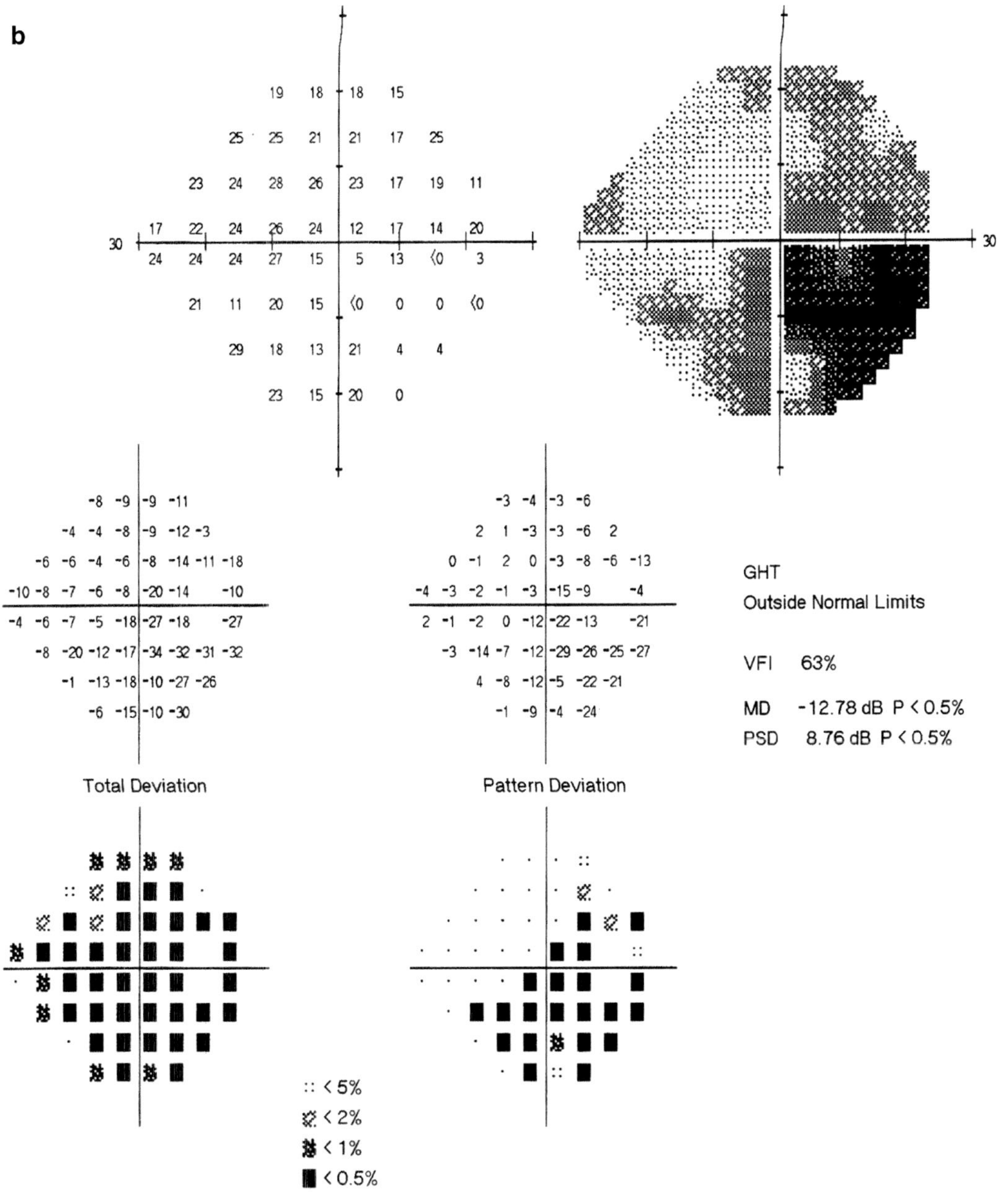

Fig. 39.3 (continued)

Full cranial MRI did not find any abnormality, and thus non-glaucomatous optic nerve cupping caused by intracranial lesions could be excluded.

39.1.3 Final Diagnosis

The final diagnosis was traumatic optic neuropathy in the right eye and physiologic large cups in both eyes.

39.1.4 Case Review

This patient was diagnosed with physiologic large cups in both eyes with optic atrophy after traumatic optic neuropathy in the right eye. The diagnosis was difficult because it was more than 20 years since the trauma occurred, and the patient failed to notice the visual impairment in the right eye earlier. Because of a thin cornea and normal intraocular pressure in both eyes and an enlarged optic cup, deepening excavation, pale color, and RNFL damage (mainly in the superior and inferior temporal quadrants) in the right eye, it might be misdiagnosed as normal tension glaucoma; C/D = 0.8 OS, and thus it would be difficult to differentiate between a physiologic large cup and a large cup from early normal tension glaucoma only based on the optic disc structure. Standardized automated perimetry was important for correct diagnosis of this patient.

39.2 Case 2

39.2.1 Case Presentation

A 26-year-old male patient complained of decreased vision without any obvious cause in both eyes for 6 years. He had no red and sore eyes, headache, pain on eye movement, or other discomforts. There was no improvement in the visual acuity after treatment in other hospitals. Histories of trauma, previous ocular diseases, or systemic diseases were denied. His maternal uncle had a similar medical history.

On examination, the UCVA was 20/28 OD and 20/25 OS. Improvement was not achieved with refraction in either eye. IOP was normal. Slit-lamp examination of his anterior segments was unremarkable. The pupil was 3 mm in diameter, and the light reflex was sensitive in both eyes. On fundus examination, the optic disc rim was pale in color, especially the temporal quadrant, the margin was distinctive, and the C/D ratio was 0.8 in both eyes. The reflection of the temporal and inferior RNFL was reduced (Fig. 39.4).

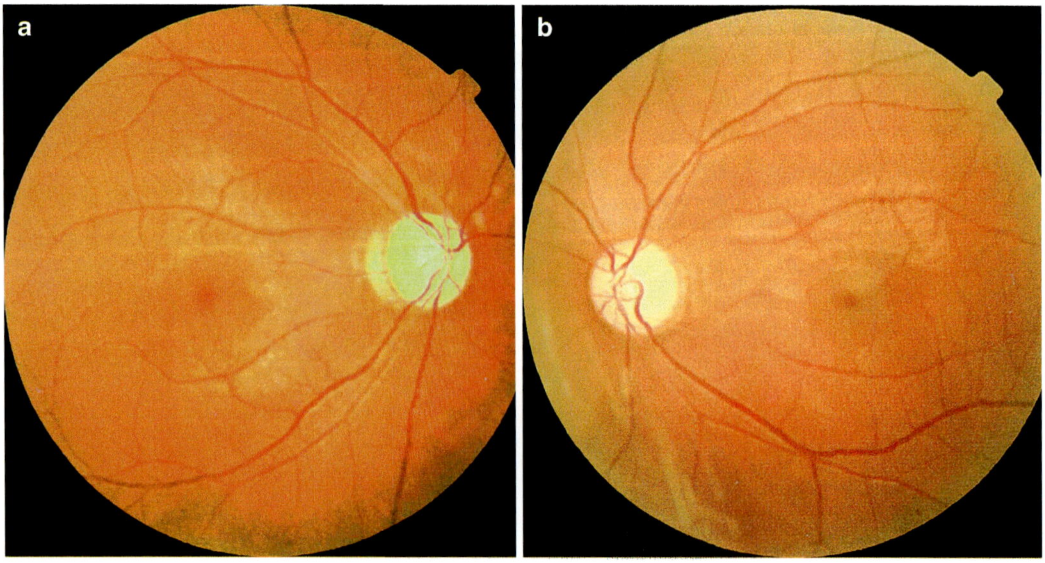

Fig. 39.4 Fundus photographs. In both eyes, the optic disc was pale in color, particularly obvious at the temporal rim, the boundary was clear, and the C/D ratio was 0.8. Panel a: right eye. Panel b: left eye

Standardized automated perimetry showed diffuse suppression and an arcuate visual field defect with its superior edge connecting to the blind spot in both eyes (Fig. 39.5).

The OCT examination revealed overall RNFL thinning in both eyes, especially in the temporal and inferior quadrants (Fig. 39.6).

Peripheral venous blood was collected for mitochondrial DNA (mtDNA) testing, which revealed 11778th nucleotide mutation, i.e., guanine (G) had mutated to adenine (A) (Fig. 39.7).

39.2.2 Final Diagnosis

The final diagnosis was Leber's hereditary optic neuropathy in both eyes.

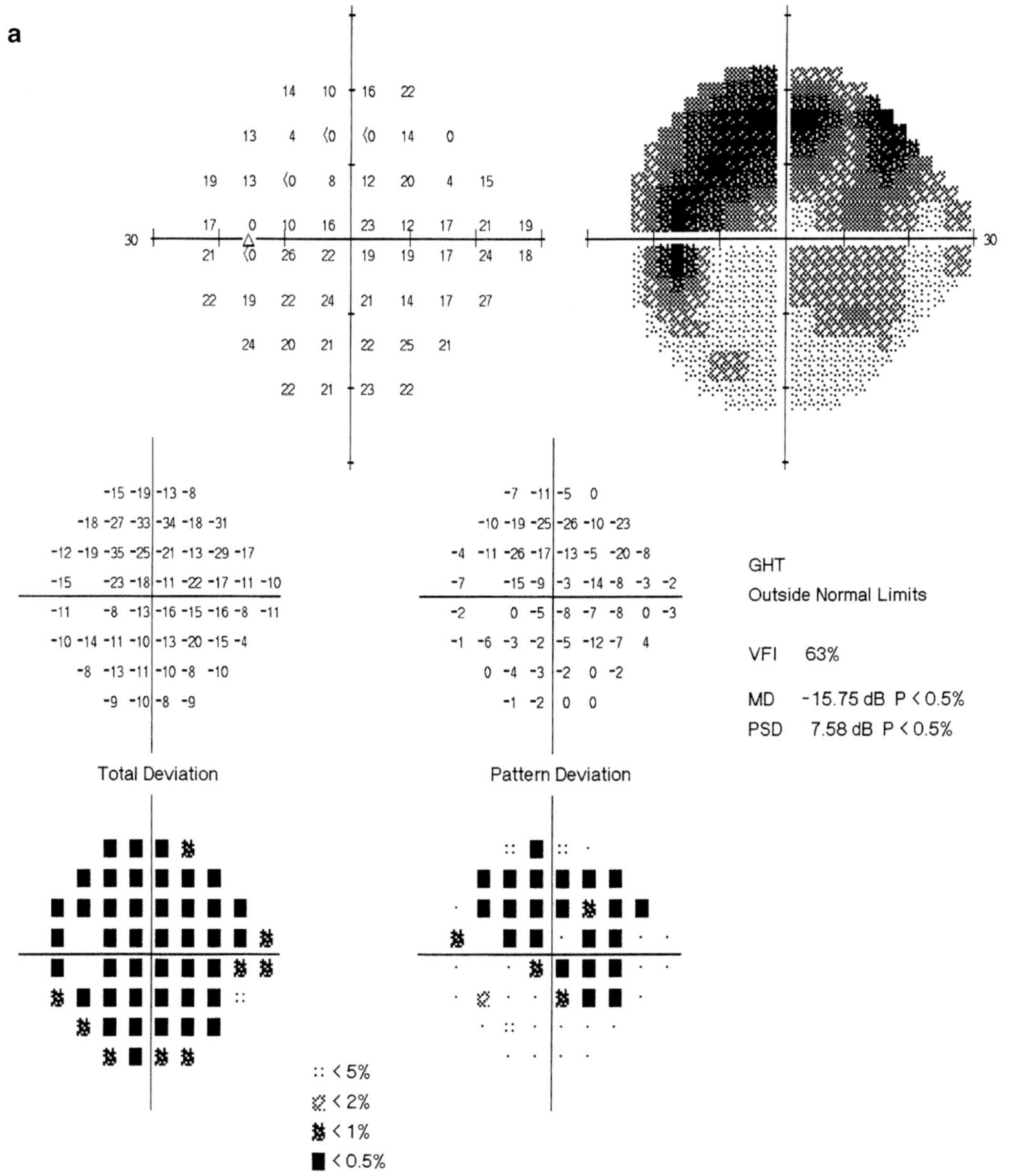

Fig. 39.5 Humphrey visual field analysis printouts. The 24-2 test showed a giant central defect extending from the blind spot in both eyes, which was the most severe in the superior quadrant. Panel a: left eye. Panel b: right eye

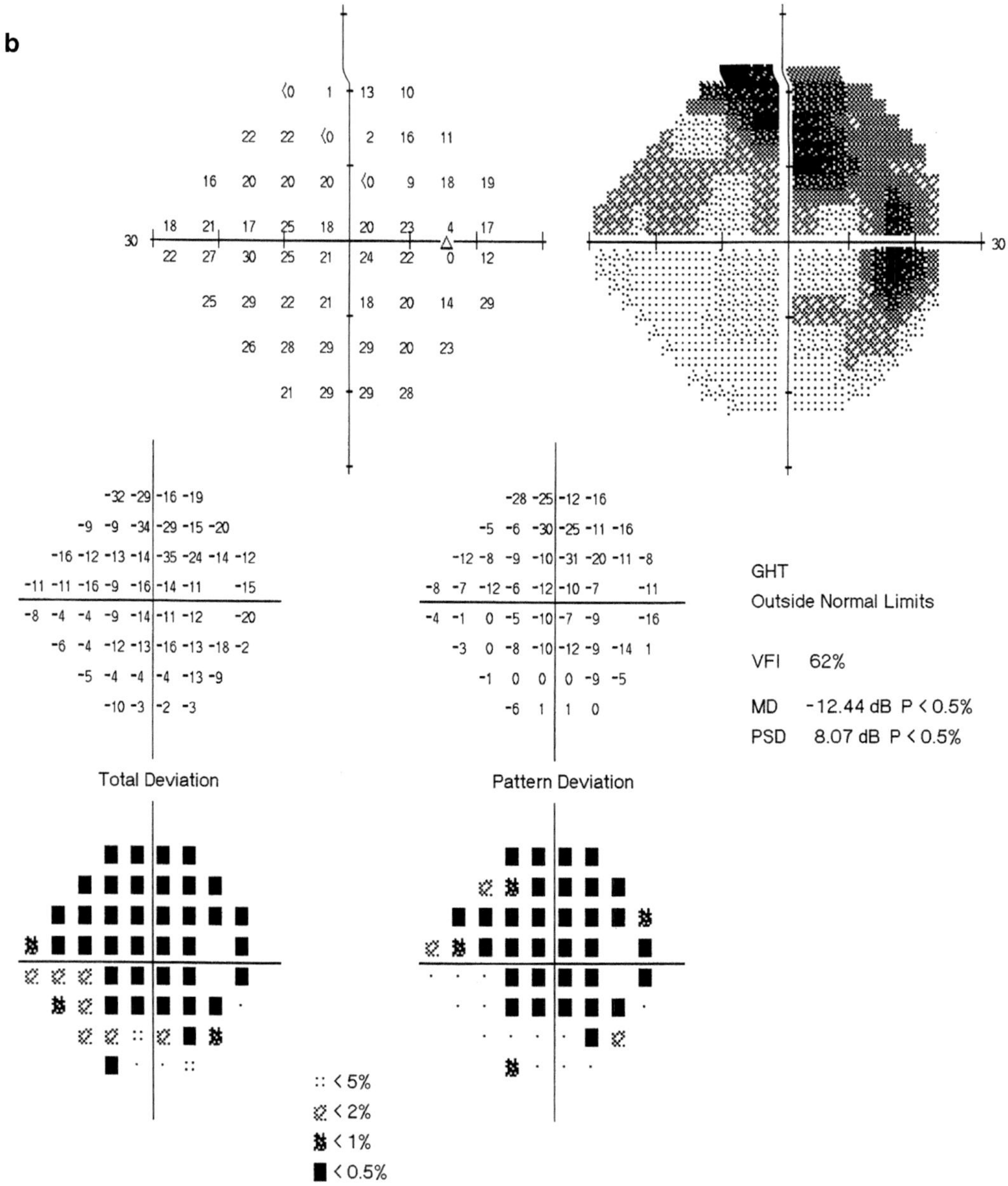

Fig. 39.5 (continued)

39.2.3 Case Review

This young patient had large optic disc cupping, which has a pale rim, especially on the temporal side, in both eyes, while the excavation was not deep. OCT also showed that temporal and inferior RNFL defects were more severe against the overall thinning of the RNFL; a superior arcuate-like defect connecting to the physiological blind spot was seen in both eyes, whereas their shape was not regular. The light sensitivity was diffusely lowered, and the central vision was also affected, which was not consistent with the typical changes in glaucoma. Given the facts that the patient was a young

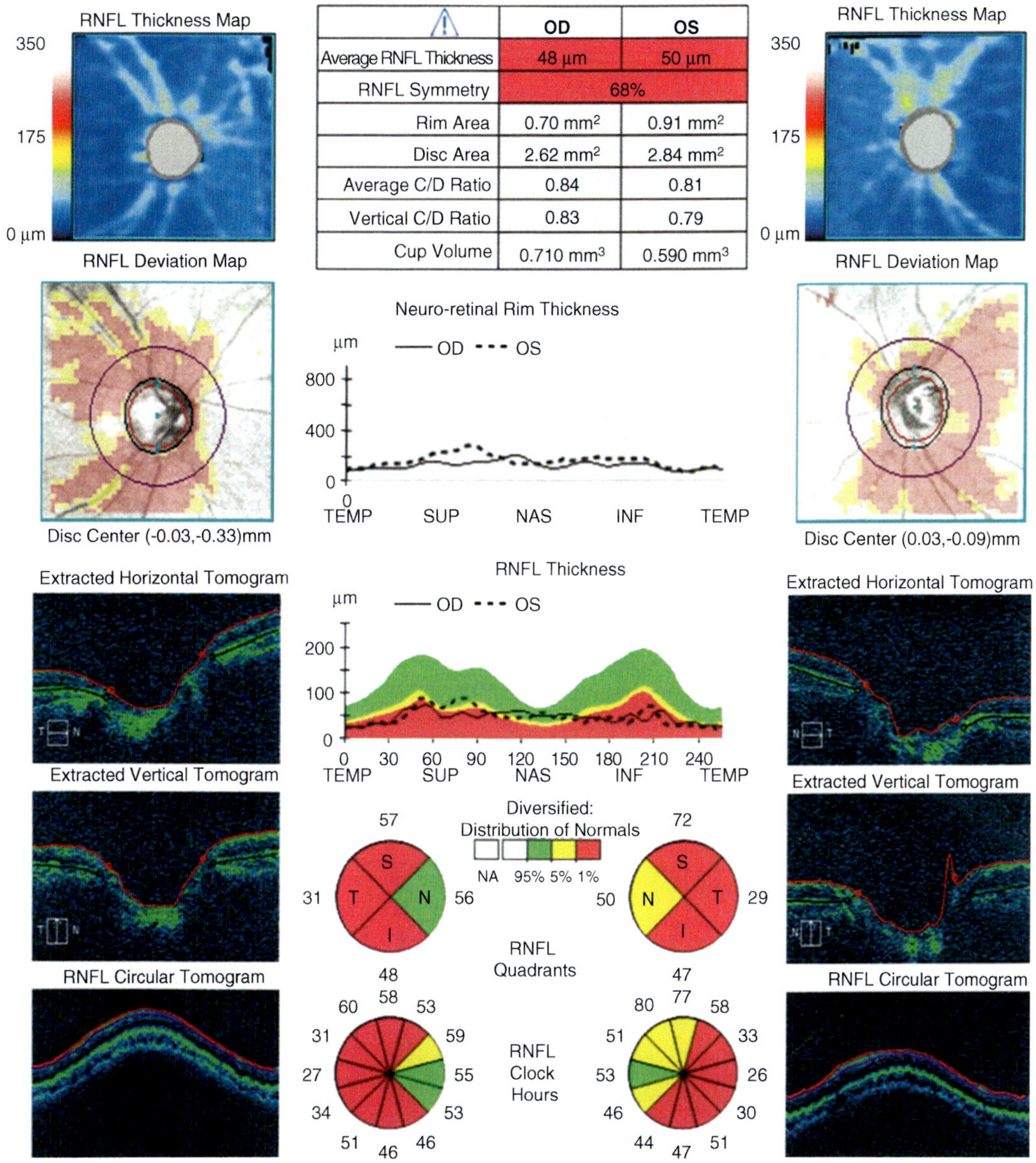

Fig. 39.6 RNFL thickness analysis printouts. Diffuse RNFL thinning occurred in both eyes, especially in the inferior quadrants

man, the onset was simultaneous in both eyes, and medications were ineffective, the diagnosis of optic neuritis was not supported. Comprehensive analysis indicated LHON was possible. The test of mtDNA with the peripheral blood showed a point mutation at site 11778, so the diagnosis was confirmed.

39.3 Discussion

The main characteristics of a glaucomatous large cup are that it is more obvious in the vertical direction, the residual neuroretinal rim is ruddy, and defects appear at superior and inferior rim and at the corresponding parts of the RNFL and

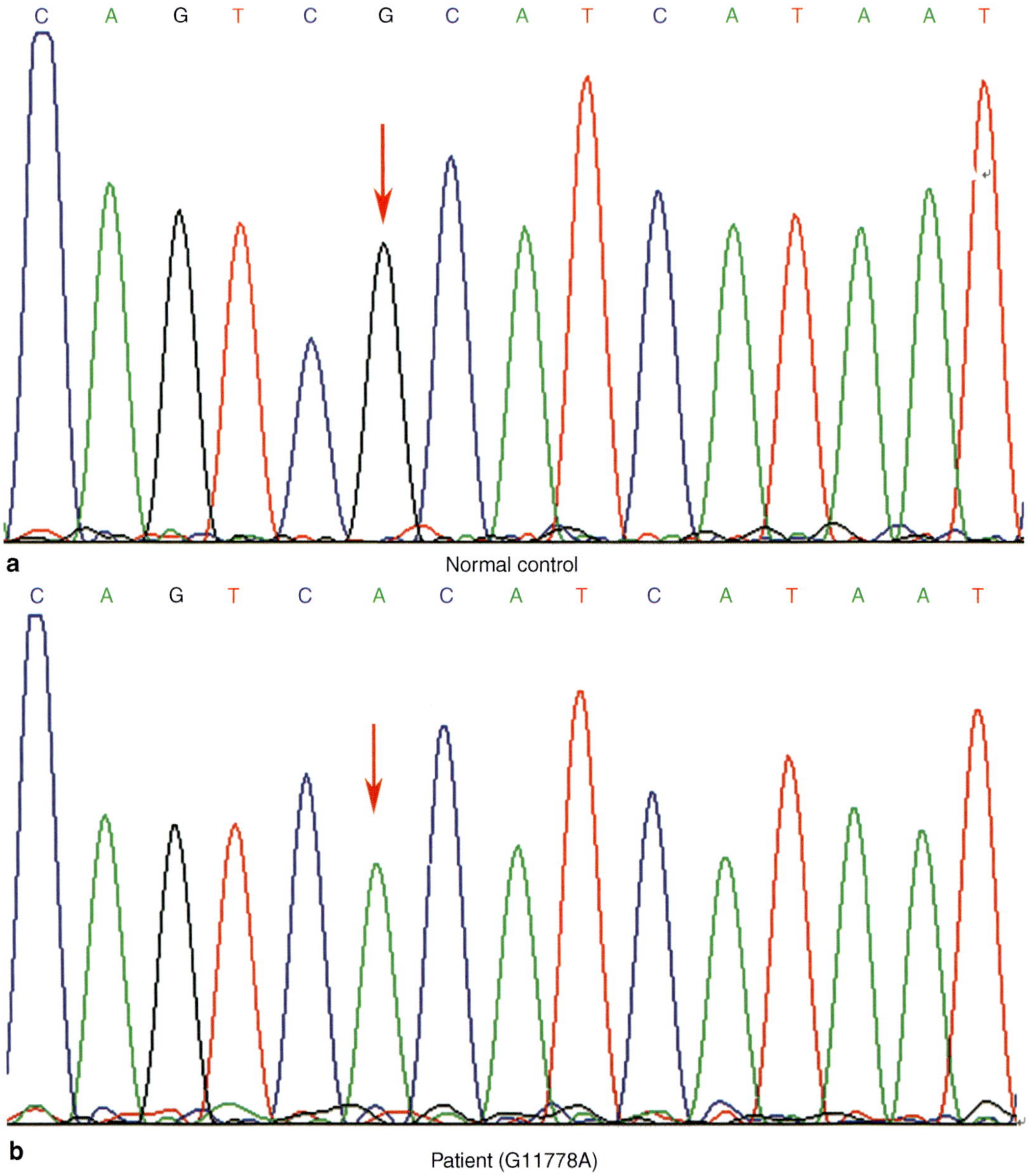

Fig. 39.7 Sequence map of the mitochondrial DNA mutation at position 11778 based on peripheral blood analysis. Panel a: signal peak image of sequencing at the mtDNA 11778 site in the control (arrow). Panel b: mutation at the mtDNA G11778A site in the patient (arrow)

visual field. The characteristic visual field changes in glaucoma can provide significant cues for diagnosis [1]. The characteristics of the visual field in glaucoma include the following: (a) a nerve fiber bundle pattern defect respecting the horizontal meridian can be found; (b) early visual field damage occurs in the Bjerrum zone and often manifests itself as a paracentral scotoma, nasal step, and an arcuate defect; (c) with the progression of disease, the arcuate defect will break through to the nasal side, leading to superior and/or inferior nasal visual field defects, as well as a annular scotoma; and (d) in the advanced phase, a tube field may appear and affect the central vision, with a visual island left on the temporal side. In Case 1, the patient had significantly decreased central vision and significant temporal damage to the visual field in the right eye; in Case 2, the patient was young and mainly experienced diffuse damage and a large central defect in the visual field. The situations of the two cases were not consistent with the characteristics of glaucomatous visual field damage, which was the key to the exclusion of normal tension glaucoma.

Clinically, a non-glaucomatous large cup is attributed to the atrophy of optic nerve fibers not caused by glaucoma and manifested as enlarged optic nerve cupping [2]. The common primary diseases include the following: (a) optic nerve diseases, such as optic neuritis, ischemic optic neuropathy, Leber's hereditary optic neuropathy, trauma, toxic optic neuropathy, etc.; (b) retinopathies, such as retinal vein occlusion, retinal artery occlusion, etc.; and (c) compression lesions and other visual pathway diseases, such as tumor in the orbital and sellar region, intracranial hemangioma, empty sella, intracranial hypertension, etc. In addition, a physiologic large cup in combination with other diseases causing optic atrophy may also have enlarged cupping of various degrees and morphologies in both eyes.

The morphology of a non-glaucomatous large cup varies with the primary diseases [2]. For example, the color of the optic cup rim in ischemic optic neuropathy is pale, but the loss of the neuroretinal rim may be not obvious; Leber's hereditary optic neuropathy often damages the papillomacular bundle; thus the color of the temporal neuroretinal rim is often pale; the sign of optic atrophy due to a compressive lesion is often diffuse pallor of the optic disc with the severity being much greater than that from neuroretinal rim tissue loss.

There is a poor correlation between the visual field defects and optic disc changes, and the damage to the central vision is serious in non-glaucomatous optic nerve cupping, while structural damage (optic cup enlargement and loss of disc rim) to the retinal nerve fibers due to glaucoma is consistent with the functional damage (visual field defects). The patients with non-glaucomatous optic nerve cupping tend to show various kinds of visual field damage, which would be associated with the primary diseases [3]. For example, the morphology of visual field damage in retinal vascular disease is associated with the vascular distribution, the morphology of visual field damage in optic neuritis is associated with the damaged nerve fibers, and the visual field damage due to optic chiasma is characterized by bilateral temporal hemianopsia. Therefore, the identification of glaucoma versus non-glaucomatous optic nerve cupping on the basis of visual field has important clinical significance.

References

1. Fengming L. Chinese ophthalmology. 2nd ed. Beijing: People's Medical Publishing House; 2005.
2. Zhang YX, Huang HB, Wei SH. Clinical characteristics of nonglaucomatous optic disc cupping. Exp Ther Med. 2014;7(4):995–9.
3. Gupta PK, Asrani S, Freedman SF, et al. Differentiating glaucomatous from nonglaucomatous optic nerve cupping by optical coherence tomography. Open Neurol J. 2011;5(1):1–7.

40 The Optic Nerve Damage and Visual Field Change in the Acute Phase of Primary Angle-Closure Glaucoma

Xiaojing Pan, Ning Fan, and Xuyang Liu

After acute onset of primary angle-closure glaucoma (PACG), it is difficult to identify the changes in the optic nerve and retina because of the tissue damage in the anterior segment. What are the characteristics of the visual field and optic nerve damage in PACG? Two cases in which the fundus changes after acute onset of PACG are quite typical are presented in this section. Although the cases are small in number, we believe they are representative based upon literature review and our observation.

40.1 Case 1

40.1.1 Case Presentation

A 33-year-old female patient complained of bulging pain and suddenly decreased vision in her left eye for 1 day. She had experienced ipsilateral headache, nausea, and vomiting. She had no history of vision loss. The patient denied a history of trauma or systemic diseases. A family history was also denied.

On examination, the uncorrected visual acuity (UCVA) was 20/20 OD and 20/200 OS. There was no improvement with refraction. Intraocular pressure (IOP) by standard Goldmann applanation tonometry was 14 mmHg OD and 56 mmHg OS. In the right eye, the cornea was transparent, the depth of anterior chamber was 2.5 CT, the peripheral anterior chamber depth was 1/4 CT, the pupil size was 3 mm, the lens was transparent, and the C/D ratio was 0.4. In the left eye, the examination showed mixed hyperemia, corneal edema, a central anterior chamber depth of 2.5 CT, a nearly closed peripheral anterior chamber angle, aqueous humor flare, an oval pupil (3.5 mm × 4.5 mm), slow direct light reflex, and loss of fundus details.

The axial length was 21.2 mm in the right eye and 20.9 mm in the left eye.

40.1.2 Final Diagnosis

The final diagnosis was primary acute angle-closure glaucoma (acute phase in the left eye and preclinical phase in the right eye).

IOP-lowering drugs were immediately administrated to the patient, including mannitol (via intravenous infusion), oral methazolamide tab-

X. Pan
Shandong Eye Institute, Qingdao Eye Hospital, Qingdao, China

N. Fan
Shenzhen Eye Hospital, Shenzhen University, Shenzhen, China

X. Liu (✉)
Xiamen Eye Center of Xiamen University, Xiamen, China

Shenzhen Eye Hospital, Shenzhen University, Shenzhen, China

N. Wang et al. (eds.), *Optic Disorders and Visual Field*, Advances in Visual Science and Eye Diseases 2, https://doi.org/10.1007/978-981-13-2502-1_40

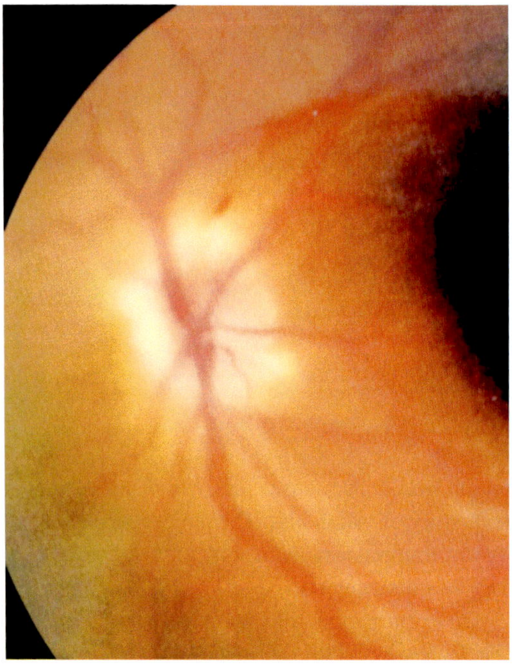

Fig. 40.1 Fundus photograph. Fundus photograph of the left eye showed multiple infarction foci surrounding the optic disc and a splinter disc hemorrhage at the supratemporal sector

lets, and topical antihypertensive and anti-inflammatory drugs. Anterior chamber puncture was performed in emergency. After the surgery, the IOP was lowered, the UCVA was 20/25 in the right eye, and the pupil size was 3 mm in diameter. Fundus examination showed optic disc edema, multiple infarction foci surrounding the optic disc, and a splinter disc hemorrhage at the supratemporal sector in the left eye (Fig. 40.1).

Standardized automated perimetry revealed diffuse light sensitivity decrease that was the most severe in the superior visual field in the left eye (Fig. 40.2).

The patient continued to receive IOP-lowering drugs and topical anti-inflammatory therapies and underwent laser peripheral iridotomy in both eyes. After 1 week of IOP control, the UCVA was 20/22, IOP was 15 mmHg, and the pupil was 3 mm in diameter in the right eye. Re-examination of the left fundus indicated that the optic disc hemorrhage had been absorbed and the optic disc edema had been relieved, but the infarction foci could still be seen, and an inferotemporal retinal nerve fiber layer (RNFL) defect could be seen (Fig. 40.3).

Re-examination of the visual field demonstrated a superior visual field defect in the left eye (Fig. 40.4).

The medication and IOP control were normal. After 3 months, re-examination showed that the UCVA was 20/22, IOP was 15 mmHg, and the pupil was 3 mm in diameter in the right eye. In addition, the optic disc was pale in color with a clear boundary, and there was an inferotemporal wedge-shaped RNFL defect. Re-examination of the visual field showed that the superior visual field defect in the left eye was almost the same as previously seen but slightly improved (Fig. 40.5).

40.2 Case 2

40.2.1 Case Presentation

A 50-year-old female patient complained of decrease in vision and bulging pain in her right eye for 1 day, which was accompanied by ipsilateral headache. She had experienced a similar onset 2 months before, which was relieved after a rest, and thus the patient did not go for diagnosis and treatment. She had undergone an antiglaucoma surgery in her left eye 5 years before and denied histories of other ocular diseases, systemic, or familial diseases.

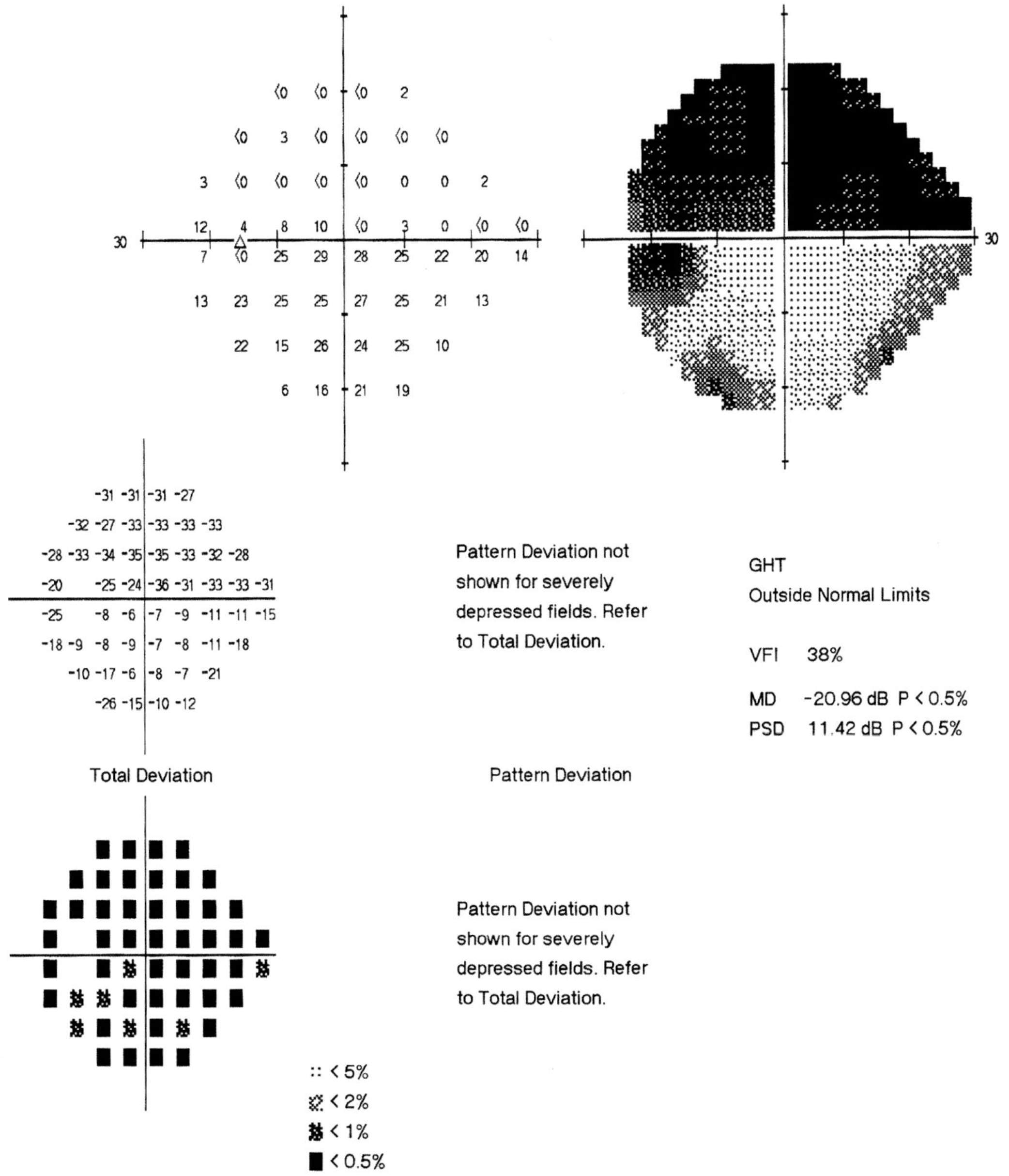

Fig. 40.2 Humphrey visual field analysis printout. The 24-2 test showed diffuse light sensitivity decrease in the left eye that was the most severe in the superior visual field

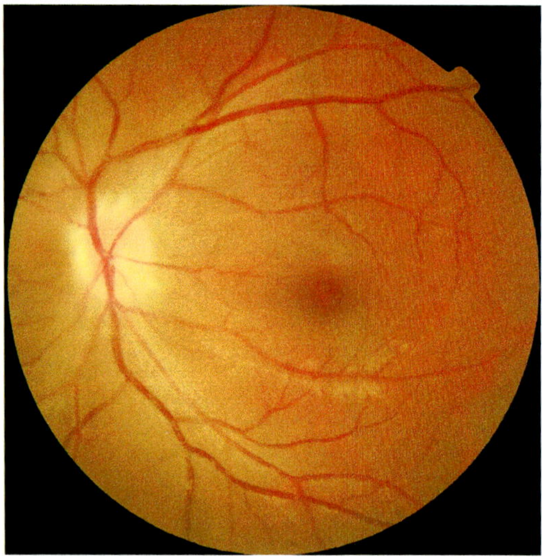

Fig. 40.3 Fundus photograph obtained during the re-examination after 1 week of IOP control. After 1 week of treatment, re-examination of the fundus showed that the optic disc edema had been relieved, but peripapillary infarction foci and an inferotemporal wedge-shaped RNFL defect could be seen

On examination, the UCVA was 20/60 in the right eye and did not improve with refraction. The UCVA was 20/28 OS, and the best corrected visual acuity (BCVA) was 20/25 OS. IOP by standard Goldmann applanation tonometry was 61 mmHg OD and 15 mmHg OS. In the right eye, there were mixed hyperemia and corneal edema, the depth of anterior chamber was 3 CT, the angle of peripheral anterior chamber closed, the pupil was 3.5 mm in diameter, the direct light reflex was sluggish, the crystalline lens was cloudy, and the fundus was unclear. In the left eye, there was no congestion in the conjunctiva, the superior filtrating bleb was diffuse and slightly elevated, the cornea was transparent, the depth of anterior chamber was 3 CT, the incision around the superior iris was unobstructed, the pupil was 3 mm in diameter, the crystalline lens was cloudy, the C/D ratio was 0.3, and the optic disc was pink in color with a distinctive boundary.

40.2.2 Final Diagnosis

The final diagnosis was primary angle-closure glaucoma (acute phase in the right eye; post-antiglaucoma surgery phase in the left eye).

IOP-lowering drugs were administrated to the patient immediately, including intravenous infusion of mannitol, oral methazolamide tablets, ocular hypertensive eye drops, and anti-inflammatory drugs. Anterior chamber puncture was performed in emergency. After the surgery, the IOP was lowered, the UCVA was 20/28, and the pupil was 2 mm in diameter in the right eye. Fundus examination showed optic disc edema and a few temporal bleeding points in the right eye (Fig. 40.6).

Standardized automated perimetry showed a ring visual field defect in the right eye (Fig. 40.7).

The patient underwent trabeculectomy after IOP of the right eye was under control. The IOP could be maintained in the normal range without any medications after surgery. After 1 month, the re-examination of the visual field showed that the ring visual field defect was the same as previously observed.

40.3 Discussion

The two patients mentioned above both had typical symptoms and signs of the acute phase of PACG, and thus the diagnosis was definite; the time from disease onset is 1 day, and active IOP-lowering therapies, including medication, laser, and surgery, were given, thereby having the IOP controlled, yet perimetry and funduscopy indicated that sharp increase in IOP caused significant damage to the optic nerve and retina. This kind of damage and its mechanism are significantly different from those of primary open-angle glaucoma (POAG): edema, infarction foci, and hemorrhagic foci could be seen in the optic disc, and although a nerve fiber bundle induced defect is seen in the visual field, it occurs simultaneously with diffuse decrease in light sensitivity.

In case of acute onset of PACG, the primary cause of optic disc edema is occlusion of the lamina cribrosa, where the nerve fiber axons could not expand due to the presence of dense connective tissue, and continuous influx of axoplasm causes swelling; retinal ganglion cells (RGCs) could not tolerate the blockage of axoplasm delivery, and thus necrosis occurs. Secondly,

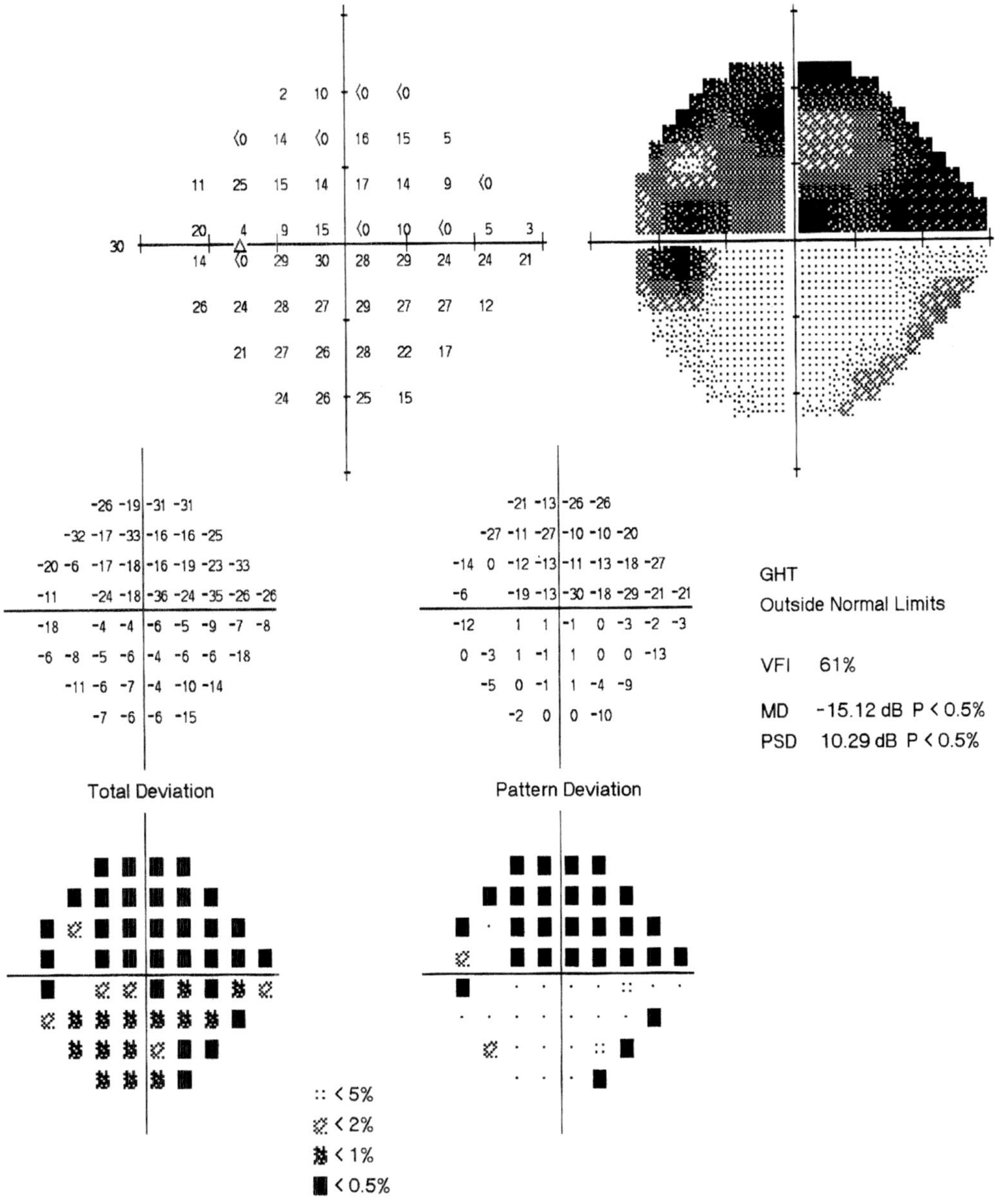

Fig. 40.4 Humphrey visual field analysis printout obtained during the re-examination after 1 week of IOP control. The 24-2 test showed a superior visual field defect in the left eye

acute increase in IOP might cause compression of the lamina cribrosa tissue, leading to distortion and dislocation of it, and the resultant shear force could also block the flow of axoplasm, leading to optic nerve damage [1, 2]. These inferences might explain the significant edema and infarction foci around the optic disc in Cases 1 and 2.

In addition, acute increase in IOP could cause change in the local hemodynamics in the optic disc. Local blood supply in the optic disc was from the central retinal artery and the short posterior ciliary artery. In case of acute PACG, sharp increase in IOP causes compression of the vessels in the anterior area of the lamina cribrosa and

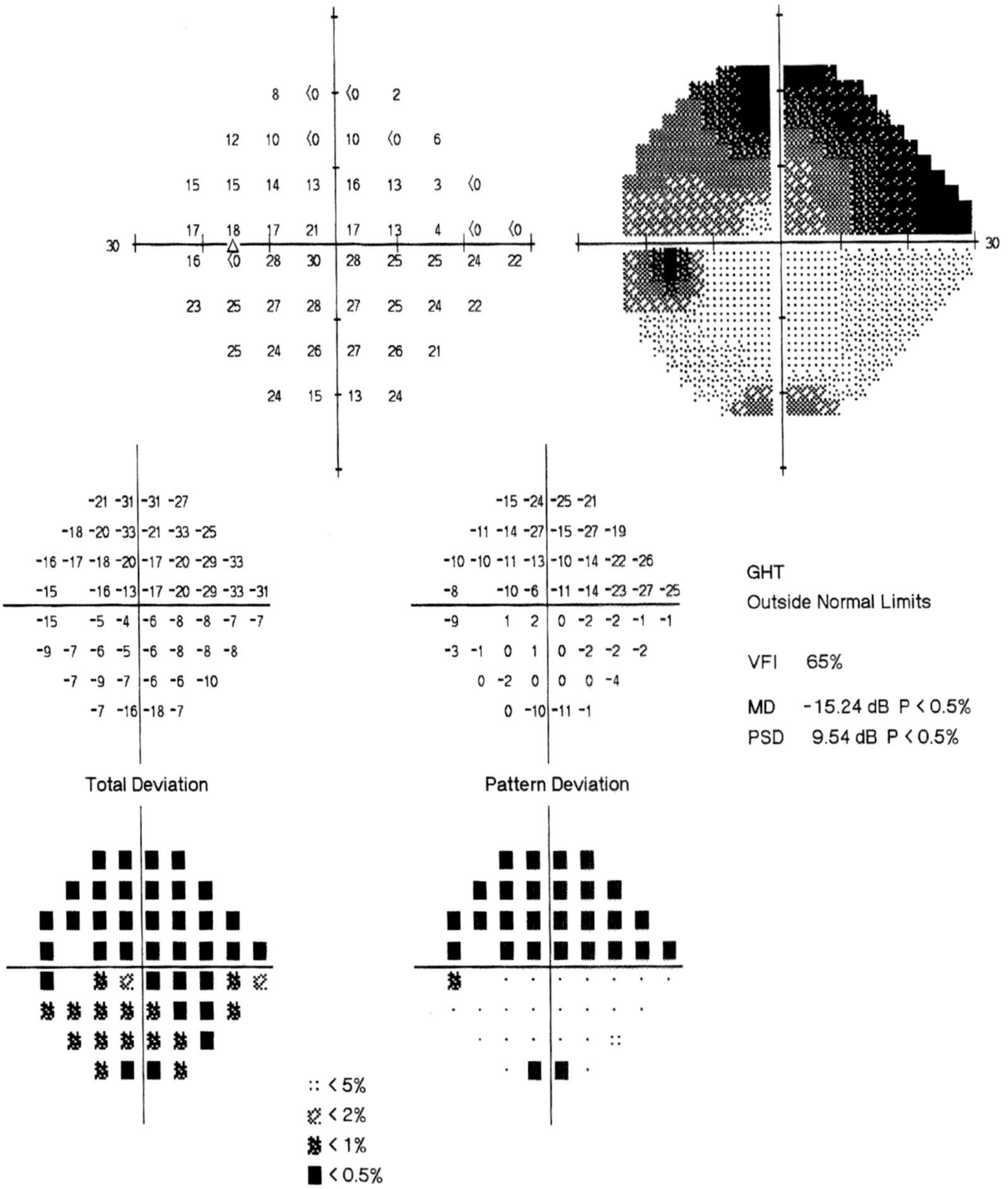

Fig. 40.5 Humphrey visual field analysis printout obtained during the re-examination after 3 months of IOP control. The 24-2 test of the visual field showed that the superior visual field defect in the left eye was almost the same as previously seen but slightly improved

less blood flow through the optic disc, which disturbs the nutrition and normal physiological function of the axons in the lamina cribrosa; decreased blood supply also impacts the capillary delivery of nutrients into astrocytes; ischemia-reperfusion injury would occur on controlling IOP, leading to irreversible ischemia-hypoxia-reperfusion injury in the surface capillaries in the optic disc and local retinal nerve fibers [3, 4], so bleeding (Case 2) and RNFL damage could be seen around the optic disc clinically. The ocular vessels of the patients with acute increase in IOP

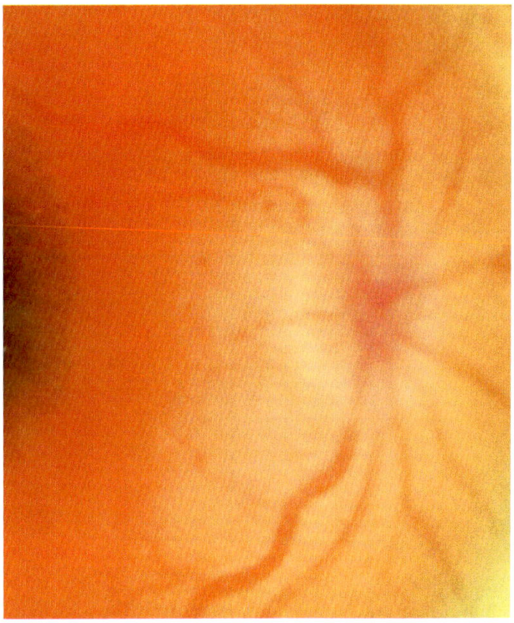

Fig. 40.6 Fundus photograph. It showed optic disc edema and a few temporal bleeding points

also had abnormal autoregulation, and some vessels had organic lesions, such as lumen stenosis and occlusion, vascular wall degeneration, and necrosis, leading to increased vascular resistance and abnormal regulation. Therefore, in case of acute PACG, retinal nerve fibers around the optic disc would be mainly injured [5], and the resultant visual field defect is still characterized by a nerve fiber bundle induced defect, such as the superior visual field defect and ring visual field defect in Cases 1 and 2.

For the damage of acute PACG, Fig. 40.8 illustrated on the cellular level the damage mechanisms of the acute tissue ischemia and acute inflammation induced by acute increase in IOP as well as the tissue ischemia-reperfusion injury after the IOP was controlled [6].

Being different from POAG, would acute PACG cause damage to the retina? Anatomically, the retina is divided into ten layers, while the blood supply of the inner five layers and outer five layers is from the central artery system and choroidal vascular system, respectively. The retinal central vascular system is a terminal artery and has no anastomosis with other vascular systems. The main branches of the central retinal artery are distributed in the retinal nerve fiber layers, and small branches from them are distributed in all the inner five layers in the retina. The angles between these branches and trunks are right angles. The supply vessels in the retinal inner nuclear layer and inner plexiform layer were the most distal branches of retinal central arterial capillaries. In acute high IOP, the anatomic site of the most severe ischemia should be the retinal inner nuclear layer, inner plexiform layer, and ganglion cell layer, and thus these three layers would have the most severe injury under ischemia [7–9].

Therefore, the early injury to the inner nuclear layer and inner plexiform layer of the retina would be significant after acute PACG. Although clinical evidences provided by examinations, such as ERG and OCT scan of the macula lutea, were limited, the diffuse decrease in the light sensitivity in early visual field was found in these two patients, indicating damaged retinal function. This required further investigation.

For the damage to the visual field and optic disc due to acute PACG, we still have many problems. For example, there are also such manifestations in non-arterial anterior ischemic optic neuropathy (NAION) as bleeding, edema and even infarction foci in the fundus, and arcuate and flabellate visual field defects connecting with the blind spot caused by RNFL damage. This is very similar to the manifestation of acute PACG. So what are the differences and similarities in the pathological mechanism between the two diseases? We found that most visual field defects occur in the superior quadrant of the central visual field after PACG, although the number of cases observed was quite small. What are the reasons for this? What is the pathophysiological basis of this visual field damage? What is the outcome of visual field damage after IOP is controlled? What are the differences and similarities between the mechanisms of ischemic damage in PACG, POAG, and NAION, as the main change in the optic disc after acute PACG is that the color of the neuroretinal rim tissue became white, which is similar to that in NAION rather than POAG? What is the relationship between the visual field damage and the peak IOP value and

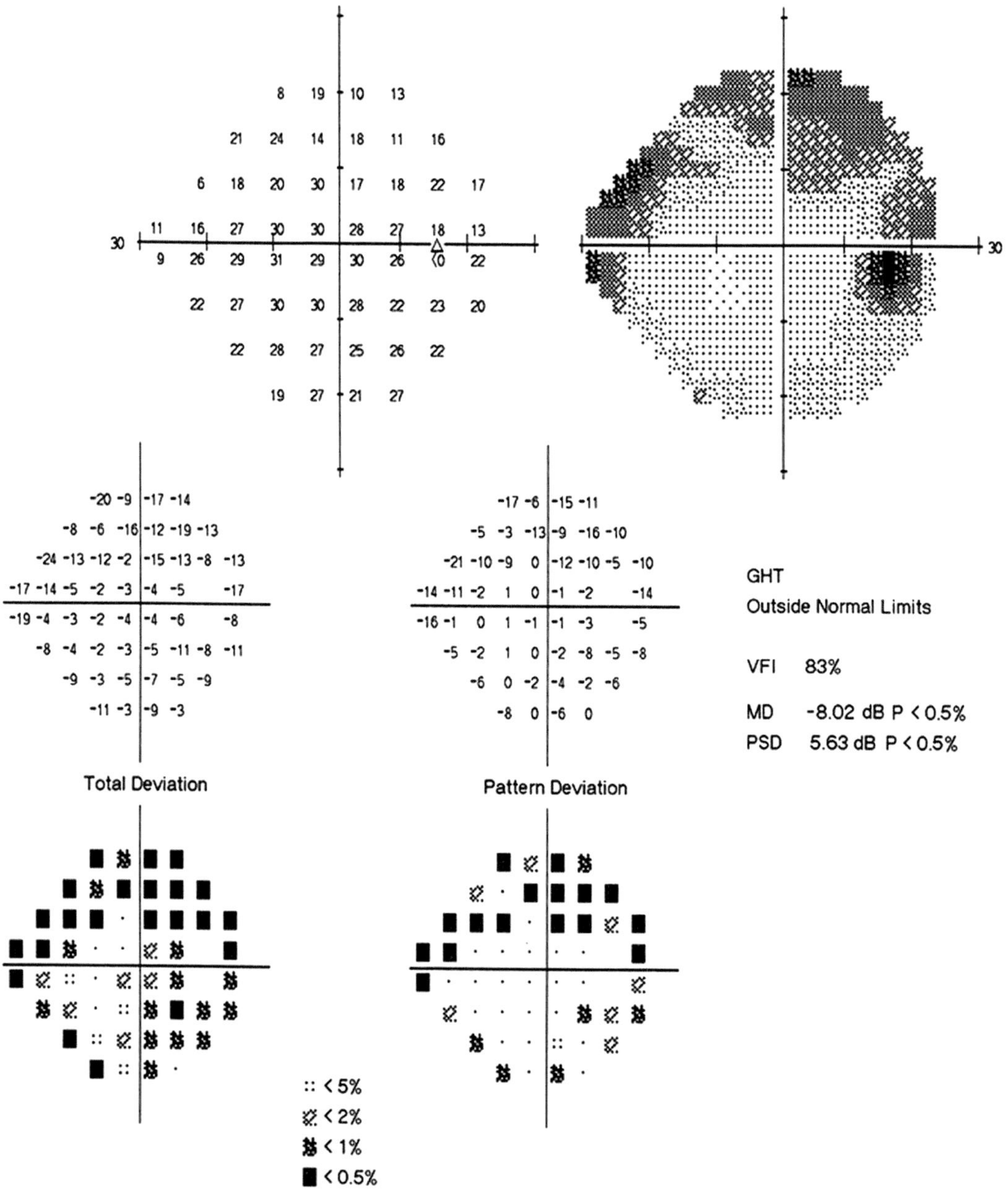

Fig. 40.7 Humphrey visual field analysis printout. The 24-2 test showed ring visual field defects in the right eye

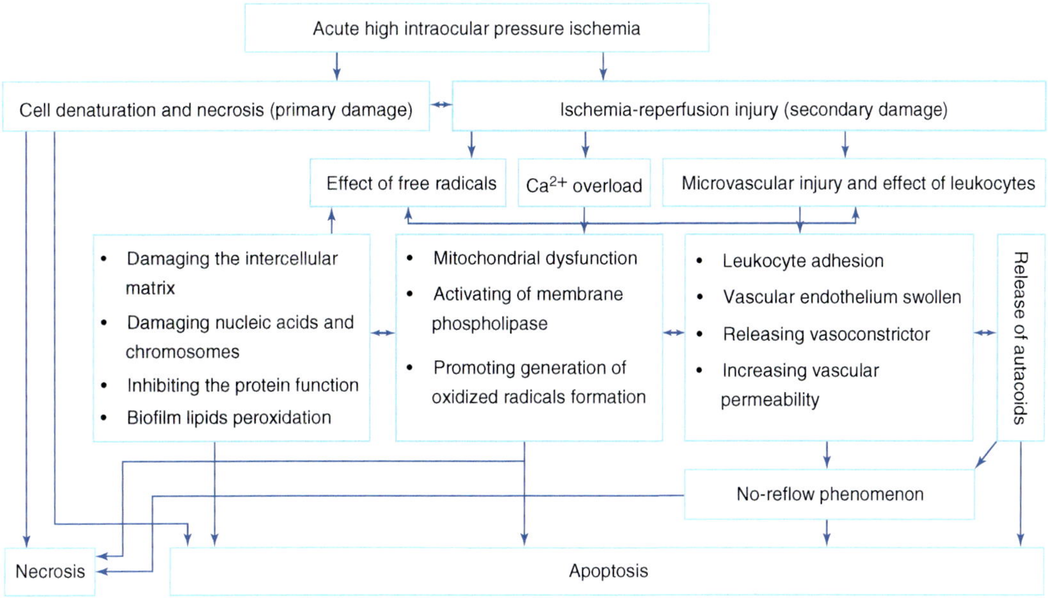

Fig. 40.8 A schematic overview of the mechanism of tissue damage in the acute phase of acute primary angle-closure glaucoma

its duration time in acute PACG? Is there any damage threshold? All these questions require prospective, large sample size studies for answers and confirmation.

References

1. Zhou W. Clinical glaucoma. 2nd ed. Beijing: People's Medical Publishing House; 1999.
2. Garcia-Valenzuela E, Shareef S, Walsh J, et al. Programmed cell death of retinal ganglion cells during experimental glaucoma. Exp Eye Res. 1995;61(1):33–44.
3. Neufeld AH. New conceptual approaches for pharmacological neuroprotection in glaucomatous neuronal degeneration. J Glaucoma. 1998;7(6):434–8.
4. Kapin MA, Doshi R, Scatton B, et al. Neuroprotective effects of eliprodil in retinal excitotoxicity and ischemia. Invest Ophthalmol Vis Sci. 1999;40(6):1177–82.
5. Aung T, et al. The visual field following acute primary angle closure. Acta Ophthalmol Scand. 2001;79(3):298–300.
6. Abott CJ, Choe TE, Lusardi TA, et al. Evaluation of retinal nerve fiber layer thickness and axonal Transport 1 and 2 weeks after 8 hours of acute intraocular pressure elevation in rats. Invest Ophthalmol Vis Sci. 2014;55(2):674–87.
7. Agoumi Y, Sharpe GP, Hutchison DM, et al. Laminar and prelaminar tissue displacement during intraocular pressure elevation in glaucoma patients and healthy controls. Ophthalmology. 2011;118(1):52–9.
8. Liu X, Li M, Zhong Y, et al. The damage patterns of retinal nerve fiber layer in acute and chronic intraocular pressure elevation in primary angle-closure glaucoma. Eye Sci. 2011;26(3):154–60.
9. Xie M, Fan N, Liu X, et al. Advance in the damage and mechanism of optic nerve in acute angle-closure glaucoma. Int Rev Ophthalmol. 2015;39(4):247–52.

41 Is It Real Glaucomatous Visual Field Loss?

Xiaojing Pan, Ning Fan, and Xuyang Liu

The diagnosis of glaucoma and the therapeutic efficacy evaluation of this disease rely on the characteristic optic nerve damage and visual field defect. Aggravation of glaucoma should be first considered when progression of glaucomatous visual field loss is noticed. However, when visual field progression cannot be explained by optic disc change, the underlying reasons should be analyzed. Two cases are described in this section.

41.1 Case 1

41.1.1 Case Presentation

A 76-year-old female complained that the visual field in the left eye had narrowed for about 2 weeks. The patient had been diagnosed with "glaucoma and narrow angle" at another hospital 6 years before, and her both eyes had been administrated bimatoprost, brimonidine tartrate, and brinzolamide to lower intraocular pressure (IOP), and YAG laser peripheral iridotomy had been performed in both eyes. On follow-up half a month before, her visual field defect in the left eye progressed. The highest IOP by standard Goldmann applanation tonometry was measured as 19 mmHg OD and 18 mmHg OS. She had a 20-year history of diabetes mellitus, and her blood glucose level was controlled with medication. She had a history of right bundle branch block for the last 4 years. The patient denied histories of hypertension and cerebrovascular diseases.

On examination, the uncorrected visual acuity (UCVA) was 20/40 OD and 20/40 OS. IOP by noncontact tonometry was measured as 11.5 mmHg OD and 9.5 mmHg OS. In both eyes, the cornea was transparent with no keratic precipitates, the central anterior chamber was shallow, and the depth of the peripheral anterior chamber was 1/4CT in the presence of iridotomy. The C/D ratio was 0.7 OD and 0.8 OS. No abnormality was found in the macula.

Gonioscopy showed large radi of angle closure without indentation in both eyes; with indentation, peripheral anterior synechiae were observed with almost fully open angles.

Half a month before, standardized automated perimetry had shown an inferior paracentral defect in the right eye and an inferior arcuate defect extending from the blind spot in the left eye (Fig. 41.1).

X. Pan
Shandong Eye Institute, Qingdao Eye Hospital, Qingdao, China

N. Fan
Shenzhen Eye Hospital, Shenzhen University, Shenzhen, China

X. Liu (✉)
Xiamen Eye Center of Xiamen University, Xiamen, China

Shenzhen Eye Hospital, Shenzhen University, Shenzhen, China

N. Wang et al. (eds.), *Optic Disorders and Visual Field*, Advances in Visual Science and Eye Diseases 2, https://doi.org/10.1007/978-981-13-2502-1_41

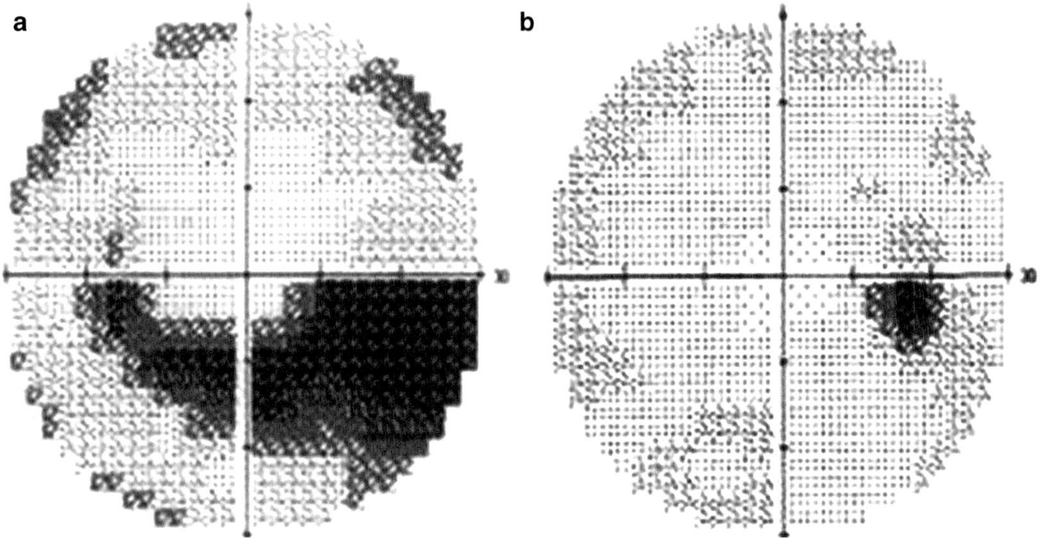

Fig. 41.1 Grayscale maps of Humphrey visual field assessment. Panel a: the 30-2 test showed an inferior arcuate defect in the left eye. Panel b: an inferior paracentral defect in the right eye was shown

The patient had experienced further narrowing of the left visual field accompanied by symptoms of headache and nausea. Re-examination showed tunnel vision; however, IOPs were normal in both eyes.

41.1.2 Case Analysis

Given the process of diagnosis and treatment of the patient's glaucoma, mixed glaucoma was considered (combined primary open-angle glaucoma and primary angle-closure glaucoma). As the patient had good control of IOP, we could not attribute the rapid visual field loss from an arcuate defect to tunnel vision within half a month to glaucoma progression.

On follow-up, the patient had gradually worsening headache which was severe and accompanied by delirium. Urgent CT showed cerebral hemorrhage, intracranial hematoma, and cerebral herniation (Fig. 41.2). The patient was transferred to neurosurgery without delay, where successful management was achieved.

41.1.3 Final Diagnosis

The final diagnosis was glaucoma in both eyes, cerebral hemorrhage, and cerebral hernia.

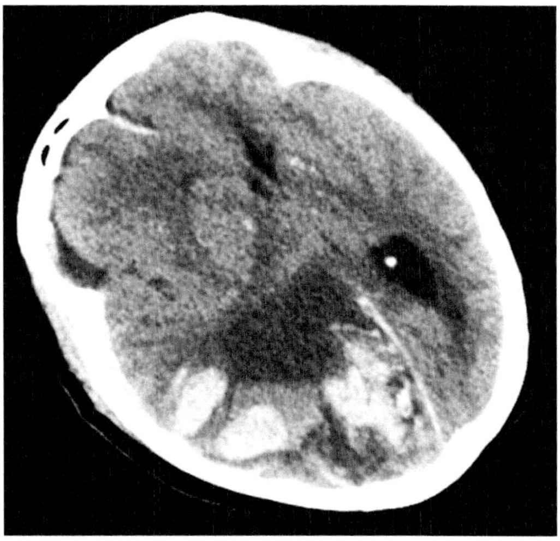

Fig. 41.2 Cranial CT image. It showed intracranial hematoma in the right temporal lobe and occipital lobe, peripheral tissue edema, and cerebral hernia

41.1.4 Case Review

The patient's presenting complaint of restricted visual fields and the typical glaucomatous changes observed in the optic nerve head led to the diagnosis of glaucoma. During management, the visual field defect in the left eye worsened, which was immediately attributed to glaucoma progression. Previous gonioscopy showed that the angle was mostly closed in both eyes without indentation, and the anterior chamber was significantly shallow, which might lead to the consideration of acute angle-closure glaucoma, given the symptoms of headache and nausea; the sudden progression to tunnel vision defect might be attributed to old age and poor compliance during acute onset of angle-closure glaucoma. Therefore, it was impossible not to consider glaucoma as the diagnosis. Confusingly, the patient had neither anterior segment changes nor raised IOP. The patient developed neurological symptoms with gradually worsening headache and delirium. Cranial CT showed intracranial hemorrhage and cerebral herniation. The patient was transferred to neurosurgery for urgent management so as to prevent further deterioration.

41.2 Case 2

Antoine Labbe

41.2.1 Case Presentation

A 65-year-old female patient complained of progressive constriction of the visual field in her right eye. She had been diagnosed with pigmentary glaucoma (early stage) and paracentral scotoma in this eye 3 years before. The patient had been using IOP-lowering drugs such as Xalatan, and the IOP was controlled, and there was no progression in the visual field defect during follow-up.

On examination, the UCVA was 20/20 OU. In both eyes, the cornea was transparent, and the anterior chambers, pupils, and lenses were normal. A Krukenberg's spindle was seen in the right eye, and no iris transillumination defects were seen. The C/D ratio was 0.4 in both eyes. The neuroretinal rim color was normal in both eyes, and the reflection of the superior retinal nerve fiber layer (RNFL) in the right eye was absent (Fig. 41.3).

Gonioscopy showed a wide and open angle in both eyes; the pigment of the trabecular meshwork in the right eye and the left eye was Grade IV and Grade I, respectively.

Central corneal thickness was 580 μm OD and 590 μm OS.

The OCT results revealed that the thickness of the RNFL reduced superiorly in the right eye and at 12 o'clock in the left eye; the ganglion cell layer in the macula of the right eye thinned with a large superior area involved, and the thickness of ganglion cell layer (GCL) in the macula of the left eye was normal (Fig. 41.4).

An inferior arcuate defect was seen in the visual field of the right eye and the visual field in the left eye was normal (Fig. 41.5).

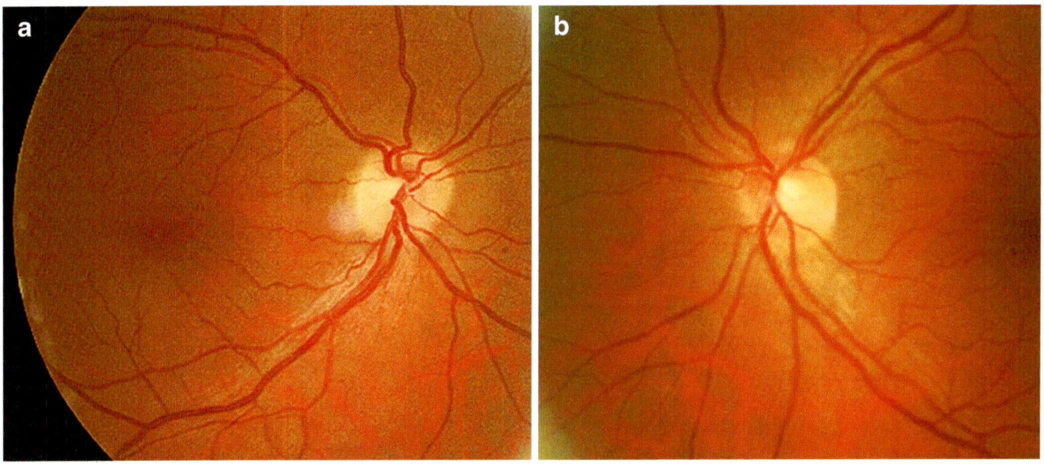

Fig. 41.3 Fundus photographs. Fundus photographs showed that the C/D was 0.4, and the neuroretinal rim was pink in color in both eyes, and a superior RNFL defect was seen in the right eye. Panel a: right eye. Panel b: left eye

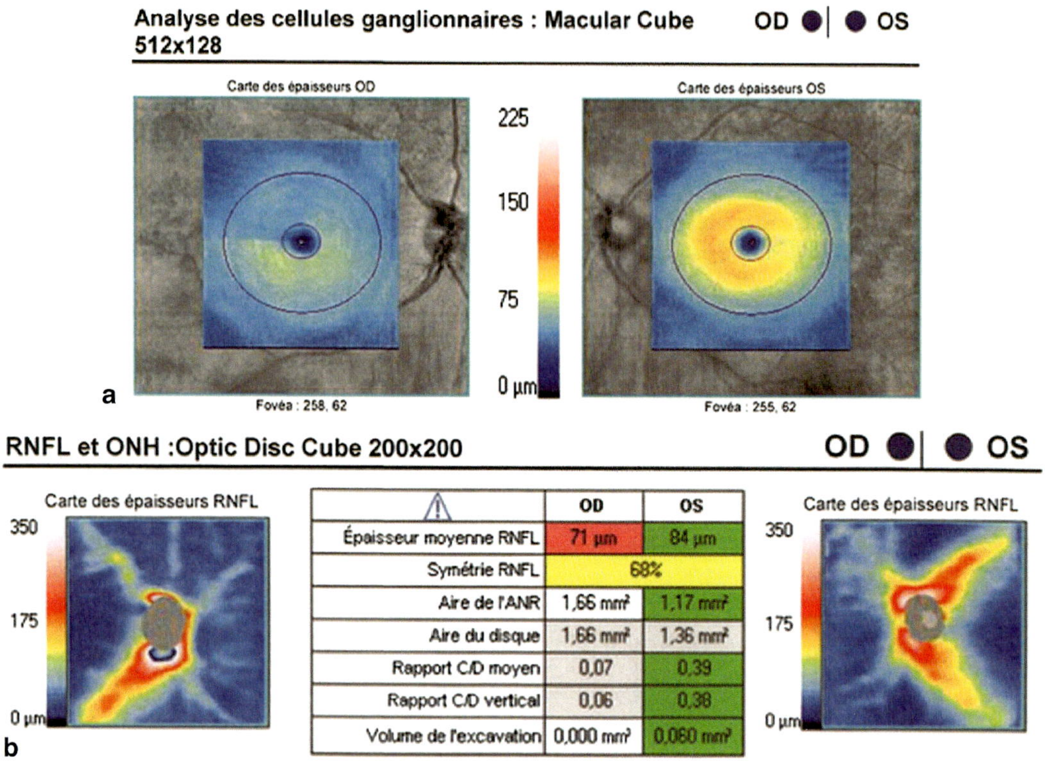

Fig. 41.4 OCT scans of the optic disc and macula. Panel a: the GCL in the macula of the right eye thinned, and the thickness of the GCL in the macula of the left eye was normal. Panel b: the thickness of the superior RNFL in the right eye and at 12 o'clock in the left eye reduced significantly

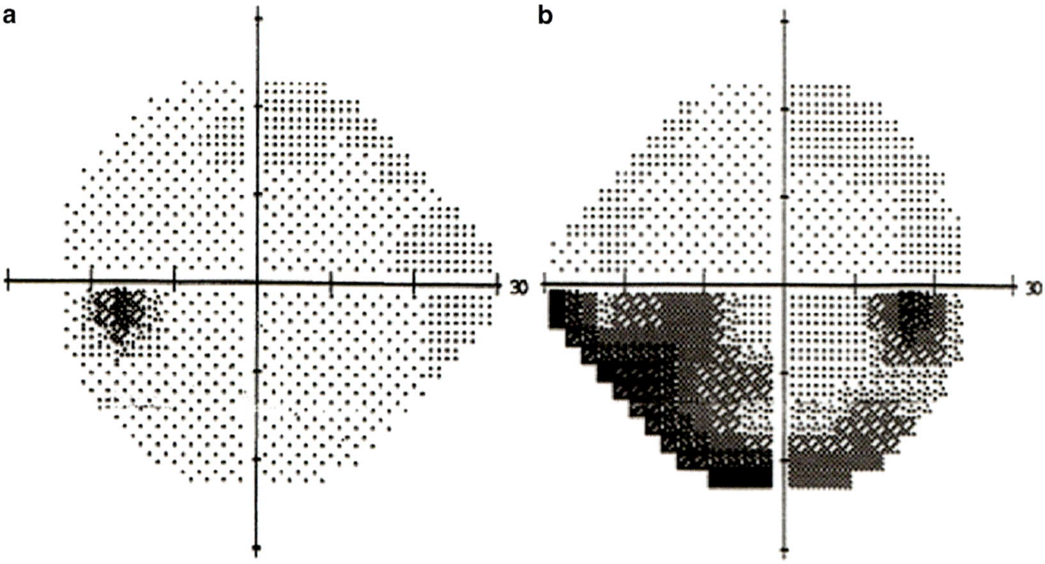

Fig. 41.5 Grayscale maps of Humphrey visual field assessment. The 24-2 test showed a normal left eye (Panel a) and an inferior arcuate defect in the visual field of the right eye (Panel b)

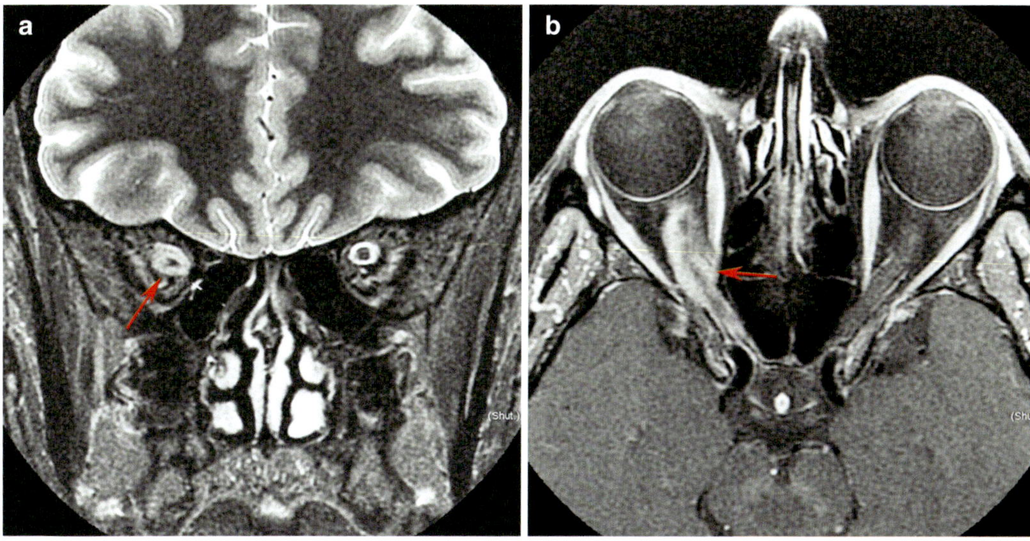

Fig. 41.6 Cranial MRI images. Panel a: the coronal T2-weighted image with fat suppression showed right optic nerve thickening, circular thickening of the peripheral optic nerve sheath, and isointensity (red arrow). Panel b: the axial T1-weighted contrast-enhanced image showed that the right optic nerve sheath was moderately enhanced and was tram-track like (red arrow)

41.2.2 Case Analysis

This patient had previous diagnosis of "pigmentary glaucoma" with the visual field change of "a paracentral defect"; examination (including anterior chamber angle) supported this diagnosis. The patient received drug treatment to control IOP, and the visual field did not progress or change. However, the patient complained of a significantly narrowed visual field in the right eye that occurred recently. Re-examination showed an inferior arcuate defect in the right eye. OCT showed that the RNFL and GCL damage was consistent with visual field manifestation. Was the visual field change caused by glaucoma progression?

Although the visual field signs, including the arcuate defect, matched that of the changes in the thicknesses of the RNFL and GCL, glaucoma progression could not explain the following: the patient had regular administration of IOP-lowering drugs for a long time and had good control of IOP; there were no corresponding changes in the optic disc and disc rim; and OCT showed superior and temporal diffuse RNFL damage and thinner ganglion cell complex (GCC) in the macular region. Did other comorbidities cause the rapid deterioration of the visual field? We chose cranial MRI for screening.

Cranial MRI showed optic nerve sheath meningioma in the right eye (Fig. 41.6).

41.2.3 Final Diagnosis

The final diagnosis was pigmentary glaucoma and optic nerve sheath meningioma in the right eye.

41.2.4 Case Review

The visual field damage caused by this optic nerve sheath meningioma may be confused with glaucomatous visual field changes. After analysis of the morphology of the optic disc and neuroretinal rim as well as the control of IOP, we found that optic nerve sheath meningioma was the underlying cause.

41.3 Discussion

Glaucoma is a group of diseases characterized by optic nerve atrophy and visual field defects, and the characteristic optic disc changes correspond with the RNFL defects and visual field deficits. These are very important for the assessment of glaucoma progression.

When glaucoma patients have worsened visual field damage, we should firstly evaluate whether the morphology and characteristics of visual field changes are consistent with those of glaucoma, i.e., whether visual field damage is consistent with the distribution and course of the RNFL, and whether glaucomatous optic disc damage is consistent with RNFL damage. When IOP is controlled well and the change of the optic disc is not significant but the visual field damage significantly worsens, we should consider diseases other than glaucoma.

The patient in Case 1 narrowly escaped danger and this teaches us an important lesion. The visual field change in glaucoma is gradual, and any rapid changes in a short period of time may indicate the presence of other pathologies. Previous gonioscopy showed that most of the angle was closed in both eyes without indentation, and the anterior chamber was significantly shallow, which might lead to the consideration of acute angle-closure glaucoma, considering that the patient had symptoms of headache and nausea; a sudden tunnel vision field defect may be related to old age and poor compliance in case of acute angle-closure glaucoma. However, there were no significant changes in IOP and fundus. The underlying pathology may be missed if one only considers glaucoma as the diagnosis. This also applies to Case 2. Case 2 was glaucoma with optic nerve sheath meningioma. The tumor originated from the arachnoid epithelial cells in the optic nerve sheath and grew around the optic nerve, which compressed the optic nerve and led to decreased vision or blindness in the patient. The optic nerve sheath meningiomas at different sites may cause different types of visual field loss, such as peripheral visual field defects, fascicular visual field defects, and paracentral or central defects. In general, the visual field loss caused by optic nerve sheath meningioma progresses slowly [1, 2]. However, the patient had "recent" accelerated visual field change with "stable" IOP control as monitored through long-term follow-up in Case 2; the reason might be related to the backward extension of the tumor and the involvement of the optic canal's inner segment. Due to anatomical factors, tumor at this site significantly compresses the optic nerve and causes worsening of the visual field in a short period of time, which is consistent with literatures.

In conclusion, when such visual field changes and original glaucomatous visual field changes overlap, we should look for the underlying pathology by differentiating the patterns of visual field loss caused by different conditions.

References

1. Luo Q, Li L, Chen J, et al. Study on optic nerve sheath meningioma and immunohistochemistry. Chin J Ophthalmol. 2013;49(6):526–30.
2. Kim SM, Lee J, Joe SG. Acute-onset altitudinal visual field defect caused by optic canal meningioma. J Clin Neurol. 2015;11(4):404–6.

Optic Neuropathy: Cassava Poisoning?

42

Xiaojing Pan, Ning Fan, and Xuyang Liu

When a middle-aged male patient presented with painless vision loss, a pale optic disc, and predominantly papillomacular bundle damage in both eyes for unknown reasons, Leber's hereditary optic neuropathy and other diseases that may cause optic atrophy in both eyes should be ruled out at first, and furthermore, the history of toxin and drug exposure should be taken into consideration to exclude the possibility of toxic optic neuropathy.

42.1 Case

Antoine Labbe

42.1.1 Case Presentation

A 37-year-old male patient complained of blurred vision in both eyes for several months. He denied histories of previous ocular and systemic diseases, trauma, and familial diseases.

On examination, the best corrected visual acuity (BCVA) was 20/33 OU. Intraocular pressure (IOP) was 14 mmHg OD and 17 mmHg OS. No abnormality was found in the anterior segment of either eye. Fundus examination showed that, in both eyes, the optic disc had a clear boundary, the temporal neuroretinal rim was pale in color, and the depression in the optic cup was deep. The C/D ratio was 0.8 OD and 0.7 OS, and no abnormality was noted in the macula (Fig. 42.1). Gonioscopy showed a wide and open anterior chamber angle in both eyes without any pigmentation. The central corneal thickness was 590 μm OD and 575 μm OS.

The OCT results showed that the temporal and inferotemporal sectors of retinal nerve fiber layer (RNFL) became thinner in the right eye, and the superotemporal and inferotemporal sectors of RNFL became thinner in the left eye (Fig. 42.2). OCT scans of the macula showed no abnormal findings.

Standardized automated perimetry with the 24-2 test showed central defects extending from the blind spot in both eyes (Fig. 42.3); the 10-2 test showed central defects that were the most severe in the inferotemporal area in both eyes (Fig. 42.4).

X. Pan
Shandong Eye Institute, Qingdao Eye Hospital, Qingdao, China

N. Fan
Shenzhen Eye Hospital, Shenzhen University, Shenzhen, China

X. Liu (✉)
Xiamen Eye Center of Xiamen University, Xiamen, China

Shenzhen Eye Hospital, Shenzhen University, Shenzhen, China

N. Wang et al. (eds.), *Optic Disorders and Visual Field*, Advances in Visual Science and Eye Diseases 2, https://doi.org/10.1007/978-981-13-2502-1_42

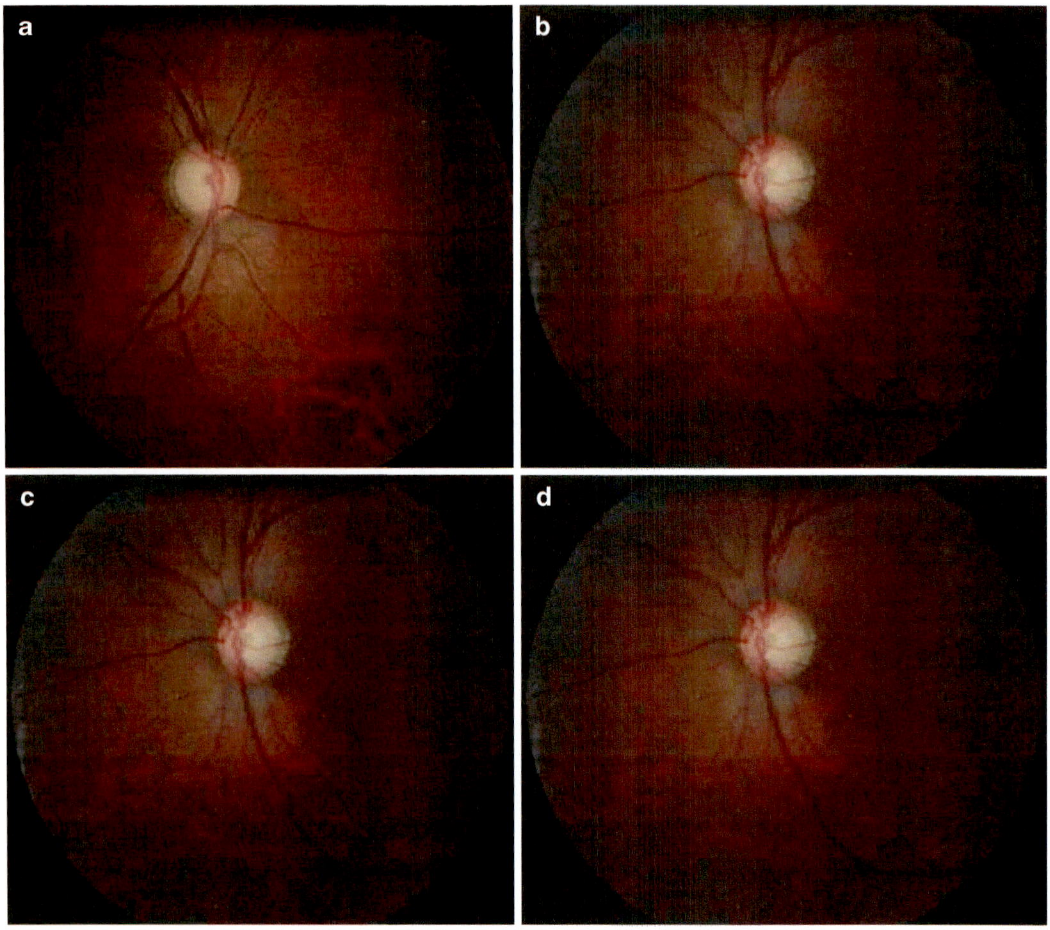

Fig. 42.1 Fundus photographs. The C/D ratio was 0.8 OD and 0.7 OS, the depression was deep, and the temporal neuroretinal rim was pale in color. Panels a, c: right eye. Panels b, d: left eye

42.1.2 Case Analysis

The patient, a middle-aged man, complained of slightly decreased vision in both eyes for several months. He denied a history of trauma. Eye examination showed temporal pale color in the optic disc and red color in the superior and inferior neuroretinal rim in both eyes, the C/D ratio was 0.8 OD and 0.7 OS, and the IOP was in normal range. Routine 24-2 threshold perimetry showed a central defect connecting to the physiological blind spot in both eyes. The 10-2 threshold perimetry showed central visual field defects that predominantly affected the inferior temporal area. OCT showed that the temporal (superior and inferior) RNFL became thinner and excluded abnormal morphology of the retina in the macular region. All these structural and functional examinations indicated that the lesion of both eyes was predominantly papillomacular bundle damage. Therefore, the following diagnoses were considered: (a) hereditary optic neuropathy, such as Leber's disease; (b) toxic optic neuropathy, such as drug, tobacco, alcohol, etc.; (c) sellar area and intracranial lesions, such as space-occupying or inflammatory lesion at the chiasm, steal syndrome, etc.; (d) inflammatory and ischemic optic neuropathy; and (e) normal tension glaucoma (NTG). The patient's vision decreased slowly, which did not support Leber's disease; the pat-

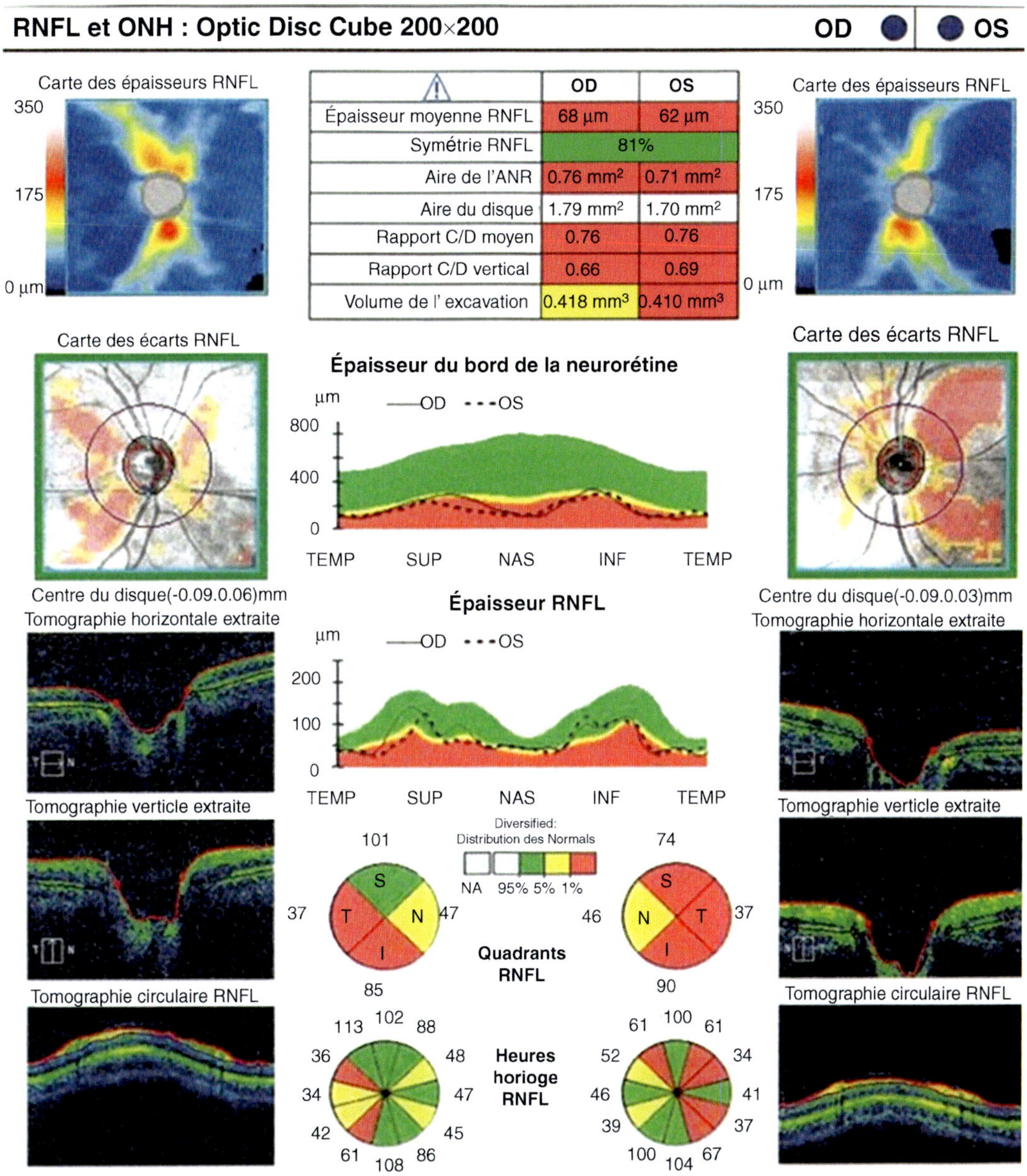

Fig. 42.2 OCT RNFL thickness analysis printout. The temporal and inferotemporal sectors of RNFL became thinner in the right eye. The superotemporal and inferotemporal sectors of RNFL became thinner in the left eye

tern of visual field loss, which was roughly bilaterally symmetrical, and the absence of pain on eye movement did not support inflammatory or ischemic optic neuropathy; the neuroretinal rim change was predominantly in the temporal quadrant, the central vision was affected and the central corneal thickness was not thin, which did not support NTG.

The test of mitochondrial DNA did not showed any mutation. Cranial and pituitary MRI did not show any abnormalities.

A review of his medical history revealed longtime consumption of cassava. After excluding the exposure to other toxicants and drugs, we determined that the patient had chronic cyanide-poisoning optic neuropathy.

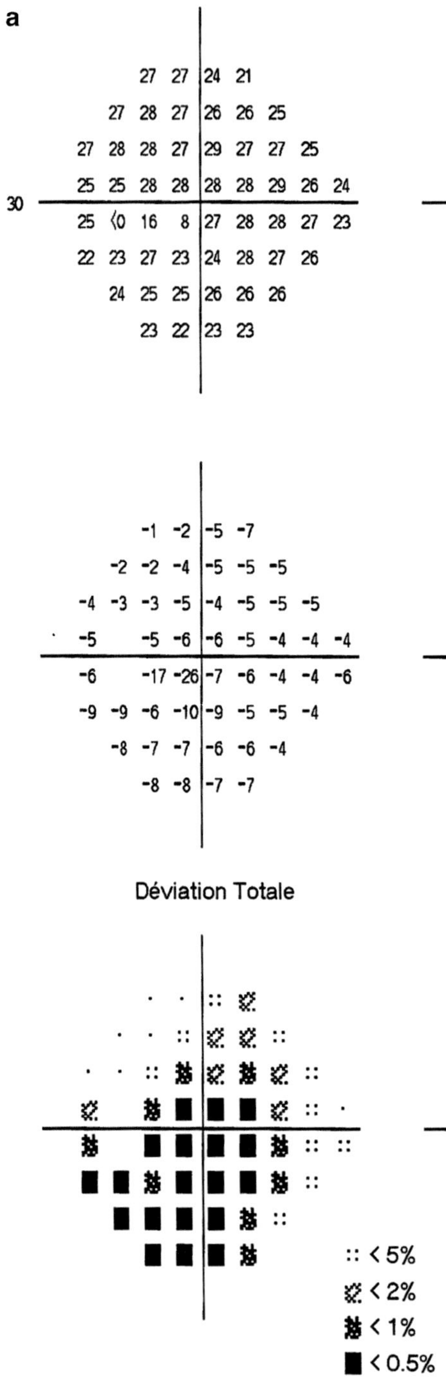

Fig. 42.3 Humphrey visual field printouts. The 24-2 test showed a central scotoma extending from the blind spot in each eye. Panel a: left eye. Panel b: right eye

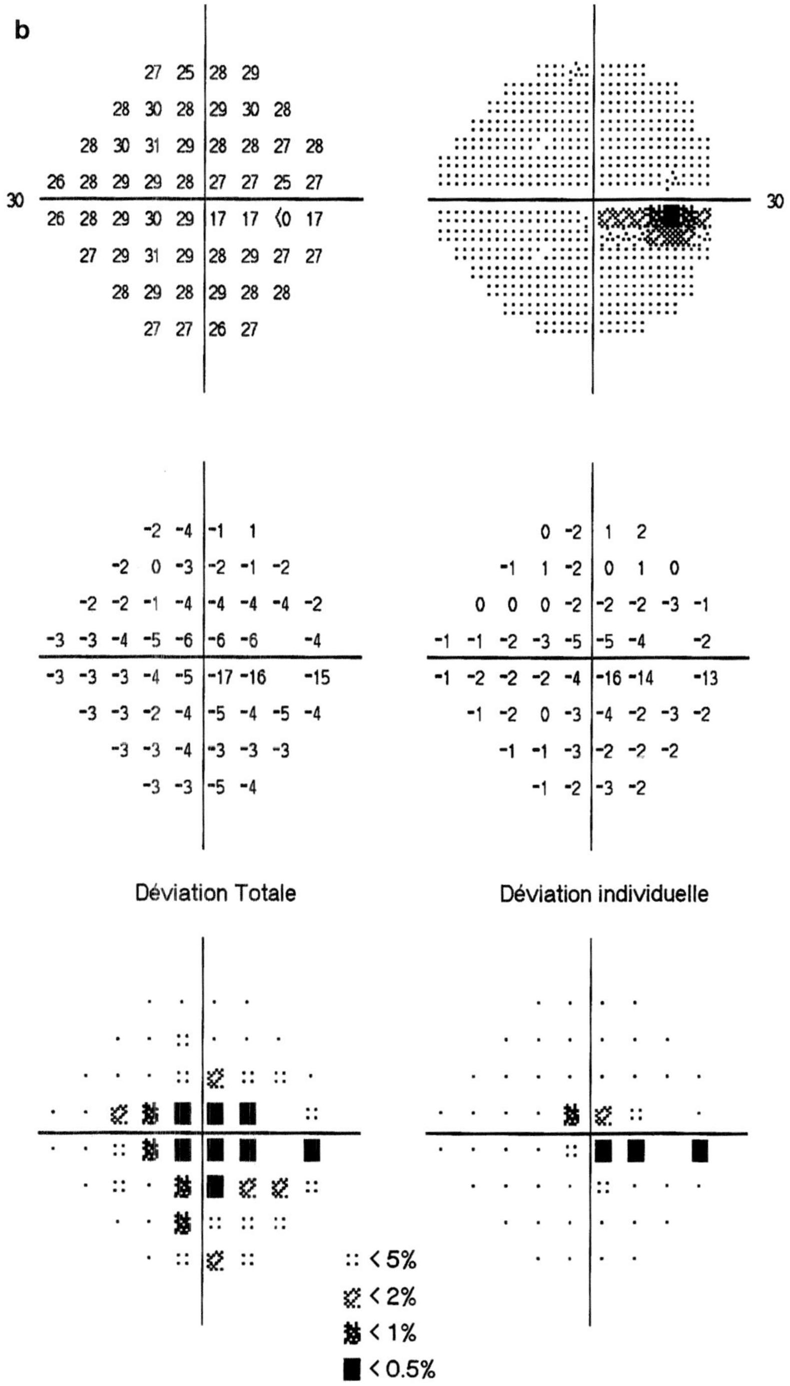

Fig. 42.3 (continued)

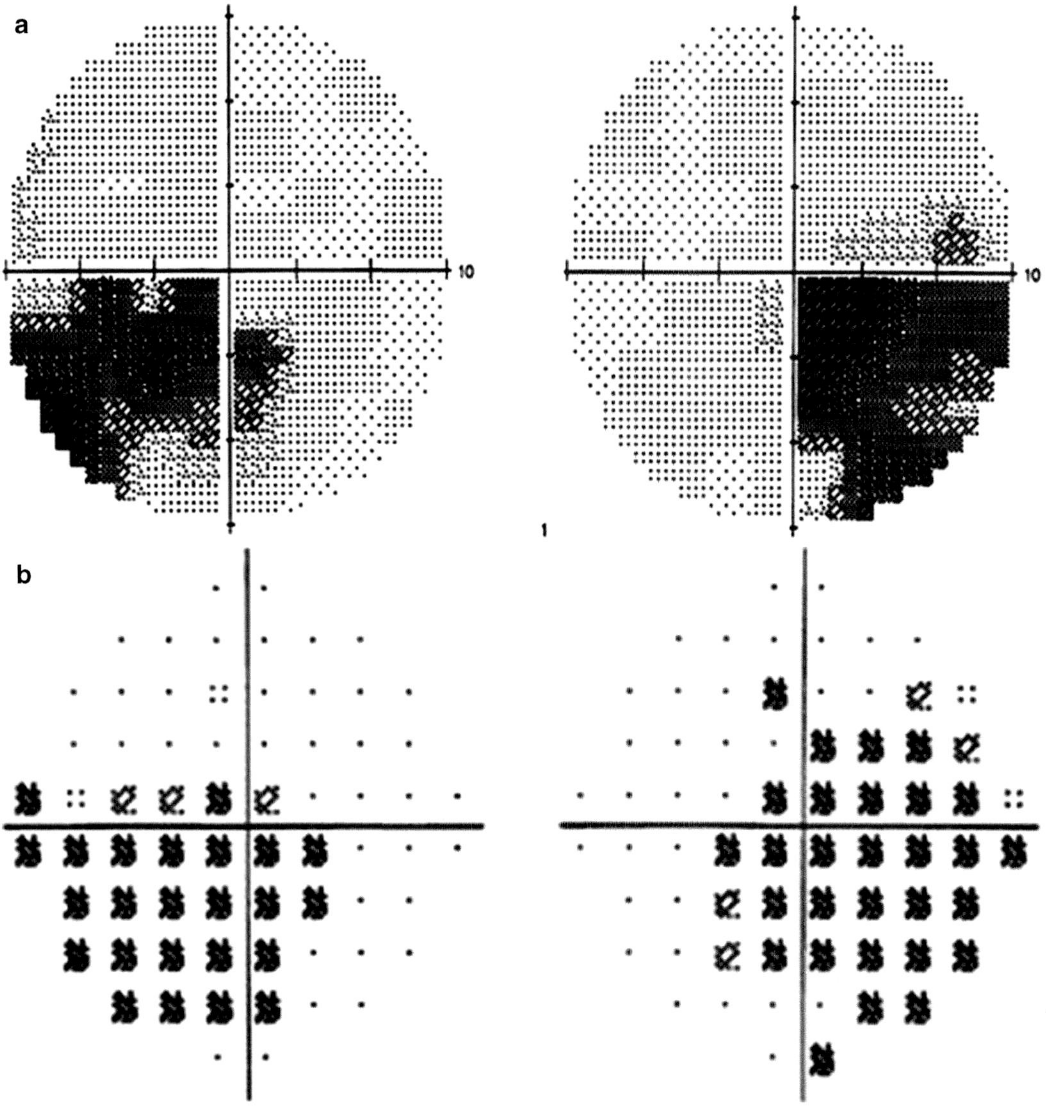

Fig. 42.4 Grayscale maps and pattern deviation probability maps of Humphrey visual field assessment. The 10-2 test showed a central scotoma predominantly affecting the inferotemporal visual field in each eye. Panel a: grayscale maps of both eyes. Panel b: pattern deviation probability maps of both eyes

42.1.3 Final Diagnosis

The final diagnosis was chronic cyanide-poisoning optic neuropathy (cassava poisoning) in both eyes.

42.2 Discussion

Cyanide poisoning can be attributed to longtime exposure to chemical products containing cyanide and excessive intake of foods rich in cyanoglycosides, such as cassava, bitter almonds, *Ginkgo biloba*, and peach kernel. The decomposition of foods containing cyanoglycosides produces hydrocyanic acid, and then the cyanide ion of the hydrocyanic acid binds to the iron ion in cytochrome oxidases and inactivates the respiratory enzyme, leading to cellular oxidation disorder and subsequent edema and necrosis. Intake of a large amount at one time may result in salivation, dizziness, headache, nausea, vomiting, palpitation, and weakness. Severely affected patients could have confusion, hypopnoea and secondary unconsciousness, corectasis, absence of light reflex, and death due to diaphragm paralysis or cardiac arrest. Chronic and long-term low-dose exposure mainly causes neurological toxicosis. Because of its complex function, the nervous system consumes a large amount of oxygen and reserves a small amount of energy, and thus it is very sensitive to hypoxia. Longtime accumulation of hydrocyanic acid may cause anoxic injury to neural tissues, for which the ocular manifestations include pale optic discs and optic atrophy. Since more blood supply in the optic disc goes to the nasal side than the temporal side, the temporal side is more sensitive to hypoxia than the nasal side. As a result, disc pallor in the temporal neuroretinal rim appears earlier and more significantly, and superior temporal and inferior temporal RNFL thinning should be differentiated from the manifestations of glaucomatous optic nerve damage [1–3].

Another differential diagnosis is tobacco-toxic optic neuropathy. Tobacco-toxic optic neuropathy is an optic neuropathy attributed to excessive smoking or excessive intake of tobacco-containing dust. Middle-aged and elderly patients who are users of smoked tobacco, cigar, chewing tobacco, or who smoke cigarette in the morning with overnight fasting are often affected. Tobacco-toxic optic neuropathy often involves the papillomacular bundle, and its pathological change is the degeneration of retinal ganglion cells, especially the vacuolated denaturation of cells in the macular region and the degeneration of the papillomacular bundle. Tobacco-toxic optic neuropathy is characterized by its long course and slow onset [1–3]. The patients would note gradual decrease of vision in both eyes, more significantly at dusk or in dark environment, and their eyes would be especially insensitive to red. Most patients experience achromatism. Because of the central scotoma, the patients would feel the vision is poorer under intense light. Funduscopy with red-free light shows obscure papillary macular nerve fibers and disappearance of foveal reflex; the patients with a long-standing disease may have pale color in the temporal disc rim.

The typical visual field change in tobacco-toxic optic neuropathy is a defect between the central fixation point and the physiological blind spot. This defect is dumbbell-shaped, and one or two regions within the scotoma have especially severe loss, and they are called the "core" of the defect. The case in this section and tobacco-toxic optic neuropathy are both cyanide poisoning in nature, and thus their visual field changes are similar (this patient denied a history of significant tobacco exposure).

Therefore, when a dumbbell-shaped scotoma in the visual field is found in a patient with decreased vision in both eyes, chronic cyanide poisoning should be considered [4–6]. The treatment of cyanide-toxic optic neuropathy is the same as that of general toxic optic neuropathy, which is predominantly accelerating the metabolism of cyanide and reducing intake of cyanide. Firstly, the patient should stop intaking relevant food or keep away from the circumstances rich in cyanide. Tobacco and alcohol consumption should be strictly prohibited. And the patient should be given mecobalamin therapy with vitamins B6 and B1; the highly effective detoxification drug 5% sodium thiosulfate at 30–40 mL, i.v., qd, with 12–20 times as a course of treatment; and oral cysteine at 4 g, qd, for 4–6 months. Symptomatic supportive therapies, such as vasodilation and microcirculation improvement, can also be added.

References

1. Vaughan D. Vaughan & Asbery's general ophthalmology (Translated by Zhao Guiqiu). 16th ed. Beijing: People's Health Press; 2006.
2. Peking Union Medical College Hospital. Routine ophthalmic diagnosis and treatment. 2nd ed. Beijing: People's Health Press; 2013.
3. Foroozan KLB. Optic nerve disorders (Translated by Xu Jun, Yang Qingsong and Ma Kai). Beijing: People's Medical Publishing House; 2014.
4. Liu X, Li S. Chronic toxicity of cyanate in eyes. J Ocul Trauma Occup Dis. 1993;15(5):501–5.
5. Liu X, Li S. Carbamylation of human lens gamma-crystallins: relevance to cataract formation. Yan Ke Xue Bao. 1993;9(3):136–42.
6. Adamolekun B. Neurological disorders associated with cassava diet: a review of putative etiological mechanisms. Metab Brain Dis. 2011;26(1):79–85.

43 The Visual Field Changes and Outcomes in Hepatitis B-Associated Optic Neuritis

Xiaojing Pan, Ning Fan, and Xuyang Liu

The clinical studies of hepatitis B-associated optic neuritis are limited, and the visual field changes are very important for its diagnosis and treatment. This section makes a preliminary exploration on its pathogenesis, clinical manifestation, treatment, and outcome through a case with reference to the literature.

43.1 Case

43.1.1 Case Presentation

A 27-year-old female patient complained of pain on eye movement and progressive loss of vision in both eyes for 10 days. Blurred vision had occurred in both eyes 10 days before and aggravated gradually. The symptoms peaked on day 5 and were accompanied by mild pain on eye movement. The blurred vision improved within the last 3 days. Since the patient was not pregnant after getting married for 3 years, she received an oral "traditional Chinese medicine" (the details were unknown) for infertility, and liver dysfunction was found 2 months later.

Physical examination showed that the blood pressure was 110/80 mmHg. She was conscious and fluent in speaking and had symmetric facial wrinkles, no tongue deviation, normal limb muscular strength and muscular tone, no ataxia, normal bilateral pinpoint pain sensation, and symmetric tendon reflex. Bilateral pathological signs were not elicited.

On examination, the uncorrected visual acuity (UCVA) was 20/60 in the right eye, and the left eye had a vision of finger counting. The visual acuity did not improve after myopic correction. The pupil was 4 mm in diameter in both eyes, and relative afferent pupillary defect (RAPD) was positive in the left eye. Fundus examination showed that, in both eyes, the optic disc was pink in color with a blurred margin. The distribution of vessels was normal, the retina was flat, and the reflection of the macular fovea was barely visible (Fig. 43.1). Both eyes were in normal position and exhibited normal eye movement.

Craniocerebral MRI revealed that the intensity of DWI signals in the posterior segment of the optic nerve increased on both sides, which suggested the possibility of optic neuritis in both eyes. No abnormal signal was seen in the brain parenchyma.

X. Pan
Shandong Eye Institute, Qingdao Eye Hospital, Qingdao, China

N. Fan
Shenzhen Eye Hospital, Shenzhen University, Shenzhen, China

X. Liu (✉)
Xiamen Eye Center of Xiamen University, Xiamen, China

Shenzhen Eye Hospital, Shenzhen University, Shenzhen, China

N. Wang et al. (eds.), *Optic Disorders and Visual Field*, Advances in Visual Science and Eye Diseases 2, https://doi.org/10.1007/978-981-13-2502-1_43

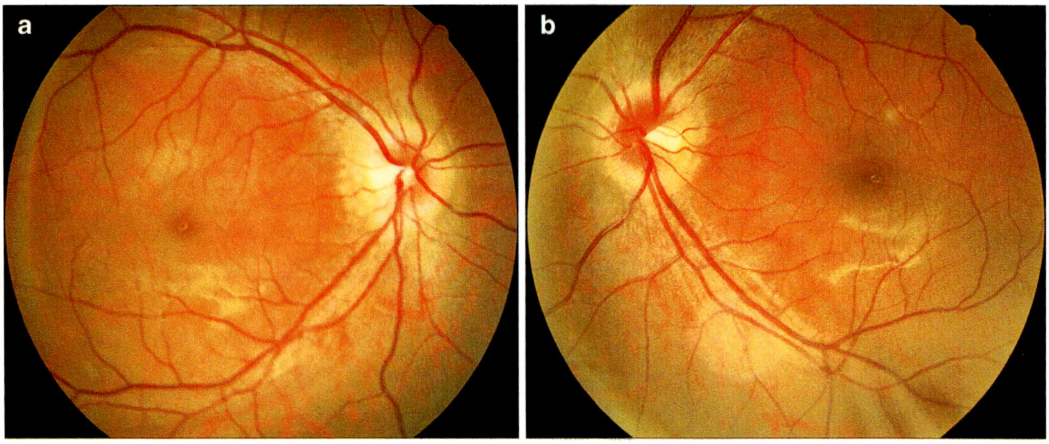

Fig. 43.1 Fundus photographs. In both eyes, the optic disc was pink in color with a blurred margin. The distribution of vessels was normal, the artery/vein ratio was 2:3, and the retina was flat. Panel a: right eye. Panel b: left eye

Liver function tests showed that alanine aminotransferase (ALT) was 760 U/L, glutamic-oxalacetic transaminase (AST) was 264 U/L, direct bilirubin (DBIL) was 17.8 μmol/L, and total bilirubin (TBIL) was 32.4 μmol/L. HBV-DNA was also tested, and the result was 1.48 × 105 IU/mL.

The OCT of the macula in both eyes revealed a relatively normal morphology (Fig. 43.2).

Standardized automated perimetry showed residual visual field only on the superonasal side in the right eye (Fig. 43.3), and the visual acuity was too poor to be examined in the left eye.

F-VEP testing showed the waveform of F-VEP was not elicited in the left eye, and the latency of each wave was prolonged in the right eye (Fig. 43.4) examination printouts.

Relevant examinations were further made after admission, including an examination for the six indicators of HBV: HBcAb (+), HBeAb (+), HBeAg (+), HBsAg (+), ANA + dsDNA + ENA + autoimmune hepatitis series (−), and ANCA (−). The results excluded autoimmune diseases and other systemic infectious diseases. Lumbar puncture was also performed, and it showed the CSF pressure was 180 mmH_2O, and the routine examination showed negative results. The biochemical test revealed the following results: chloride 115.9 mmol/L, glucose 4.92 mmol/L, albumin 13.5 mg/dL, and OB (oligoclonal band)/MBP (myelin basic protein)/24 h IgG synthesis (−), which excluded optic neuritis caused by intracranial infection, intracranial tumor, and noninfectious demyelinating diseases. Given the medical history and signs of the patient, optic neuritis due to active hepatitis B was considered for both eyes.

43.1.2 Final Diagnosis

The final diagnosis was hepatitis-associated optic neuritis in both eyes.

At the time of this presentation, the patient was with hepatitis in active phase with a high viral load, and administration of steroid might increase viral replication rate and result in fulminant hepatitis, which is life threatening. Therefore, anti-hepatitis drugs (entecavir), hepatinica, and immunoglobulin (IV) were administered.

While the patient was admitted and received antiviral therapies to control hepatitis, the progressive loss of vision led to no light perception in both eyes.

Re-examination 10 days after antiviral treatment showed an HBV-DNA of 1.15 × 105 IU/mL, which was significantly decreased than

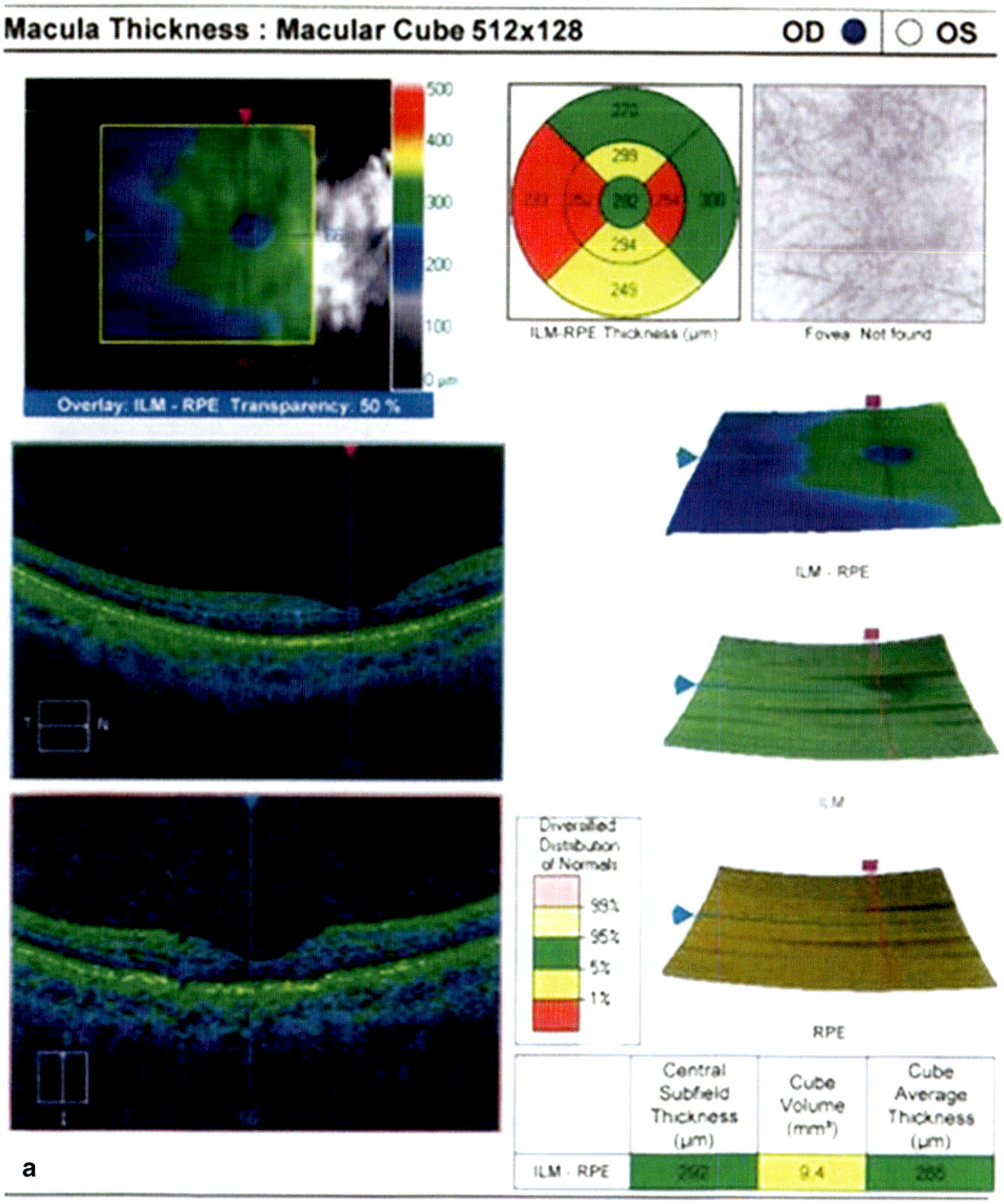

Fig. 43.2 OCT macula thickness analysis printouts. OCT showed normal morphology of the macula in both eyes. Panel a: right eye. Panel b: left eye

before. The patient continued anti-hepatitis treatment with concomitant intravenous methylprednisolone 1000 mg/day × 3 days, 500 mg/day × 3 days, 250 mg/days × 3 days, and 120 mg/day × 3 days and then changed to oral steroid.

After the steroid therapy began, the visual acuity gradually improved. On the tenth day of steroid therapy, re-examination showed visual acuities in the right eye and left eye were 1.5 and 0.5, respectively. Re-examination of the visual

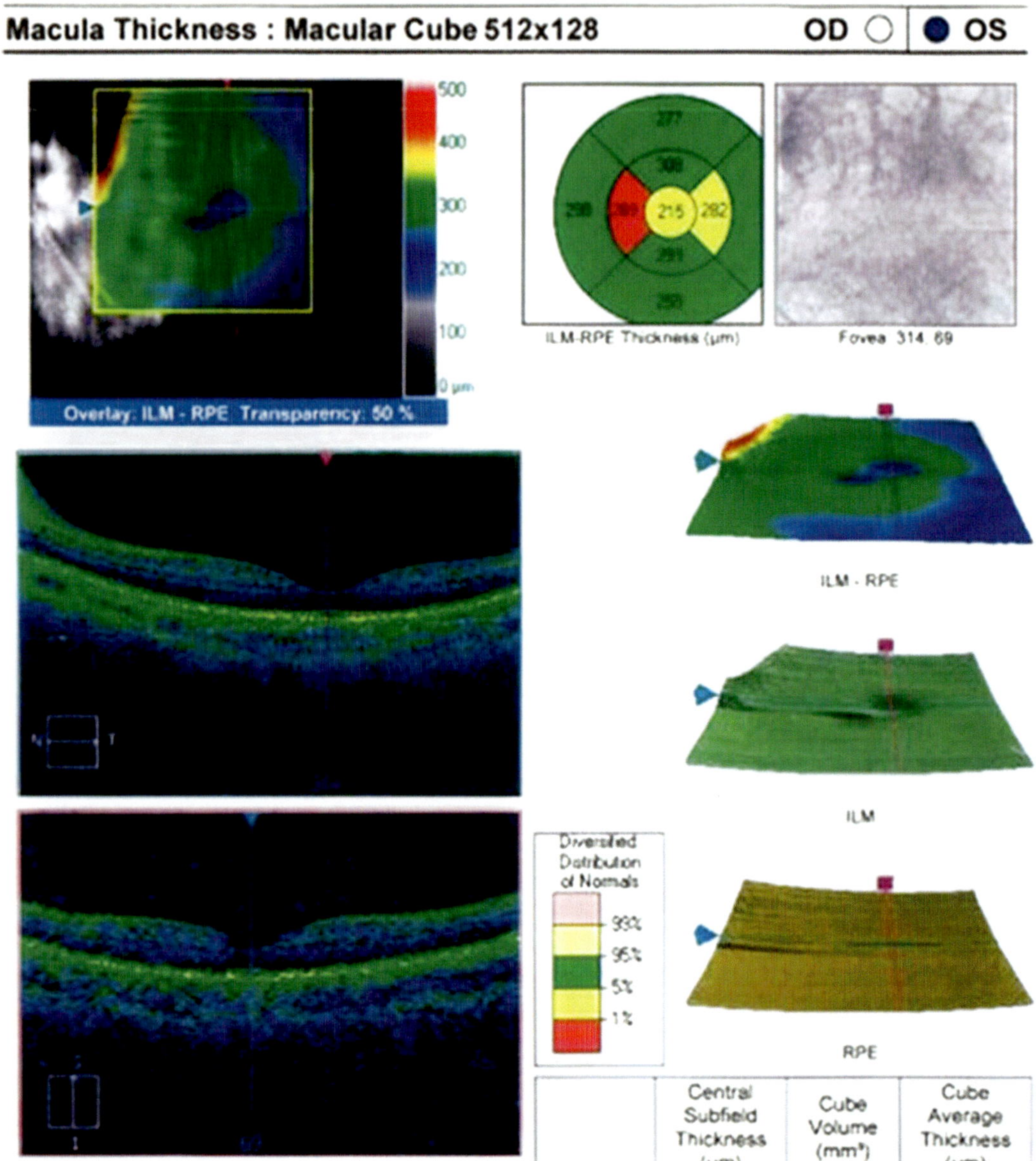

	Central Subfield Thickness (µm)	Cube Volume (mm³)	Cube Average Thickness (µm)
ILM - RPE	215	9.7	270

Fig. 43.2 (continued)

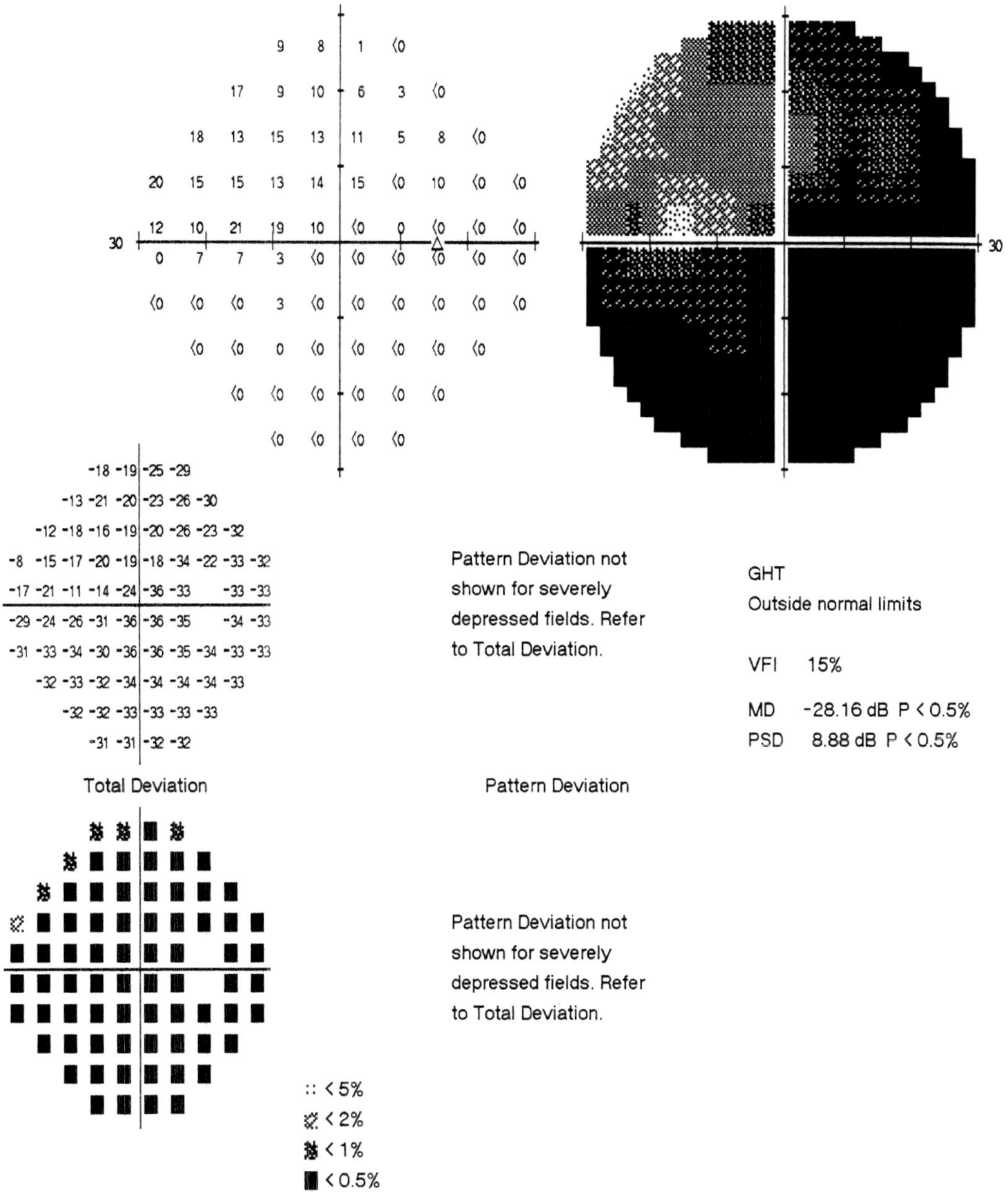

Fig. 43.3 Humphrey visual field analysis printout. The 30-2 test showed only residual visual field on the superonasal side and significant decrease of light sensitivity in the right eye

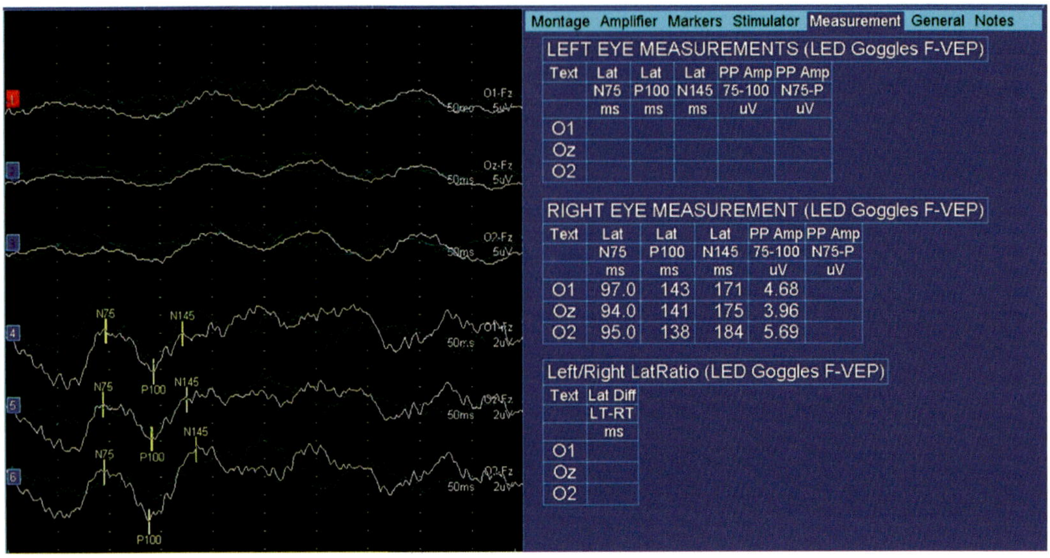

Fig. 43.4 F-VEP examination printouts. The F-VEP of both eyes showed that no waveform was elicited in the left eye, and the latency of each wave was prolonged in the right eye

field with a Humphrey analyzer showed that the sensitivity reduced globally in both eyes, and superior and inferior temporal arcuate defects were observed in the visual field of the left eye (Fig. 43.5). Fluorescence fundus angiography (FFA) of both eyes showed retinal vasculitis in both eyes and obstruction of the superior branch of the retinal artery in the left eye. Follow-up visit after 1 month of treatment showed significantly increased visual acuity than before (Fig. 43.6). Follow-up visit after half a year of treatment, the patient felt that both her visual acuity and visual field recovered to the level before the onset of the disease (Fig. 43.7).

43.1.3 Case Review

The patient was a young female with illness that was acute in onset and rapid in progression and ran a monophasic course. At its worst, the patient experienced complete loss of vision in both eyes, and the visual field examination showed diffuse loss in both eyes. The patient developed the typical symptoms and signs of optic neuritis, such as pain on eye movement and optic disc edema. Cranial MRI indicated possible optic neuritis. F-VEP examination showed that no waveform was elicited in the left eye, and the latencies of each wave in the right eye extended. Based on these, the patient was diagnosed with optic neuritis.

Then the patient received autoimmune-related antigen tests and diagnostic lumbar puncture. The optic neuritis caused by autoimmune diseases, intracranial infection, craniocerebral space-occupying lesion, and noninfectious demyelinating diseases were excluded.

Given the medical history that the patient underwent liver function tests at another hospital for abdominal discomfort a week before she experienced ocular symptoms and the test indicated impaired liver function and significantly increased HBV viral load, we considered infectious or infection-related optic neuropathy due to acute active hepatitis.

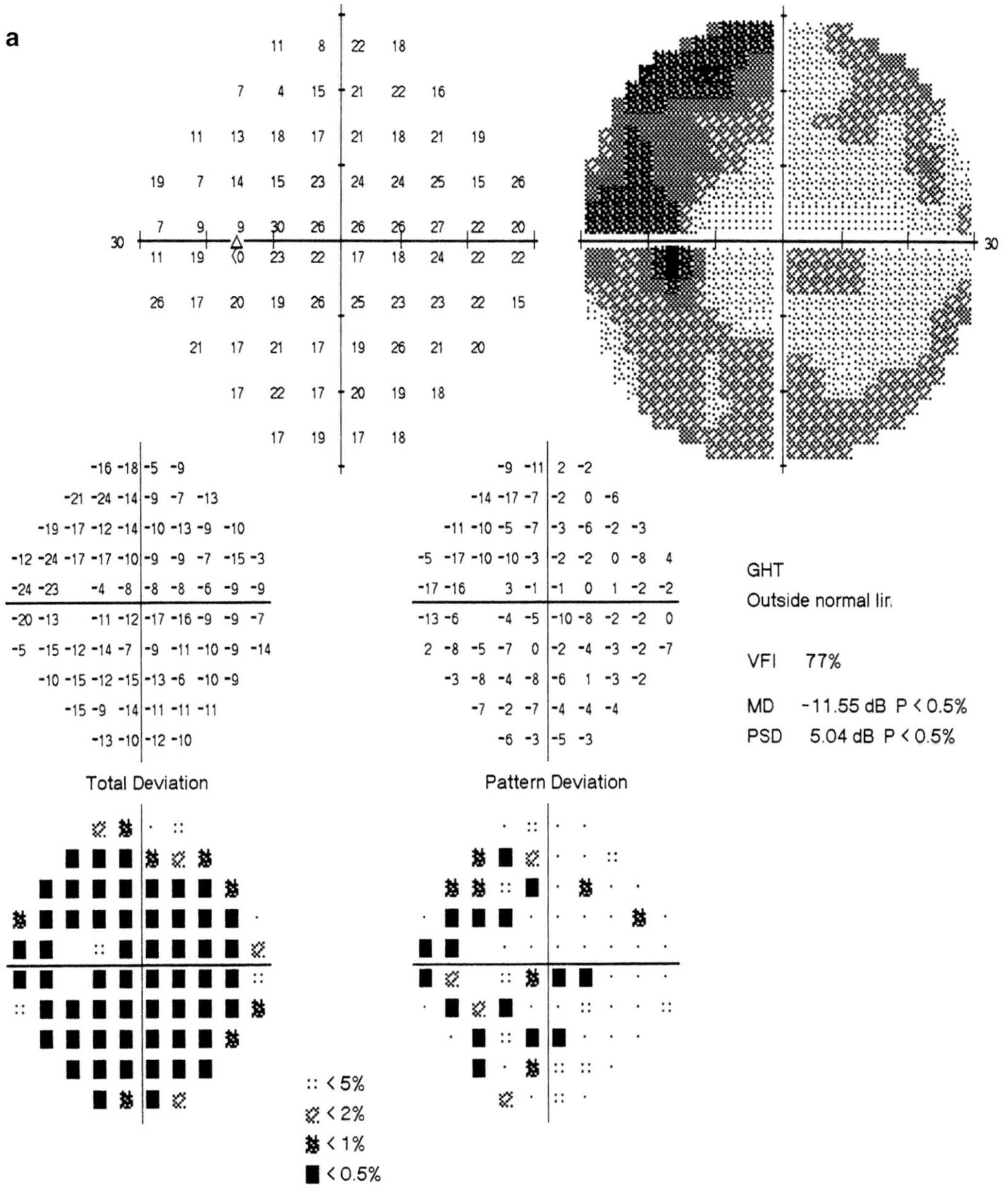

Fig. 43.5 Humphrey visual field analysis printouts on the tenth day of steroid therapy. The 30-2 test showed generalized reduction of sensitivity in both eyes and supratemporal and inferotemporal arcuate scotomas in the left eye. Panel a: left eye. Panel b: right eye

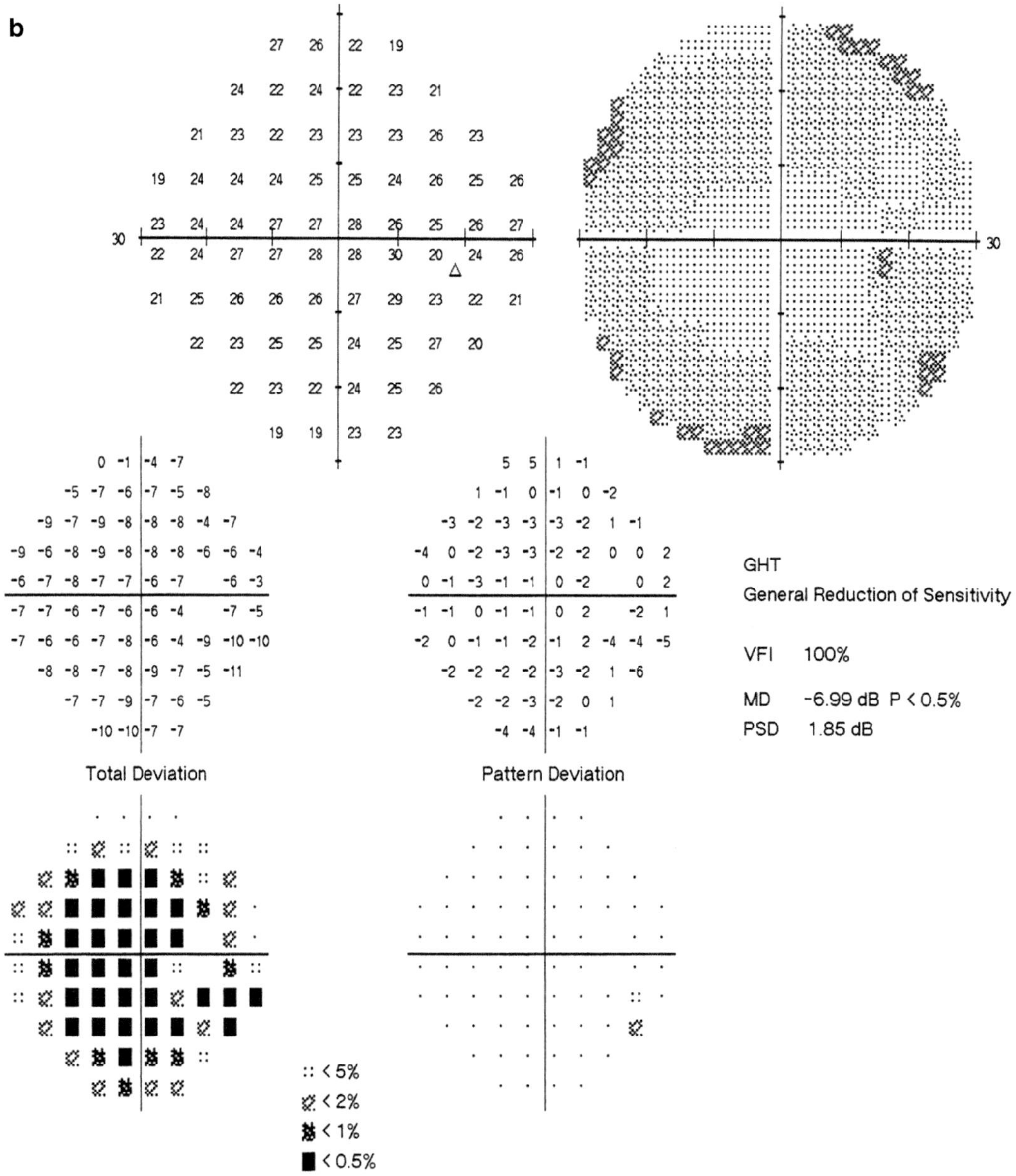

Fig. 43.5 (continued)

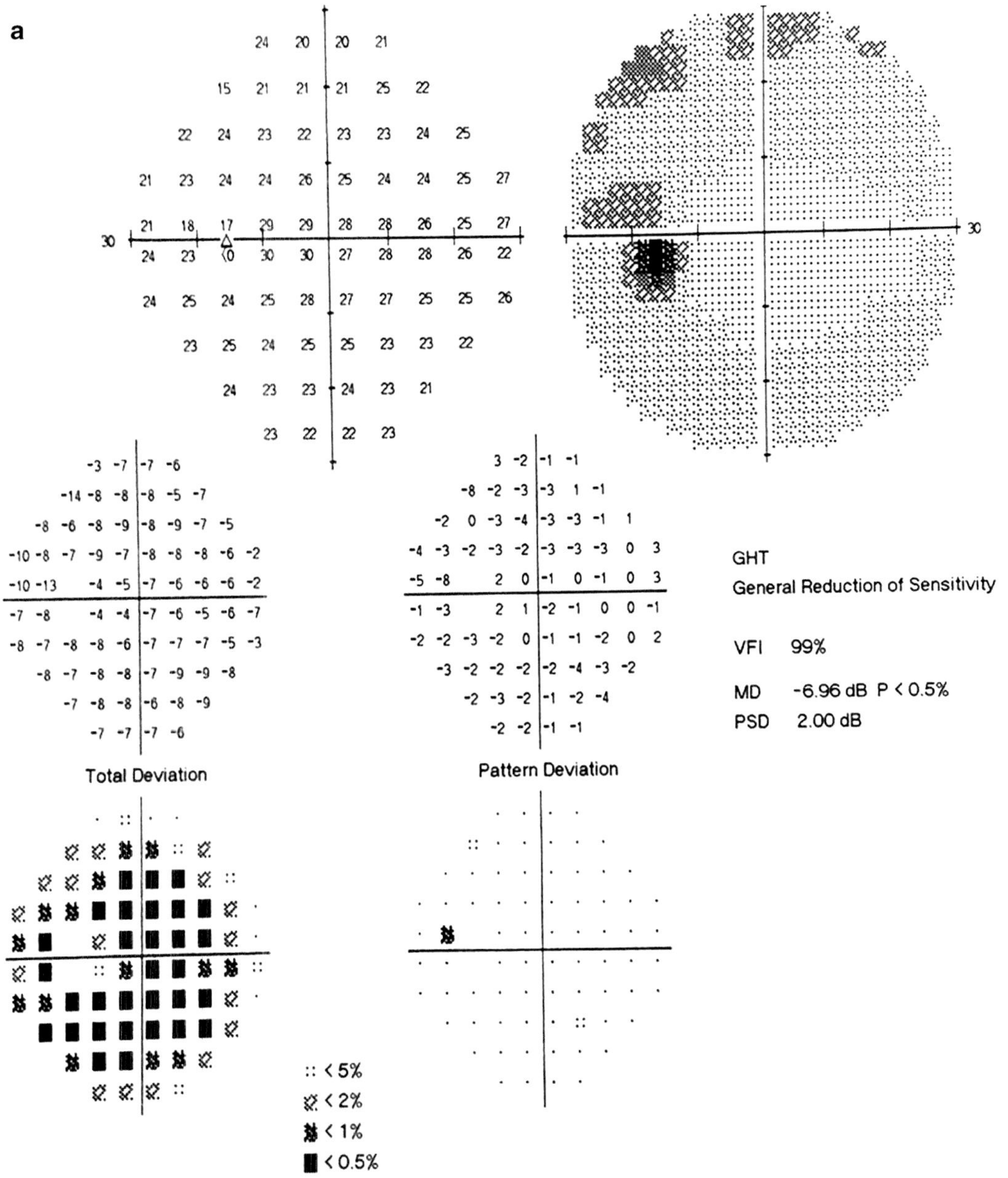

Fig. 43.6 Humphrey visual field analysis printouts after 1 month of intravenous glucocorticoid therapy. The 30-2 test showed increased visual field sensitivity when compared to that seen previously in both eyes. Panel a: left eye. Panel b: right eye (low reliability)

b

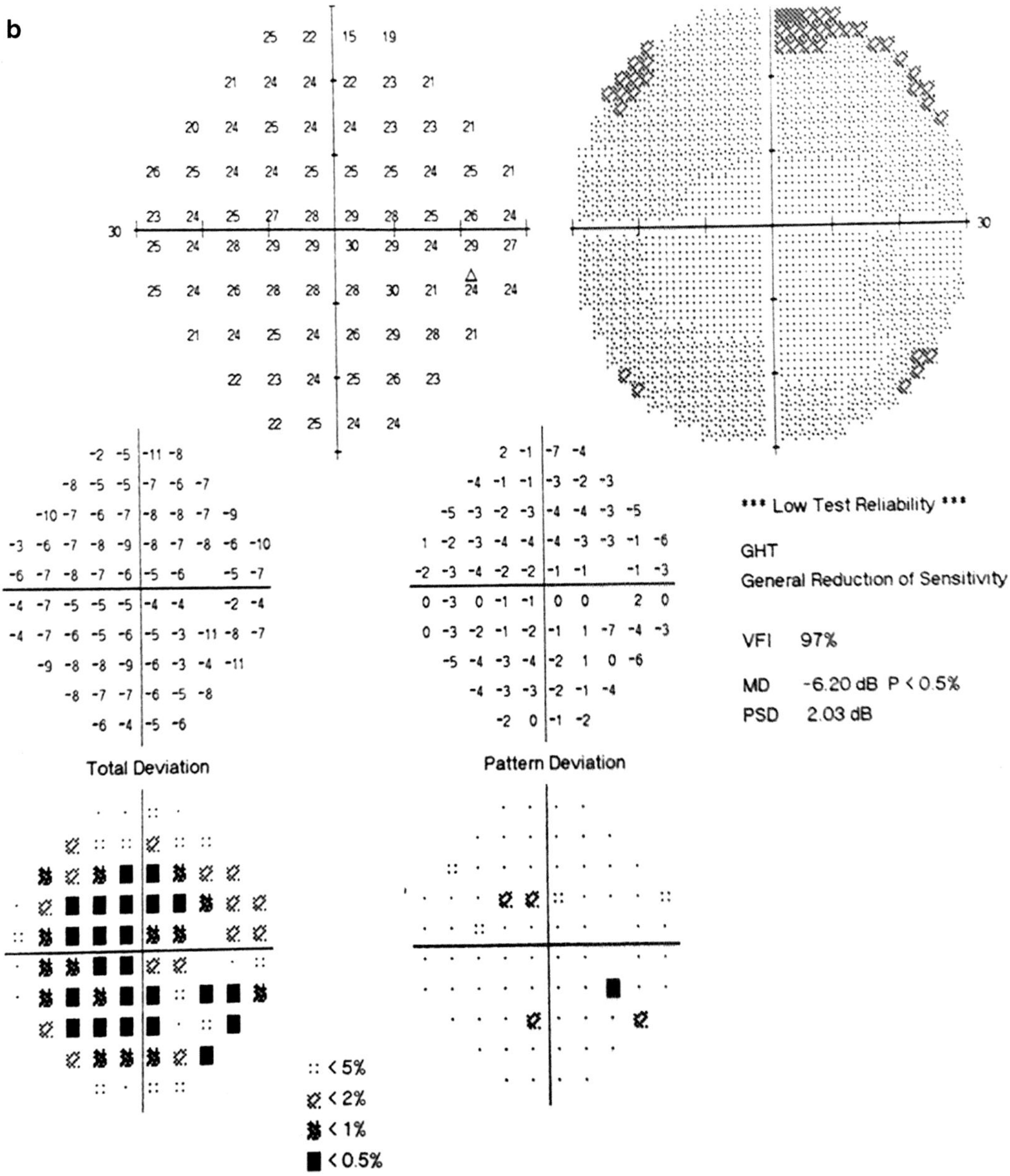

Fig. 43.6 (continued)

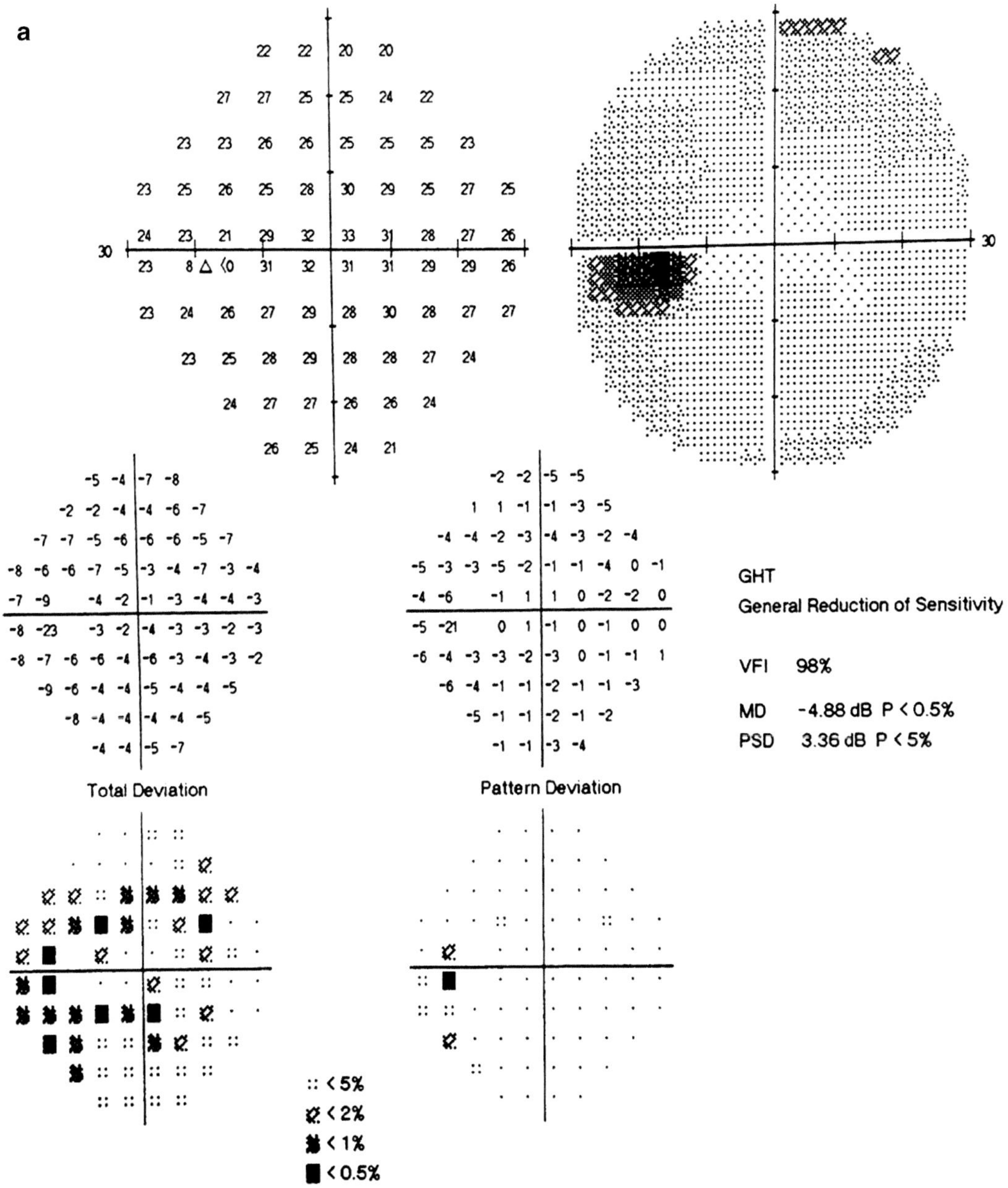

Fig. 43.7 Humphrey visual field analysis printouts after 6 months of intravenous glucocorticoid therapy. The 30-2 test strategy showed mild decrease of light sensitivity in both eyes. Panel a: left eye. Panel b: right eye (low reliability)

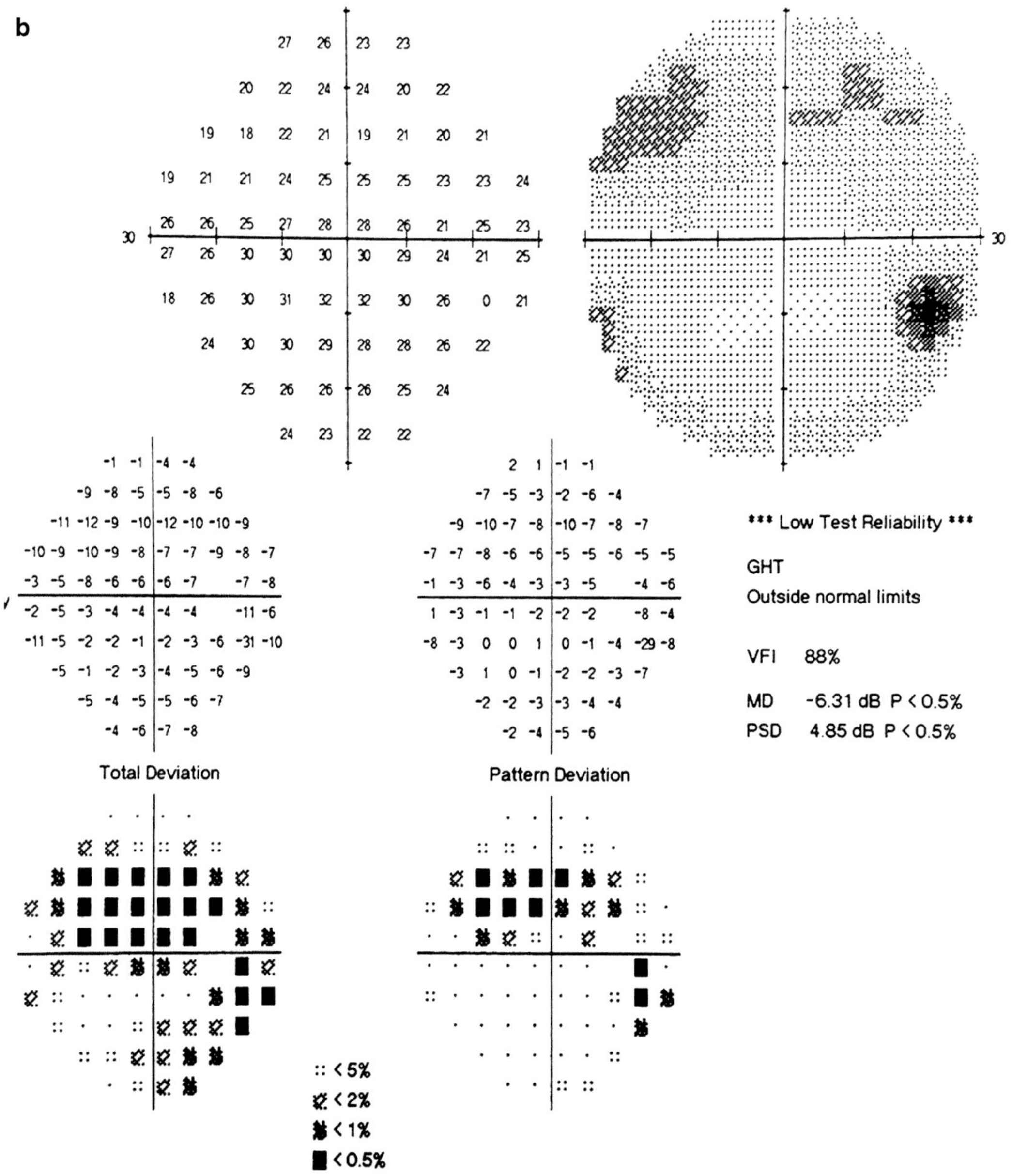

Fig. 43.7 (continued)

43.2 Discussion

Optic neuritis could be divided into the following types: idiopathic optic neuritis associated with multiple sclerosis or optic neuromyelitis, infection-related optic neuritis, and inflammatory optic neuropathy. Infection-related optic neuritis is rare clinically, for which the pathogenesis is not clear, but it is associated with bacterial and viral infection. A preliminary exploration on the pathological mechanism of HBV-associated optic neuritis in this patient is made as below.

The extrahepatic injury in hepatitis B is mainly caused by immune complexes, and the extrahepatic manifestations included serum sickness-like response (polyarteritis nodosa), membranous glomerulonephritis, and infantile papular acrodermatitis (Gianotti-Crosti syndrome). Approximately 1–10% of infected persons have these manifestations. Serum sickness-like response occurs in the early phase of acute hepatitis B, usually before the development of jaundice. Clinical characteristics of serum sickness-like response include fever, rash, and polyarteritis. This symptom may disappear rapidly after jaundice, but it can also be seen in the acute phase of hepatitis. In patients with acute necrotizing arteritis (polyarteritis nodosa), approximately 30–50% are carriers of HBV.

Hepatitis B virus (HBV) infection and the immunhistopathological mechanism play an important role in the pathogenesis of polyarthritis nodosa (PAN). PAN is a non-granulomatous vasculitis characterized by segmental inflammation and necrosis of small and medium arteries. It predominantly invades small and medium arteries with a segmental distribution and often occurs in the aortic bifurcation and spreads distally [1].

Peripheral nerve diseases are common in PAN (50–80%), and about 20–30% cases experience skin damage manifested as painful erythematous subcutaneous nodules. It appears in clusters along the arteries. ANCA is not commonly positive (<20%). Angiography shows microangioma and/or vascular stenosis. Biopsy of small and medium artery walls reveals cellular infiltration. The diagnostic criteria of polyarteritis nodosa presented by the American Rheumatism Association in 1990 included the following: (a) weight loss since disease onset ≥4 kg; (b) livedo reticularis on the skin; (c) testicular pain or tenderness not due to infection, trauma, or other reasons; (d) myalgia, lethargy, or lower limb haphalgesia; (e) mononeuritis or polyneuropathy; (f) diastolic pressure ≥90 mmHg; (g) increased creatinine and urea nitrogen; (h) HBsAg or HbsAb (+); (i) arteriography shows visceral artery infarction or aneurysm formation (except for arteriosclerosis, fibromuscular dysplasia, or other inflammatory reasons); and (j) biopsy of small and medium artery wall shows infiltration of granulocyte or mononuclear cell in the artery wall. Patients who meet three out of the ten criteria can be considered as having polyarteritis nodosa. Among these, biopsy and arteriography are very important for diagnosis [1].

This patient had optic neuritis in both eyes and was HbsAg (+); fluorescence fundus angiography showed retinal vasculitis in both eyes and obstruction of the superior branch of the retinal artery in the left eye. All of these were consistent with the diagnosis criteria of polyarteritis nodosa as listed above. Preferred drug for the treatment of polyarteritis nodosa was glucocorticoid. In this case, the symptoms were rapidly relieved after glucocorticoid treatment. Therefore, this patient had hepatitis B-related optic neuritis, and the basis of the pathological injury was polyarteritis nodosa due to HBV.

The patients with infectious or infection-related optic neuritis usually have acute and subacute onset. Single eye or both eyes may be involved. Its manifestations include optic disc inflammation, retrobulbar optic neuritis, neuroretinitis, or optic perineuritis. The prognosis varies greatly with the pathogens and severity of infection. Some types of infectious optic neuritis spontaneously resolve (such as optic papillitis and optic perineuritis), or when the disease is not serious, early diagnosis and targeted antibiotic treatment can lead to good recovery of visual function; in cases such as infectious optic neuritis caused by treponema pallidum or *Mycobacterium tuberculosis* or other severe infection, recovery may not be made without timely treatment. The recovery of visual acuity in most patients with infection-related optic neuritis is good [2, 3].

In this case of hepatitis B-related optic neuritis, the visual acuity and visual field after treatment had recovered to the premorbid level. However, globally, clinical diagnosis and management of hepatitis B-related optic neuritis are guided by only a limited number of case reports. There is a severe lacking of large prospective studies upon which clinical practice guidelines can be drafted and followed [4, 5].

The author retrospectively investigated optic neuritis related to viral hepatitis in 20 patients from Neuro-ophthalmology of Tongren Ophthalmology Hospital, including 18 patients with chronic hepatitis B and 2 patients with chronic hepatitis C. Of these, 13 patients had single-eye involvement at onset (65%), and 16 patients had a monophasic disease course (80%). Twenty-seven eyes were affected by optic nerve damage, and optic disc edema (n = 14, 52%) was common; based on the worst recorded visual acuity during the course of the disease, 19 eyes (70%) had a best corrected visual acuity <20/200. Visual field changes were predominantly inferior visual loss (ten eyes, 50%). All patients were followed for 3 months after glucocorticoid therapy, and the visual acuity of 3 eyes (11%), 4 eyes (15%), 12 eyes (44%), and 8 eyes (30%) completely recovered, significantly improved, improved, and had no change, respectively. All these results indicated that the visual acuity damage was serious in patients with optic neuritis and viral hepatitis. Some patients had completely recovered visual acuity after glucocorticoid therapy; visual field testing was of high clinical significance in assessing disease severity and monitoring treatment outcome.

References

1. Chinese Medical Association of Rheumatology. Guideline for the diagnosis and treatment of polyarteritis nodosa. Chin J Rheumatol. 2011;15(3):192–3.
2. Zhu L, Lu H, Yan R, et al. Clinical studies of optic neuritis with viral hepatitis. Chin J Ophthalmol. 2012;48(5):428–31.
3. The Neuroophthalmology Group of Ophthalmology Branch in Chinese Medical Association. Expert consensus on the diagnosis and treatment of optic neuritis. Chin J Ophthalmol. 2014;2014(6):459–63.
4. Trepo C, Guillevin L. Polyarthritis nodosa and extrahepatic manifestations of HBV infection: the case against autoimmune intervention in pathogenesis. J Autoimmun. 2001;16(3):269–74.
5. Zhao S, Chen T, Peng C, et al. The putative acceleration of optic neuritis when combined with chronic hepatitis B. J Neurol Sci. 2015;358(1–2):207–12.

Brucella Encephalitis and Optic Neuropathy

44

Xiaojing Pan, Ning Fan, and Xuyang Liu

Neurological brucellosis is a relatively rare complication of brucella infection, while ocular involvement is even rarer. Clinically, we have been confronted with the patients who had visual function decrease in both eyes as the initial symptom.

44.1 Case

44.1.1 Case Presentation

A 25-year-old male patient complained of paroxysmal amaurosis in both eyes that had occurred half a year before and worsened in the last month, accompanied by progressive vision loss, headache, and fever. The patient had "encephalitis" when he was a child, from which he recovered with no sequela. He had a history of contact with cows and sheep as well as suspected tuberculosis patients.

On eye examination, the uncorrected visual acuity (UCVA) was 20/40 in the right eye, and the left eye had a vision of finger counting. No improvement was seen with the pinhole test. In both eyes, the cornea was transparent, the anterior chamber was clear, the pupil size was 3 mm in diameter, the direct light reflex was present, and the density of lens increased. Fundus examination showed the optic disc congestion and edema, as well as tortuous and dilated retinal veins in both eyes (Fig. 44.1). Both eyes were in normal position and showed normal eye movement.

Neurological examination showed symmetric facial wrinkles, neck stiffness, normal limb muscular strength and muscular tension, no ataxia, bilateral normal pinpoint sensation, and symmetric tendon reflex but no nystagmus. The bilateral pathological signs were not induced.

Standardized automated perimetry showed that the light sensitivity was decreased or even lost in the right eye (Fig. 44.2), and the visual acuity was too poor to be examined in the left eye.

The F-VEP results revealed that the latency of the P2 wave in the left eye was longer when compared to that in the right eye, and the P2 wave was normal in the right eye.

X. Pan
Shandong Eye Institute, Qingdao Eye Hospital, Qingdao, China

N. Fan
Shenzhen Eye Hospital, Shenzhen University, Shenzhen, China

X. Liu (✉)
Xiamen Eye Center of Xiamen University, Xiamen, China

Shenzhen Eye Hospital, Shenzhen University, Shenzhen, China

N. Wang et al. (eds.), *Optic Disorders and Visual Field*, Advances in Visual Science and Eye Diseases 2, https://doi.org/10.1007/978-981-13-2502-1_44

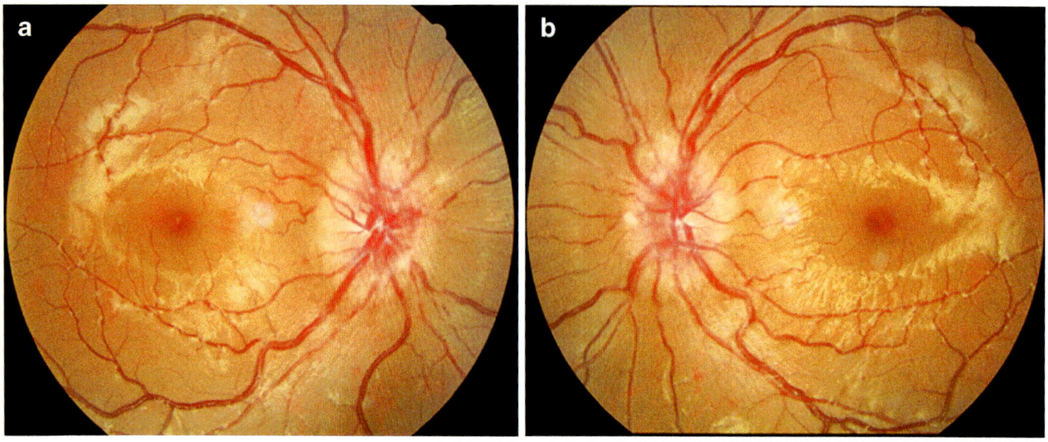

Fig. 44.1 Fundus photographs. The optic disc was congestion and edema, and the retinal veins showed tortuous and dilated in both eyes. Panel a: right eye. Panel b: left eye

Further systemic examination indicated the following:

Full blood examination showed the white blood cell count was 4.62×10^9/L, neutrophils accounted for 41.8%, and lymphocytes accounted for 44.2%; urinalysis, erythrocyte sedimentation rate, immunology, tumor markers (AFP, CEA, SCC, CYFRA21-1, CA19-9, and T-PSA), rheumatoid panel (ASO, RF, and CRP), HLA-B27, Quanteferon, fungal-D glucan, cardiolipin antibody, and TB-DNA-PCR test showed negative results.

With lung CT, the tree-in-bud sign was suspected, and the possibility of pulmonary tuberculosis was not excluded.

Paranasal sinus CT revealed nasal septum deviation and bilateral inferior turbinate enlargement. No other significant abnormalities were observed.

Craniocerebral MRI displayed thickened and enhanced meninges around the bone platform and in the left middle cranial fossa. These were likely to be inflammatory lesions. A partially empty sella was noted (Fig. 44.3); brain CT venogram (CTV) showed right sigmoid sinus stenosis. Positron emission tomography (PET) did not show significant metabolic hotspots.

Lumbar puncture showed an opening pressure of >330 mmH_2O, and biochemistry and cytology tests showed WBC 236×10^6/L, glucose 2.6 mmol/L, chloride 106.5 mmol/L, protein 339.8 mg/dL, CD4+, CD20−, and Ki67−, which indicated that no tumor cells were present. Cerebrospinal fluid X-pert, five viruses PCR (HBV, HCV, Syphilis TP, HIV, and CMV), common bacterial staining, ink staining, and acid-fasting staining all gave negative results.

Based on these tests, the patient was highly suspected of having infectious meningitis. Given the previous history of contact with sheep, the pathogen was considered to be brucella. A further Wright's agglutination test showed positive results, and thus the diagnosis was Brucella meningitis.

44.1.2 Final Diagnosis

The final diagnosis was optic neuropathy in both eyes and brucella meningitis.

The patient was administered with rifampicin, doxycycline, and ceftriaxone for two 8-week courses with a 2-week break in between. After the treatment, the UCVA was 1.0 in the right eye, and the UCVA in the left eye corresponded to a

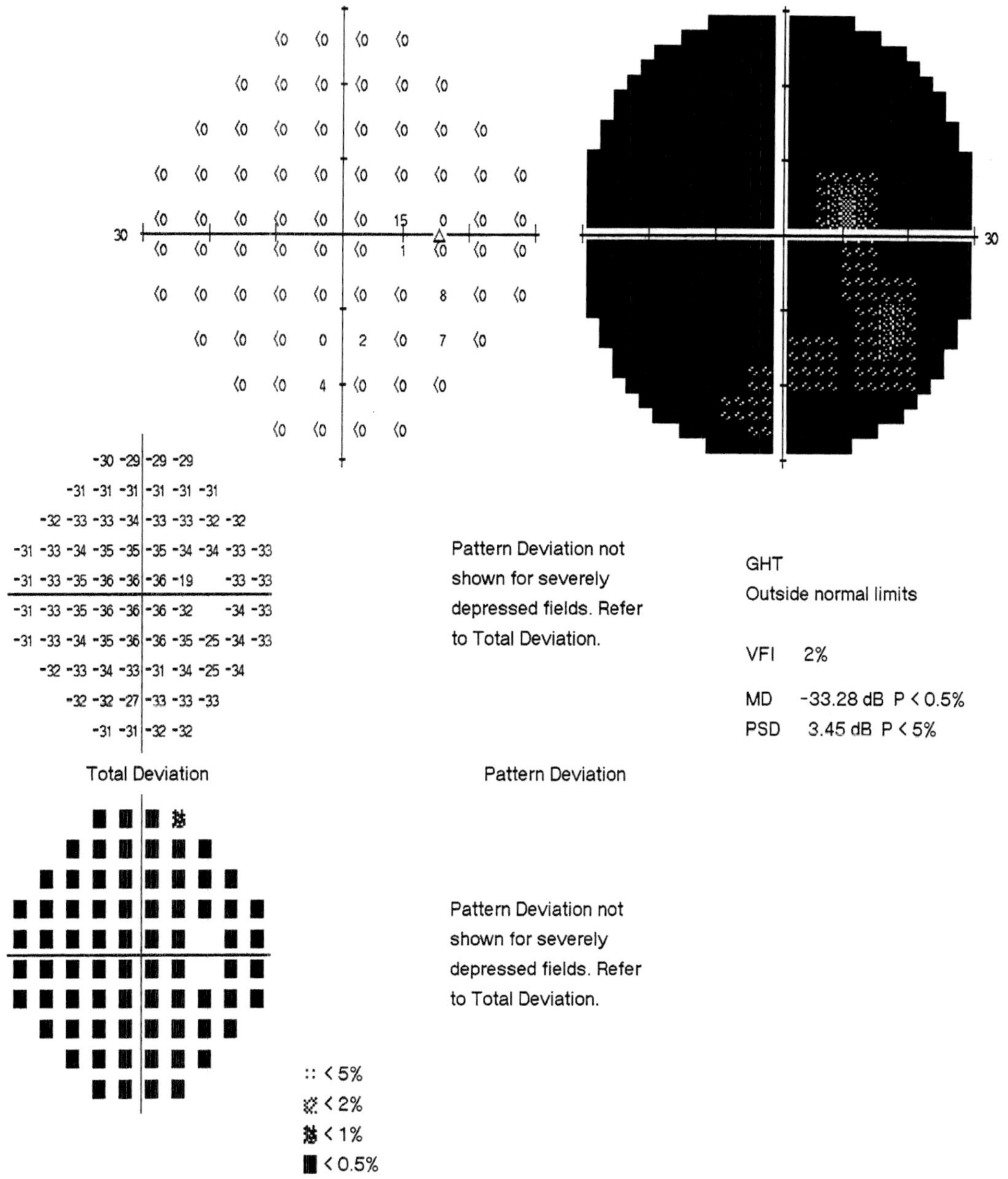

Fig. 44.2 Humphrey visual field analysis printout. The 30-2 test revealed that the light sensitivity was deceased significantly or even lost

vision of finger counting at a distance of 50 cm. The optic disc edema evidently resolved and the color became pale in both eyes.

Re-examination of the right visual field showed that the light sensitivity had significantly improved after the treatment (Fig. 44.4).

Fig. 44.3 Cranial MRI image. After T1W1-enhanced scan, thickened and enhanced meninges around the bone platform and in the middle cranial fossa were displayed (yellow arrow)

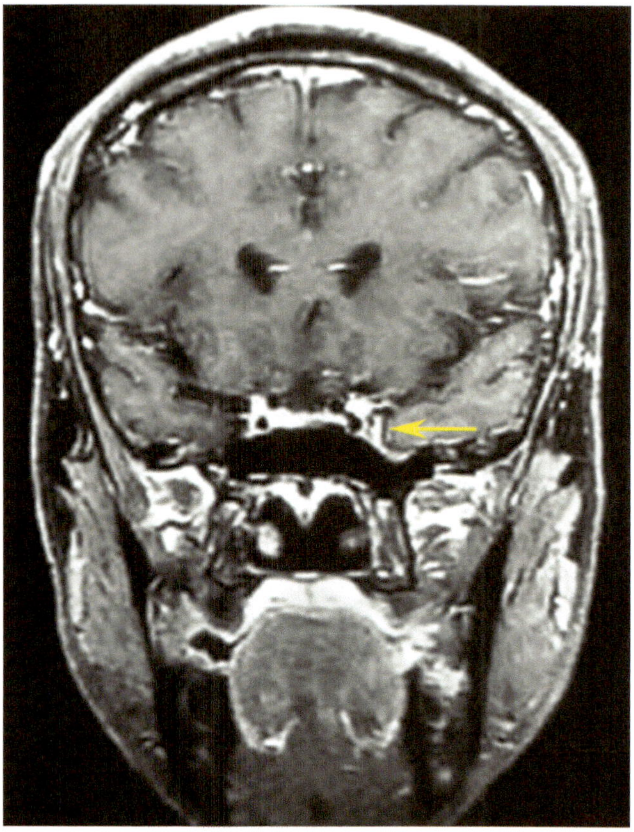

44.2 Discussion

Brucellosis is an infectious zoonotic disease. The disease has a variety of clinical manifestations, including prolonged fever, hyperhydrosis, lethargy, hepatosplenomegaly and lymphadenopathy, joint pain, and neuralgia, as well as some rare manifestations, such as abscess, sacroiliac arthritis, pneumonia, endocarditis, and epididymo-orchitis [1]. When brucellosis involves the nervous system, it is usually manifested as meningitis, encephalitis, radiculitis, and myelitis, and the symptoms of meningeal irritation may appear, such as headache, vomiting, and neck stiffness. The common neurological symptoms include irritability, dystrophy, myasthenia, disorientation, neck stiffness, peripheral nerve injury, etc. The pathogenesis may be that brucella infection causes cerebral meningeal adhesions, which influences cerebrospinal fluid circulation, leading to increased intracranial pressure; or brucella infection causes inflammatory lesion of the cranial nerve vasa vasorum; or brucella infection directly involves the cranial nerves [2].

The ocular symptoms caused by neurological brucellosis are usually attributed to the increased intracranial pressure transduced to Schwalbe's spaces through the subarachnoid space, thus increasing the pressure in Schwalbe's spaces and compressing the central retinal vein, which blocks the outflow and leads to edema of the optic disc [3, 4]. Clinical manifestations include damage of various severities to the visual acuity and visual field. In some patients, oculomotor nerve (CNIII) is affected, which is manifested as diplopia, strabismus and ptosis, etc. Since nervous involvement is usually manifested as blood circulatory disorder, most patients experience amaurosis fugax in the early phase; with the extended time and worsened severity of optic nerve compression, the frequency of amaurosis fugax increases, which often indicates serious optic nerve damage. Peripheral visual field damage often

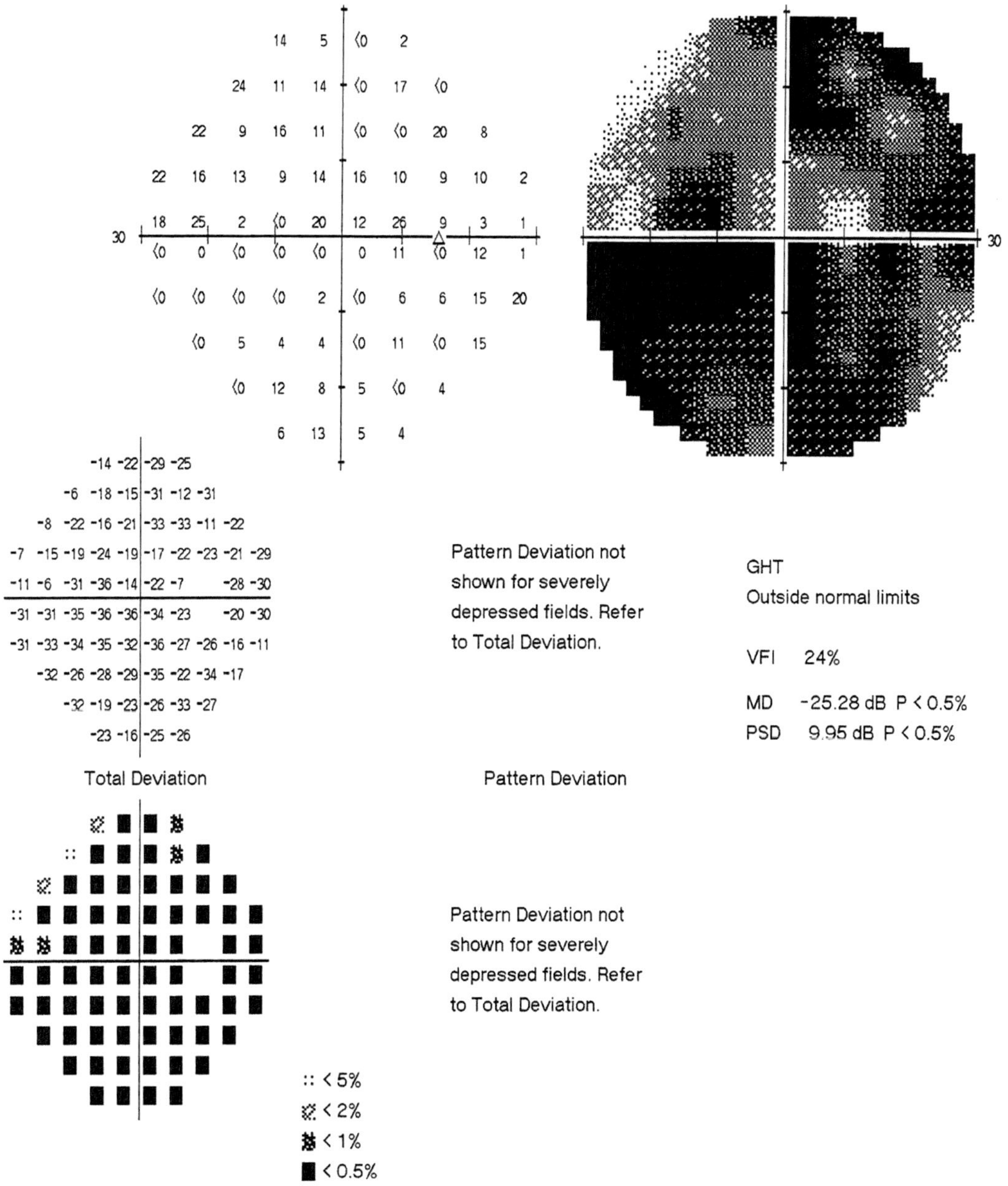

Fig. 44.4 Humphrey visual field analysis printout. The 30-2 test showed that the light sensitivity had significantly improved after the treatment

occurs before central vision damage. Most of visual field changes are manifested as diffuse decrease in light sensitivity of both eyes [5].

The ocular symptoms caused by neurological brucellosis are not specific. When the patient has vision loss, it should be differentiated with other infectious, demyelinating, autoimmune-related optic neuropathy and retinal diseases. The differentiation with the neurological abnormality caused by other pathogens mainly depends on cerebrospinal fluid examination. The cerebrospinal fluid changes in the neurological complications of brucellosis are similar to the early changes in viral meningitis, i.e., protein levels and cell (mainly lymphocytes) numbers slightly increase, and both glucose and chloride levels are normal; in the late phase, both glucose and chloride levels in cerebrospinal fluid decrease, similar to the situation in tuberculous meningitis; but cerebrospinal fluid etiological DNA-PCR, virological test, and cytological and biochemical examinations are useful to exclude other types of central nervous system infections and tumor-related diseases [2]. Most demyelinating optic neuritis cases exhibit acute painful loss of vision in one eye. VEP and MRI examinations can detect demyelinating changes of optic nerve, and some patients with optic neuromyelitis-related optic neuritis may possess positive serum aquaporin antibodies. Autoimmune-related optic neuropathy is often secondary to systemic autoimmune diseases, such as systemic lupus erythematosus and sarcoidosis. Abnormal autoimmune indicators may accompany symptoms and signs of optic nerve injury. In cases of retinopathy, metamorphopsia may occur, and lesions involving the macula can usually be detected through careful fundus examination. Combined with systemic and eye examination and comprehensive pathologic investigations, detailed history of epidemiology can help to reach the diagnosis of neurological brucellosis.

Brucella mainly propagates in human reticuloendothelial cells. Brucellosis is resistant to treatment and prone to relapse. The principle of treatment is to intervene early with a combination of antibiotics, sufficient dosage, with adequate treatment duration, and prolong the treatment if necessary. Antibiotics should have good intracellular and central nervous system penetration. Currently, the baseline therapy is doxycycline + rifampin, which are used in combination with any one of aminoglycosides, ceftriaxone, and quinolones, i.e., a triple therapy. In the chronic phase, tetracycline and rifomycins are usually used. Some patients need two to three treatment courses. For concomitant meningitis, low-dose steroid and symptomatic treatment of dehydration can be provided in addition to antibacterial treatment. This patient was not cured after one course of combination therapy and improved after the second course, with the vision of the left eye slightly improved and residual visual field defects found in both eyes.

References

1. K Ose S, Serin Senger S, Akkoglu G, et al. Clinical manifestations, complications and treatment of brucellosis; evaluation of 72 cases. Turk J Med Sci. 2014;44(2):203–20.
2. Guven T, Ugurlu K, Ergonol O, et al. Neurobmcellosis: clinical and diagnostic features. Clin Infect Dis. 2013;56(10):1407–12.
3. Li Q, Dai F, Zhu L, et al. Analysis of the clinical characteristics of nervous brucellosis with eyes involved. Chin J Ophthalmol. 2015;51(12):896–900.
4. Abd Elrazak M. Brucella optic neuritis. Arch Intern Med. 1991;151(4):776–8.
5. Tunç M, Durukan H. Bilateral severe visual loss in brucellosis. Ocul Immunol Inflamm. 2004;12(3):233–6.

The Diagnostic Process of a Patient with Bilateral Physiological Blind Spot Enlargement

45

Xiaojing Pan, Ning Fan, and Xuyang Liu

In a "slender" female with an enlarged physiological blind spot in both eyes, bilateral optic disc edema was observed during ophthalmologic examination, and intracranial pressure increase was also found during neurologic consultation, but the head MRI showed no abnormality. Was the condition benign intracranial hypertension? What enlightenment did the full blood examination give us? What was the culprit?

45.1 Case

45.1.1 Case Presentation

A 24-year-old female patient complained of blurred vision in her left eye for 1 month because of fatigue and emotional stress. She had peripheral orbital pain and occasional nausea. No headache or vomiting was reported. The symptom of blurred vision worsened gradually, but no fixed dark shadow in front of eyes or pain on eye movement was present. The patient denied amaurosis fugax, tinnitus, double vision, or numbness or weakness in the extremities. The abovementioned symptoms briefly improved after the patient was given steroid therapy at another hospital based on the diagnosis of optic neuritis. However, the blurred vision worsened once again when the steroid dose was reduced. She felt that the vision was normal in her right eye. Histories of trauma, operation, other ocular diseases, systemic diseases, or familial diseases were denied.

The patient was underweight and the blood pressure (BP) was 120/80 mmHg.

On examination, the uncorrected visual acuity (UCVA) was 20/22 OD and 20/20 OS with no improvement in visual acuity (VA) achieved with myopic correction. Intraocular pressure (IOP) was normal OU. In both eyes, no conjunctival congestion was revealed, the media was clear, the pupil was 3 mm in diameter, and the light reflex was normal. Relative afferent pupillary defect (RAPD) was negative bilaterally. Fundus examination showed the optic disc was edema with blurred margin, and the macula was edema, especially in the temporal to the optic disc in both eyes. No hemorrhage or effusion focus was found (Fig. 45.1). Both eyes were in normal position and showed normal eye movement.

X. Pan
Shandong Eye Institute, Qingdao Eye Hospital, Qingdao, China

N. Fan
Shenzhen Eye Hospital, Shenzhen University, Shenzhen, China

X. Liu (✉)
Xiamen Eye Center of Xiamen University, Xiamen, China

Shenzhen Eye Hospital, Shenzhen University, Shenzhen, China

N. Wang et al. (eds.), *Optic Disorders and Visual Field*, Advances in Visual Science and Eye Diseases 2, https://doi.org/10.1007/978-981-13-2502-1_45

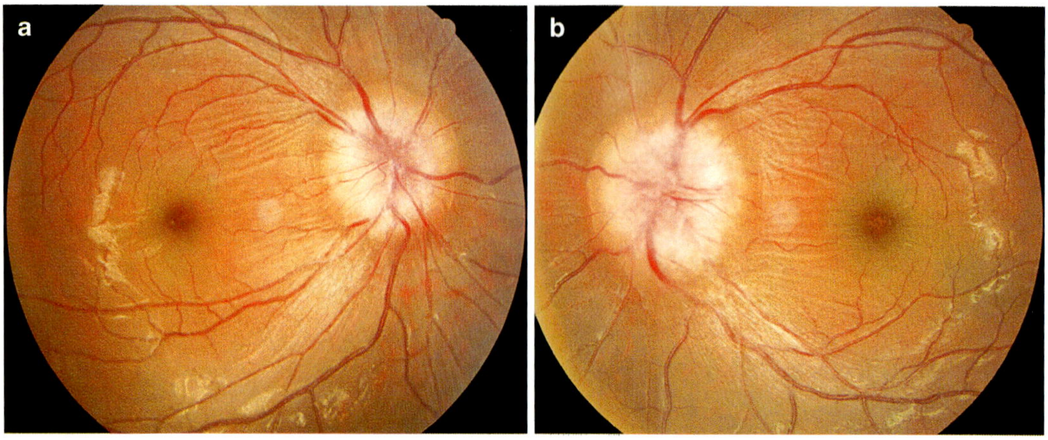

Fig. 45.1 Fundus photographs. The optic disc was edema with blurred margin; the macula was edema, especially in the temporal to the optic disc in both eyes. Panel a: right eye. Panel b: left eye

Standardized automated perimetry revealed enlarged physiological blind spots (Figs. 45.2 and 45.3).

45.1.2 Case Analysis

The patient was a young female with complaint of blurred vision in her left eye. The examination found significant optic disc edema in both eyes, and the visual field manifestation was bilateral physiological blind spot enlargement. However, the loss of vision in both eyes was mild, and no pain on eye movement was present. RAPD was negative, and no uveitis was present. Therefore, the bilateral optic disc edema was firstly considered to be caused by raised intracranial pressure. Other differential diagnoses were papillitis, optic disc vasculitis, neuroretinitis, etc. These diseases can be excluded based on medical history and clinical signs. Further head MRI and lumbar puncture were performed.

Craniocerebral MRI with plain and enhanced scans revealed no abnormality.

Lumbar puncture showed that the intracranial pressure was higher than 330 mmH_2O. Routine biochemistry, cytology, and virology were normal.

Intracranial pressure increase did occur in the patient, and it could explain the bilateral optic disc edema. However, what's the etiology? The common causes of intracranial pressure increase are intracranial tumor, inflammation, trauma, and congenital malformation. The craniocerebral MRI of the patient provided negative results, and trauma history was denied. The patient had no headache, vomiting, fever, chill, tinnitus, numbness, or weakness in the extremities. Therefore, the abovementioned possible causes could be basically excluded. So, was it idiopathic intracranial hypertension (IIH)? The time from disease onset was short, and symptoms including obesity, headache, double vision, amaurosis fugax, tinnitus, etc. were absent, which did not support IIH. Therefore, we needed to continue to look for the real cause of her raised intracranial pressure.

The full blood examination of the patient gave us an important tip, namely, significant increase of blood platelet.

A routine blood test showed WBC 18.6×10^9/L, PLT 656.0×10^9/L, LYMPH 4.64×10^9/L, MONO 1.20×10^9/L, and neutrophil 12.51×10^9/L.

Abdominal ultrasound demonstrated multiple lymph node enlargements in the inguinal regions bilaterally, and we took reactive hyperplasia into consideration. No significant abnormality was found in the liver, gallbladder, pancreas, spleen, and kidneys.

The hypercoagulable state caused by platelet increase may lead to cerebral venous sinus thrombosis in combination with factors such as fatigue and emotional stress. The cerebral venous sinus thrombosis is closely associated with intracranial pressure increase. Further cerebrovascular CT,

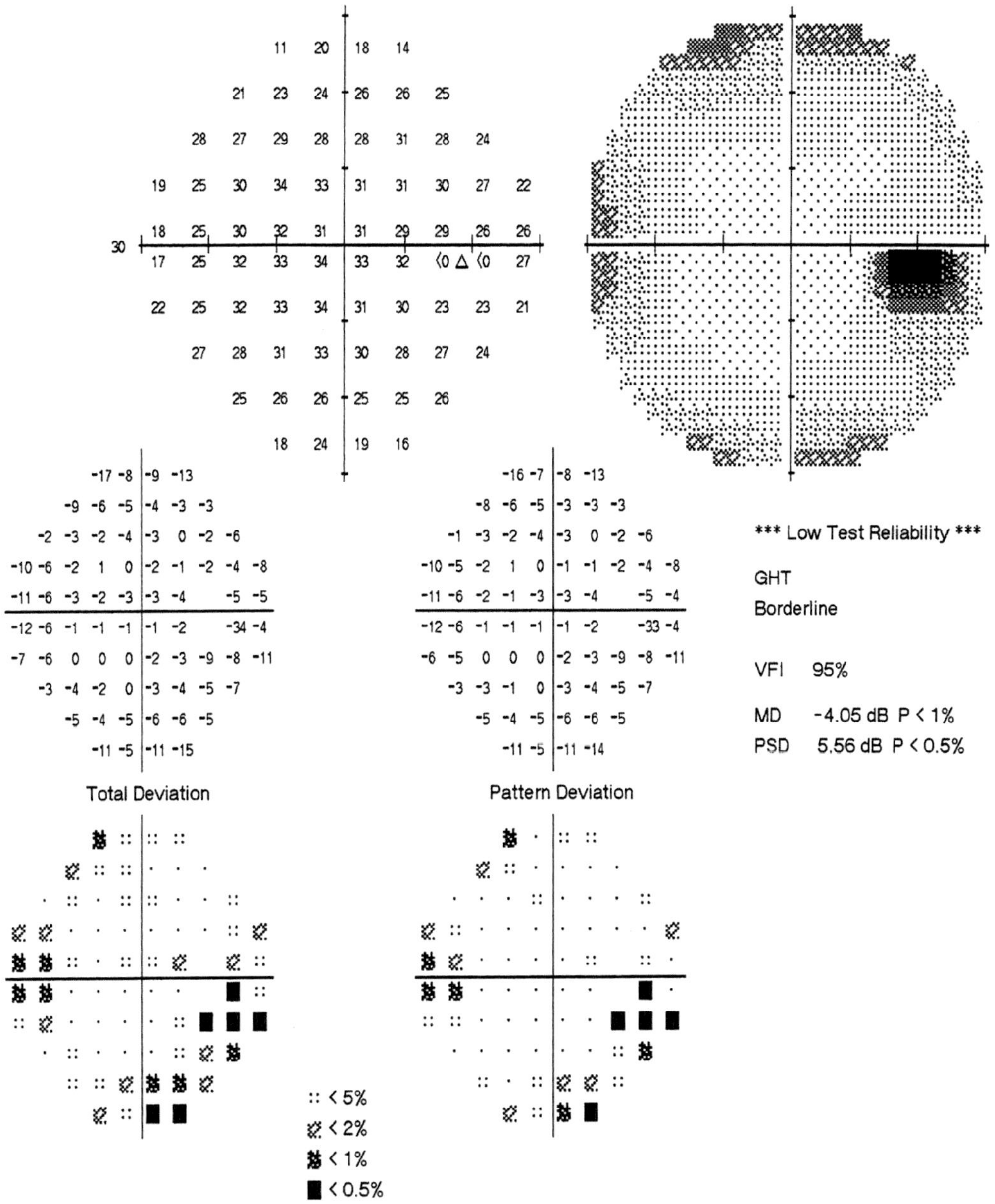

Fig. 45.2 Humphrey visual field analysis printout in the right eye. An enlarged physiological blind spot and scattered relative defects were seen (the patient's compliance was poor)

CT venography (CTV), and digital subtraction angiography (DSA) supported our deduction.

Cerebrovascular CTV revealed filling defects inside the right sigmoid sinus, and cerebral venous sinus thrombosis was suspected. Further DSA was recommended.

DSA showed thinning in the superior sagittal sinus and left transverse sinus. Left sigmoid sinus occlusion was revealed. Stenosis occurred at the junction of the right transverse sinus and sigmoid sinus (Fig. 45.4).

The platelet increase found in the patient led to the cranial venous sinus thrombosis, and the cerebral venous return was affected. Next, cerebrospinal fluid was affected, which led to intracranial hypertension and papilloedema. But what

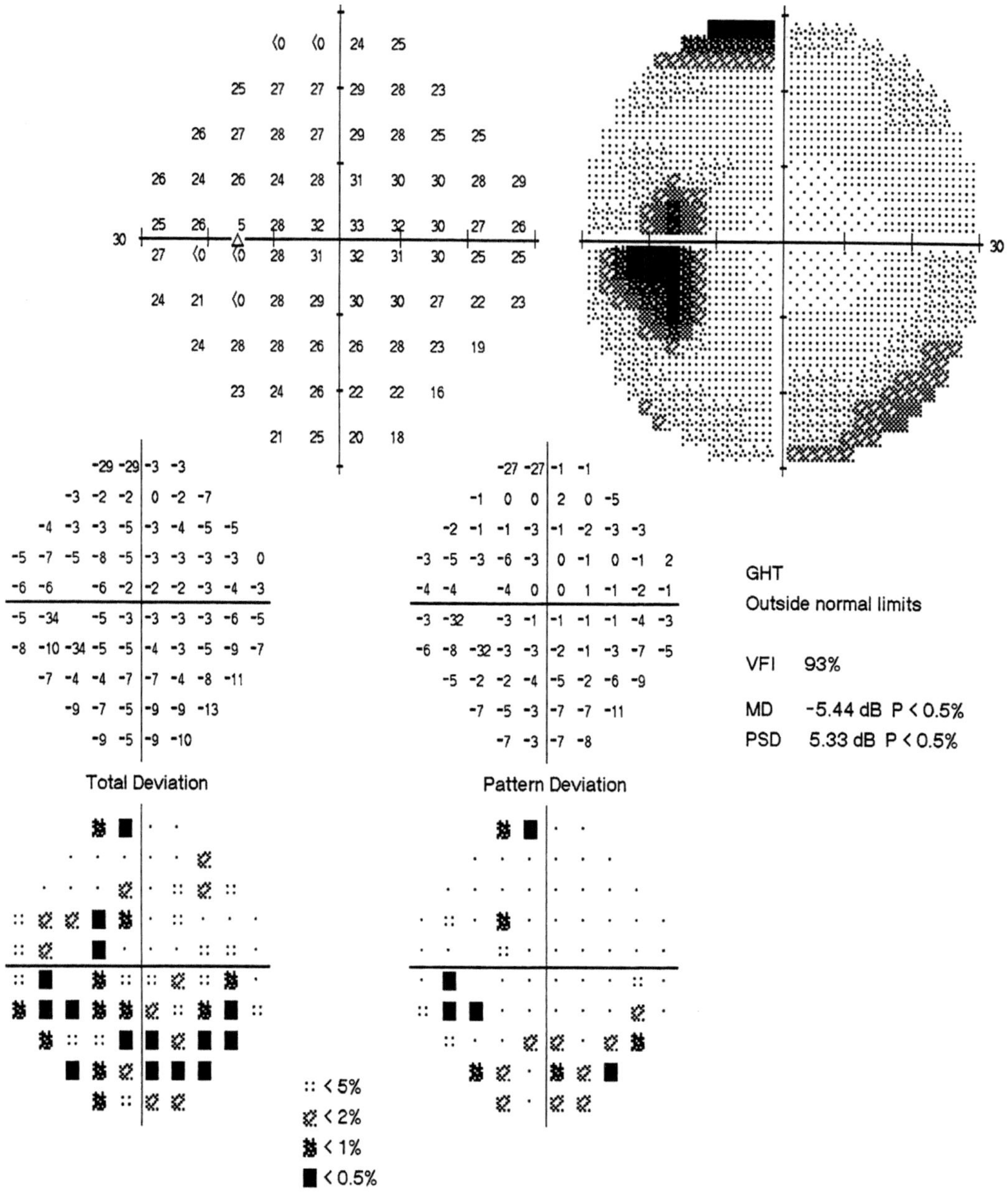

Fig. 45.3 Humphrey visual field analysis printout in the left eye. An enlarged physiological blind spot and scattered relative defects were noted

was the underlying cause of the thrombocythemia? Let's see what the pathological examination of bone marrow cells would tell us.

Morphological examination of bone marrow cells yielded the following results: (a) granular neutrophilic segmented granulocytes accounted for about 45.5% of the granulocytes and could be seen in all the remaining stages. Multi-lobulation could be noted in neutrophilic segmented granulocytes. (b) Polychromatic and orthochromatic normoblasts could be observed in erythroid cells. The morphology of mature erythrocytes was normal. (c) The proportion of lymphocytes was normal. (d) Three granular megakaryocytes were observed in the whole film, and an increased number of platelets were seen (Fig. 45.5).

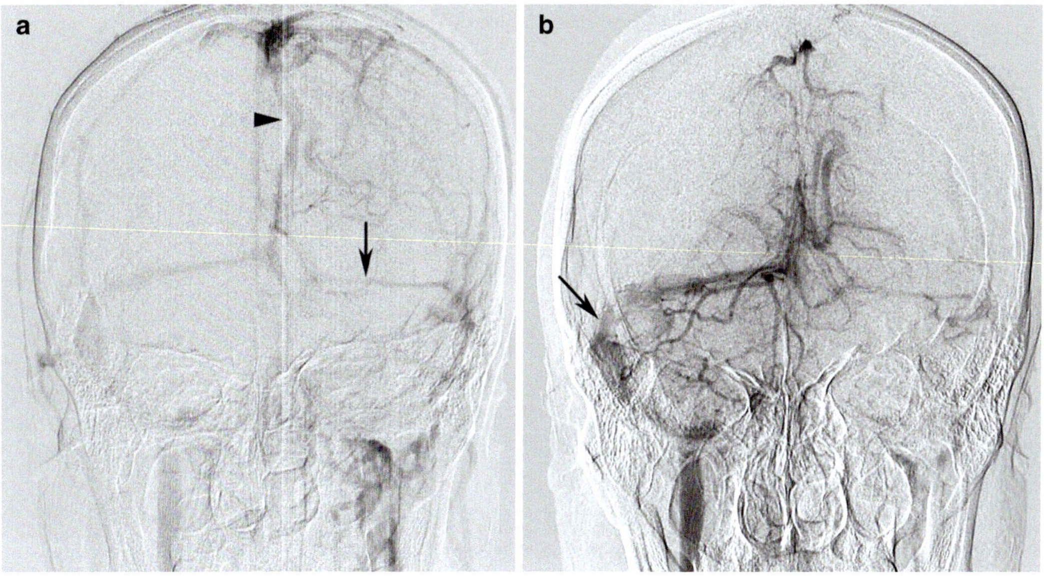

Fig. 45.4 DSA images. Panel a: left internal carotid angiography revealed thinning of the superior sagittal sinus (black triangle) and left transverse sinus (arrow) and occlusion of the left sigmoid sinus. Panel b: right internal carotid angiography revealed stenosis at the junction of the right transverse sinus and sigmoid sinus (arrow)

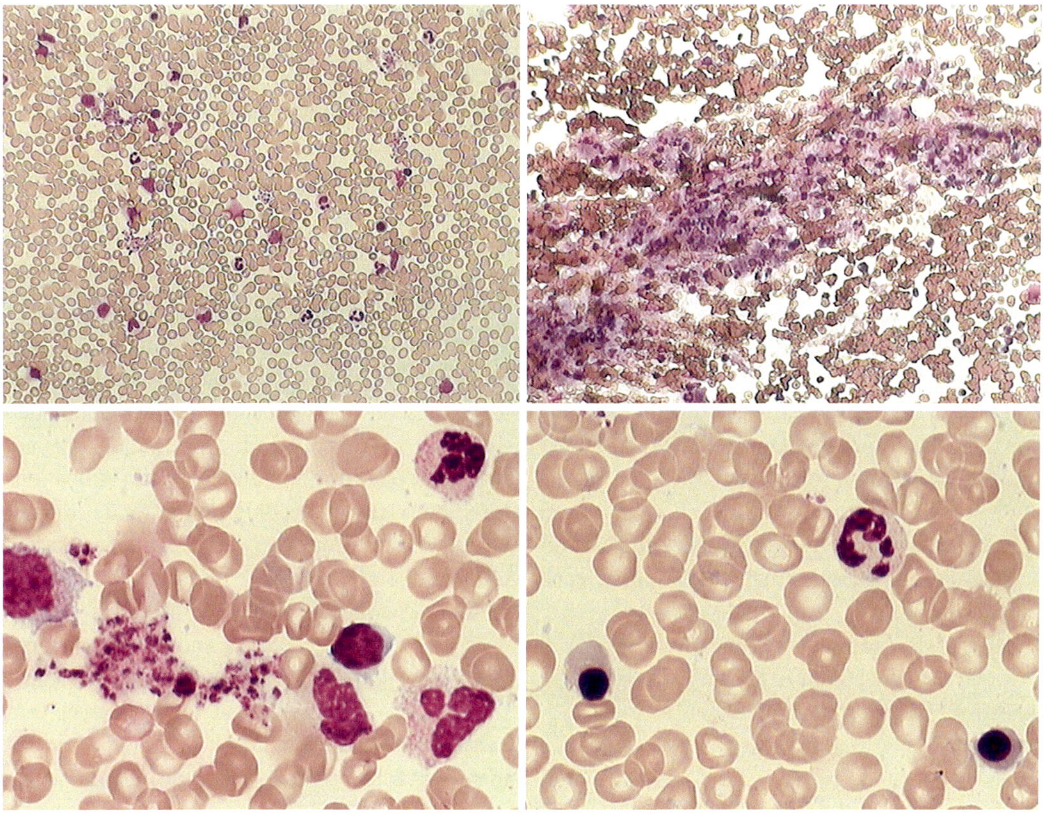

Fig. 45.5 Morphological images of the bone marrow cells

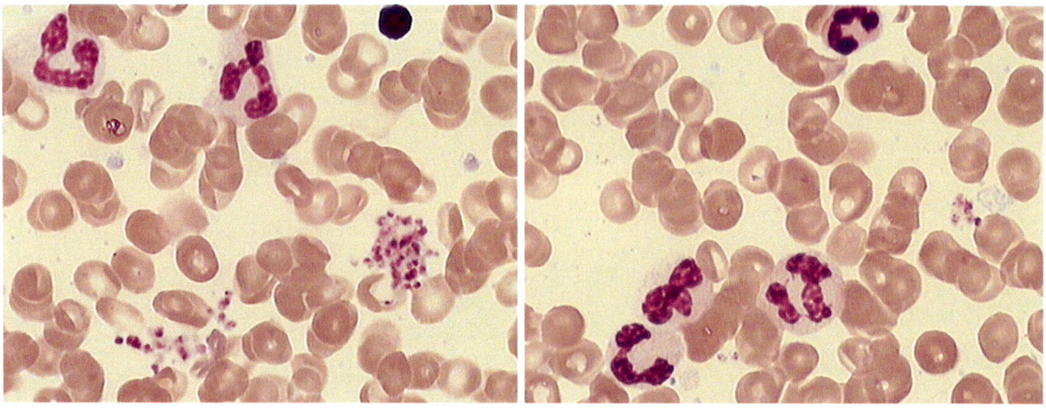

Fig. 45.5 (continued)

Pathological examination of the bone marrow showed that the bone, bone marrow, hemopoietic and adipose tissues, as well as the granulocyte-erythroblast ratio were normal. Significant hyperplasia was observed in the aggregation cells, presenting polymorphism and heterogeneity. Cluster of aggregation cells was easily found. Given these clinical results, the findings supported the diagnosis of primary thrombocytosis (IHC: CD20+ individual +, CD45RO−, CD61+, CD235a+, MPO+, Ki-67+, Fe−, Ag+, PAS−).

Bone marrow immunophenotyping disclosed that the proportion of lymphocytes (p2) was 8.13%, which was normal, and most of them were mature T lymphocytes. The proportion of myelocytes (p4) was 82.55%, which was higher than normal, and most of them were mature CD16+ and CD10+ granulocytes. The proportion of monocytes was 1.04%, and phenotyping showed no significant abnormality. The proportion of karyocytes was 1.61% (a lowered proportion), and the immature CD34+CD17+ myelocyte was 0.23% (a low proportion). The proportions of basophils and acidophils were 0.38% and 0.34%, respectively. By now, the cytologic diagnosis has become clear. Finally, let's see the gene analysis results.

Blood cells of the bone marrow were taken by bone marrow puncture to carry out genotype detection. The mutation detection at the 617th amino acid site (valine/phenylalanine) of JAK2 provided positive results. The genotype was the heterozygote of G and T. Qualitative PCR detection for mutations in exon 9 of the CALR gene was found to be negative. The gene mutation detection at the 515th amino acid site of MPL (tryptophan/leucine or tryptophan/lysine) revealed negative results.

The inquiry on the family history showed that the patient's younger brother experienced raised platelet counts with unknown causes but no diagnosis or treatment were given.

45.1.3 Final Diagnosis

The final diagnosis was bilateral optic disc edema, primary thrombocytosis, venous sinus thrombosis, and secondary intracranial hypertension.

The patient was given aspirin for antiplatelet therapy and methazolamide for reduction of cerebrospinal fluid secretion. The consultations with neurosurgeon and vascular surgeons concluded that the vision impairment of the patient was not serious at that time and there were no indications for optic nerve decompression and surgical thrombectomy. Follow-up and treatment at hematology department were recommended. The patient experienced acute loss of vision in both eyes (20/33 in the right eye and no light perception in the left eye) half a year after discharge. Optic nerve decompression for both eyes was carried out at another hospital. Vision improvement was achieved after operation, and follow-up is ongoing.

45.2 Discussion

For relatively young adult patients with bilateral optic disc edema, whose visual fields show bilateral physiological blind spot enlargement but the vision impairment is relatively mild, the most common cause is raised intracranial pressure. The causes of raised intracranial pressure include intracranial tumor, hematoma, infection, inflammation, idiopathic intracranial hypertension, etc. [1, 2]. Idiopathic intracranial hypertension is a syndrome with no apparent cause, and it often affects obese women. The common symptoms were headache and bilateral optic disc edema. The treatments mainly focus on the intracranial pressure control and symptoms alleviation. The prognosis is relatively good. The pathogenesis of idiopathic intracranial hypertension is still unclear. The etiology cannot be found in the vast majority of cases, and a small minority of patients may have autoimmune diseases, previous head trauma, endocrine diseases, drug-induced diseases, hypercoagulability, venous sinus thrombosis, etc.

The patient in this case was a young female with bilateral optic disc edema. The visual field showed bilateral physiological blind spot enlargement, but the vision impairment was relatively mild. From the perspective of ophthalmology, the ocular diseases excluded were as follows: (a) papillitis, (b) optic disc vasculitis, (c) neuroretinitis, (d) ischemic optic neuropathy, etc. Then, raised intracranial pressure was considered during the diagnostic process, and lumbar puncture carried out for the patient confirmed the suspicion. But what is the underlying cause? Idiopathic intracranial hypertension is a possible diagnosis. We found that the time from disease onset was short, and symptoms including obesity, headache, double vision, amaurosis fugax, tinnitus, etc. were not observed after careful analysis of the patient's medical history, clinical symptoms, and signs. The diagnosis of idiopathic intracranial pressure was thus not supported. The case was a diagnostic dilemma.

The most basic blood test gave us an important tip: Significant increase of platelet was shown in the patient. It meant that the patient's blood was in a hypercoagulable state, and she was prone to venous sinus thrombosis. The DSA carried out for the patient confirmed the diagnosis of venous sinus thrombosis. Secondary intracranial hypertension could occur when reabsorption via arachnoid granulations are obstructed.

The cause of platelet increase was found to be essential thrombocythemia (primary thrombocytosis) through bone marrow pathology and genotyping analysis. A heterozygous mutation was detected at the 617th amino acid site of the JAK2 gene in the patient. The answer to the riddle was finally revealed. Upon further questioning about the patient's history, it was found that the patient's younger brother also had essential thrombocythemia. The culprit turned out to be gene mutations.

As a type of myeloproliferative neoplasms (MPN), essential thrombocythemia is mainly manifested as significant hyperplasia of the megakaryocytes and granulocytes in bone marrow accompanied by the deposition of reactive fibers in the connective tissues and extramedullary hemopoiesis. The 617th valine in exon 14 of JAK2 gene was mutated into phenylalanine (V617F) causing continuous activation of JAK2 independent of cell factors, which leads to the proliferative change of bone marrow through the STAT signaling pathway and other pathways [3].

Essential thrombocythemia is a type of clonal disorder of hematopoietic cells with slow progression, and it has minimal impact on the patients' life span. The main objective of treatment is to prevent the complications of thrombosis and hemorrhage and lower the risks of myelofibrosis and leukemia transformation.

From blurred vision, physiological blind spot enlargement, eye disease exclusion, observation of intracranial hypertension, routine blood tests, cause analysis of raised platelet level, and confirmed diagnosis of venous sinus thrombosis by DSA to cytologic and genetic diagnoses of the primary diseases, the diagnostic process of the disease is interlinked. We managed to stay on the right path, and this case provided us with a lot of inspirations. Firstly, it's a successful trial on molecular diagnosis. It is no doubt that the modern analytical method is important during the process, but multidisciplinary medicine played the key role. Secondly, the author firmly believes that most diseases we face in our daily life have their molecular foundations. With the guidance of such thought, as far as this case was concerned, we did not halt our investigation when intracranial hypertension was confirmed, or when a significant platelet increase was found, or even when the analysis report of bone marrow cells was obtained. Such type of case analysis can also be found in the other chapters of this book. Churchill once said that "this is not the end. It is not even the beginning of the end. But it is, perhaps, the end of the beginning." For precision medicine, the ultimate goal is to individualize research and to develop successful treatment at a cellular and molecular level.

References

1. Chen E, Mullally A. How does JAK2 V617F contribute to the pathogenesis of myeloproliferative neoplasms? Hematology Am Soc Hematol Educ Program. 2014;2014(1):268–76.
2. Zhang X, Jing Y. A practical case analysis in Neurophthalmology Department of Beijing Tongren Hospital. Beijing: Science Press; 2010.
3. Wang Z. Advances in research of essential thrombocythemia. Chin J Hematol. 2015;36(9):802–4.

46 Optic Nerve Glioma and Diffuse Field Loss

Xiaojing Pan, Ning Fan, and Xuyang Liu

The visual field defect and optic disc findings in this case indicated optic neuropathy. However, the confirmed diagnosis of optic glioma was provided by the MRI after other optic nerve diseases and intracranial hypertension were excluded, which suggested that imaging shall be carried out at the early stage to assist with the diagnosis of optic neuropathy.

46.1 Case

46.1.1 Case Presentation

A 26-year-old female patient experienced amaurosis fugax in the right eye without any obvious cause for 4 months. The condition often occurred when the patient woke up and opened her eyes. The duration was about 30 s. She had no significant vision change, pain on eye movement, headache, dizziness, and tinnitus. She visited the local hospital for treatment and was diagnosed with optic neuritis in the right eye. Retrobulbar injection of lidocaine and dexamethasone was given for treatment, but the symptoms did not improve. The vision in the patient's right eye showed acute decrease 1 month before, and oral steroid was ineffective. The right eye progressed to no light perception after 2 weeks. The patient had visited the ophthalmology department in our hospital 20 days before for treatment and received retrobulbar injection of lidocaine, dexamethasone, and neurotrophic drugs. The vision improved slightly.

On ocular examination, the uncorrected visual acuity (UCVA) was hand motion (HM) OD with no improvement with the pinhole test. The best corrected visual acuity (BCVA) was 20/13 in the left eye. The pupils were 3 mm in diameter. Relative afferent pupillary defect (RAPD) was found to be positive in the right eye. Fundus examination showed that the optic disc was pink in color with a clear margin in the left eye and edema in the optic disc with a blurred margin and slight pallor in the right eye (Fig. 46.1). Both eyes were in normal position and showed normal eye movements.

The systemic nervous system examination showed no abnormality.

X. Pan
Shandong Eye Institute, Qingdao Eye Hospital, Qingdao, China

N. Fan
Shenzhen Eye Hospital, Shenzhen University, Shenzhen, China

X. Liu (✉)
Xiamen Eye Center of Xiamen University, Xiamen, China

Shenzhen Eye Hospital, Shenzhen University, Shenzhen, China

N. Wang et al. (eds.), *Optic Disorders and Visual Field*, Advances in Visual Science and Eye Diseases 2, https://doi.org/10.1007/978-981-13-2502-1_46

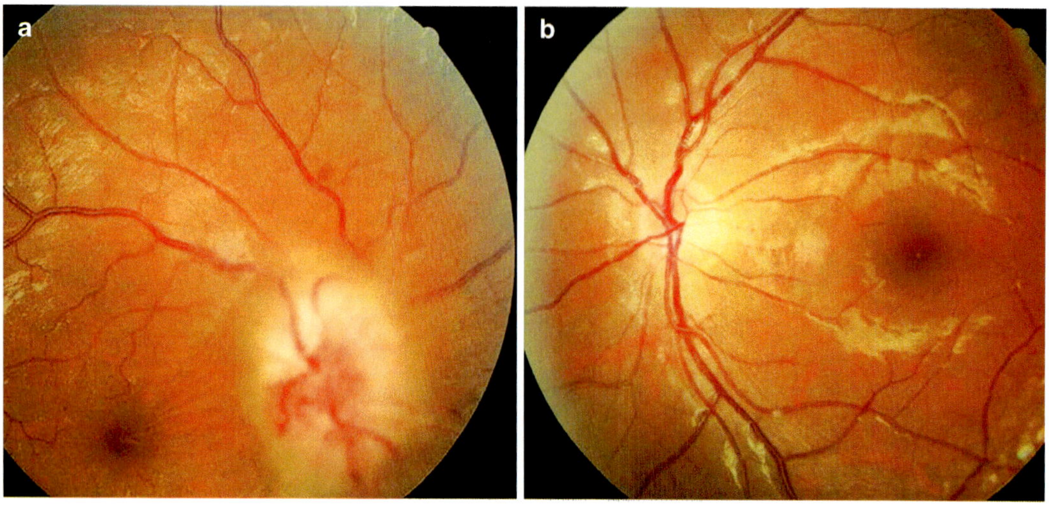

Fig. 46.1 Fundus photographs. Edema in the optic disc with a blurred margin and slight pallor was seen in the right eye. A pink optic disc with a clear boundary was noted in the left eye. Panel a: right eye. Panel b: left eye

Generalized reduction or even complete loss of light sensitivity was revealed in the right eye, and no significant abnormality was observed in the visual field of the left eye (Fig. 46.2).

The F-VEP results showed normal waveform, latency, and amplitude in the left eye. No waveform was elicited in the right eye (Fig. 46.3).

MRI showed that the intraorbital, intracanalicular, and intracranial segments of the optic nerve on the right side thickened. The boundary was clear, and no significant internal echo was revealed. Nodular change was seen in the intracranial segment. Therefore, a space-occupying lesion or optic nerve glioma to be specific was considered to be the likely cause (Fig. 46.4).

46.1.2 Case Analysis

The patient was a young female with the main manifestation of painless loss of vision in the right eye. Amaurosis fugax was firstly found at the onset of the disease, and then progressive worsening followed. There was no light perception when the disease was at its worst. Serious diffuse reduction of light sensitivity was shown in the visual field. The optic disc showed congestion, edema, and small sheetlike hemorrhage. The ocular B-ultrasound excluded the possibility of optic disc drusen, etc.

In order to exclude the possibility of benign intracranial hypertension, lumbar puncture was carried out to test the cerebrospinal fluid pressure, and a normal result was revealed (145 mmH_2O).

Head MRI (plain scan + enhanced scan) showed that the orbital segment, intracanalicular segment, and intracranial segment of the optic nerve on the right side, as well as the optic chiasm, thickened. The optic foramen in the right eye dilated. The intracranial lesion was nodular and was hyperintense on T2WI. The enhanced scan showed significant enhancement (Fig. 46.4). The findings suggested that the lesion was likely to be glioma.

The patient was then transferred to the neurosurgery department for excision of the optic nerve tumor in the right eye. The results obtained from the pathologic examination confirmed the diagnosis of optic nerve glioma (WHO Grade 1, Fig. 46.5).

46.1.3 Final Diagnosis

The final diagnosis was optic glioma in the right eye (WHO Grade I).

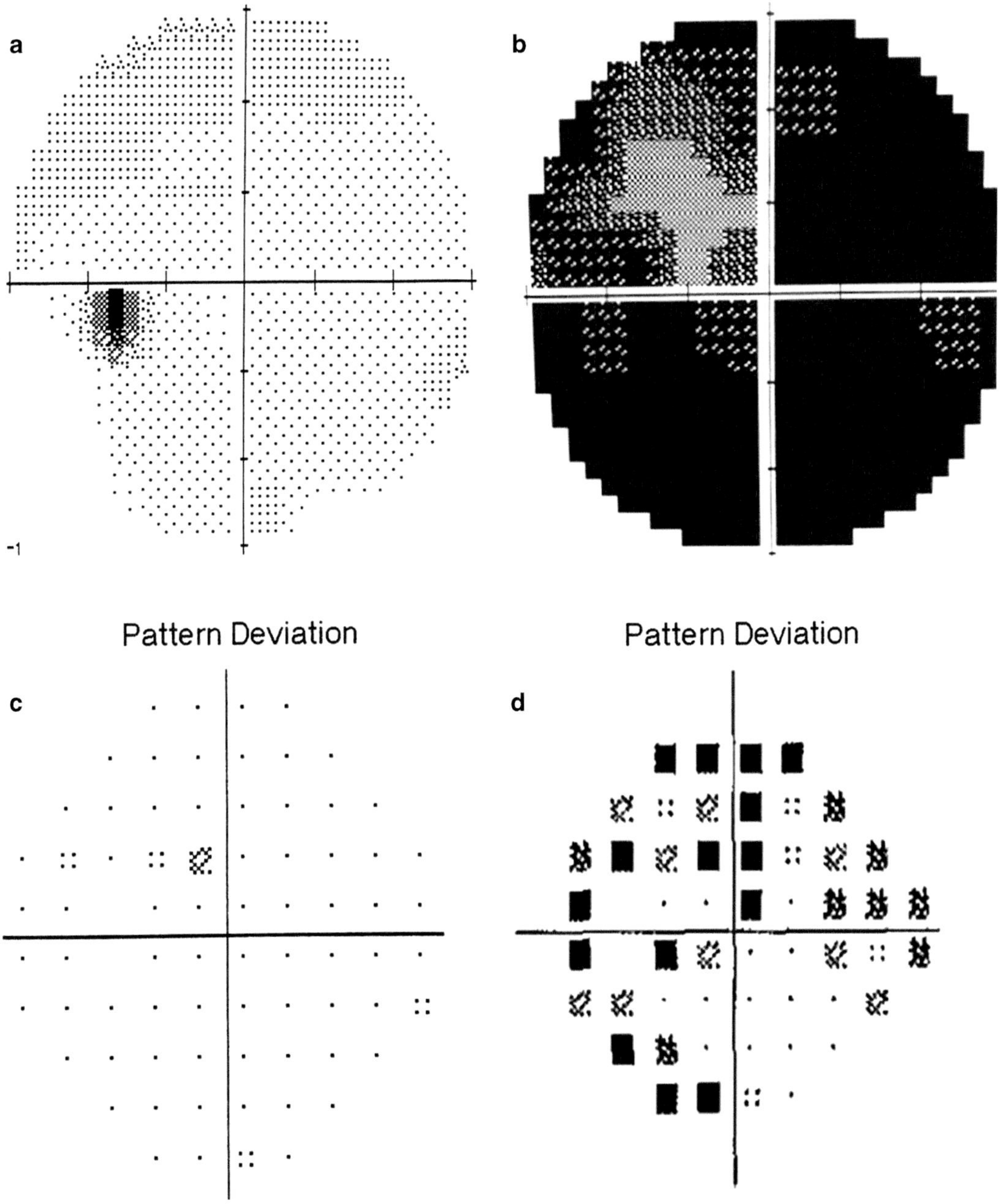

Fig. 46.2 Grayscale maps and pattern deviation probability maps of Humphrey visual field assessment. Generalized reduction or even complete loss of light sensitivity was revealed in the right eye, and the visual field was normal in the left eye. Panel a: grayscale map of the left eye. Panel b: grayscale map of the right eye. Panel c: pattern deviation probability map of the left eye. Panel d: pattern deviation probability map of the right eye

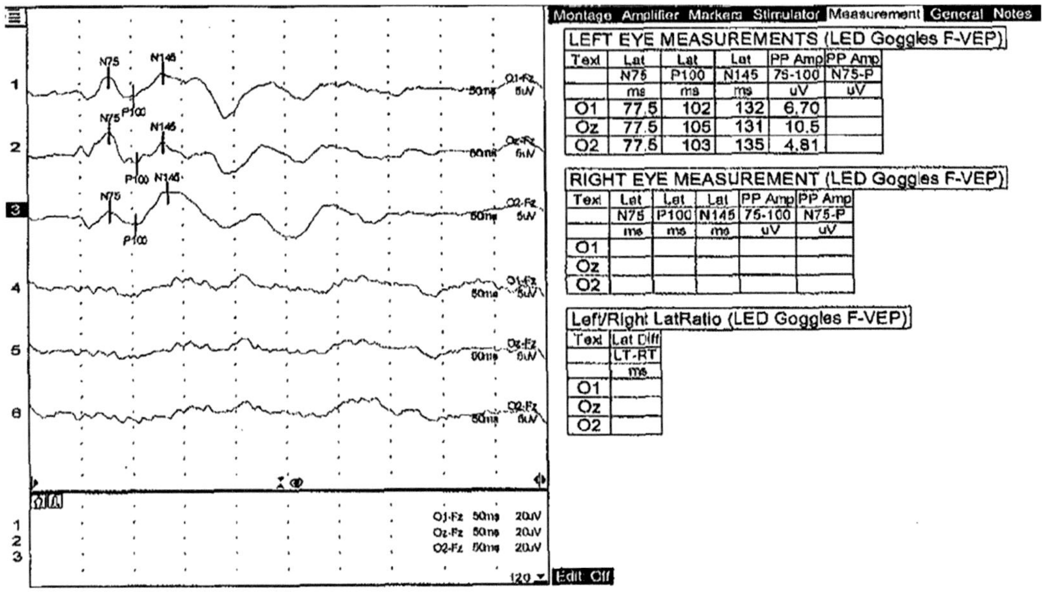

Fig. 46.3 VEP examination printouts. The waveform, latency, and amplitude of the left eye were within normal limits. No waveform was elicited in the right eye

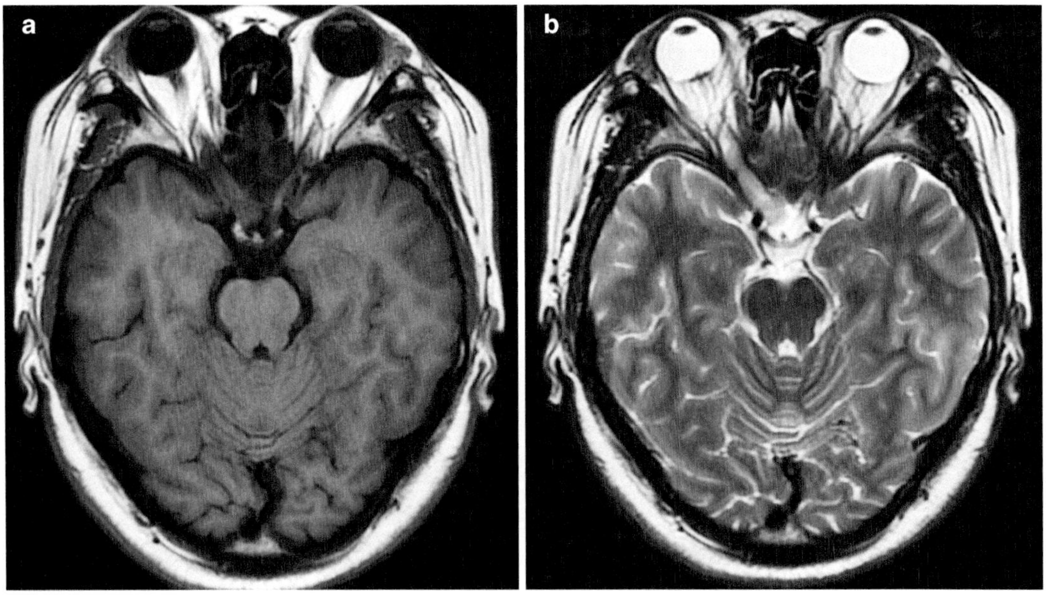

Fig. 46.4 Plain and enhanced scan images of head MRI. Panels a, b: the intraorbital, intracanalicular, and intracranial segments of the optic nerve on the right side, as well as the optic chiasm thickened. The optic foramen dilated in the right orbit. The intracranial lesion appeared nodular with isointensity on T1WI and hyperintensity on T2WI. Panel c, d: the enhanced scan showed significant enhancement

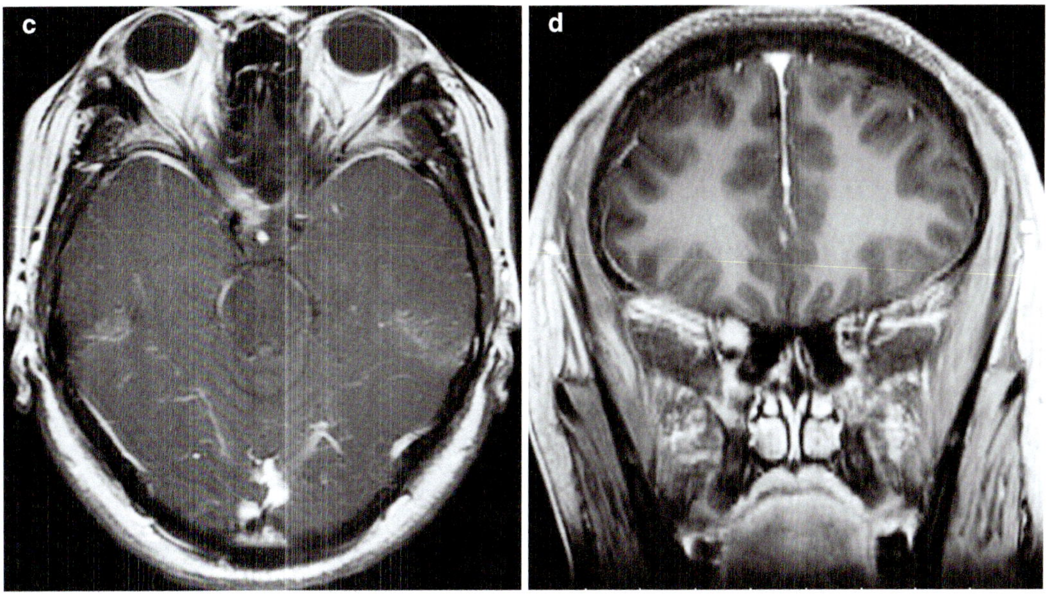

Fig. 46.4 (continued)

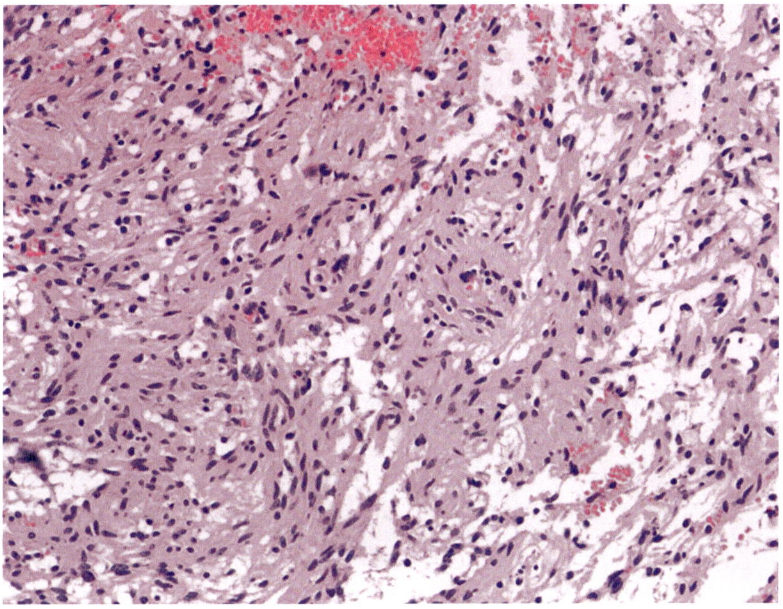

Fig. 46.5 Pathological photograph of optic glioma (WHO Grade 1). It showed the tumor tissues were comprised of an astrocyte mesh and mesenchyma rich in fibers and vessels. Immunohistochemistry yielded the following result: GFAP positive, olig-2 scattered positive, S-100 positive, vimentin positive, CD34 positive, and Ki-67 positive (0–3%)

46.2 Discussion

Optic nerve glioma, also known as gliocytoma, is a benign tumor originating from the glial cells of the optic nerve. Glial cells include astrocytes, oligodendrocytes, and microglial cells. The gliocytomas observed inside the optic nerve are almost always astrocyte gliocytomas. The primary site of the optic glioma in this case was unclear. The MRI revealed that the intraocular segment, orbital segment, intracanalicular segment, and intracranial segment of the optic nerve had tumor involvement. The optic nerve fibers are compressed first due to hyperplasia of the glial cells of the optic nerve and cause severe optic nerve injury. Therefore, vision loss and visual field defects could be rapidly detected at the early stage of the disease. The visual field defect has no fixed characteristics and is linked to the optic nerve fiber involvement. The entire optic nerve will be affected if disease progression is not inhibited [1, 2]. For instance, the visual field examination of the patient in this case showed total blindness, but only eye was affected, which suggests that the optic chiasm may not have been invaded. Corresponding visual field changes could be found if the optic chiasm and retrochiasmal visual pathway were involved.

The early manifestations of optic glioma are variable, and this disease can easily be mistaken as other optic nerve diseases. The diagnosis of this patient's condition went through several stages. It was first diagnosed as optic neuritis in the right eye at a local hospital, but the patient's manifestation was painless amaurosis fugax, which did not match the acute loss of vision that was usually found in optic neuritis. Meanwhile, her vision loss progressed to no light perception after the steroid and other treatments. These findings did not support the diagnosis of optic neuritis. Ischemic optic neuropathy and similar conditions could also be excluded. The possibility of intracranial hypertension was then considered due to the optic nerve edema. This was excluded by the normal cerebrospinal fluid pressure obtained from lumbar puncture. Blurred margin, elevation, and vascular tortuosity with small flame hemorrhage were found in the optic disc of the affected eye. The manifestations were caused by tumor invasion of the intraocular segment of the optic nerve and caused bulging of the optic nerve head toward the vitreous. Optic neuropathy was finally observed on MRI. The pathology examination carried out after the operation revealed optic glioma. The diagnosis was finally confirmed.

Imaging at an early stage is crucial for the diagnosis of optic nerve glioma and monitoring of tumor progression. One case of unilateral optic glioma had been reported in the literature, in which the optic chiasm was not involved at the time of diagnosis. The optic chiasm was invaded 1 year later, and the tumor continued to invade backward along the optic radiation and hypothalamus during the next 6 months [3]. The findings have shown that the progression of optic glioma is rapid, and prompt operation or radiotherapy after the diagnosis is necessary. Supportive treatments after operation, such as nerve growth factor therapy, are expected to restore certain visual function.

References

1. Falsini B, Chiaretti A, Rizzo D, et al. Nerve growth factor improves visual loss in childhood optic gliomas: a randomized, double-blind, phase II clinical trial. Brain. 2016;139(Pt 2):404–14.
2. Weed MC, Almeida DR, Chin EK, et al. Distinguishing optic pathway glioma and retinitis pigmentosa with visual field testing. Can J Ophthalmol. 2016;51(3):e94–6.
3. Walrath JD, Engelbert M, Kazim M. Magnetic resonance imaging evidence of optic nerve glioma progression into and beyond the optic chiasm. Ophthal Plast Reconstr Surg. 2008;24(6):473–5.

Part V

Lesions in Sellar and Parasellar Region

47 Visual Field Defects Caused by Craniopharyngioma in 34 Cases

Li Tang, Xuyang Liu, and Ning Fan

Craniopharyngioma is a common tumor in the sellar region, which accounts for 1.2–3% of the intracranial tumors. It is a benign epithelial tumor and derived from the residual squamous cells in the craniopharyngeal duct. Patients with craniopharyngioma often present a series of systemic symptoms, such as increased intracranial pressure, loss of pituitary function, and damage to the hypothalamic-pituitary axis, thus resulting in hypogonadism, growth retardation, edema, obesity, and diabetes insipidus. Some patients with craniopharyngiomas may be initially admitted to the department of ophthalmology due to decreased vision and visual field defects. This section focuses on the characteristics of visual field defects caused by the craniopharyngioma and introduces the research progresses in the pathogenesis of this disease at the molecular level.

Thirty-four cases of the craniopharyngioma with diagnosis confirmed by postoperative pathology were analyzed, including 20 males and 14 females with ages from 9 to 70 years. All the tumors were situated in the suprasellar region. There were six different types of visual field defects presented by the 34 patients before the operations, as summarized below (Fig. 47.1):

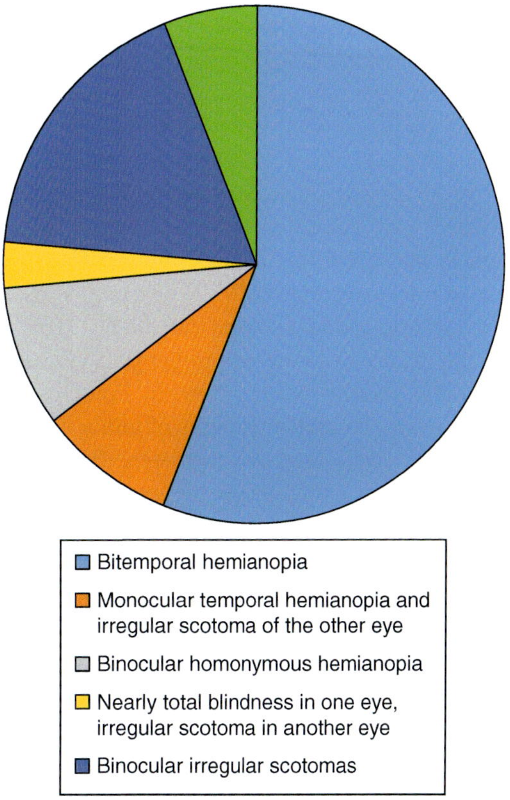

Fig. 47.1 Patterns of visual field defects in the 34 cases of craniopharyngiomas before the operations

L. Tang
West China Hospital, Sichuan University, Chengdu, China

X. Liu
Xiamen Eye Center of Xiamen University, Xiamen, China

Shenzhen Eye Hospital, Shenzhen University, Shenzhen, China

N. Fan (✉)
Shenzhen Eye Hospital, Shenzhen University, Shenzhen, China

N. Wang et al. (eds.), *Optic Disorders and Visual Field*, Advances in Visual Science and Eye Diseases 2, https://doi.org/10.1007/978-981-13-2502-1_47

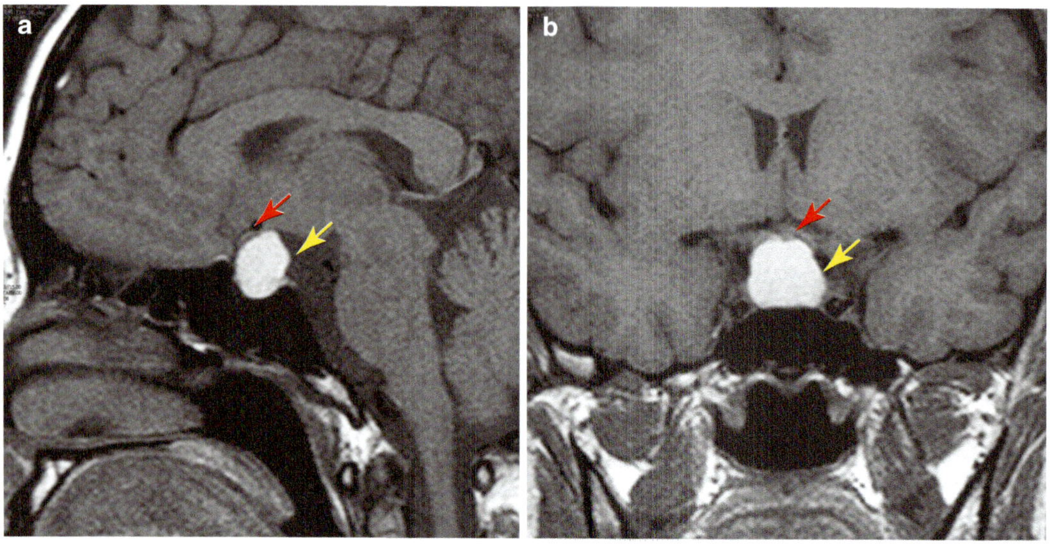

Fig. 47.2 MRI of a craniopharyngioma. It shows a suprasellar space-occupying lesion with hyperintense signals (yellow arrow). The optic chiasm (red arrow) located above the lesion is compressed. Panel a, sagittal T1 image; Panel b, coronal T1 image

Most craniopharyngiomas grow in the suprasellar and parasellar regions, mostly in the suprasellar region. The tumor body of the craniopharyngioma is soft and lobulated and has a smooth surface. The craniopharyngioma can be divided into three types: cystic tumor, solid tumor, and mixed (cystic-solid) tumor. The cranial sagittal and coronal MRI T1 of a patient with craniopharyngioma shows a high signal-occupying lesion on the suprasellar lesion, where the optic chiasm located above is compressed (Fig. 47.2). The growth patterns of tumor can be greatly varied due to its characteristics. Therefore, the location of optic chiasm compression is not the same, and hence different types of visual field damages can arise.

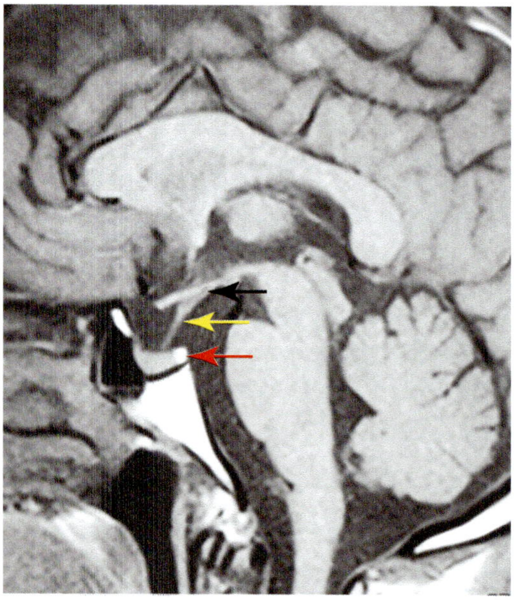

Fig. 47.3 Sagittal MRI of the optic chiasm, pituitary, and pituitary stalk. Red arrow, pituitary; yellow arrow, pituitary stalk; black arrow, optic chiasm

Firstly, to understand the visual field damages caused by the craniopharyngioma, we must be familiar with the relative position of optic chiasm and the pituitary gland. The optic chiasm is located above the pituitary (Fig. 47.3). Due to individual differences, the positions of the optic chiasm with respect to the pituitary are usually divided into three types (Fig. 47.4): (a) prefixed type, the optic chiasm is located above the tuberculum sellae, anteriorly above the pituitary. This type accounts for 3–10%; (b) normal type, the optic chiasm is centered over the sellar diaphragm. This type accounts for 75–87%; (c) postfixed type, the optic chiasm is located above the dorsum sellae, posteriorly above the pituitary. This type accounts for 7.5–17.5%. Due to the various locations of the optic chiasm, the site of

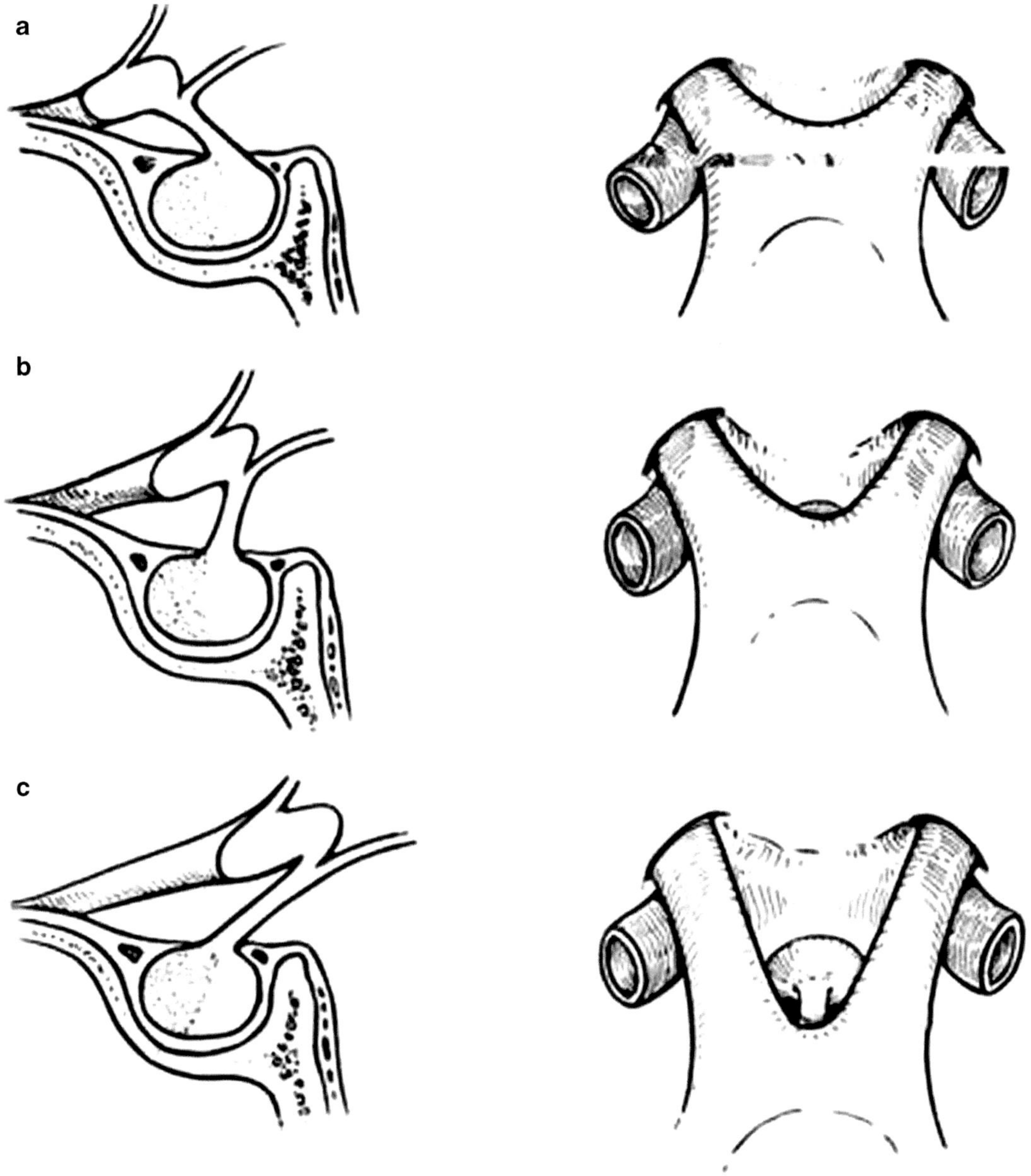

Fig. 47.4 Types of anatomic positions of the optic chiasm. Panel a, prefixed type; Panel b, normal type; Panel c, postfixed type

the optic chiasm compressed by a craniopharyngioma may also vary. For example, if the tumor compresses the central portion of the normal optic chiasm, it will result in bitemporal hemianopia. For the prefixed optic chiasm, the tumor will compress the optic chiasm and optic tract, thus resulting in total blindness in one eye and temporal hemianopia in the other eye. For the postfixed optic chiasm, the tumor may not compress the optic chiasm, and the visual field might be intact in both eyes.

Secondly, the anatomy of the chiasmic nerve fiber distribution shall be taken into consideration (Fig. 47.5). After the nerve fibers enter the optic chiasm, the distribution of fibers from different sources is shown as follows: (a) nerve fibers from the nasal retina (including nasal macula) cross the midline and enter the contralateral optic tract. The fibers

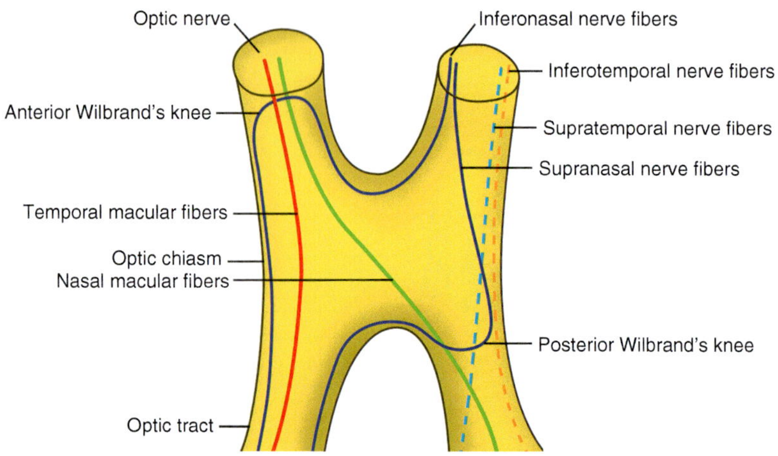

Fig. 47.5 Schematic diagram of the nerve fiber distribution of the optic chiasm

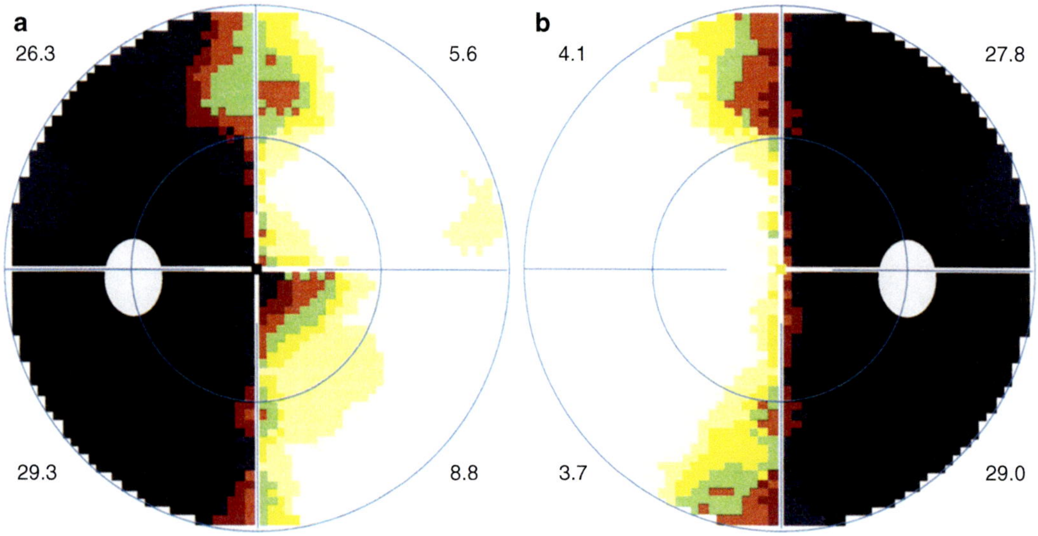

Fig. 47.6 The grayscale maps of Octopus perimeter visual field assessment. Bitemporal hemianopia was shown. Panel a, left eye; Panel b, right eye

from the inferonasal retina run along the front edge of the optic chiasm to the opposite side and form a forward curve called anterior Wilbrand's knee. Then the fibers will run along the lateral edge of the optic chiasm backward to enter the ventrolateral part of the contralateral optic tract. On the other hand, the fibers from the supranasal retina, after entering the optic chiasm, run backward into the initial part of the ipsilateral optic tract and form a backward curve, which is called posterior Wilbrand's knee. Then the supranasal fibers will run along the posterior edge of the optic chiasm and enter the dorsomedial part of the contralateral optic tract. (b) The fibers from the temporal half run backward and enter the ipsilateral optic tract. (c) Papillomacular fibers are also divided into a nasal half and a temporal half. The fibers from the nasal half cross the midline to the opposite side at the superoposterior part of the optic chiasm and then enter the contralateral optic tract. The fibers from the temporal half run backward through the lateral part of the optic chiasm and enter the ipsilateral optic tract.

47.1 Bitemporal Hemianopia

The craniopharyngioma can compress the central part of the optic chiasm and cause the typical bitemporal hemianopia (Fig. 47.6). Supratemporal visual field defects will be observed at the early stage of disease, followed by infratemporal area, and then hemianopia will appear. It presumes that the middle portion of the optic chiasm was affected from the anterior to the posterior.

47.2 Monocular Temporal Hemianopia and Irregular Scotoma in Temporal Side of the Other Eye

At the early stage of disease which results in bitemporal hemianopia, monocular temporal hemianopia and irregular scotomas in the temporal side of the other eye will be observed. It is caused by mild tumor compression on mainly one side of the central part of the optic chiasm. Supratemporal hemianopia is usually caused by anterior (ventral) lesions in the optic chiasm and can also be observed in patients with a postfixed optic chiasm. Inferotemporal hemianopia is usually caused by posterior (dorsal) lesions in the optic chiasm and can also be observed in patients with a prefixed optic chiasm (Fig. 47.7). As the tumor grows larger and compresses the central portion of the optic chiasm, whole bitemporal hemianopia will be observed at the advanced stage.

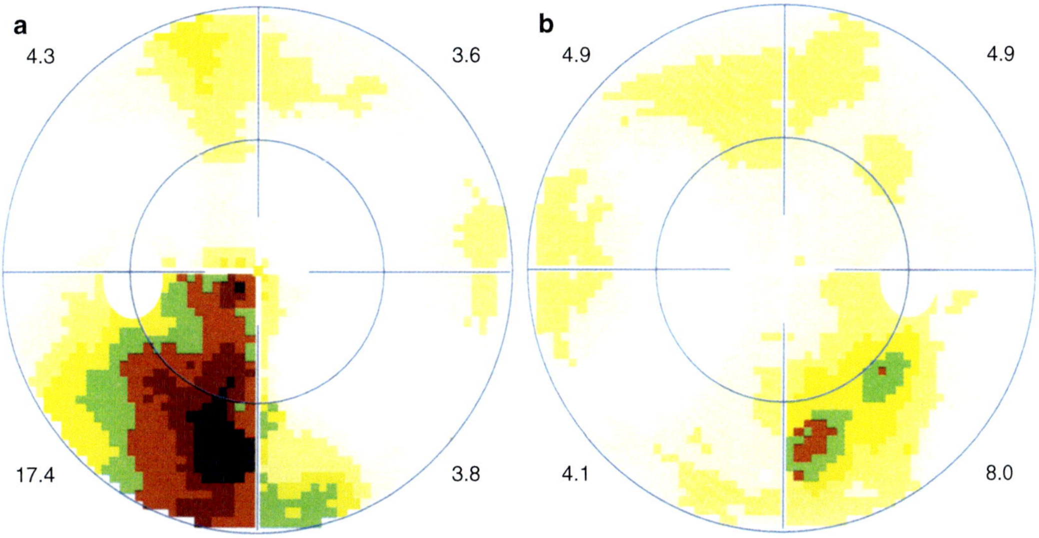

Fig. 47.7 The grayscale maps of Octopus perimeter visual field assessment. Temporal hemianopia was seen in one eye and an irregular defect was noted in the other eye. Panel a, left eye; Panel b, right eye

47.3 Binocular Homonymous Hemianopia

In this type, the tumor tends to compress one optic tract, thus damaging ipsilateral non-crossing fibers and some of the crossing fibers and also the crossing fibers from the contralateral eye. There were three patients with left homonymous hemianopia (Fig. 47.8), for whom the site of tumor compression might mainly be the right optic tract.

47.4 Nearly Total Blindness in One Eye, Irregular Scotoma in Another Eye

As shown in Fig. 47.9, one patient had nearly total blindness with a residual temporal island in the right eye, and irregular scotomas were scattered in all quadrants in the left eye, suggesting that the position of tumor compression was at the junction of the right optic nerve and the anterior

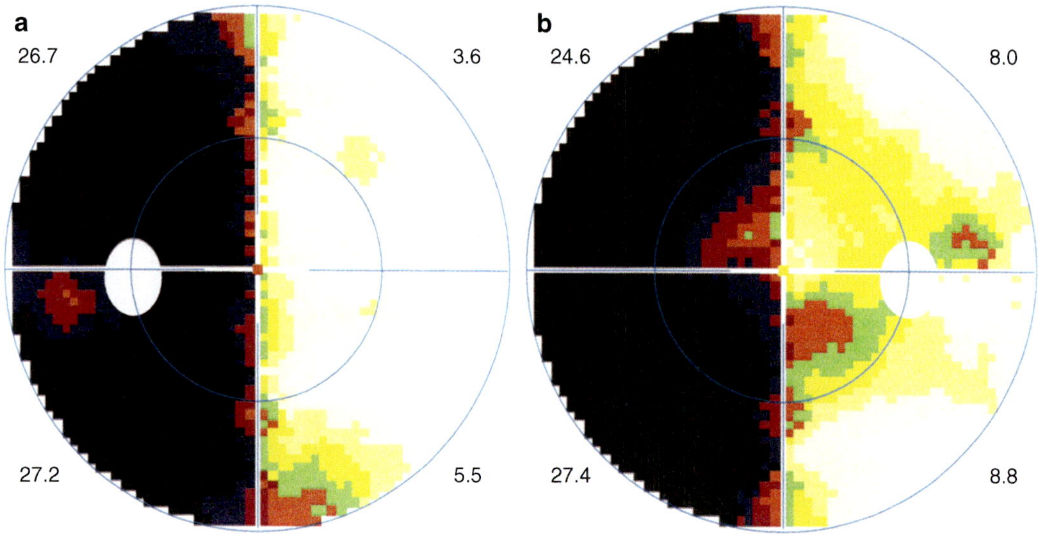

Fig. 47.8 The grayscale maps of Octopus perimeter visual field assessment. Left homonymous hemianopia was shown. Panel a, left eye; Panel b, right eye

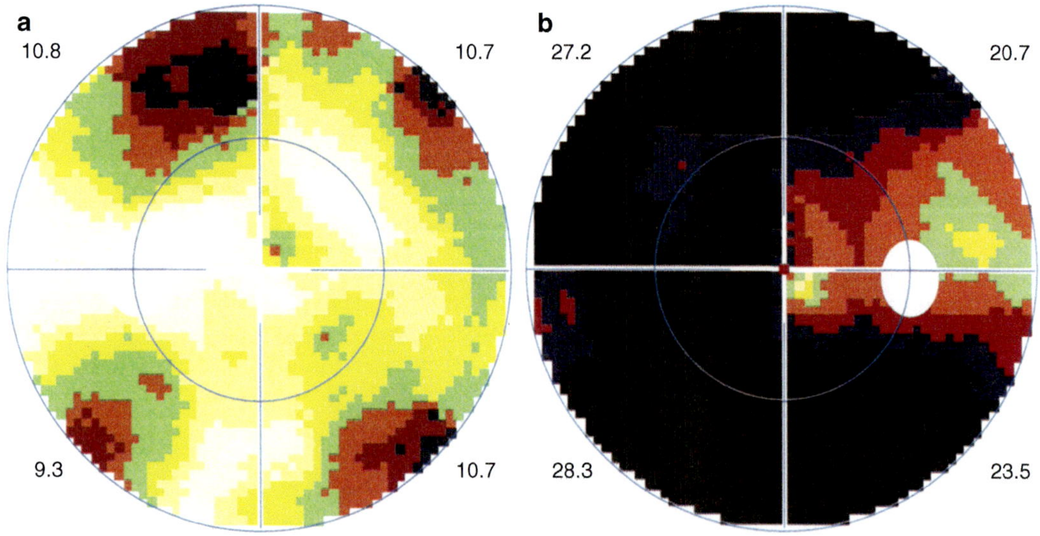

Fig. 47.9 The grayscale maps of Octopus perimeter visual field assessment. Total blindness in one eye and irregular scotomas in another eye was shown. Panel a, left eye; Panel b, right eye

chiasm (with the inferonasal nerve fibers of the retina in the left eye involved), which would be closer to the right optic nerve. With the soft texture and irregular shape of the tumor and the less concentrated force of tumor compression, it led to a special change in the visual field, as shown in Fig. 47.9. In addition, according to the temporal island of vision in the right eye, it is speculated that the damages are not serious on macular nerve fibers and a few nerve fibers from the lateral part of the retina distributed in the median and posterior chiasm of the right eye.

47.5 Binocular Irregular Scotomas

Six patients had scattered, multiple, irregularly distributed defects in the visual field of both eyes (Fig. 47.10), and the visual field defects did not respect the vertical meridian. It is presumably due to the soft texture and irregular shape of the tumor, which exerted a weak and scattered force on the optic chiasm, thus leading to a mild damage to the visual field. It may also affect the blood supply of the optic chiasm to some extent.

47.6 Normal Binocular Visual Field

Two patients had a normal visual field in both eyes (Fig. 47.11). It is speculated that the tumor had not yet affected the optic chiasm. It may also be due to the postfixed location of the optic chiasm.

We also analyzed the differences in age, sex, and tumor volume among the 34 patients with one of the six types of visual field manifestations, and no significant difference was found (p-value > 0.05 with ANOVA comparison). Table 47.1 compares tumor volume in patients with different types of visual fields. The tumor volume (V) was calculated based on the following formula: tumor volume = length × width × height (mm^3). Those values were obtained as the largest diameters of the tumor in the coronal or axial cranial MRI. There was no significant difference in tumor volume (size) among patients with different types of visual field defects. The above results further suggest that the visual field defects mainly arise from the relative position of the tumor with respect to the optic chiasm, rather than the size of the tumor.

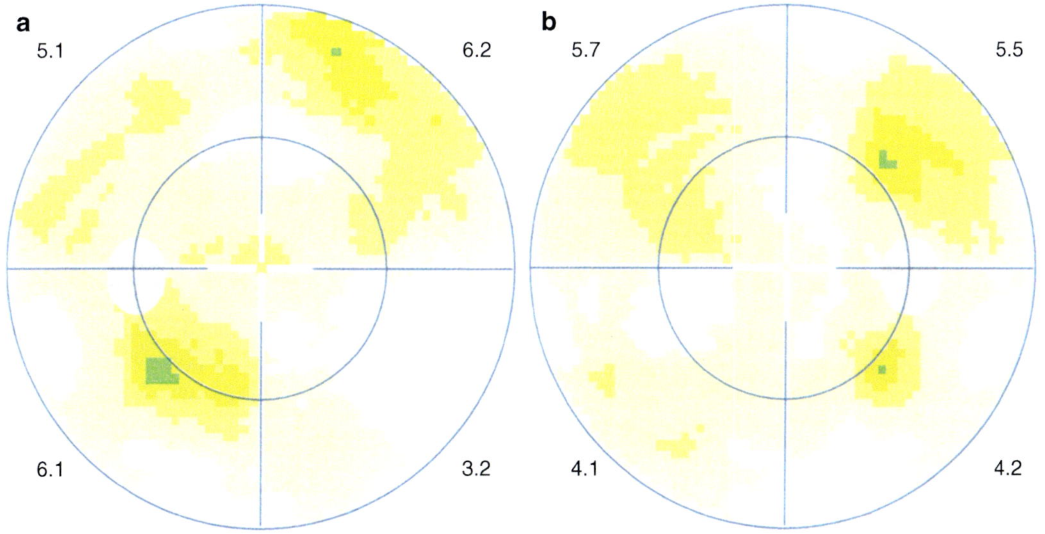

Fig. 47.10 The grayscale maps of Octopus perimeter visual field assessment. Irregular scotomas were shown in both eyes. Panel a, left eye; Panel b, right eye

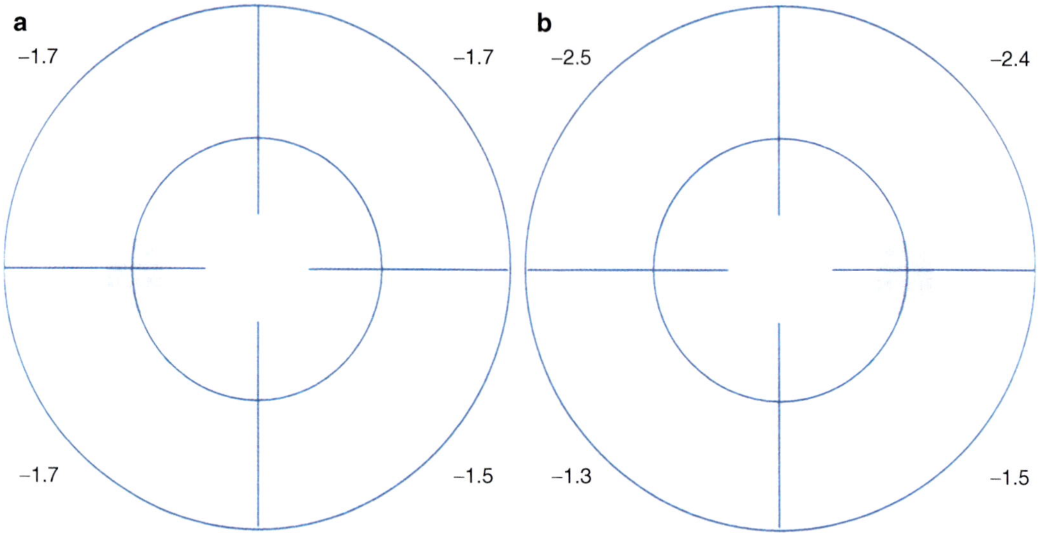

Fig. 47.11 The grayscale maps of Octopus perimeter visual field assessment. The visual field was normal in both eyes. Panel a, left eye; Panel b, right eye

Table 47.1 Comparison of craniopharyngioma tumor volume (mm^3) among patients with one of the six types of visual field defects

	Sample size	Tumor volume (M ± SD)	*P*-value[a]
Bitemporal hemianopia	19	20.4 ± 18.7	0.550
Monocular temporal hemianopia and irregular scotoma in temporal side of the other eye	3	39.0 ± 36.4	
Binocular homonymous hemianopia	3	11.6 ± 5.3	
Nearly total blindness in one eye, irregular scotoma in another eye	1	24.9	
Binocular irregular scotomas	6	25.9 ± 21.9	
Normal binocular visual field	2	9.0 ± 2.8	

[a]One-way ANOVA

47.7 Discussion

Similar to the visual field changes in pituitary tumors (see Part V, Chap. 48), the visual field manifestations of craniopharyngioma are mainly bitemporal hemianopia. The defect pattern of the visual field is related to the position of tumor compression on the optic chiasm. Due to the soft texture, irregular growth pattern, lobulated shape, and individual variations in the position of the optic chiasm with respect to the pituitary gland, there may be a variety of visual field damages; the visual field changes have no significant relationship with age, gender, or tumor volume. Clinically, for temporal visual field defects in one eye or both eyes, especially for those respecting the vertical meridian, the possibility of optic chiasm lesions should be taken into consideration; for atypical visual field changes that cannot be explained by ocular diseases, even in cases of monocular vision changes, intracranial space-occupying lesions should also be considered, and neuroimaging examinations should be done.

Compared with that of pituitary adenomas, the incidence of craniopharyngiomas peaks in two age groups, i.e., children of 5–15 years and elderly people of 45–65 years. Since the tumor body of a craniopharyngioma is soft, its growth pattern is more irregular, and it can compress the optic chiasm from above [1, 2], the types of visual field damage in craniopharyngioma are more complex and less symmetrical between the two eyes. The visual field defects without respecting the vertical meridian are more commonly seen, and it is easily misdiagnosed or neglected in clinical practice [3, 4]. Visual field defects caused by pituitary adenomas will be elaborated in the next section.

At present, craniopharyngioma is mainly treated by surgical operations. However, due to the lack of specific symptoms at the early stage, a definitive diagnosis is often only obtained when tumors become larger; since the location where the tumor grows is quite deep, the surgical operation is not only supposed to completely remove the tumor to prevent its recurrence but also to avoid damage to important tissues around the tumor, and thus the surgery is quite difficult and has many complications. In addition, hypopituitarism after craniopharyngioma removal is common and can be life-threatening. Once craniopharyngioma recrudesces, as it is not sensitive to either radiotherapy or chemotherapy, the treatment would be more troublesome.

Fortunately, in recent years, international research has made significant progress regarding the genes related to this disease [5–7]. Studies have demonstrated that 14–50% of adult craniopharyngiomas are squamous papillary craniopharyngiomas, mainly caused by gene mutations in exon 3 of the BRAF gene. BRAF, one of the most important oncogenes in human, is a major activating factor of extracellular signal-regulated kinases/mitogen-activated protein kinase signaling pathway. Therefore, BRAF inhibitors, such as dabrafenib, and mitogen-activated protein kinase signaling pathway inhibitors, such as trametinib, can be used for targeted therapy in patients with such mutations.

The craniopharyngiomas in other adults and most children are adamantinomatous craniopharyngiomas, some of which are related to CTNNB1 gene mutations. The CTNNB1 gene encodes β-catenin, which mainly mediates intercellular adhesion and participates in gene expression. As a multifunctional protein, β-catenin is widely found in various types of cells and plays important regulatory roles in the proliferation, differentiation, and apoptosis of these cells. Abnormal expression of CTNNB1 protein associated with adamantinomatous craniopharyngiomas can lead to over-activation of the WNT (wingless-type MMTV integration site family members) signaling pathway, which may be one of the important molecular biological mechanisms underlying the pathogenesis of craniopharyngiomas.

References

1. Miller NR. Walsh & Hoyt's clinical neuro-ophthalmology: the essentials. Translated by Zhang Xiaojun and Wei Wenbin. Beijing: Science Press; 2009.
2. Yi T, Shihui W. You Siwei basis and clinical progress of visual pathway diseases. Beijing: People's Medical Publishing House; 2010.
3. Rowe F. Visual fields via the visual pathway. 2nd ed. Boca Raton: CRC; 2016.
4. Savino PJ, Danesh-Mayer HV. Neuro-ophthalmology. 2nd ed. Tianjin: Tianjin Science and Technology Translation Publishing House; 2015.
5. Lubuulwa J, Lei T. Pathological and topographical classification of craniopharyngiomas: a literature review. J Neurol Surg Rep. 2016;77(3):e121–7.
6. Cohen LE. Update on childhood craniopharyngiomas. Curr Opin Endocrinol Diabetes Obes. 2016;23(4):339–44.
7. Brastianos PK, Santagata S. Endocrine tumors: BRAF V600E mutations in papillary craniopharyngioma. Eur J Endocrinol. 2016;174(4):R139–44.

48 Visual Field Analysis of 371 Cases with Pituitary Adenoma

Li Tang, Xuyang Liu, and Ning Fan

Pituitary adenoma (PA) is one of the most common tumors occurring in the sella turcica. It mainly arises from the anterior lobe of the pituitary gland (adenohypophysis). The pituitary adenoma arising from neurohypophysis is rare. Patients with pituitary adenoma may present with symptoms of endocrine dysfunction or with neurologic space-occupying symptoms. Some patients initially go to the Department of Ophthalmology due to decreased vision and visual field defects caused by the optic chiasm compression [1].

48.1 Case Presentation

Three hundred seventy-one patients diagnosed with pituitary adenoma by postoperative pathological evaluation were enrolled in the study. One hundred twenty-nine cases, accounting for 34.8% of all patients, showed visual field defects examined before the surgery. Among these 129 cases, there were 85 cases of binocular visual field defects and 44 cases of monocular visual field defects (Fig. 48.1).

Figure 48.2 demonstrates the craniocerebral coronal T1-weighted contrast-enhanced MRI scan of a patient, which indicates the space-occupying lesions in the sellar region. The lesions

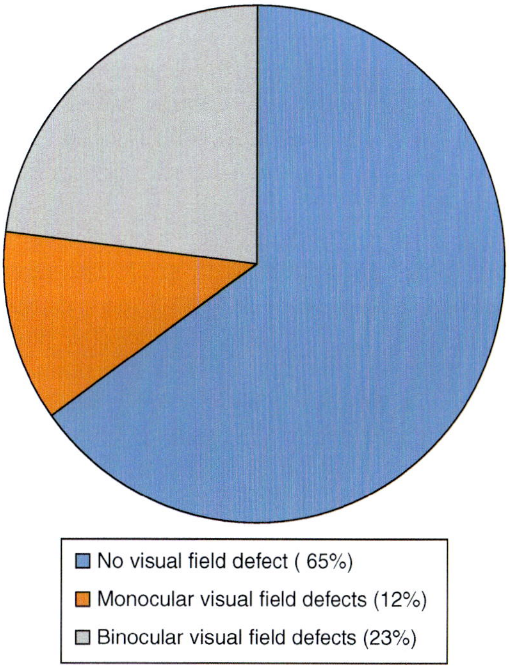

Fig. 48.1 Preoperative visual field condition in 371 cases of pituitary adenoma

L. Tang
West China Hospital, Sichuan University, Chengdu, China

X. Liu
Xiamen Eye Center of Xiamen University, Xiamen, China

Shenzhen Eye Hospital, Shenzhen University, Shenzhen, China

N. Fan (✉)
Shenzhen Eye Hospital, Shenzhen University, Shenzhen, China

N. Wang et al. (eds.), *Optic Disorders and Visual Field*, Advances in Visual Science and Eye Diseases 2, https://doi.org/10.1007/978-981-13-2502-1_48

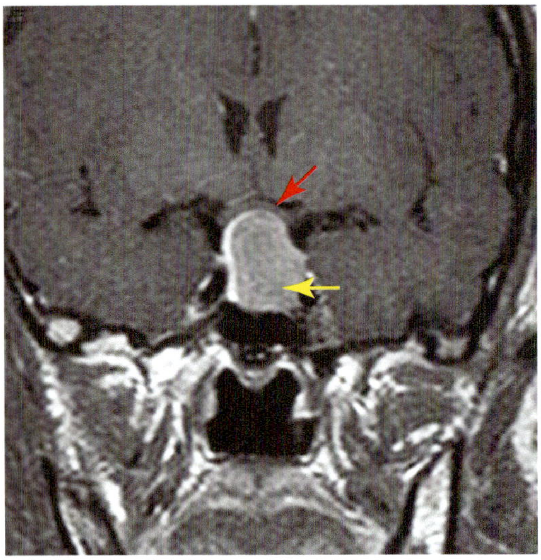

Fig. 48.2 Coronal MRI image. A contrast-enhanced T1-weighted scan disclosed space-occupying lesions in the sellar region (slight enhancement, yellow arrow), which had broken through the sellar diaphragm and compressed the optic chiasm from below (red arrow)

showed a slight enhancement and had broken through the sellar diaphragm, exhibiting the hourglass sign (the pituitary adenoma grows toward the suprasellar area but is restricted by the sellar diaphragm, hence forming a dumbbell shape on the coronal MRI. This is called the hourglass sign). It compressed the optic chiasm from below.

In these 129 patients, there were 61 males and 68 females aged from 15 to 77. The mean age of the patients was 43.2 ± 10.5 years; among them, there were 79 cases of suprasellar pituitary adenomas, 44 cases of intrasellar pituitary adenomas, 2 cases of parasellar pituitary adenomas, 3 cases of intra-suprasellar pituitary adenomas, and 1 case of intra-parasellar adenomas (Fig. 48.3).

We have analyzed the anatomic relationship between the optic chiasm and the pituitary gland in the previous chapter. Based on the positions of the optic chiasm with respect to the pituitary that are divided into three types (prefixed, normal, and postfixed optic chiasmata) and the distribution of nerve fibers in the optic

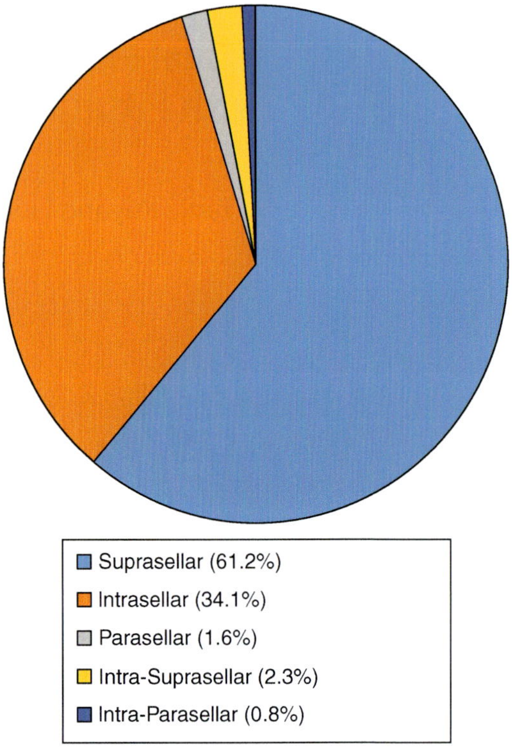

Fig. 48.3 The growth site of 129 cases of pituitary adenomas with preoperative vision defect

chiasm, we can have a preliminary understanding of the visual field defects caused by damage to the optic chiasm, optic nerve, and optic tract from space-occupying lesions in the sellar region. Similar to that of craniopharyngiomas, when the upward growth of pituitary adenoma pushes up the sellar diaphragm or breaks through the sellar diaphragm to reach the sellar region, it may compress or oppress the optic chiasm and may even cause dislocation of the optic chiasm, thus causing visual field damage. Visual impairments can be triggered by a pituitary adenoma when it grows in the sellar region or the parasellar area, pushes the pituitary and the sellar diaphragm upward, and consequently causes compression on the optic chiasm and its surrounding tissues [2, 3].

The common presentations of visual field defects before surgical treatment of pituitary adenomas in the 129 cases include the following:

48.1.1 Binocular Supratemporal Quadrantanopia (Fig. 48.4)

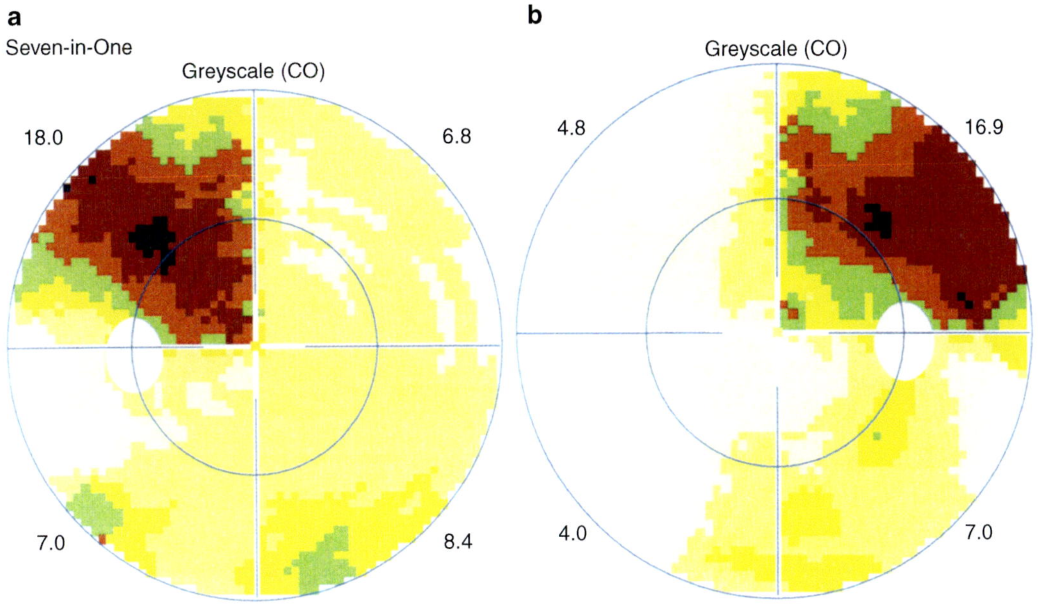

Fig. 48.4 The grayscale maps of Octopus perimeter visual field assessment. Binocular supratemporal quadrantanopia was shown. Panel a, left eye; Panel b, right eye

48.1.2 Non-Quadrantic Bitemporal Hemianopsia (Fig. 48.5)

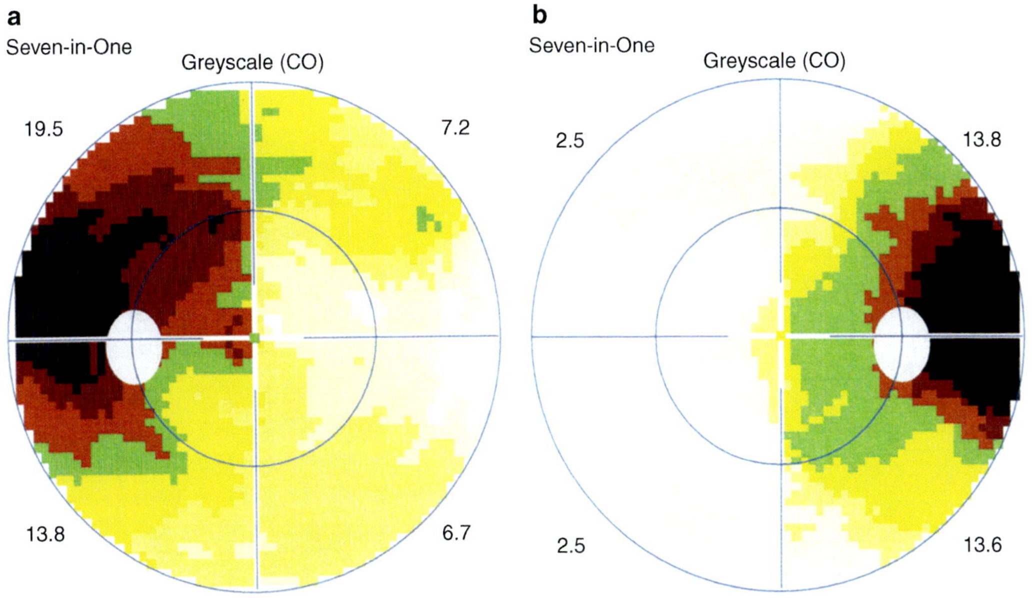

Fig. 48.5 The grayscale maps of Octopus perimeter visual field assessment. Bitemporal non-quadrantic hemianopsia was shown. Panel a, left eye; Panel b, right eye

48.1.3 Vertical Bitemporal Hemianopsia (Fig. 48.6)

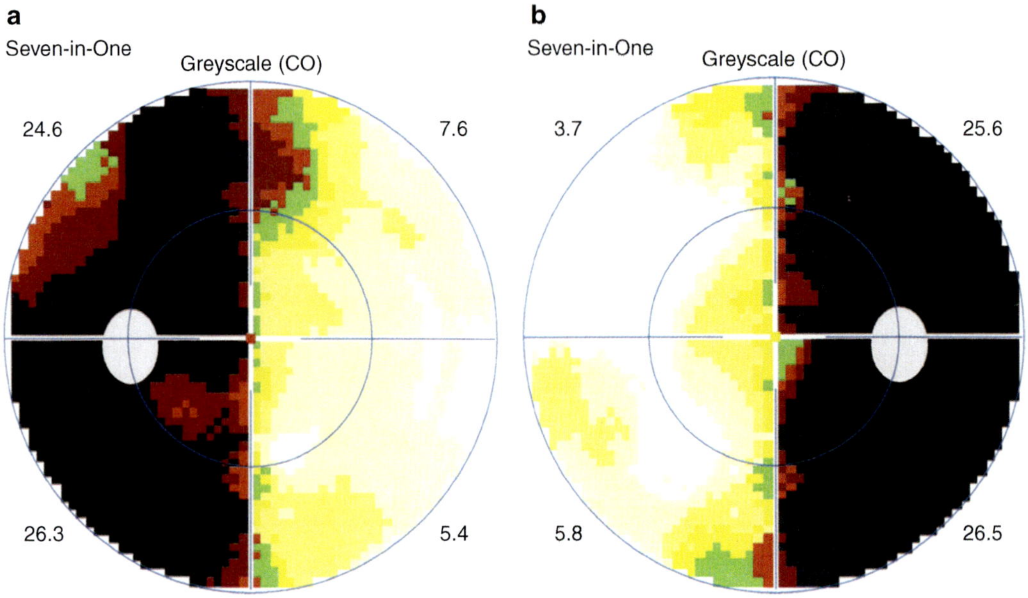

Fig. 48.6 The grayscale maps of Octopus perimeter visual field assessment. Vertical bitemporal hemianopsia was shown. Panel a, left eye; Panel b, right eye

48.1.4 Bitemporal Hemianopsia Extending Across the Midline and Affecting the Nasal Visual Field (Fig. 48.7)

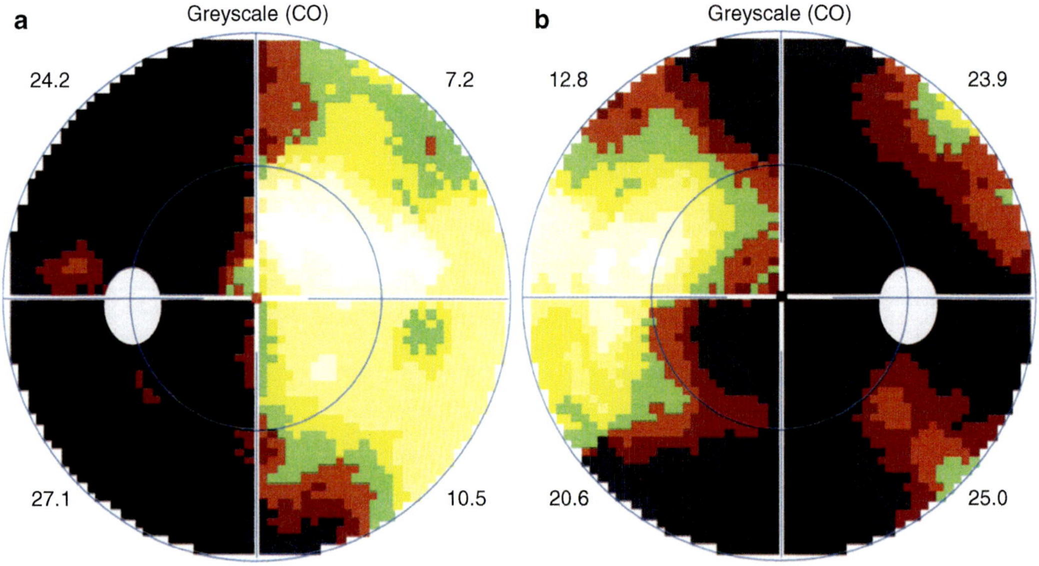

Fig. 48.7 The grayscale maps of Octopus perimeter visual field assessment. Bitemporal hemianopsia extending across the midline and affecting the nasal visual field was shown. Panel a, left eye; Panel b, right eye

48.1.5 Residual Supranasal Tubular Visual Field in Both Eyes (Fig. 48.8)

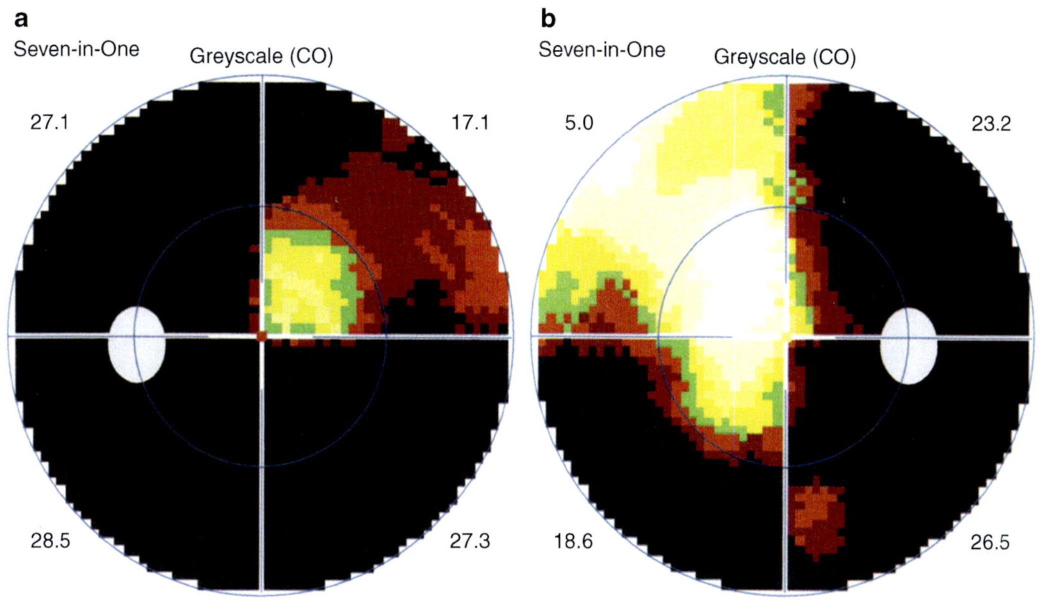

Fig. 48.8 The grayscale maps of Octopus perimeter visual field assessment. A residual supranasal tubular visual field was shown in both eyes. Panel a, left eye; Panel b, right eye

48.1.6 Binocular Homonymous Hemianopsia (Fig. 48.9)

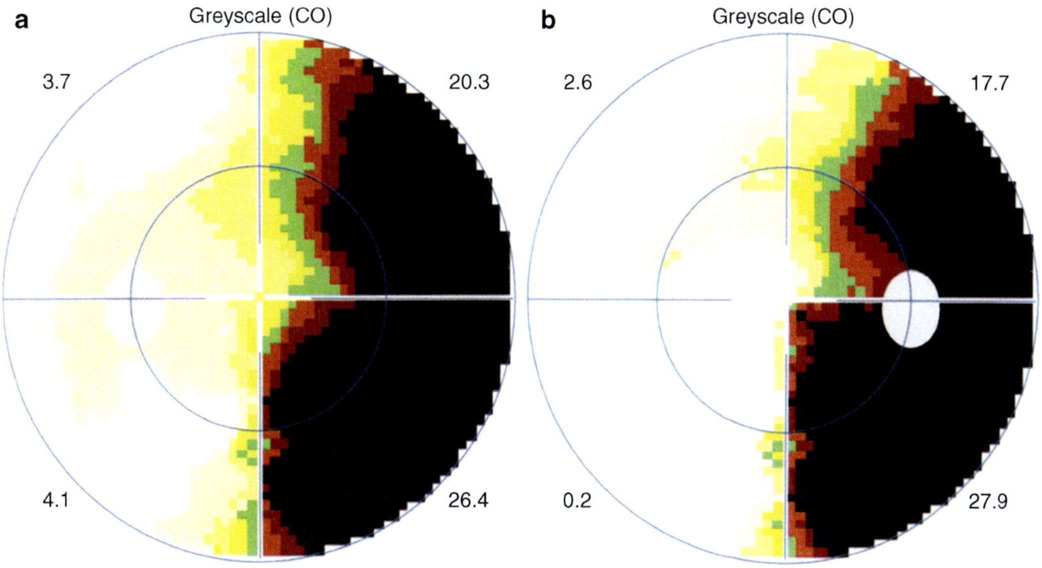

Fig. 48.9 The grayscale maps of Octopus perimeter visual field assessment. Binocular homonymous hemianopsia was shown. Panel a, left eye; Panel b, right eye

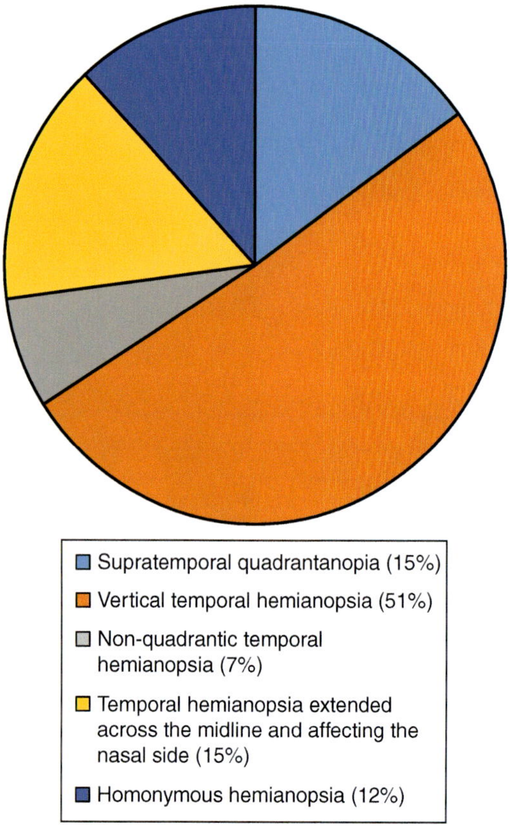

Fig. 48.10 Characteristics of binocular symmetric visual field defects caused by pituitary adenomas

Binocular visual field defects were determined in 85 patients, symmetrical visual field defects were determined in 73 patients, and asymmetrical visual field defects were determined in 12 patients.

Symmetrical visual field damage include the following five presentations (Fig. 48.10): bilateral supratemporal quadrantanopia (11 cases), vertical bitemporal hemianopsia (37 cases), non-quadrantic bitemporal hemianopsia (5 cases), bitemporal hemianopsia extended across the vertical midline and affecting the nasal visual field (11 cases, including 3 cases of residual supranasal tubular visual field in both eyes), and binocular homonymous hemianopsia (9 cases).

The most common characteristic symmetric visual field defects usually begin in the upper temporal sector, gradually develop to the temporal side, then break through the midline and affect the inferior nasal visual field, and finally produce a residual superior nasal tubular visual field. It indicates that the optic chiasm damage starts from the ventral medial (anterior knee of Wilbrand), gradually spreads to the entire middle portion of the optic chiasm and the posterior knee of the optic chiasm, and then further extends to both sides of the optic chiasm. Once the scotoma extends across the vertical midline, the difference between the eyes becomes obvious (Fig. 48.5), which suggests that multiple sites of the optic chiasm may be compressed and oppressed by the tumor in the advanced stage.

For non-quadrantic bitemporal hemianopsia, it is presumably because of the compression at the posteromedial optic chiasm, thus resulting in damage to the macular nerve fibers in the optic disc. For binocular homonymous hemianopsia, it is presumably because of the damage to the nerve fibers of the optic tract at one side behind the optic chiasm. It may also occur in patients with a prefixed chiasm.

Of the 44 patients with monocular visual field damage, 31 had vertical temporal hemianopsia, 5 had quadrantic temporal defects, and 2 had non-quadrantic temporal defects. In three

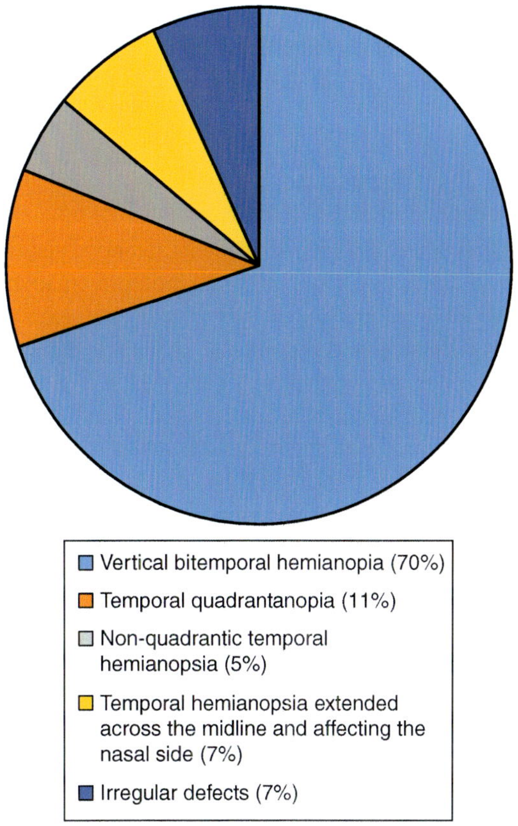

Fig. 48.11 Characteristics of monocular visual field defects caused by pituitary adenomas

patients, the temporal hemianopsia extended across the midline and affected the nasal visual field. Three patients had irregular defects (Fig. 48.11).

Temporal visual field defects are still the most common presentation in patients with monocular defects, which is determined by the anatomic relationship between the pituitary adenomas and the chiasm. Tumors grow upward and would most often compress the nerve fibers in the central portion of the optic chiasm. This suggests that the possibility of space-occupying pituitary lesions should be considered for patients with temporal visual field defects, even with monocular defects.

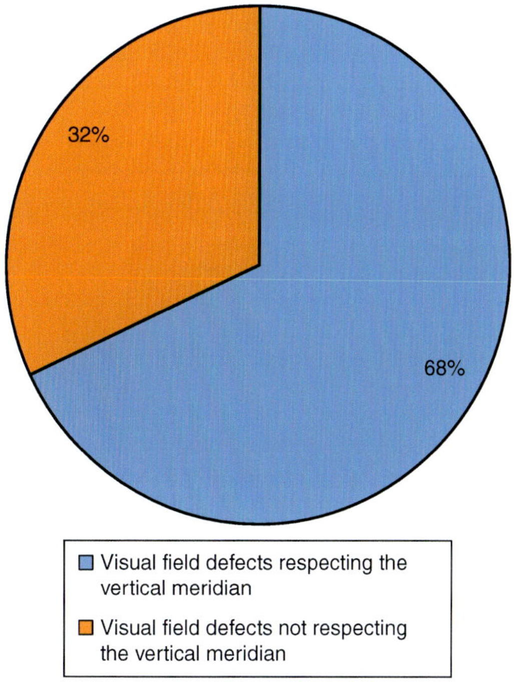

Fig. 48.12 Vertical meridian characteristics of visual field defects caused by pituitary adenomas

There were 214 eyes (129 patients) with visual field defects. According to the presentation of visual field defects, they can be divided into the following:

1. Visual field defects respecting the vertical meridian were found in 145 (68%, Fig. 48.12) eyes. One hundred thirty-six eyes (94%) had

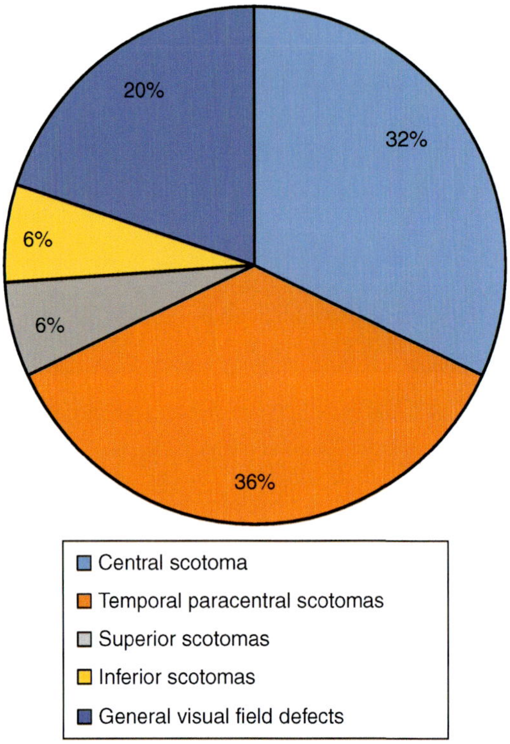

Fig. 48.13 Characteristics of visual field damage not respecting the vertical meridian caused by pituitary adenomas

temporal defects (including 22 eyes with damage breaking through the vertical meridian and affecting the nasal side), and only 9 eyes (6%) had nasal visual field defects. According to the results, temporal hemianopsia was the most common defect caused by pituitary adenomas.

2. Visual field defects not respecting the vertical meridian was found in 69 (32%, Fig. 48.13) eyes. Twenty-two eyes had central defects, 25 eyes had temporal paracentral defects, 4 eyes had superior defects, 4 eyes had inferior defects, and 14 eyes had diffuse depressions. It is speculated that these atypical visual field defects were due to the mild tumor compression of the optic chiasm and the individual differences in the relative position between the optic chiasm and the pituitary gland. It is noteworthy that, in these patients with such atypical visual field defects, the proportion of temporal central scotomas was still high.

48.2 Discussion

According to this group of patients, temporal visual field defects were the most common presentation caused by pituitary adenomas. Usually, the characteristic visual field is binocular symmetric defects respecting the vertical meridian, which begin in the upper temporal sector, gradually develop to the temporal side, then extend across the midline and affect the inferior nasal visual field, and finally turned into residual superior nasal tubular visual field or even blindness. It indicates that the optic chiasm damage starts from the ventral medial, gradually spreads to the entire middle portion of the optic chiasm, and then further extends to both sides of the optic chiasm. A variety of atypical changes in the visual field can be observed due to normal variation and individual differences in the anatomic relationship between the optic chiasm and pituitary gland/pituitary tumor, such as binocular homonymous hemianopsia, irregular defects, central defects, and monocular defects. Temporal visual field defects are still the most common presentation in patients with monocular defects or paracentral defects, indicating that the central part of the optic chiasm is the common location of compression or oppression by pituitary adenomas.

We further evaluated the associations between visual field damage presentations and the pituitary adenoma volume (Table 48.1). The tumor volume (*V*) is calculated based on the following formula: tumor volume = length × width × height (mm^3). Those values were obtained as the largest diameters of the tumor in the coronal or axial cranial MRI. The mean sensitivity (MS) is the arithmetic average of the light sensitivity obtained at each checkpoint in the 24-2 testing with an Octopus perimeter. The unit of MS is dB. For patients with binocular visual field damage, the MS values of their right eyes were analyzed. For

Table 48.1 Comparison of tumor volumes and MS values among three common types of visual fields in patients with pituitary adenomas

	Quadrantic temporal hemianopsia	Vertical temporal hemianopsia	Tubular visual field	*p*-value
Tumor volume (mm^3)	33,821.0 ± 63,403.2	21,528.0 ± 16,327.1	27,272.0 ± 28,108.0	0.75[a]
MS value (dB)	21.44 ± 4.06	15.45 ± 4.38	10.82 ± 5.09	0.00[b]

[a]Kruskal-Wallis *H* test
[b]One-way ANOVA

patients with monocular defects, the MS values of their affected eyes were analyzed.

The homogeneity analysis for variance of the tumor volume in the three groups was done by the Levene method. The statistical value was 3.529, $p = 0.034$. The variance in the three groups could be considered heterogeneous at the level of $\alpha = 0.10$. After Kruskal-Wallis H test for the comparison of multiple independent samples, X2 = 0.58, $p = 0.75$. The difference of tumor volume in the three groups was not significant at the level of $\alpha = 0.05$. The variance of homogeneity analysis of the MS value in the three groups was done by the Levene method, which yielded a statistical value of 0.375, $p = 0.689$. The variance in the three groups could be considered homogeneous at the level of $\alpha = 0.10$. Using a completely randomized analysis of variance, $F = 27.11$, $p = 0.00$. The differences of the average MS values in the three groups could be considered statistically significant at the level of $\alpha = 0.05$. Through the paired SNK test for multiple independent samples, the MS value of the quadrantic hemianopsia group was then considered as higher than that of the temporal vertical hemianopsia group, and the MS value of the temporal vertical hemianopsia group was higher than that of the tubular visual field group, at the level of $\alpha = 0.05$.

The results of statistical analysis shows that, as an indicator to measure the effect of mechanical compression on the sellar region by the tumor, there was a weak correlation between tumor volume and the visual field impairments by pituitary adenoma.

At the same time, this result also supports our previous speculation about the sequence of visual field damage caused by pituitary adenomas, i.e., the visual field defects in both eyes begin in the upper temporal sector, gradually develop to the temporal side, then extend across the midline and affect the inferior nasal visual field, and finally produce a residual superior nasal tubular visual field. The progression of visual field impairments was accompanied by visual acuity loss.

Sometimes, the visual field defects can get better or completely resolve if the bitemporal hemianopsia is mild and the patient has undergone a successful operation without delay. The patient shown below is an example. Perimetry before surgical treatment of pituitary adenoma showed bitemporal hemianopsia, more severe in the left eye (Fig. 48.14); MRI showed space-occupying lesions in the sellar region compressing the optic chiasm superiorly (Fig. 48.15).

Perimetry and MRI were done 1 month after the surgical treatment of pituitary adenoma showed normal view fields (Fig. 48.16). MRI showed a mildly enlarged pituitary that did not reach the optic chiasm (Fig. 48.17).

Usually pituitary tumors, such as adenomas, are soft, and thus their damage to the optic chiasm is sometimes not entirely due to mechanical compression but also related to the tumor's interference with the blood supply to the optic chiasm [4]. After the surgical operation relieving the compression, the blood supply to the optic chiasm would be improved, so visual field defects would also be improved. This could be compared with the pituitary microadenoma and steal syndrome to be reported in the following section (see Part V, Chap. 49).

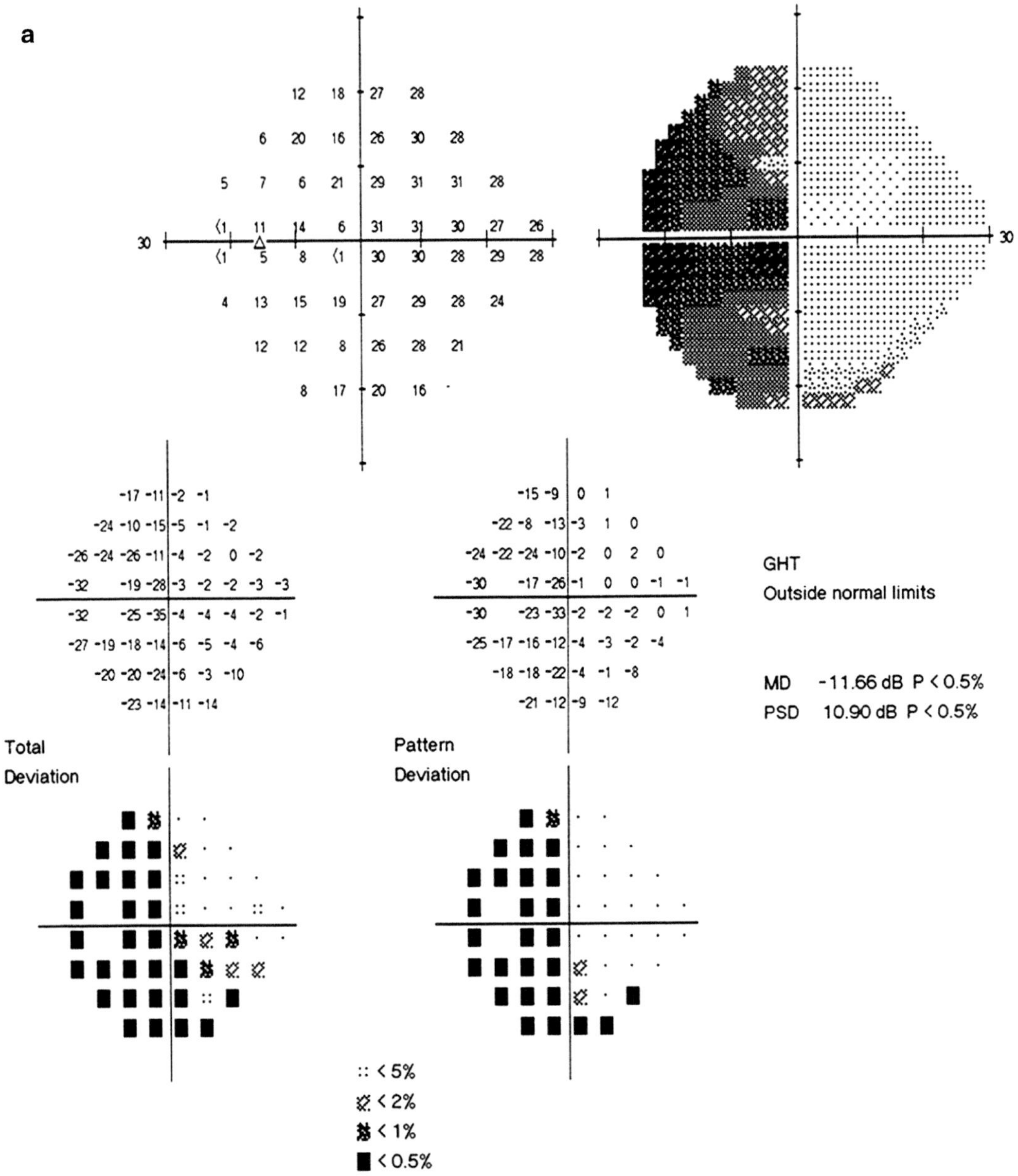

Fig. 48.14 Humphrey visual field analysis printouts. Panel a, temporal hemianopsia in the left eye; Panel b, temporal visual field defect in the right eye respecting the vertical meridian

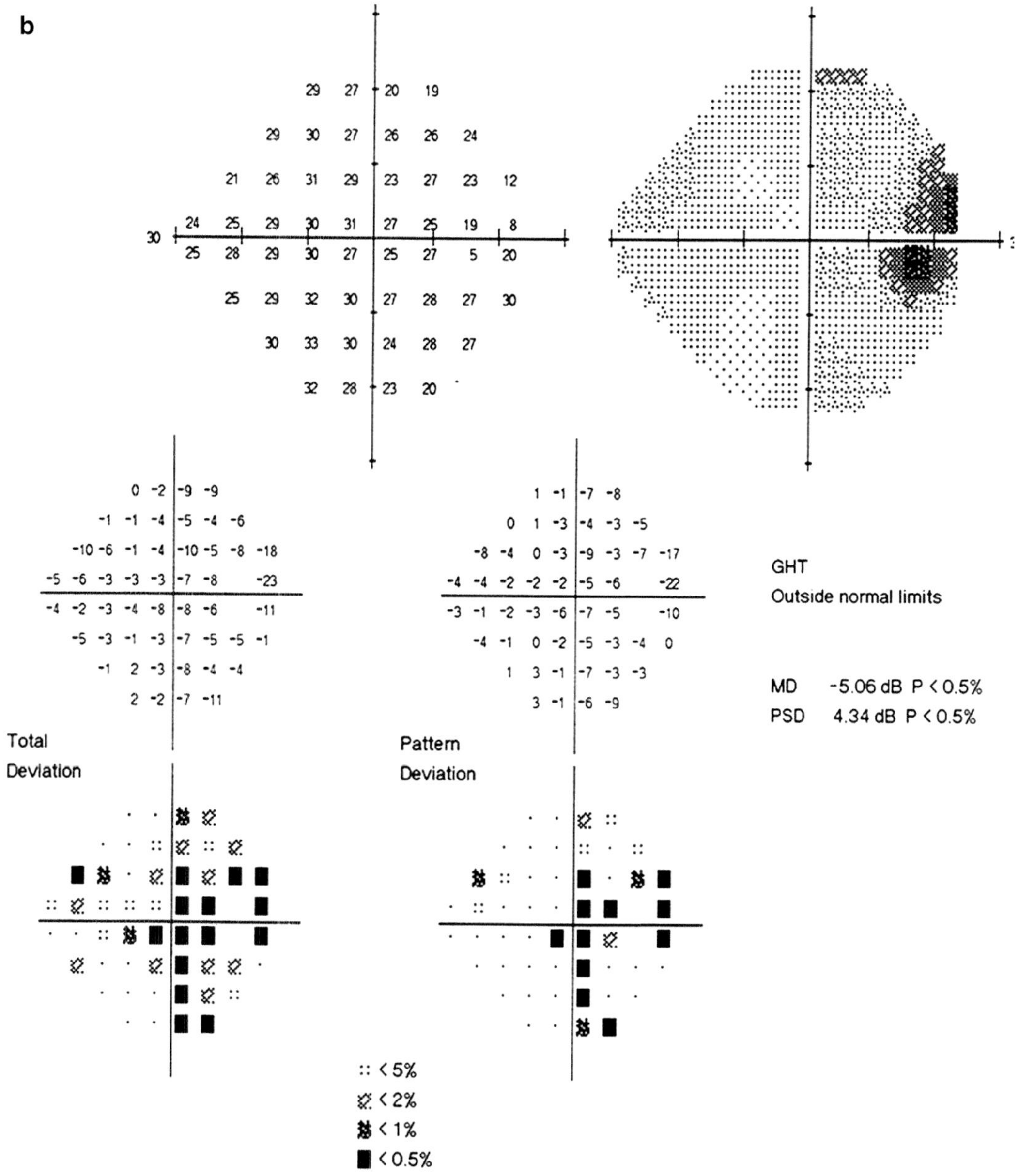

Fig. 48.14 (continued)

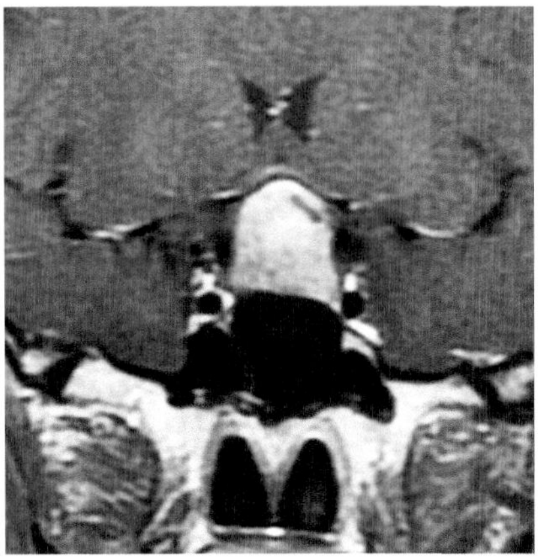

Fig. 48.15 Preoperative MRI of pituitary tumor. Enhanced T1 shows occupying lesions in the sellar region which broke through the sellar diaphragm and compressed the optic chiasm superiorly

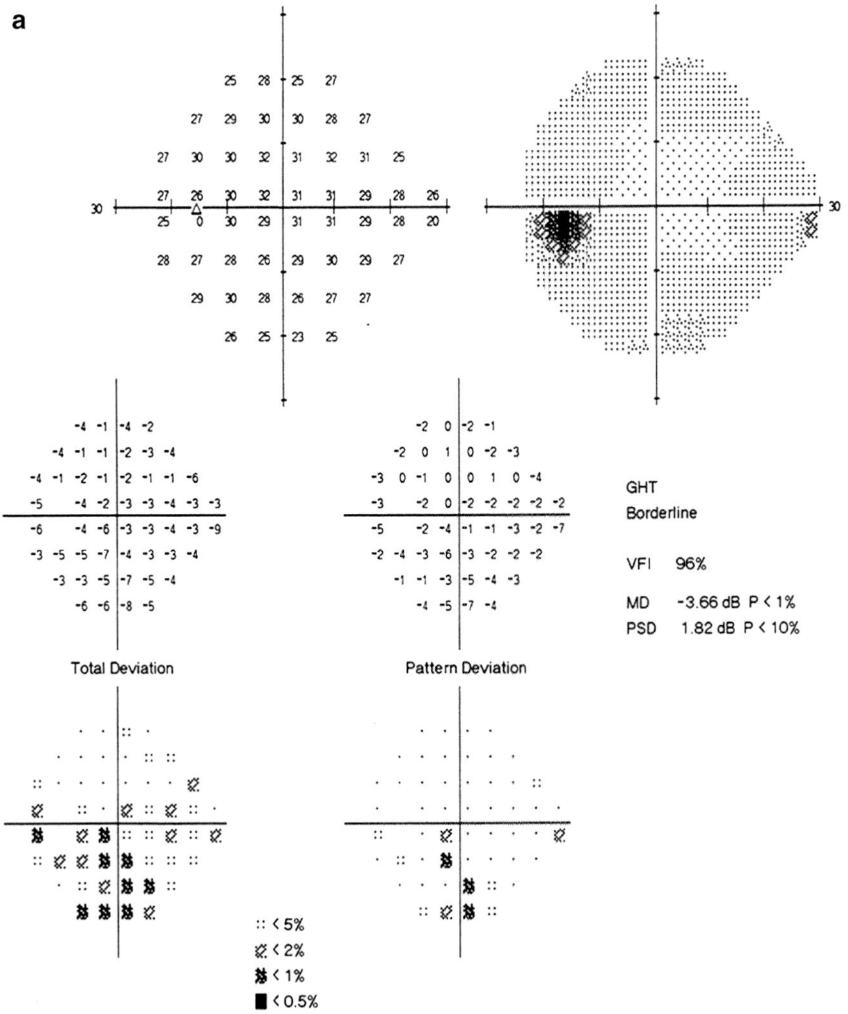

Fig. 48.16 Postoperative visual field. A normal visual field was shown in both eyes. Panel a, left eye; Panel b, right eye

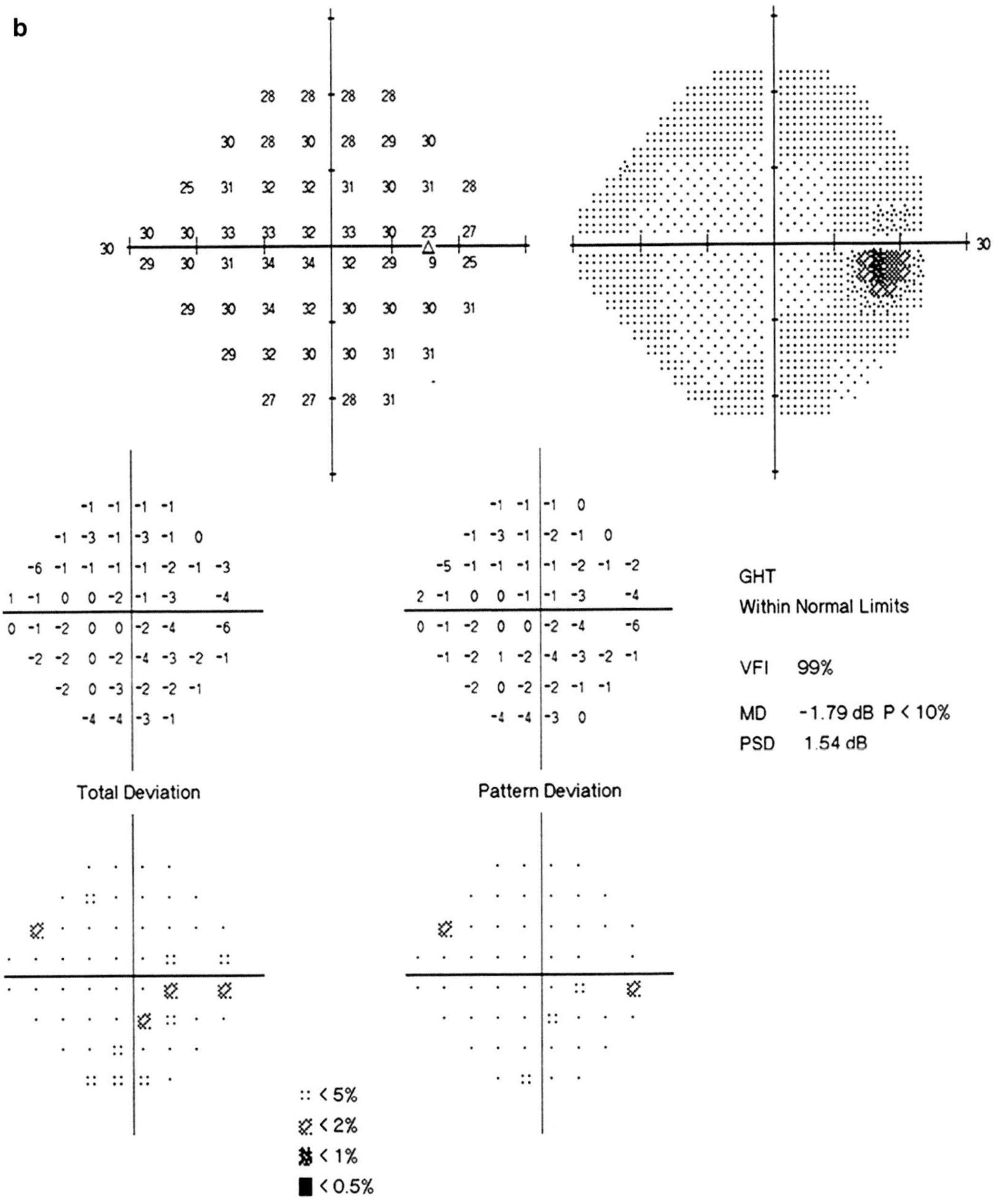

Fig. 48.16 (continued)

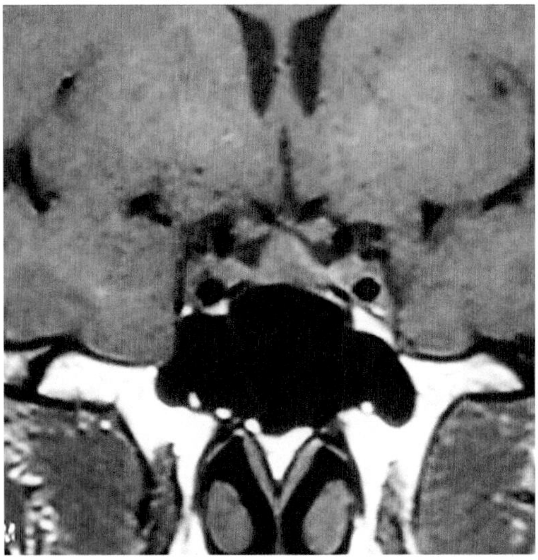

Fig. 48.17 Postoperative MRI of pituitary tumor. Coronal MRI showed a slightly enlarged pituitary with an irregular shape, which had less homogeneous internal signal and uneven enhancement. It did not reach the optic chiasm

References

1. Yi T, Shihui W, Siwei Y. Basis and clinical progress of visual pathway diseases. Beijing: People's Medical Publishing House; 2010.
2. Rowe F. Visual fields via the visual pathway. 2nd ed. Boca Raton: CRC; 2016.
3. Savino PJ, Danesh-Mayer HV. Neuro-ophthalmology. 2nd ed. Tianjin: Tianjin Science and Technology Translation Publishing House; 2015.
4. Guozhen H. Pituitary neoplasm. 1st ed. Beijing: Military Science Publishing House; 2004.

49 Pituitary Microadenomas and Artery Steal Syndrome

Li Tang, Xuyang Liu, and Ning Fan

Compression of the optic chiasm usually results in typical bitemporal visual field loss. However, a small tumor, like pituitary microadenoma, was not big enough to compress the optic chiasm but might also be able to cause bitemporal visual field defects. What are the underlying reasons?

49.1 Case 1

49.1.1 Case Presentation

A 49-year-old female patient had been diagnosed with glaucoma without complain of eye pain, blurred vision, or headache 1 year before and was treated with brimonidine tartrate eye drops for both eyes twice a day. The peak value of 24-h intraocular pressure (IOP) was lower than 15 mmHg before treatment. Histories of trauma, other ocular and systemic diseases, and familial diseases were denied; systemic evaluation was unremarkable.

On ophthalmological examination, the uncorrected visual acuity (UCVA) was 20/20 (OU). IOP by standard Goldmann applanation tonometry was measured as 10 mmHg OD, 11 mmHg OS. Central corneal thickness was 515 μm OD and 520 μm OS. Slit-lamp examination of her anterior segments was unremarkable. Fundus examination revealed that the cup-to-disc ratio was 0.85 with the superior and inferior rim narrowed in the right eye, and the cup-to-disc ratio was 0.7 with normal disc rim in the left eye. There was no significant change in either optic nerve compared to 1 year before (Fig. 49.1).

The visual field test done 1 year before showed a superior scotoma and nasal step in both eyes (Fig. 49.2). Current visual field test revealed that the supratemporal visual field defects got better, while the nasal step scotomas remained the same as previously seen (Fig. 49.3).

Pituitary MRI indicated that there was no obvious change in the size and location of the pituitary microadenoma when compared to those seen 1 year before (Fig. 49.4).

Pituitary hormone tests revealed within normal limits.

L. Tang
West China Hospital, Sichuan University, Chengdu, China

X. Liu
Xiamen Eye Center of Xiamen University, Xiamen, China

Shenzhen Eye Hospital, Shenzhen University, Shenzhen, China

N. Fan (✉)
Shenzhen Eye Hospital, Shenzhen University, Shenzhen, China

N. Wang et al. (eds.), *Optic Disorders and Visual Field*, Advances in Visual Science and Eye Diseases 2, https://doi.org/10.1007/978-981-13-2502-1_49

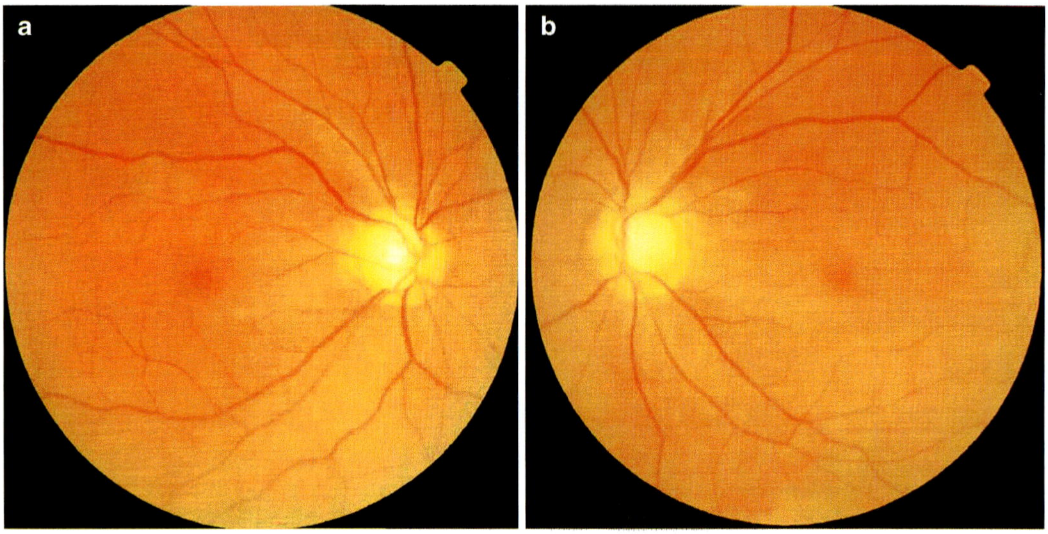

Fig. 49.1 Fundus photographs. Panel a: The cup-to-disc ratio was 0.85 in the right eye, with the superior and inferior rim narrowed. Panel b: The cup-to-disc ratio was 0.7 in the left eye, with a deepened disc cup and normal rim

49.1.2 Final Diagnosis

The final diagnosis was NTG OU, pituitary microadenoma, and superior hypophyseal artery steal syndrome.

49.2 Case 2

49.2.1 Case Presentation

A 64-year-old female complained of blurred vision in both eyes for more than 2 months, with the left eye being more severe. No other discomforts such as eye pain, visual loss, floaters, or headache were noticed. Histories of trauma, other ocular and systemic diseases, and familial diseases were denied; systemic evaluation was unremarkable.

On ophthalmological examination, the UCVA was 20/17 OD and 20/22 OS, and no improvement was achieved with refractive correction in either eye. IOP by standard Goldmann applanation tonometry was measured as 24 mmHg OD and 26 mmHg OS. Slit-lamp examination of her anterior segments was unremarkable. The C/D ratio was 0.55 OD and 0.6 OS. The foveal reflex was normal in both eyes.

The central corneal thickness was 566 μm OD and 565 μm OS.

Standardized automated perimetry showed a supratemporal defect in the right eye and a superior altitudinal defect in the left eye. The visual field defect in the supratemporal quadrant was more serious than that in the supranasal quadrant. Central scotomas were noticed on the temporal side of the fixation in both eyes (Fig. 49.5).

Pituitary MRI showed a pituitary gland that was slightly enlarged on the left side, indicating the presence of a microadenoma. However, the optic chiasm was not directly compressed (Fig. 49.6).

Pituitary hormone test results are within normal limits.

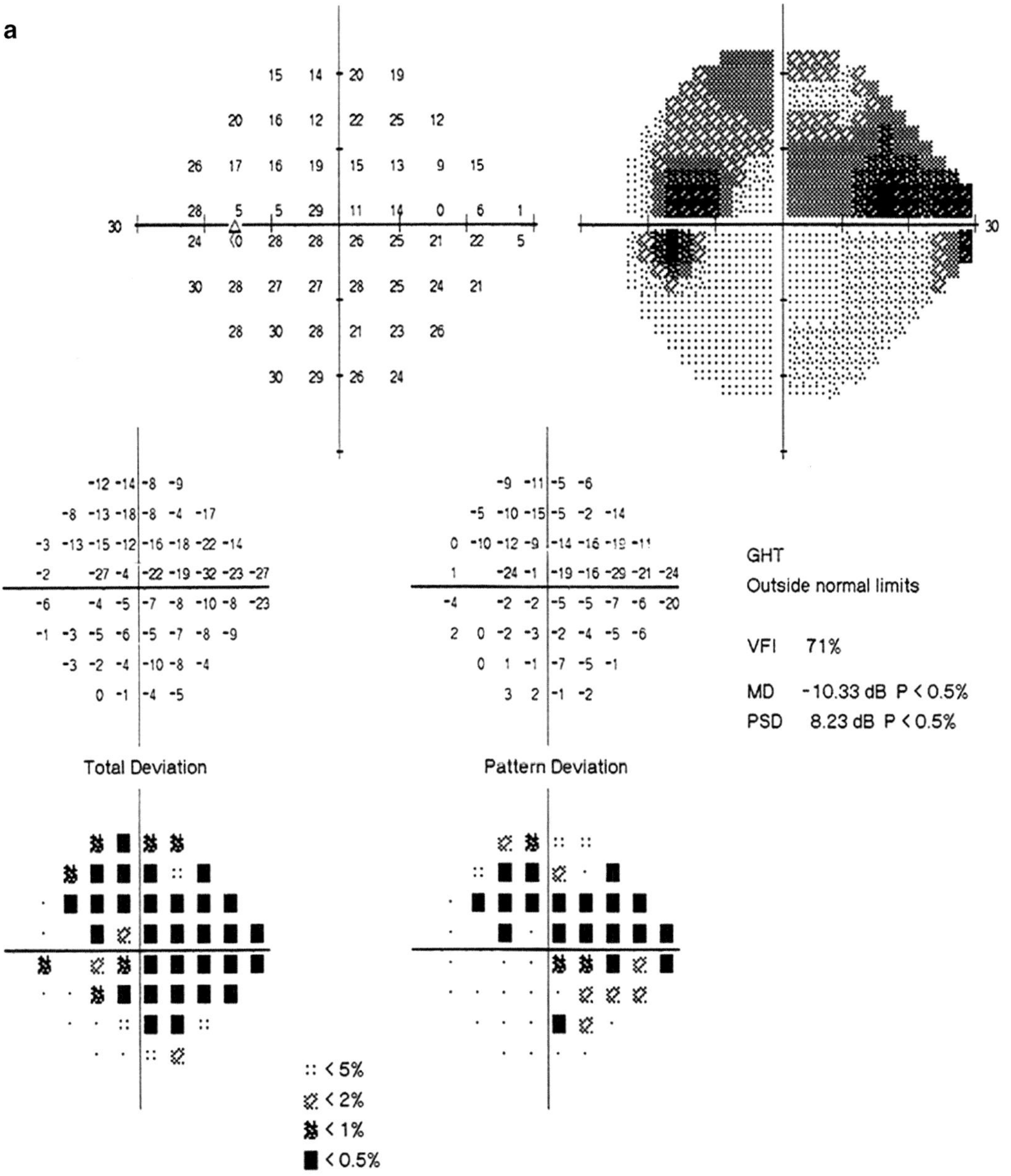

Fig. 49.2 Humphrey visual field analysis printouts obtained 1 year before. The 24-2 test showed a superior scotoma and nasal step in both eyes. Panel a, left eye; Panel b, right eye

b

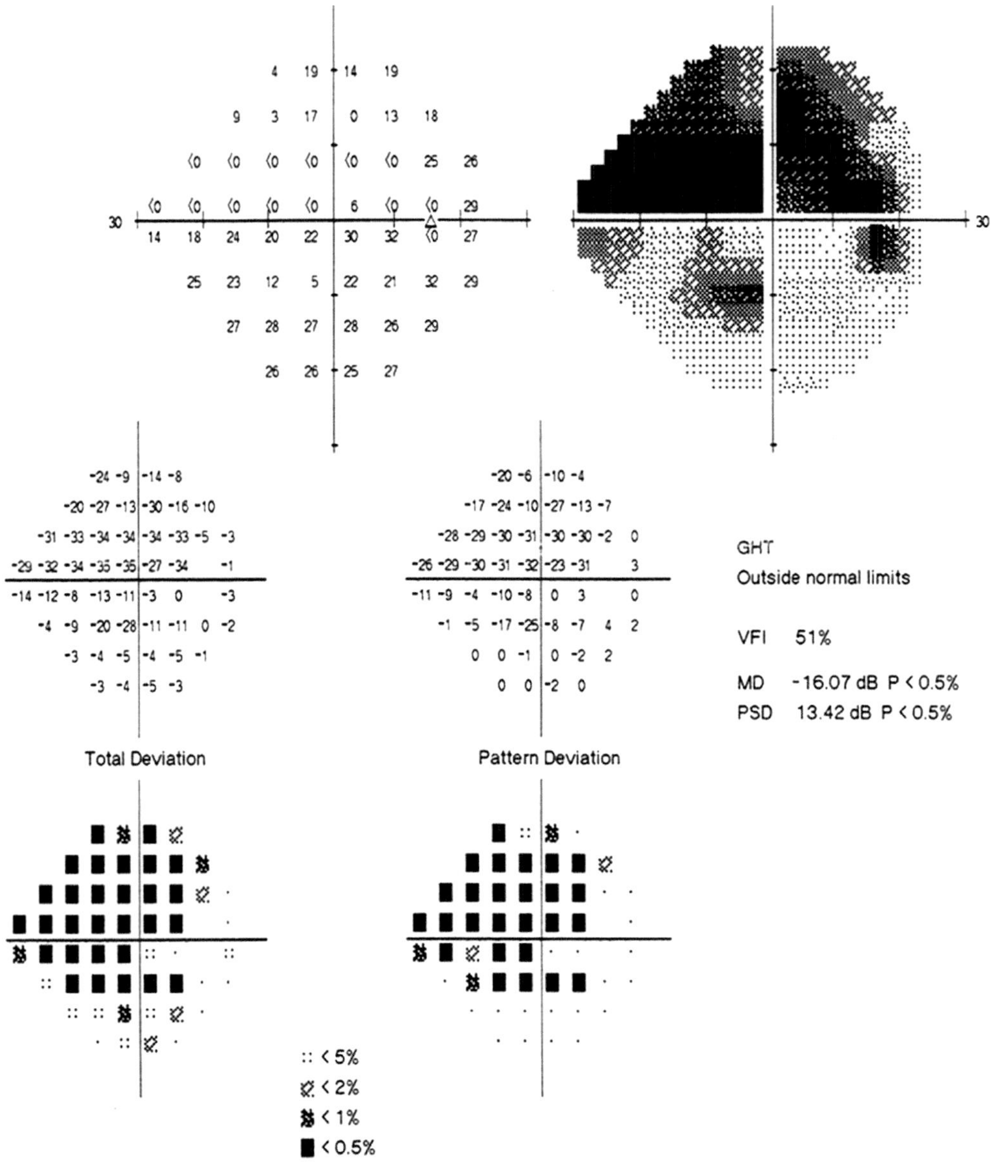

Fig. 49.2 (continued)

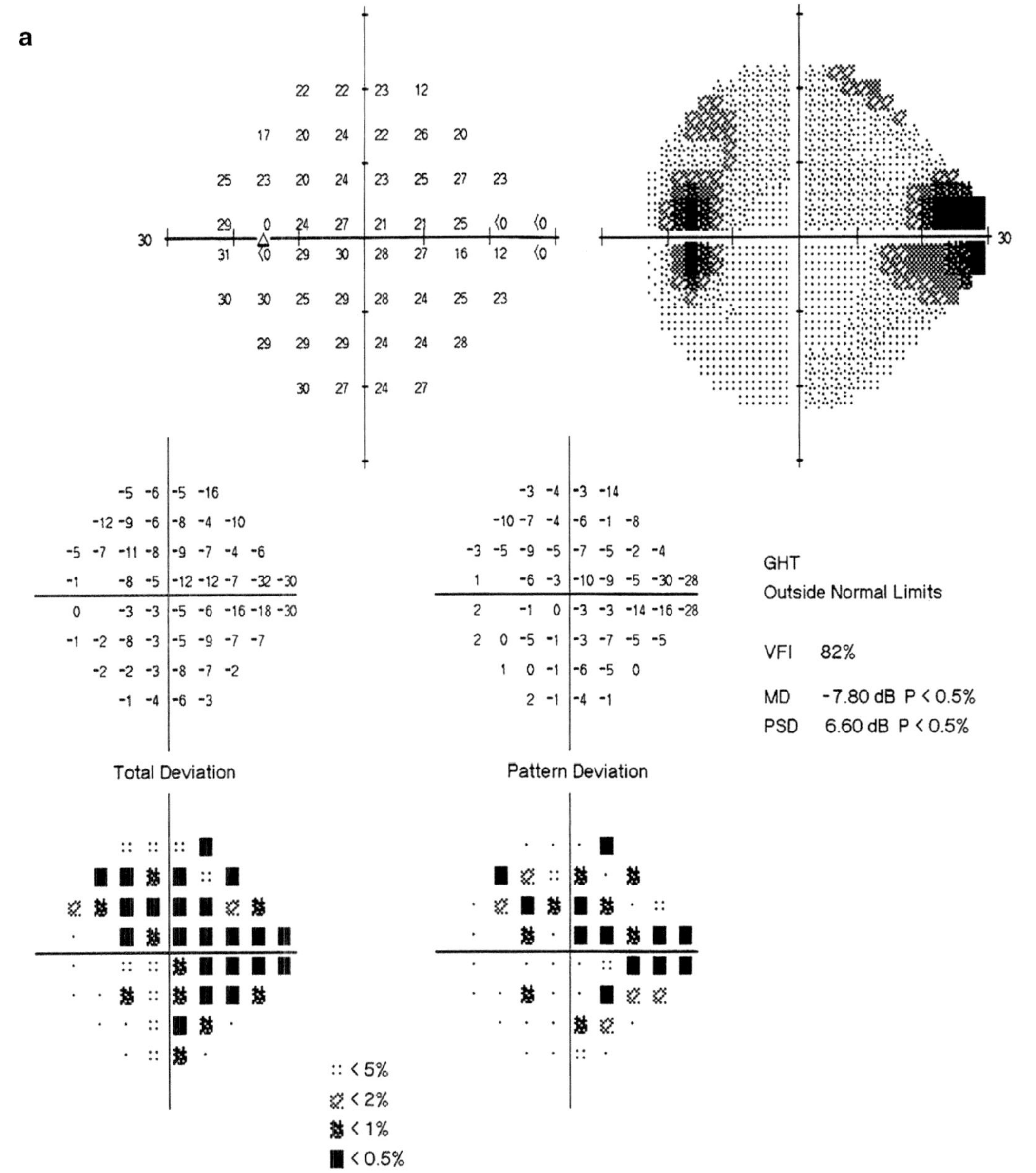

Fig. 49.3 Humphrey visual field analysis printouts obtained recently. The 24-2 test showed that the supratemporal visual field defects got better, while the nasal step scotomas remained the same as previously seen. Panel a, left eye; Panel b, right eye

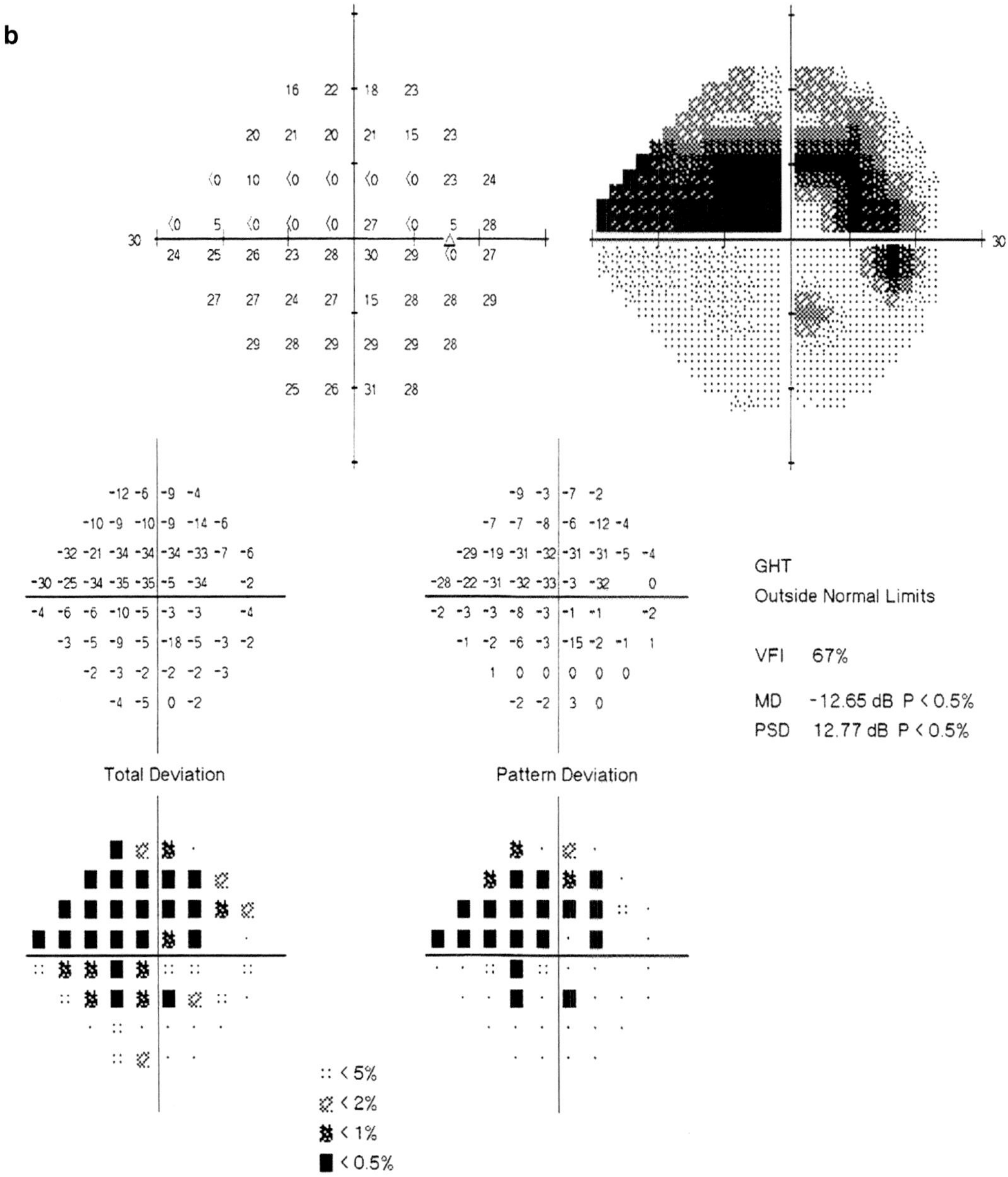

Fig. 49.3 (continued)

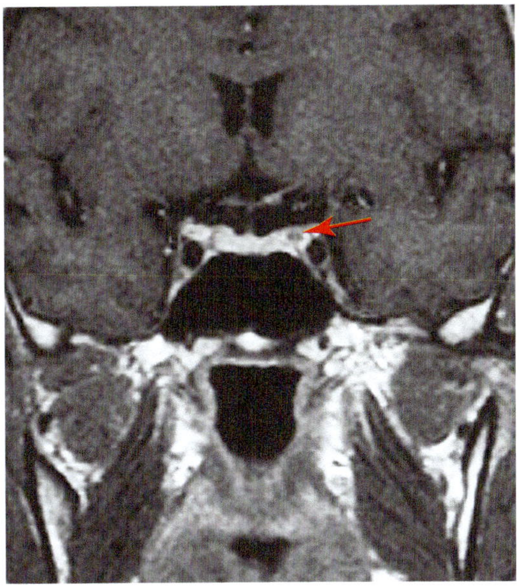

Fig. 49.4 Pituitary MRI image. A microadenoma (red arrow) was noted

49.2.2 Final Diagnosis

The final diagnosis was pituitary microadenoma, superior hypophyseal artery steal syndrome, and suspected glaucoma in both eyes.

49.3 Discussion

As early as 1884, Vossius found that binocular temporal hemianopia is a specific visual field defect of pituitary tumor as a result of the direct compression of the optic chiasm by the tumor. However, a pituitary microadenoma is even not big enough to touch the sellar diaphragm, and therefore it is impossible for it to compress the optic chiasm. What is the pathological cause of bitemporal visual field defects in pituitary microadenoma?

A brief review of the anatomical relationship between the pituitary and the optic chiasm is helpful. The meninges under the optic chiasm tightly

Fig. 49.5 The grayscale maps of Octopus perimeter visual field assessment. Supratemporal visual field defects and central scotomas temporal to the fixation were seen in both eyes, and the supranasal visual field was involved in the left eye. Panel a, right eye; Panel b, left eye

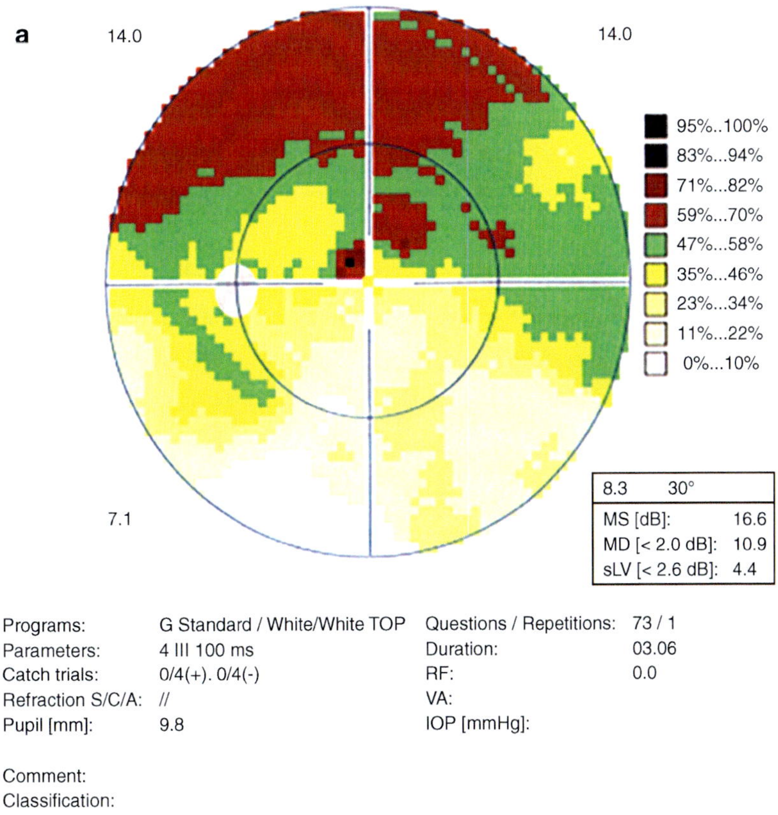

Fig. 49.5 (continued)

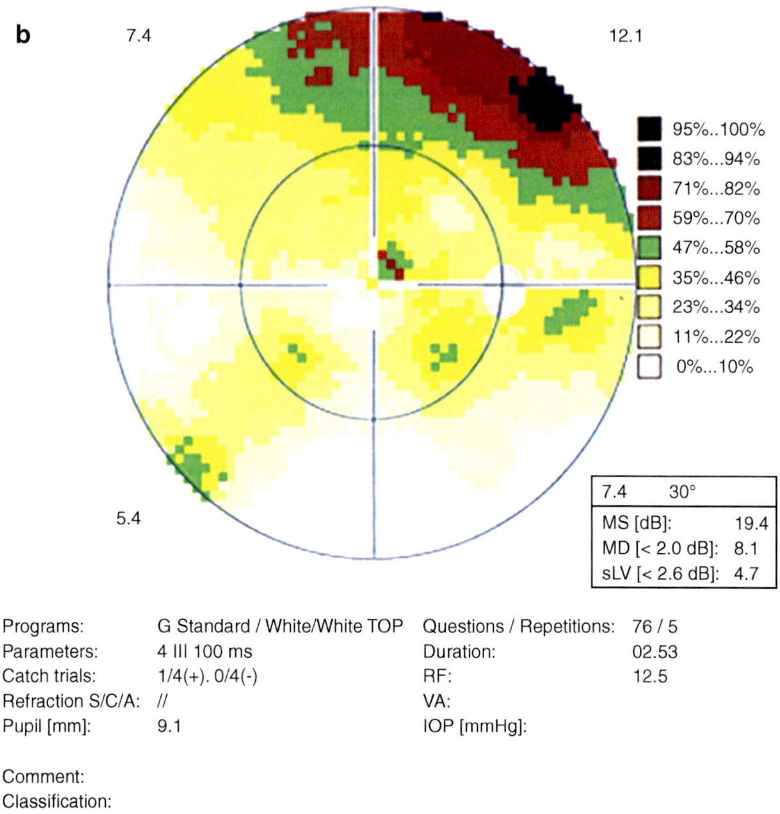

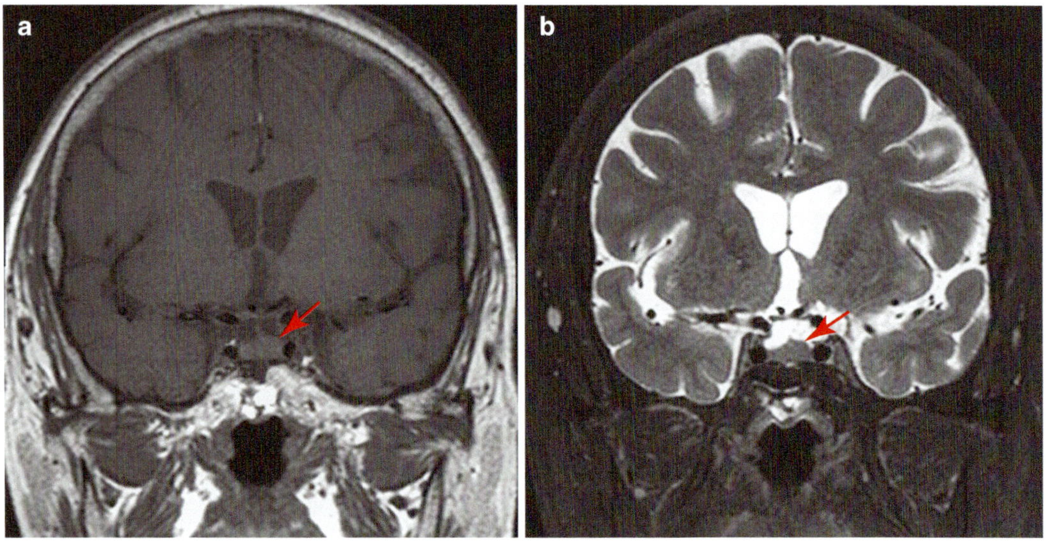

Fig. 49.6 Pituitary MRI image. Panel a: Coronal T1 showing a pituitary gland that was slightly enlarged on the left side than that on the right side, indicating the presence of a microadenoma (red arrow); Panel b, coronal T2

attach to the sphenoid crest, the tuberculum sellae, and the pituitary fossa. The hypothalamus is just above and adjacent to the optic chiasm. The pituitary is located in the pituitary fossa below the optic chiasm. The distance between the dorsum sellae and optic chiasm is about 10 mm (Fig. 49.7).

The blood supply for both the optic chiasm and pituitary is from the basilar artery rings (the circle of Willis). The optic chiasm crosses the circle of Willis at 45-degree angle upward from the front to the back. Lao et al. [1] studied the blood supply of the optic chiasm in 85 cases by the method of scanning electron microscopy (SEM) following intravascular ink infusion with tissue transparentization and vascular casting. The research found that the chiasm receives many small blood vessels from the neighboring circle of Willis, including the internal carotid, anterior cerebral artery, anterior communicating artery, posterior communicating artery, and branching arterioles from the middle cerebral artery, most of which form the superior hypophyseal artery (Fig. 49.8). The blood sup-

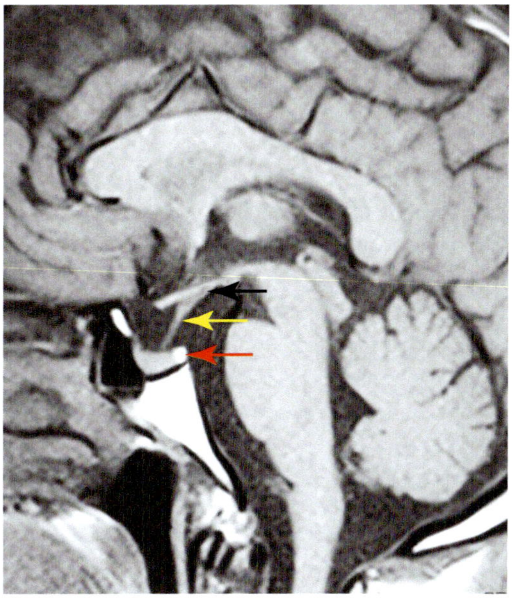

Fig. 49.7 MRI image of the normal pituitary. The black arrow indicates the optic chiasm, the yellow arrow indicates the hypophyseal stalk, and the red arrow indicates the pituitary

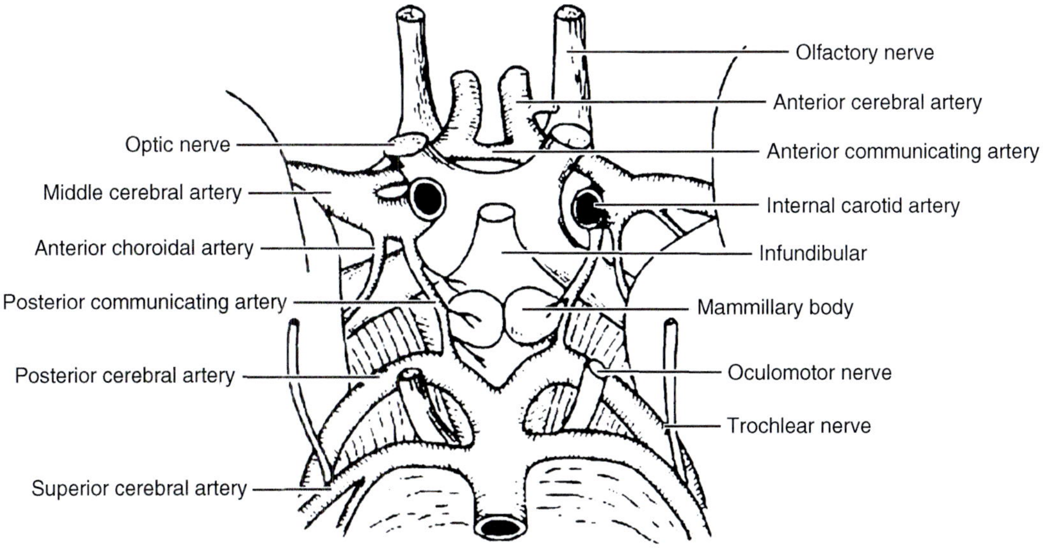

Fig. 49.8 Anatomical diagram of the circle of Willis and optic chiasm

ply is mainly from the internal carotid artery and anterior cerebral artery. In addition, the branches of these arterioles form two anastomosis networks around the anterior angles of the optic chiasm and the inferior infundibulum, respectively. Small branches derived from these two anastomosis networks run to the pia mater on the surface of the optic chiasm and again form a pial network before entering the parenchyma of the optic chiasm. The capillary networks in the lateral part of the optic chiasm have more anastomoses, smaller meshes, and higher density in a back-to-forth longitudinal arrangement penetrated by branches of arterioles, whereas those in the middle part of the optic chiasm have less anastomoses, bigger meshes, and lower density in a left-to-right horizontal arrangement hardly penetrated by any arterioles. Most importantly, capillaries in the middle part are formed by the convergence of the ends of small vessels, and most of them are lateral capillaries that turn abruptly from a longitudinal arrangement to a horizontal one. Therefore, the middle part of the optic chiasm is one of the weak points of blood supply [2–4] (Fig. 49.9).

The blood supply to the optic chiasm is provided by the circle of Willis (which is composed

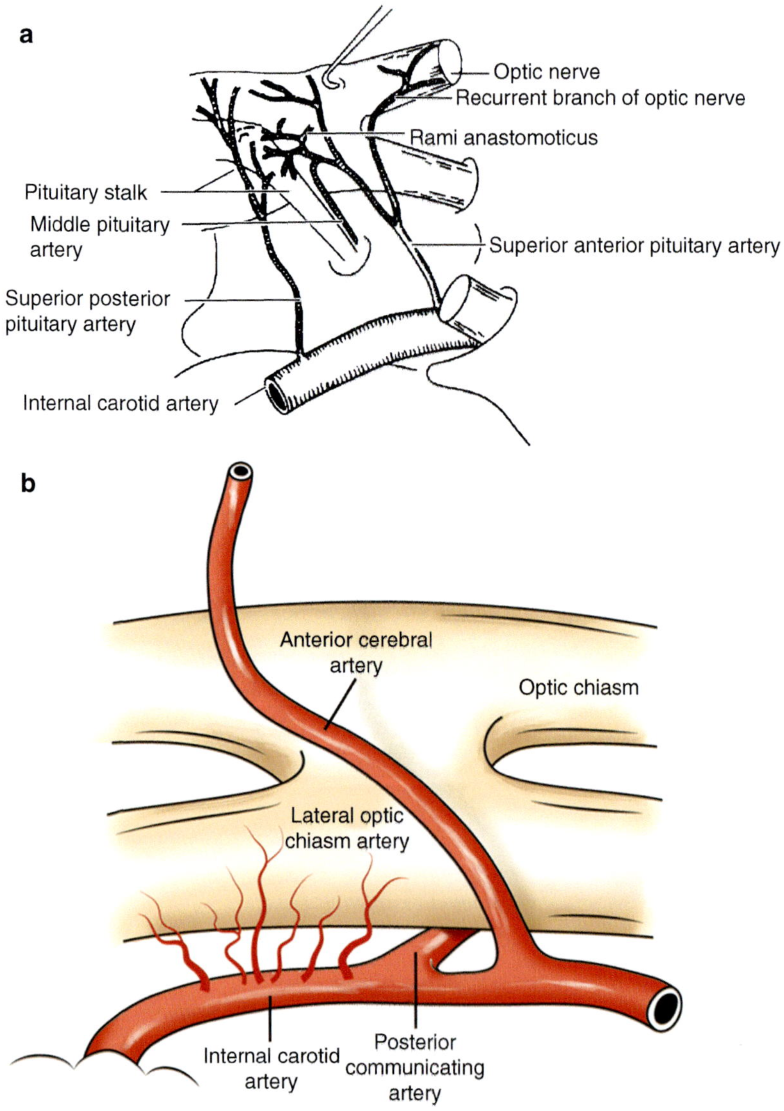

Fig. 49.9 Schematic diagram of the capillary networks located in the middle part and lateral part of the optic chiasm. Panel a: the capillary networks in the lateral part of the optic chiasm have more anastomoses, smaller meshes, and higher density in a back-to-forth longitudinal arrangement; the capillary networks in the middle part of the optic chiasm have less anastomoses, bigger meshes, and lower density in a left-to-right horizontal arrangement. Panel b: the capillary networks in the lateral part of the optic chiasm penetrated by branches of arterioles; the capillary networks in the middle part hardly penetrated by any arterioles

of the internal carotid artery, the anterior cerebral artery, and the anterior and posterior communicating arteries) and branching arterioles from the middle cerebral artery (most of which form the superior hypophyseal artery).

The chiasmic nerve fiber distribution is also very important (Fig. 49.10). We have already discussed this part in detail in the third section of the first chapter, so we will not repeat that here.

The fibers from the inferonasal retina cross the midline to the opposite side at the inferoanterior part of the optic chiasm and then enter the contralateral optic tract. The fibers from the supranasal retina cross the midline to the opposite side at the posterior part of the optic chiasm and then enter the contralateral optic tract. The nerve fibers from the temporal half of the retina in both eyes run backward and enter the ipsilateral optic tract; the fibers from the nasal half of the macular in both eyes cross the midline to the opposite side near the posterior edge at the supracentral part of the optic chiasm and then enter the contralateral optic tract, respectively. The fibers from the temporal half of the macula in both eyes run backward through the lateral part of the optic chiasm and enter the ipsilateral optic tract, respectively.

Based on the anatomy as discussed above, we can analyze the mechanism of bitemporal visual field defects caused by pituitary microadenoma—the "steal blood phenomenon" [3] (Fig. 49.11). Being different from a pituitary adenoma, due to relatively active metabolism and hyperplastic growth of a pituitary microadenoma, the neoplastic tissue may usually need

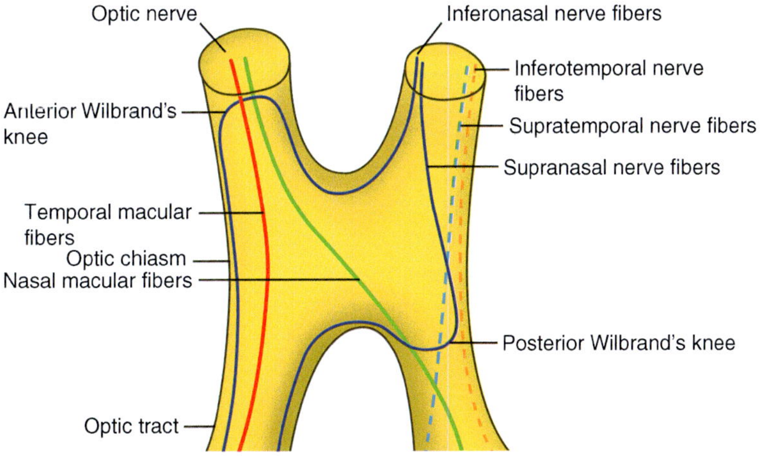

Fig. 49.10 Schematic diagram of the nerve fiber distribution of the optic chiasm

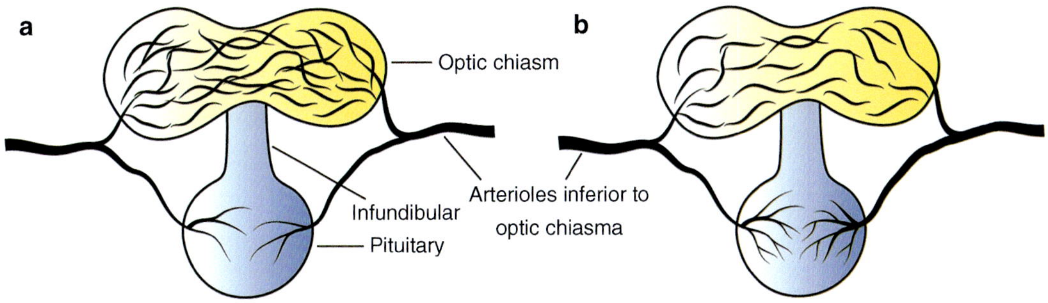

Fig. 49.11 Schematic diagrams for pituitary microadenoma and artery steal syndrome. Panel a: Normal blood supply to the pituitary and the optic chiasm. Panel b: When microadenomas undergo proliferation, the blood volume they require exceeds the normal; consequently, pituitary microadenoma will "steal" blood from the blood vessels that simultaneously supply the optic chiasm, resulting in blood supply insufficiency in the optic chiasm

more blood supply and therefore "overdraw" flood flow from the chiasma and infundibulum; in other words, when microadenomas undergo proliferation, the blood volume they require exceeds that normally needed, and consequently, pituitary microadenoma will "steal" blood from the blood vessels that simultaneously supply the optic chiasm, interfering with the normal blood supply to the optic chiasm. In this way, blood supply insufficiency occurs in the weak point of microcirculation existing in the middle part of the optic chiasm, which is also extremely sensitive to ischemia 4. Nerve fibers from the nasal retina are distributed throughout the middle part of the optic chiasm, and thus bitemporal visual field defects are the result. According to the characteristics of the visual field defects in the two cases, i.e., supratemporal visual field defects and temporal central scotoma in both eyes, it is suggested that the impairment of the optic chiasm caused by "arterial steal" affects the inferonasal retina near the macula and nasal macula.

If the ischemia in the middle part of the optic chiasm was of short duration and the damages were mild, the impairment of the optic chiasm may be improved with the requirement of blood supply reduced and compensation from the collateral circulation in pituitary microadenomas established, and the visual field defect may be improved consequently. We speculated this to be the reason for the visual field defects improvement during follow-up in Case 1.

This is also the difference between artery steal syndrome and bitemporal hemianopsia due to direct tumor compression. Unfortunately, there is currently rare direct imaging evidence supporting the artery steal syndrome.

From these two cases, we also learned that, if the visual field defects cannot be explained by the initial diagnosis (glaucoma), or its progression is inconsistent with the visual field defect caused by glaucoma, the possibility of other diseases should be taken into consideration. If necessary, the diagnosis should even be modified or doubted. In the other chapters of this book, glaucoma combined with retinal diseases, other optic neuropathy, and intracranial lesions will be presented and discussed.

References

1. Lao Y, Gao H, Zhong Y. Vascular architecture of the human optic chiasma and bitemporal hemianopia. Chin Med Sci J. 1994;9(1):38–44.
2. Kidd D. The optic chiasm. Handb Clin Neurol. 2011;102:185–203.
3. Wang N, Xie L, Cui H. Analysis on clinical diagnosis and treatment of ocular disease cases. Beijing: People's Medical Publishing House; 2011.
4. Li X, Lei T, Li L. Research progress and clinical significance of pituitary anatomy. Chin J Clin Neurosurg. 2006;11(4):251–3.

50 Monocular Visual Field Defects Caused by Sellar Mass

Li Tang, Xuyang Liu, and Ning Fan

Due to the particularity of the lesions and the individual differences of anatomical structures, tumors in the sellar region or anterior cranial fossa sometimes can also cause visual field defect such as monocular hemianopsia and total blindness, which are easily misdiagnosed or overlooked.

50.1 Case 1

50.1.1 Case Presentation

A 32-year-old male patient complained of acute vision loss in his right eye 2 years before without any cause. No other discomforts such as red eye or pain were reported. The histories of trauma, systemic diseases, and familial diseases were also denied. He had been diagnosed with optic neuropathy in the right eye before and had been taking microcirculation-enhancing drugs and neurotrophic drugs, but the symptom was not improved.

On ophthalmological examination, the UCVA was 20/200 OD and 20/20 OS. The BCVA was also 20/200 in his right eye. IOP was normal OU. In both eyes, slit-lamp examination of his anterior segments was unremarkable, and the pupil was 3 mm in diameter in both eyes. In the right eye, the relative afferent pupillary defect (RAPD) was positive, and the optic disc was pale in color with a C/D ratio of 0.6, but the cup depression was not deep. In the left eye, the optic disc was pink in color with a clear margin, and the C/D ratio was 0.3. No abnormalities were found in the retina in both eyes. Ocular motility examination was unremarkable in both eyes.

Visual field test showed generalized reduction of sensitivity in the right eye, while the left eye was normal (Fig. 50.1).

L. Tang
West China Hospital, Sichuan University, Chengdu, China

X. Liu
Xiamen Eye Center of Xiamen University, Xiamen, China

Shenzhen Eye Hospital, Shenzhen University, Shenzhen, China

N. Fan (✉)
Shenzhen Eye Hospital, Shenzhen University, Shenzhen, China

N. Wang et al. (eds.), *Optic Disorders and Visual Field*, Advances in Visual Science and Eye Diseases 2, https://doi.org/10.1007/978-981-13-2502-1_50

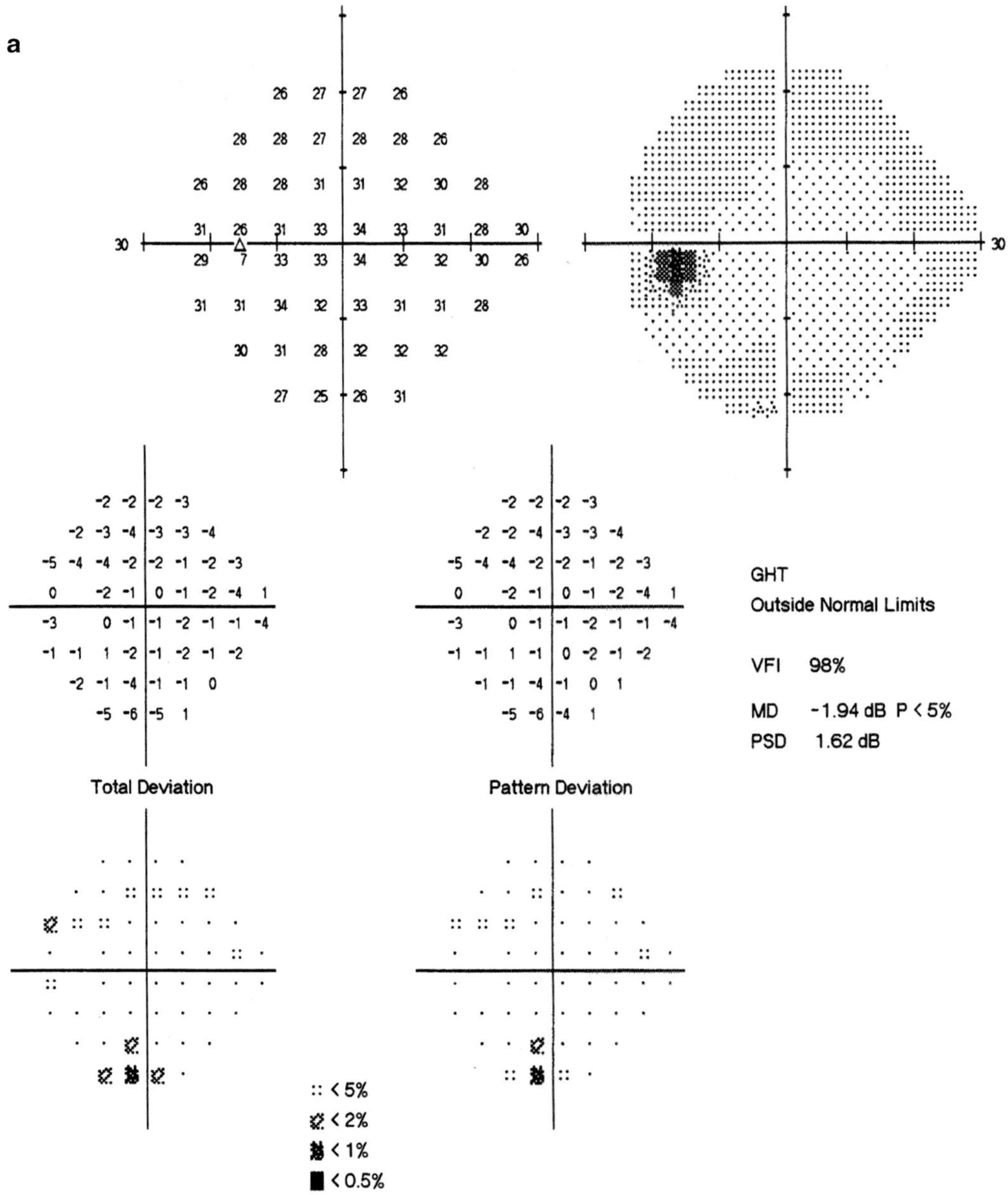

Fig. 50.1 Humphrey visual field analysis printouts. Panel a: The 24-2 strategy showed that the left eye was normal. Panel b: General reduction of sensitivity was noticed in the right eye

VEP examination revealed that the P100 waveform was severely abnormal in both amplitude and latency in the right eye, while the P100 waveform was normal in the left eye.

Brain MRI showed parasellar space-occupying lesions on the right side. The lesions were located outside the brain and were attached to the middle cranial fossa. The imaging diagnosis was sphenoid ridge meningioma (Fig. 50.2).

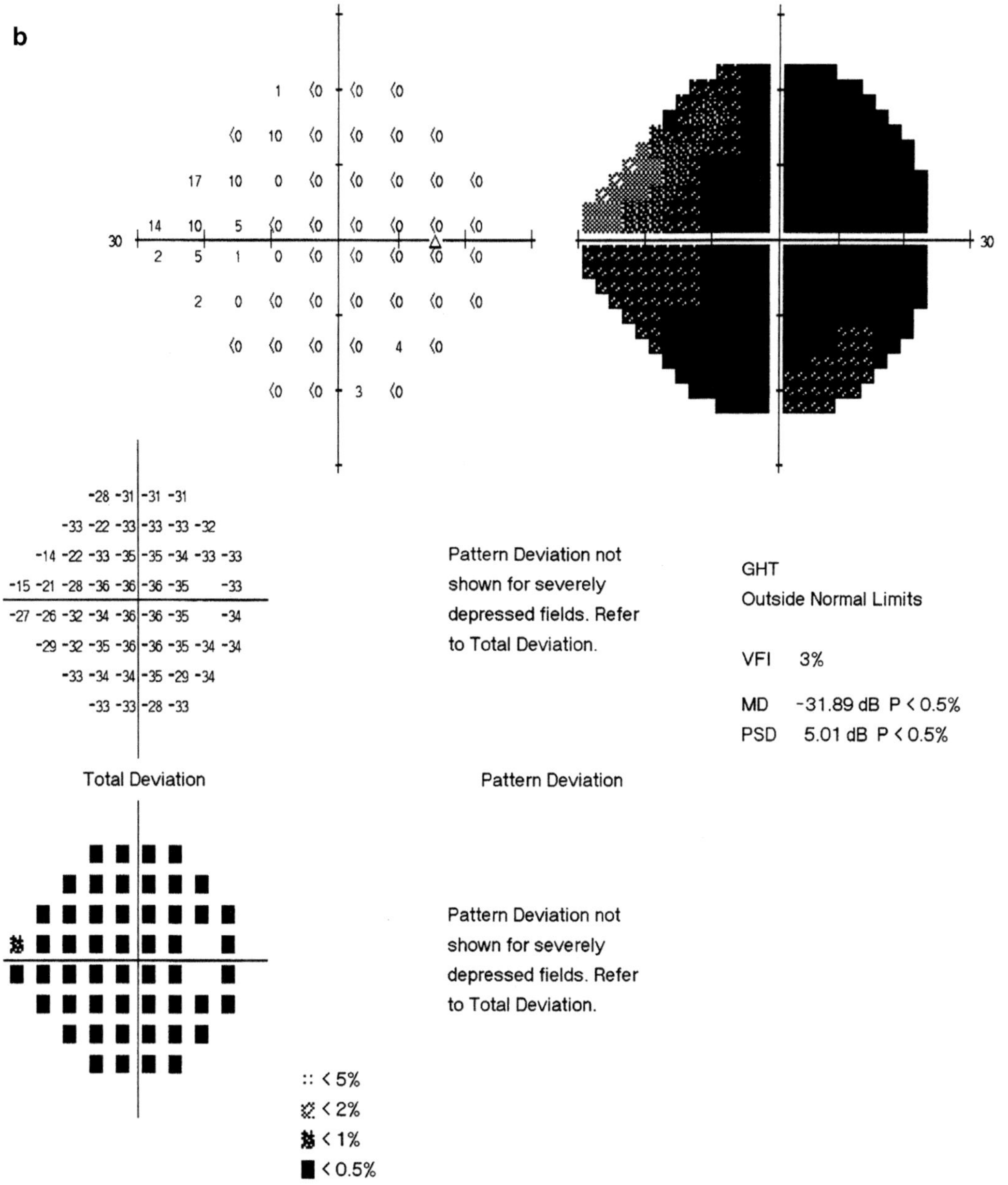

Fig. 50.1 (continued)

50.1.2 Final Diagnosis

The final diagnosis was right sphenoid ridge meningioma and optic atrophy in the right eye.

50.1.3 Case Review

The patient was a young male with an acute monocular visual acuity decrease for 2 years. His trauma history and past systemic history

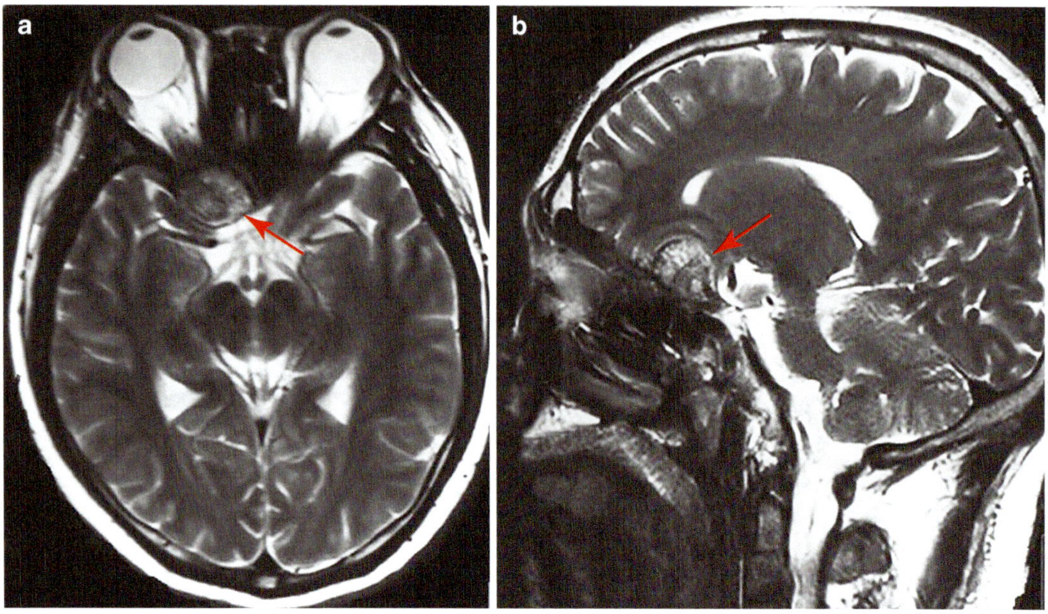

Fig. 50.2 The visual field and MR images of the patient with sphenoid ridge meningioma. The red arrows indicate the parasellar space-occupying lesions on the right side in the axial and sagittal T2WI images of craniocerebral MRI

were denied. Ocular examination showed severe impairment of visual functions and general reduction of sensitivity in the visual field. The positive ophthalmologic signs included RAPD, enlarged optic cup not caused by glaucoma, and abnormal VEP waveforms in the affected eye. Therefore, the common causes of optic atrophy of the right eye were considered to be the following: (a) primary demyelinating optic neuritis; (b) optic neuropathy caused by infection, inflammation, and ischemia; and (c) Leber's disease. According to the outcome of the disease and systemic examination, infection, inflammation, and ischemia were ruled out. Leber's disease was ruled out for no mutations were found in the mitochondrial DNA screening for the three high incidence loci of Leber's disease. What was the real cause of optic atrophy and whether the contralateral eye would also be involved or not? The patient and his families are very worried about these problems.

Brain MRI showed that the patient's sphenoid ridge meningioma, which was located in the front edge of the parasellar area, compressed the right optic nerve, resulting in visual impairment of the right eye and general visual field defects [1].

50.2 Case 2

50.2.1 Case Presentation

A 66-year-old female complained of vision loss without redness and pain in her left eye for 6 months. There was no obvious trigger for the disease onset. History of trauma and familial history were denied; systemic evaluation was unremarkable. She had been diagnosed with "ischemic optic neuropathy in the left eye" and received medications in another hospital. However, there was no improvement in the visual acuity of her left eye.

On ophthalmological examination, the UCVA was 20/32 OD and 20/80 OS. No improvement was achieved with refractive correction in either eye. IOP was normal OU. In both eyes, the pupil was 3 mm in diameter, round, and equally reactive to light; the lens presented mild cortical opacity. In the right eye, the optic disc was pale in color with a clear margin, and a normal C/D ratio (0.4), while in the left eye, the optic disc was pink, with a clear margin and a normal C/D ratio (0.4). The morphology and distribution of retinal blood vessels were normal in both eyes.

Humphrey visual field perimetry showed temporal visual field defects, and the superior visual field defect had crossed the meridian involving the nasal visual field in the left eye. The visual field in the right eye was normal (Fig. 50.3a).

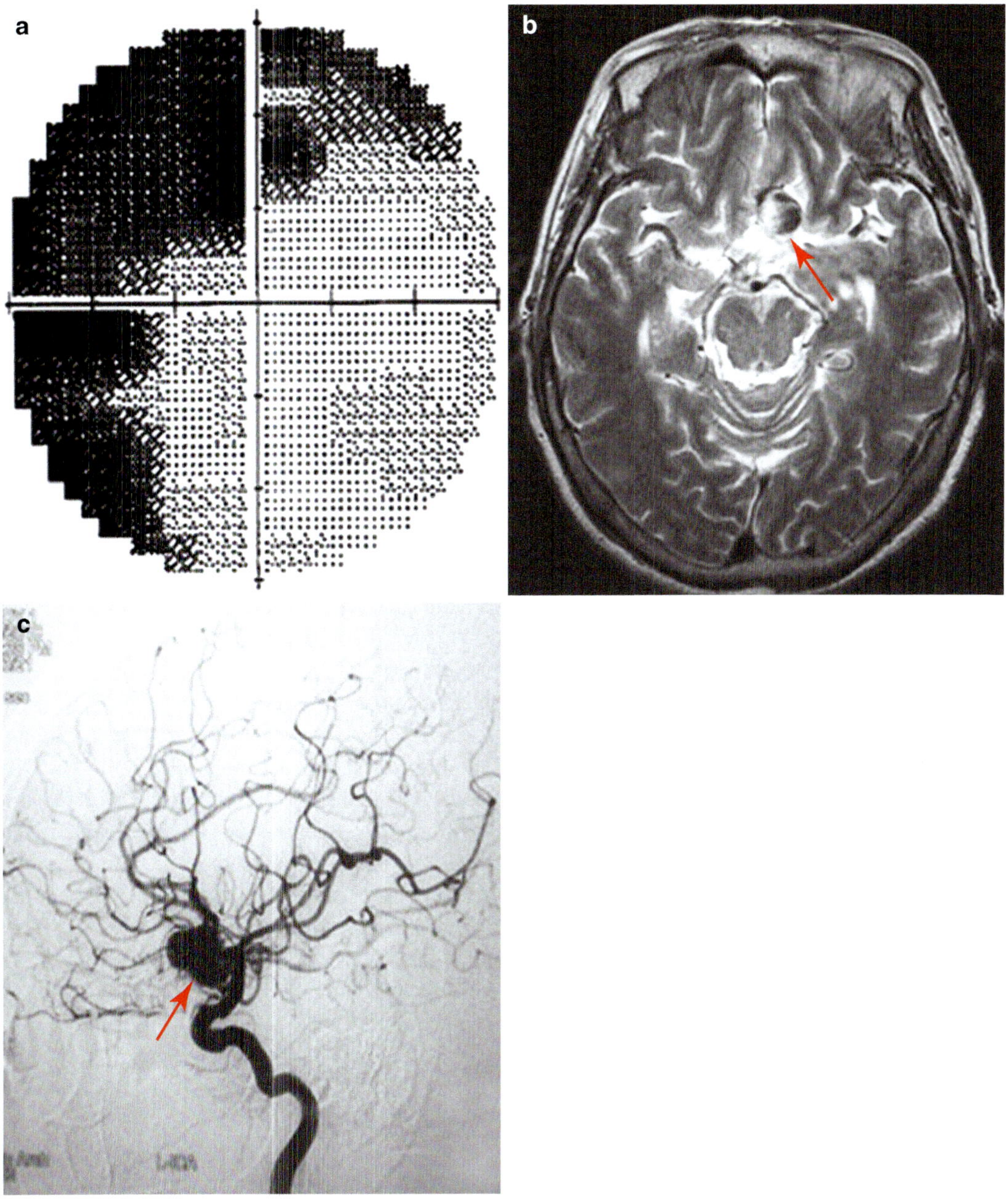

Fig. 50.3 Humphrey visual field grayscale map and imaging results. Panel a: The 30-2 test showed temporal and supranasal visual field defects in the left eye. Panel b: An ovoid abnormal signal was seen in the left side of suprasellar region in the T2WI axial image of cranial MRI (red arrow). Figure c: DSA image showed aneurysm of the anterior communicating artery (red arrow)

Brain MRI: Axial T2WI showed an ovoid abnormal signal on the left suprasellar region. Hemangiomas were considered (Fig. 50.3b). Digital subtraction angiography (DSA) showed aneurysm in the anterior communicating artery (Fig. 50.3c).

50.2.2 Final Diagnosis

The final diagnosis was aneurysm of the left anterior communicating artery and optic atrophy in the left eye.

50.2.3 Case Review

This patient was an elderly woman complaining of progressive decrease of vision in one eye for 6 months. The visual field defect was a monocular temporal defect, and the superior visual defect had crossed the meridian involving the nasal visual field. It was easily misdiagnosed as ischemic optic neuropathy or optic neuritis. Intracranial space-occupying lesions were found by neuroimaging examination, and the final diagnosis was aneurysm in the anterior communicating artery as confirmed by DSA.

Aneurysm of anterior communicating artery can not only directly compress the optic nerve and the optic chiasm because they are located proximally but also change the hemodynamics, then interfering with the blood supply to the proximal optic nerve or the optic chiasm. The hematomas that occur after the aneurysm ruptures will also compress the optic nerve and the optic chiasm. In this patient, the cause of visual impairment was considered to be related to the former two reasons, namely, the direct compression on the left optic nerve fibers by the aneurysm of the anterior communicating artery and the blood supply insufficiency in the left optic nerves caused by the aneurysm.

Fortunately, the aneurysm in this patient was found before its rupture, and a minimally invasive surgical operation was performed to remove the aneurysm with subsequent recovery of the compressed optic nerves and improvement of the blood supply to the optic chiasm, thus preventing further damage to the optic nerves.

50.3 Case 3

50.3.1 Case Presentation

A 34-year-old female patient complained of vision loss in her right eye without any obvious cause for 5 days. No discomforts such as red and orbital pain upon eye movement were noted. History of trauma, personal history, and familial history were denied. Review of systemic evaluation noted a history of headache and menopause for more than 2 months.

On ophthalmological examination, the UVCA was 20/400, and the BVCA was 20/200 with refractive correction (−1.25DS) OD; the UVCA was 20/200 and the BVCA 20/20 with refractive correction (−1.50DS) OS. IOP was normal in each eye; the pupil was about 3 mm in diameter in each eye; there was a positive RAPD in the right eye; the lens was clear, the optic disc was pink in color with a clear margin and a C/D ratio of 0.4, and the retina was flat with normal reflex in both eyes.

Standardized automated perimetry showed temporal hemianopia in the right eye, involving the inferonasal visual field (Fig. 50.4a). The visual field in the left eye was normal (Fig. 50.4b).

Brain MRI examination revealed a solid mass in the suprasellar region with a size of about 2.5 cm × 2.0 cm × 2.2 cm. Its signal was significantly enhanced (Fig. 50.4c).

After consultation with endocrinologist and neurologist, the impression was pituitary prolactinoma.

50.3.2 Final Diagnosis

The final diagnosis was pituitary prolactinoma and optic chiasm disorder.

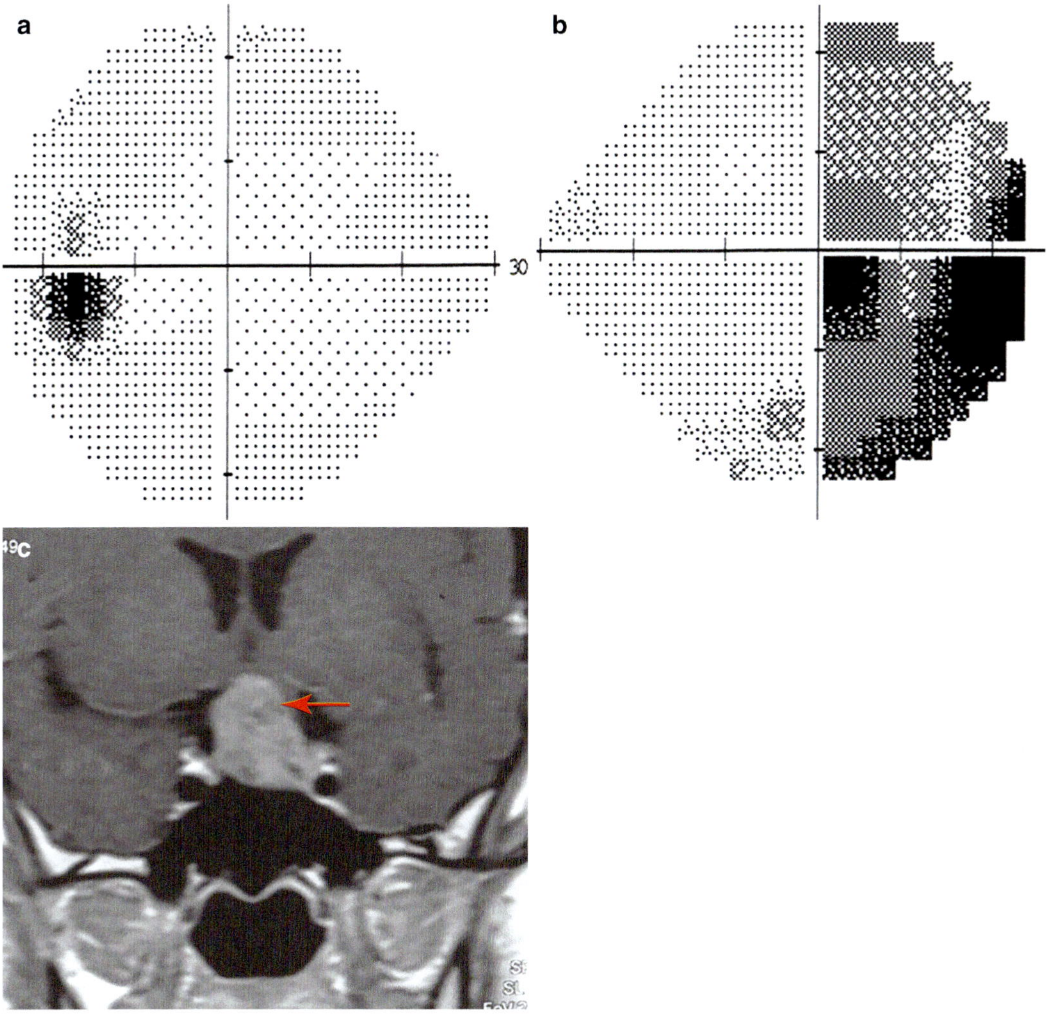

Fig. 50.4 Humphrey visual field grayscale maps (the 24-2 test strategy) and MR images. Panel a: The visual field in the left eye was normal; Panel b: Temporal hemianopsia was shown in the right eye; Panel c: Significantly enhanced space-occupying lesions were seen in the coronal T1WI image of craniocerebral MRI (arrow)

50.3.3 Case Review

The visual deficits associated with intracranial space-occupying lesions depend on the relative position of the tumor with respect to the optic nerve, the optic chiasm, and postchiasmal visual pathway, as well as the growth direction of the tumor, etc. Although this patient showed monocular visual field damage, the vertical meridian was respected. Given the systemic symptoms of amenorrhea and headache, the possibility of pituitary adenoma could be considered. However, it is rare for such a huge solid mass (around 2.5 cm × 2.0 cm × 2.2 cm) to affect the visual field of one eye only. The MR images showed that the tumor growing from lower left to upper right had broken through the sellar diaphragm, compressing the optic chiasm. But the visual field finding was only temporal vertical hemianopsia in the right eye, the reason for which was not clear. Maybe the optic chiasm of the patient is closer to the back, while the tumor is closer to the right, and thus the visual impairment aroused from the compression of the nasal cross-fibers of the right optic nerve.

50.4 Discussion

Tumors in the sellar region often cause binocular vision loss and visual field defects, especially the temporal hemianopsia by direct compression of the optic chiasm in different directions or "artery steal syndrome" (see Chap. 49 in Part V). However, asymmetry in visual field abnormalities or even monocular defects were also noted, which may be attributed to the special distribution of the crossing fibers and non-crossing fibers, the displacement between the optic chiasm and the surrounding tissues, the individual differences, and so on. As suggested by the above cases, for patients with various optic neuropathy lesions and optic atrophy without clear causes, especially for those not responding to treatments, intracranial space-occupying lesions should be ruled out, even if only one eye is affected. For patients with temporal visual field defects and hemianopsia respecting the vertical meridian, intracranial and sellar region lesions should be considered.

In addition, only visual deficits without any general discomforts can be found at the early stage of space-occupying lesions in the sellar region because the brain tissues and ventricle remain intact [2, 3]. In such cases, if the space-occupying lesions can be found early by ophthalmologists and handled with corresponding treatment, serious complications can be avoided, and mild visual field damage may improve and resolve. However, some absolute visual field defects may not be improved and may even continue to deteriorate after the operation or other treatments. Monitoring the visual field progression is of great significance during follow-up.

References

1. Jiao Y, Yan Z, Che S, et al. Relationship between the pathological features of intracranial meningioma and its locations. Chin J Clin Neurosurg. 2014;19(12):723–5.
2. Tang Z, Yuan Y. The effect of sellar tumor on visual field. Int Rev Ophthalmol. 2010;34(3):198–201.
3. Solomon AE, Tataranu L, Ciubotaru V, et al. Pituitary apoplexy: clinical features, management and outcome. Clinical study and review of the literature. Roman Neurosurg. 2015;22(1):69–77.

51 Any Visual Field Change Has Reasons: A Case of Glaucoma Combined with Internal Carotid Artery Malformation

Li Tang, Xuyang Liu, and Ning Fan

Any visual field change has reasons. Therefore, when the visual field defect cannot be explained by the known reasons, the underlying pathogenesis should be analyzed.

51.1 Case

51.1.1 Case Presentation

A 65-year-old male patient complained of gradual vision loss in both eyes for more than 4 years had been aggravating in the past 2 years. No discomforts such as eye sore, red eyes, pain, or eye floaters were noted. Trauma history, past ocular history, personal history, and family history were all denied, and the systemic evaluation was unremarkable.

On ophthalmological examination, the BCVA was 20/80 with refractive correction (−4.75DS) OD and 20/40 (−4.25DS) OS. Color vision test showed protanomaly in both eyes. IOP measured by Goldmann applanation tonometry was 16 mmHg OU. Slit-lamp examination of his anterior segments was unremarkable, and the pupil was 2.5 mm in diameter, round, with negative RAPD in both eyes. Fundus examination showed lacquer cracks in both eyes, with no foveal reflex, and the C/D ratio was 0.85 OD and 0.7 OS (Fig. 51.1).

Standardized automated perimetry showed a superior and nasal arcuate scotoma extending from the blind spot in the right eye, an inferior arcuate scotoma extending from the blind spot, and a superior peripheral visual field defect in the left eye (Fig. 51.2).

51.1.2 Case Review

The patient had moderate myopia with lacquer cracks and myopic crescent. The optic disc changes of the right eye were characterized by superior and inferior notching of the rim with the inferior notching being more serious, bayoneting of blood vessels, and healthily rosy residual nasal disc rim, which were all consistent with glaucomatous optic cupping. The visual field loss of the right eye was caused by

L. Tang
West China Hospital, Sichuan University, Chengdu, China

X. Liu
Xiamen Eye Center of Xiamen University, Xiamen, China

Shenzhen Eye Hospital, Shenzhen University, Shenzhen, China

N. Fan (✉)
Shenzhen Eye Hospital, Shenzhen University, Shenzhen, China

N. Wang et al. (eds.), *Optic Disorders and Visual Field*, Advances in Visual Science and Eye Diseases 2, https://doi.org/10.1007/978-981-13-2502-1_51

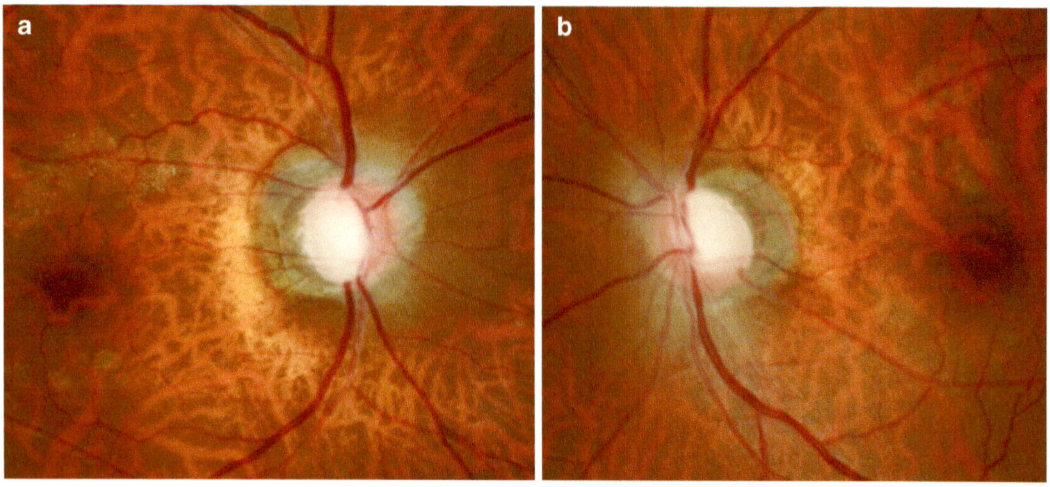

Fig. 51.1 Fundus photographs. Lacquer cracks were seen in both eyes. Panel a: The C/D ratio was 0.85 in the right eye. Panel b: The C/D ratio was 0.7 in the left eye

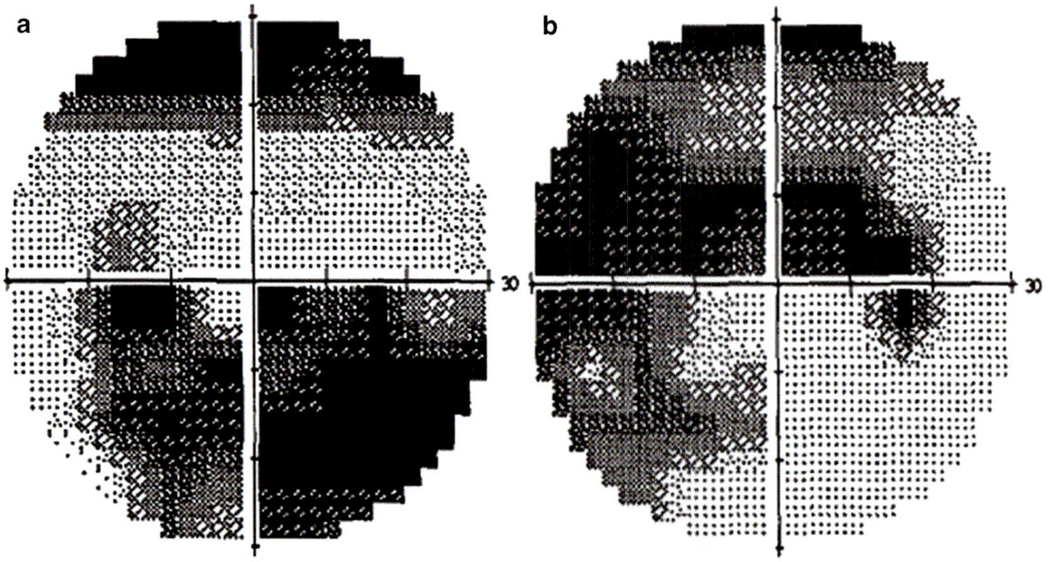

Fig. 51.2 The grayscale maps of Humphrey visual field assessment. Panel a: The inferior arcuate scotoma extending from the blind spot and the superior peripheral visual field defect in the left eye. Panel b: The superior and nasal arcuate scotoma extending from the blind spot in the right eye

the superior and nasal arcuate scotoma extending from the blind spot, conforming with the diagnosis of normal tension glaucoma (NTG). The optic disc assessment in the left eye is a tilted disc, superior notching of the rim, bayoneting of blood vessels, and healthily rosy residual nasal and inferior disc rim. The visual field loss was caused by the inferior arcuate scotoma extending from the blind spot. These clinical evidence also supported the diagnosis of NTG.

In this patient, glaucomatous optic nerve damage was severe, and the inferior arcuate scotoma in the left eye and the superior arcuate scotoma and nasal defects in the right eye were consistent with the changes in the optic discs, respectively. But the superior defects of both eyes (more severe in the left eye), which were confirmed to be not caused by upper eyelid overlapping, could not be explained by glaucomatous defects. Is there any other explanation?

The cranial MRI examination revealed abnormalities. The T1-weighted fat suppression image of the cranial MR (Fig. 51.3) showed that the anterior geniculate body and supraclinoid segment of the internal carotid artery were significantly tortuous on both sides (red arrow), and the optic chiasm (and the intracranial optic nerve) showed compressive deformation and elevation. The abnormalities were more obvious on the left side (yellow arrow).

Instead of glaucomatous defects, the underlying causes of the superior visual field defects of both eyes were optic chiasm compression by malformed internal carotid arteries. The malformed internal carotid arteries compressed the intracranial segment of the optic nerve when it entered the optic chiasm. At this location, the inferior nasal and inferior temporal retinal nerve fibers originally running along the lateral side of the optic nerve had moved below the optic nerve, causing superior visual field defects of both eyes. The compression was more severe on the left side, so the visual field defect of the left eye was worse.

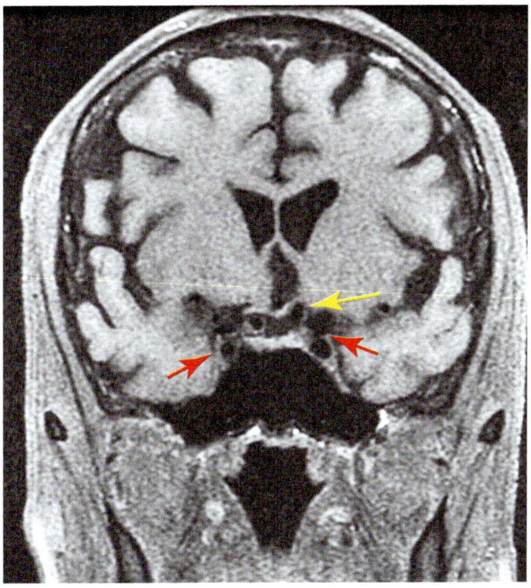

Fig. 51.3 Cranial MRI image. The T1-weighted fat suppression image showed that the anterior geniculate body and supraclinoid portion of the internal carotid arteries are significantly tortuous on both sides (red arrow), and the optic chiasm (and the intracranial optic nerve) showed compressive deformation and elevation. The abnormalities were more obvious on the left side (yellow arrow)

51.1.3 Final Diagnosis

The final diagnosis was normal tension glaucoma in both eyes and internal carotid artery malformation.

51.2 Discussion

In differential diagnosis of normal tension glaucoma (NTG), compressive lesions of the intracranial anterior visual pathway must be considered. Quite a number of patients who suffer from compressive lesions of the anterior visual pathway were clinically diagnosed with NTG [1, 2]. In a study by Trobe, among 8 (27%) of 30 eyes with compressive optic neuropathy were misdiagnosed as glaucoma because of a change that resembled glaucomatous optic disc cupping; in another study, 13 (44%) of 29 non-glaucomatous optic atrophy cases were misdiagnosed as glaucoma. In the current case, the optic chiasm compression by malformed internal carotid arteries is easy to be misdiagnosed as glaucoma with the absence of imaging examinations.

Therefore, for patients who might be with NTG in the physician's primary impression, a cranial MRI examination is necessary. The detection rate of intracranial lesions in patients with NTG is far greater than that in the general population.

In this case, the major visual field defects of both eyes matched the visual field manifestations of rim tissue loss. However, the changes in the superior visual field of both eyes can be easily overlooked or mistaken for eyelid overlapping. When the visual field is difficult to be interpreted by glaucomatous optic nerve damages, we should analyze the visual field carefully to find the underlying causes.

In this case, magnetic resonance imaging analysis revealed the malformation of the internal carotid arteries, which compressed the optic nerves as they entered the optic chiasm. At this location, the inferior nasal and inferior temporal retinal nerve fibers originally running along the lateral side of the optic nerve had moved below the optic nerve. Therefore there were superior visual field defects in both eyes. The compression was more severe on the left side, so the visual field defect of the left eye was worse (Figs. 51.4 and 51.5).

Regarding the treatment for this patient, currently there is no safe way to relieve the compression, as the compression was caused by the deformed internal carotid arteries. For the

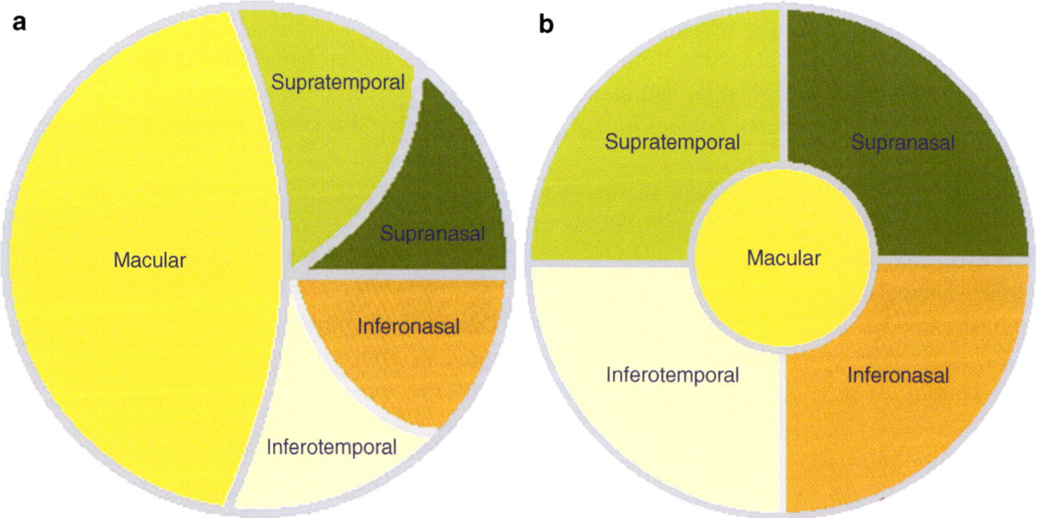

Fig. 51.4 Schematic diagram of the optic nerve fiber distribution in the optic disc and before entering the optic chiasm. Panel a: Distribution of optic nerve fibers in the optic disc of the right eye: macular fibers were on the temporal side. The supratemporal and supranasal fibers are on the upper side; the inferotemporal and inferonasal fibers are on the lower side. Panel b: Distribution of optic nerve fibers in the right eye before they enter the optic chiasm in a coronal view: macular fibers had moved to the center, supratemporal and supranasal fibers had moved to the upper side, and inferotemporal and inferonasal fibers had moved to the lower side

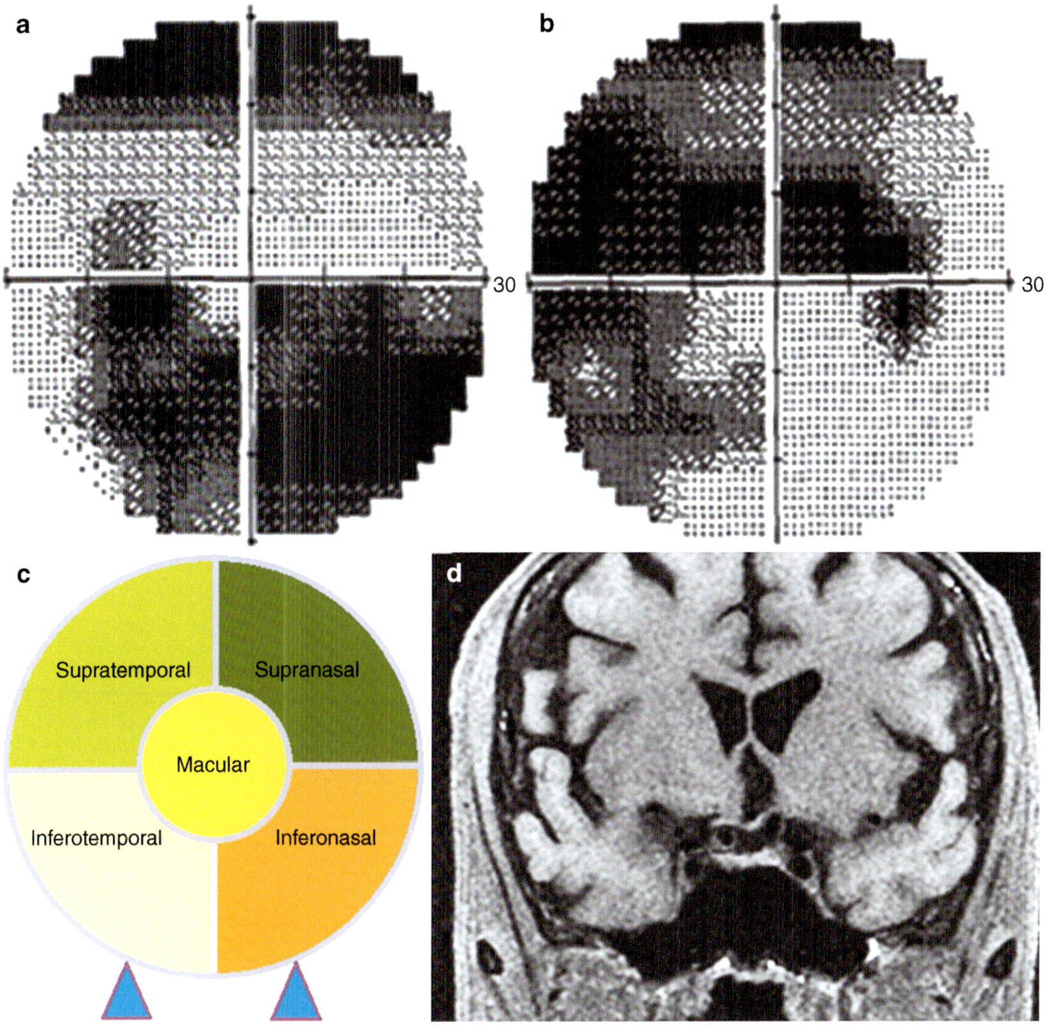

Fig. 51.5 Schematic diagram of the superior visual field damage and optic nerve compression in this patient. The diagram showed the relationship between the superior visual field defects of both eyes and the distribution of fibers before the optic nerve entered the optic chiasm, as well as their relationship with lesion sites. The diagram mainly illustrates the lesions in the superior visual field in both eyes (blue triangles). The compression on the left side was more severe, so the superior visual field defects in the left eye were worse than those in the right eye

damage to the optic nerve, intraocular pressure reduction, optic nerve nutrition, circulation improvement, and other therapies might be administered. In addition, paying attention to cardiovascular health is very important. Along with regular follow-up, low-salt and low-fat diets are suggested.

References

1. Yang T. Clinically-oriented neurotomy. Beijing: Peking Union Medical College Press; 2002.
2. Liu X, Liu Y, Liu J, et al. Histological changes and mechanisms of intracranial optic nerve compression by internal carotid. J Anat. 2006;29(5):627–30.

Binasal Hemianopsia

52

Li Tang, Xuyang Liu, and Ning Fan

Binasal hemianopsia is a rare type of visual field defect. In this section, we will introduce two cases of empty sella and review related literature, with the aim of finding the characteristics and clinical implications of binasal hemianopsia.

52.1 Case 1

52.1.1 Case Presentation

A 51-year-old male complained of progressive painless vision loss in the right eye without any obvious trigger for about 1 year. He had not seen a doctor or received treatment. Histories of trauma and other ocular and systemic diseases were denied; systemic evaluation was unremarkable. On ophthalmological examination, the UCVA was 20/33, and the BCVA was 20/20 with refractive correction (+1.50 DC × 170) OD; the UCVA was 20/22, and the BCVA was 20/20 with refractive correction (+0.50DS + 1.25 DC × 175) OS. IOP by standard Goldmann applanation tonometry was measured as 12 mmHg OU. In both eyes, the anterior segment was normal, the pupil was 3 mm in diameter, and the direct response to light was normal. Fundus examination showed that, in both eyes, the optic disc was swollen and pink in color, with scattered hemorrhage. The retinal veins were slightly tortuous and the arteriovenous ratio was 1:2. No foveal reflex was noticed (Fig. 52.1).

Standardized automated perimetry showed symmetrical inferonasal quadrantanopia and enlargement of the physiological blind spot in both eyes (Fig. 52.2).

The MRI examination revealed a slightly enlarged pituitary fossa filled with cerebrospinal fluid on the T1-weighted sagittal image. The pituitary gland had become flattened, and its superior rim showed an arc-shaped concave. These were consistent with the diagnosis of empty sella (Fig. 52.3). No significantly abnormal signs were seen on the intracranial MRA image.

OCT showed a normal macula in both eyes (Fig. 52.4).

According to the retinal nerve fiber layer (RNFL) thickness measurement by OCT, the peripapillary RNFL thickness significantly increased in both eyes and could not be autoanalyzed by the computer, which suggested severe edema in the retinal nerve fiber layer (Fig. 52.5).

L. Tang
West China Hospital, Sichuan University, Chengdu, China

X. Liu
Xiamen Eye Center of Xiamen University, Xiamen, China

Shenzhen Eye Hospital, Shenzhen University, Shenzhen, China

N. Fan (✉)
Shenzhen Eye Hospital, Shenzhen University, Shenzhen, China

N. Wang et al. (eds.), *Optic Disorders and Visual Field*, Advances in Visual Science and Eye Diseases 2, https://doi.org/10.1007/978-981-13-2502-1_52

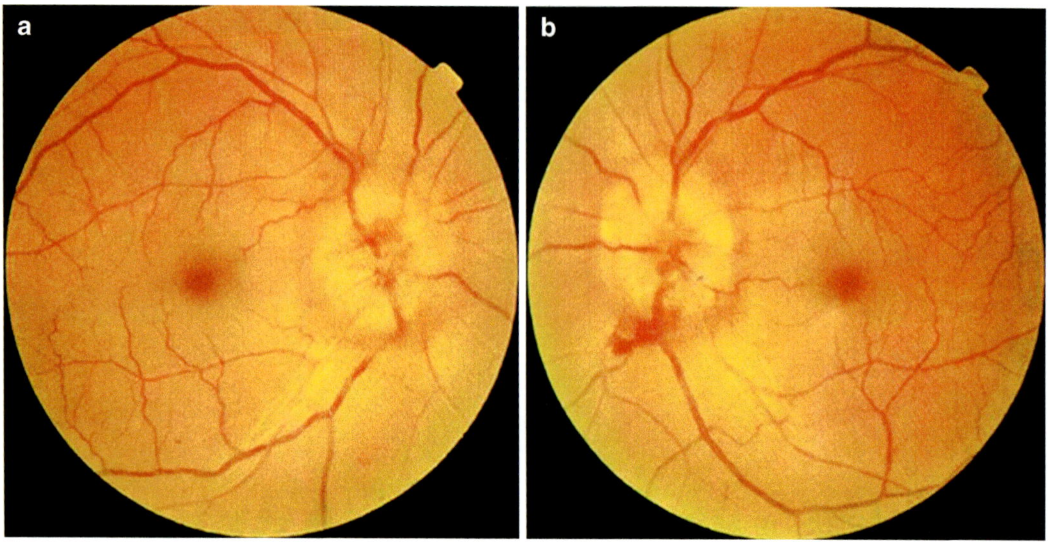

Fig. 52.1 Fundus photographs. The optic disc was swollen and pink in color in both eyes. Scattered hemorrhage was seen. Panel a, right eye; Panel b, left eye

FFA revealed diffuse telangiectasis on the surface of the edematous optic disc in both eyes and flaky hemorrhage blocking the fluorescence in the inferior optic disc of the left eye. Minimal dye leakage was seen over time. Late-phase angiography showed hyperfluorescent staining of the disc associated with blurred margins (Fig. 52.6).

52.1.2 Final Diagnosis

The final diagnosis was optic neuropathy in both eyes and empty sella.

52.1.3 Case Review

It was not difficult to make the diagnosis of optic neuropathy for binocular optic disc edema and hemorrhage in this patient, but what is the underlying cause? The visual field gives us important hints: the enlargement of the physiological blind spots in both eyes may be produced by optic disc diseases; however, symmetric binocular inferior nasal quadrant defects are uncommon, which may be associated with the empty sella. Please refer to the discussion in this section.

52.2 Case 2

52.2.1 Case Presentation

A 40-year-old female complained of floaters in both eyes for 1 month. No vision loss, eye pain, red eyes, and headache were noticed. Histories of trauma, other ocular diseases, systemic diseases, and familial diseases were denied. On ophthalmological examination, the UCVA was 20/25 OU, with no improvement achieved with refrac-

a

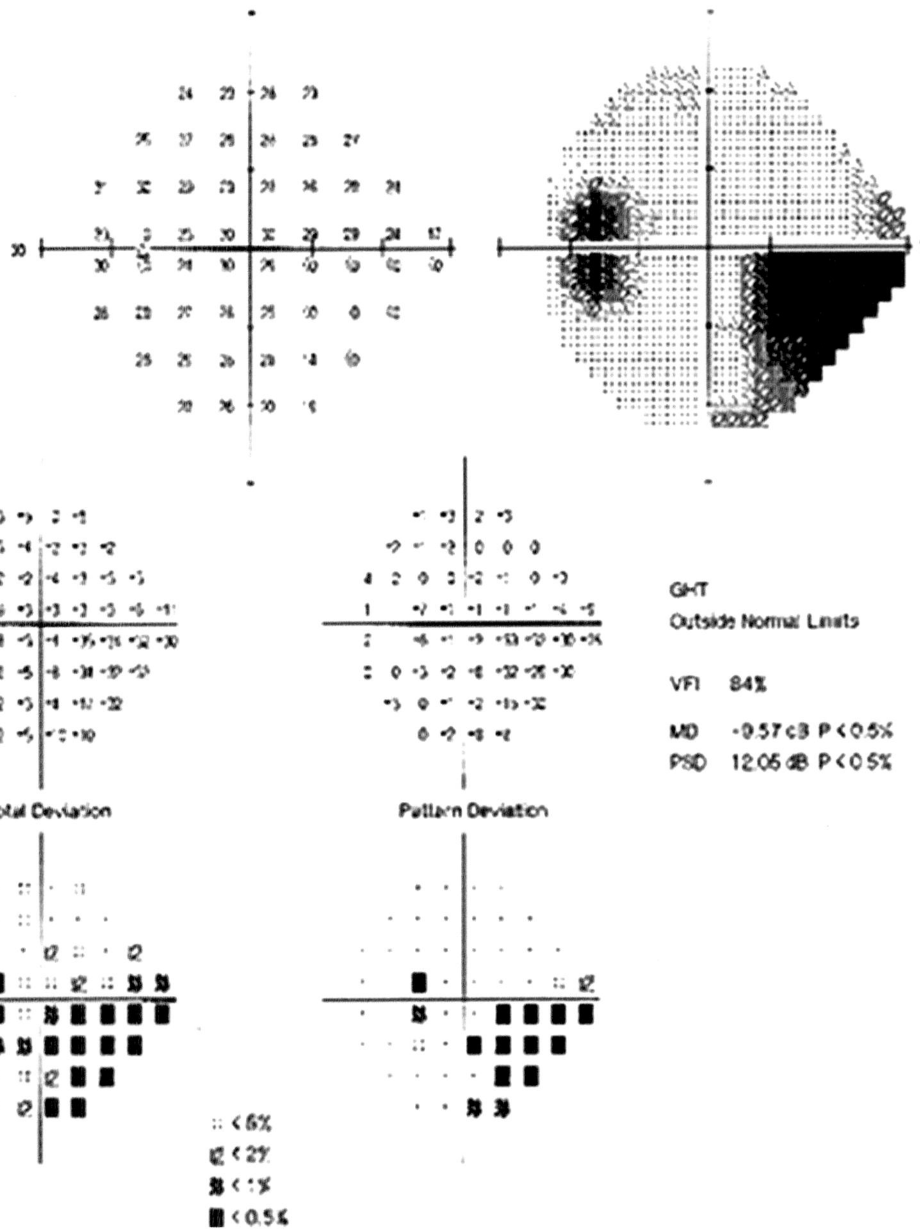

Fig. 52.2 Humphrey visual field analysis printouts. The 24-2 test showed symmetrical inferonasal quadrantanopia and enlargement of the blind spot in both eyes. Panel a, left eye; Panel b, right eye

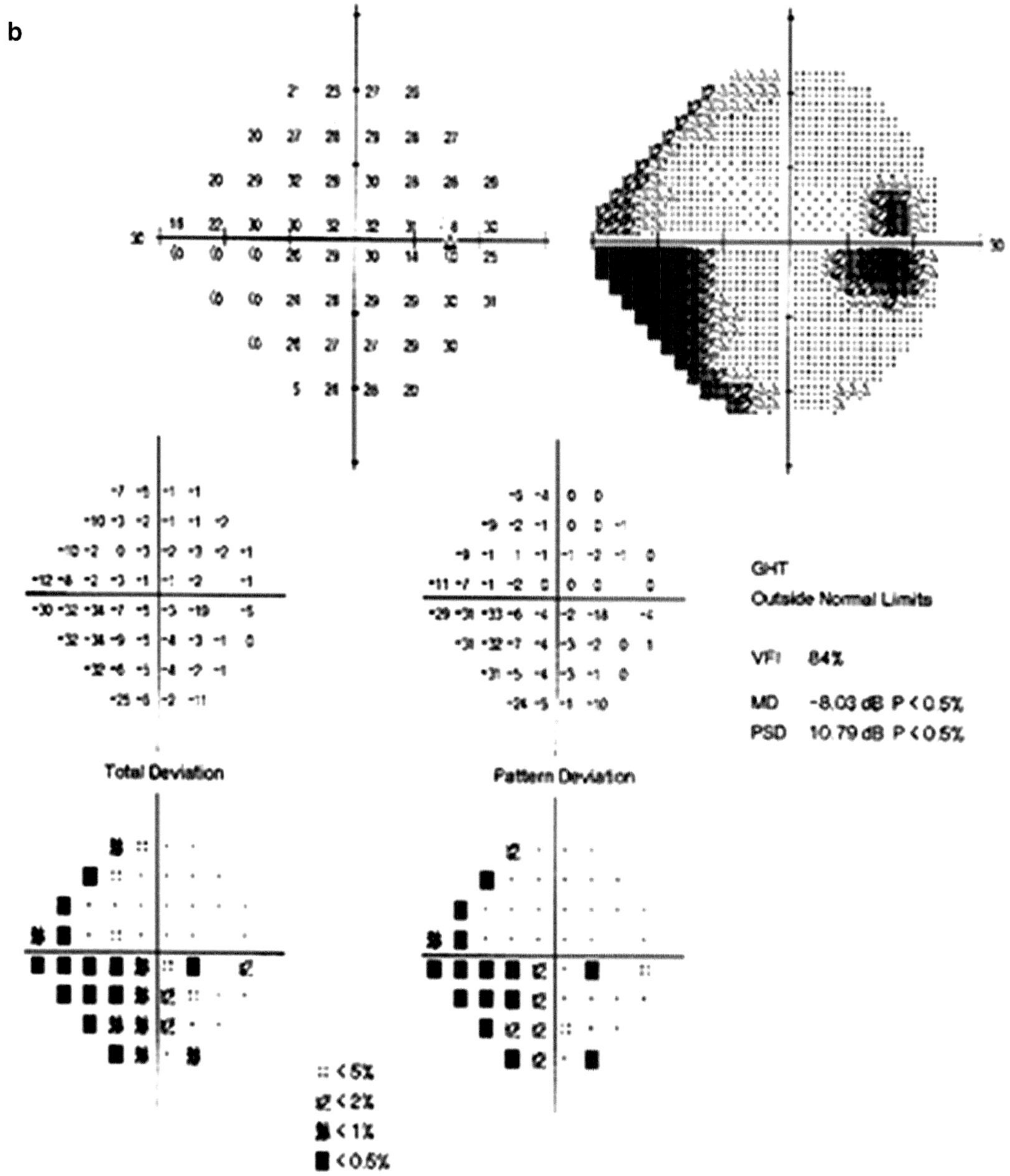

Fig. 52.2 (continued)

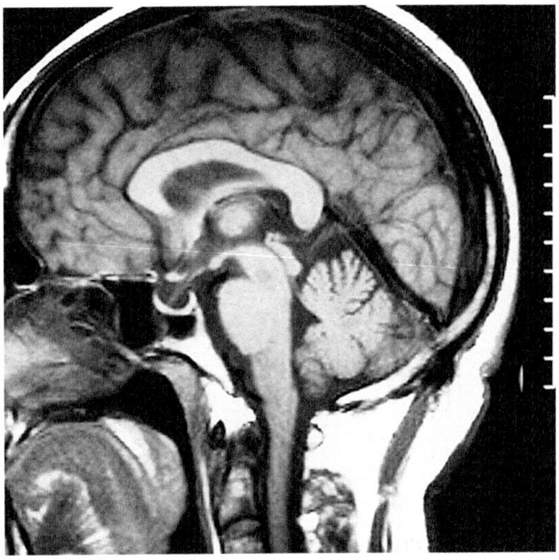

Fig. 52.3 Head MRI image. A lightly enlarged pituitary fossa filled with cerebrospinal fluid in the fossa was seen on the image. The pituitary gland became flattened and its superior rim showed an arc-shaped concave

tive correction. IOP by standard Goldman applanation tonometry was measured as 32 mmHg OD and 25 mmHg OS. In both eyes, the cornea was transparent, the anterior chamber was deep, the pupil was 3 mm in diameter, and direct response to light was normal. Fundus examination showed the C/D ratio was 0.75 OD and 0.5 OS.

Standardized automated perimetry revealed nasal visual field defects in both eyes (Fig. 52.7).

52.2.2 Case Analysis

The 40-year-old female patient complained of floaters in both eyes for 1 month. The examination showed elevated intraocular pressure, a deep anterior chamber, and an enlarged cup/disc ratio in both eyes. The first impression was primary open-angle glaucoma (POAG) suspect. Further examination of the visual field showed binasal visual field defects, which was not consistent with the typical glaucomatous visual field changes, and therefore we should consider diseases other than glaucoma.

Orbital MRI showed normal optic nerves without compression in both eyes; long T1 and long T2 signals suggested that the sella was filled with cerebrospinal fluid, consistent with the characteristics of empty sella (Fig. 52.8).

52.2.3 Final Diagnosis

The final diagnosis was primary open-angle glaucoma suspect and empty sella in both eyes.

52.2.4 Case Review

This 40-year-old female patient complained of floaters in both eyes for 1 month. A diagnosis of POAG suspect was made by the elevated intraocular pressure, deep anterior chamber, and enlarged cup/disc ratio in both eyes. However, the changes in the visual fields were not consistent with glaucomatous optic nerve damage, and empty sella was proven by brain MRI. There was no direct relationship between empty sella and POAG.

52.3 Discussion

Binasal hemianopsia usually results from two discrete lesions located in the temporal retina in both eyes or on both sides of the optic chiasm

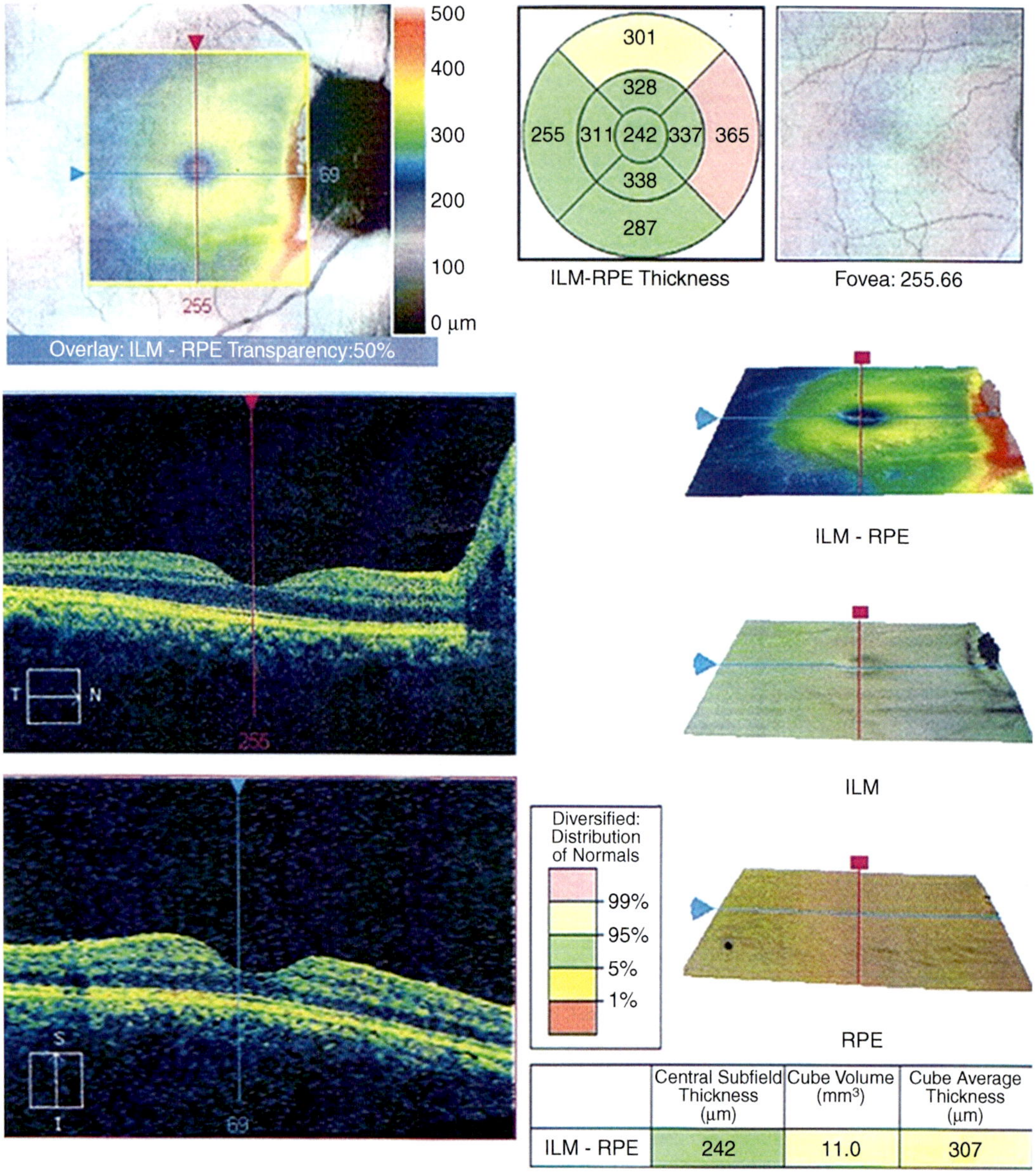

Fig. 52.4 OCT macular thickness analysis printouts. The macula morphology was normal in both eyes. Panel a, right eye; Panel b, left eye

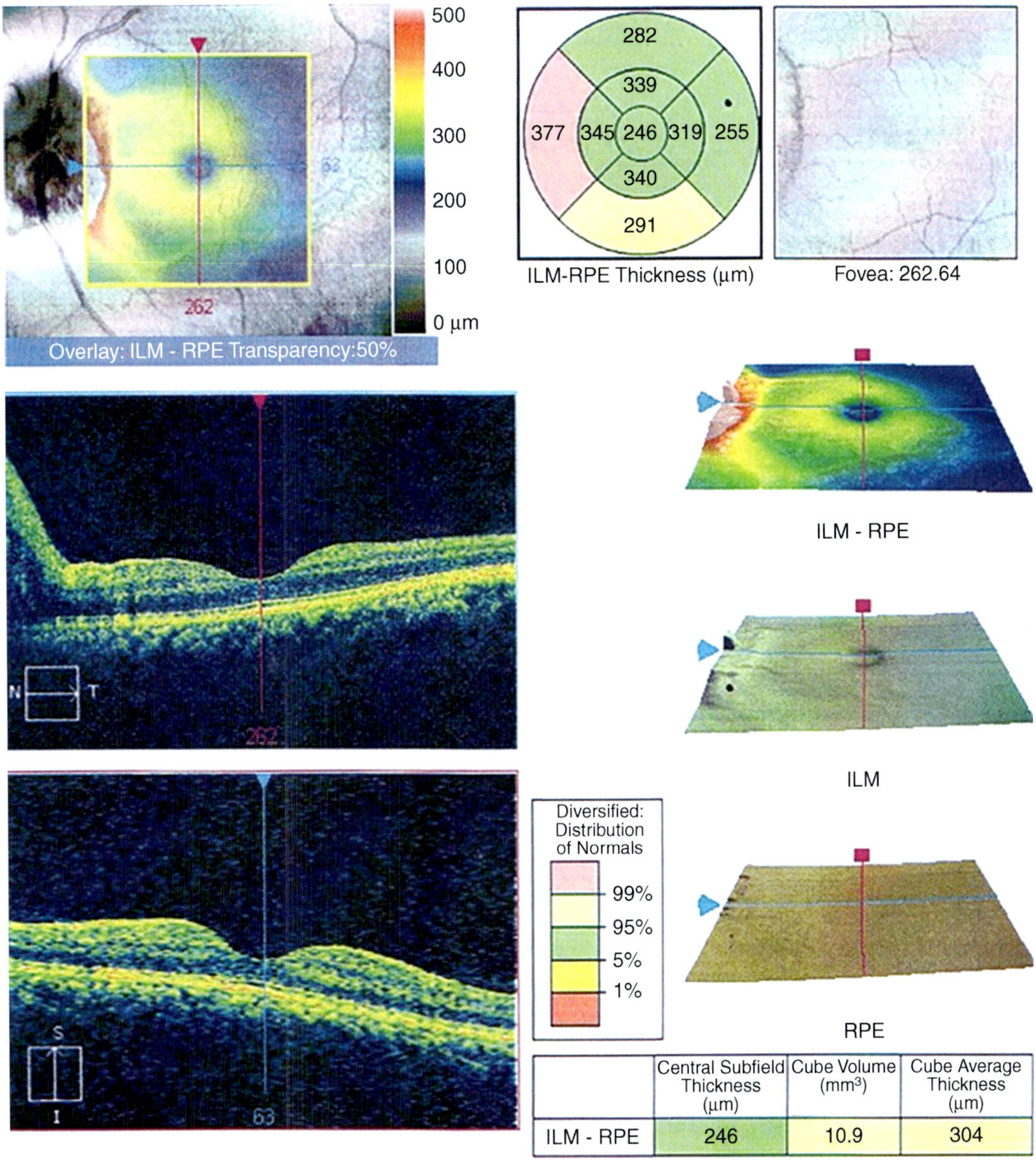

Fig. 52.4 (continued)

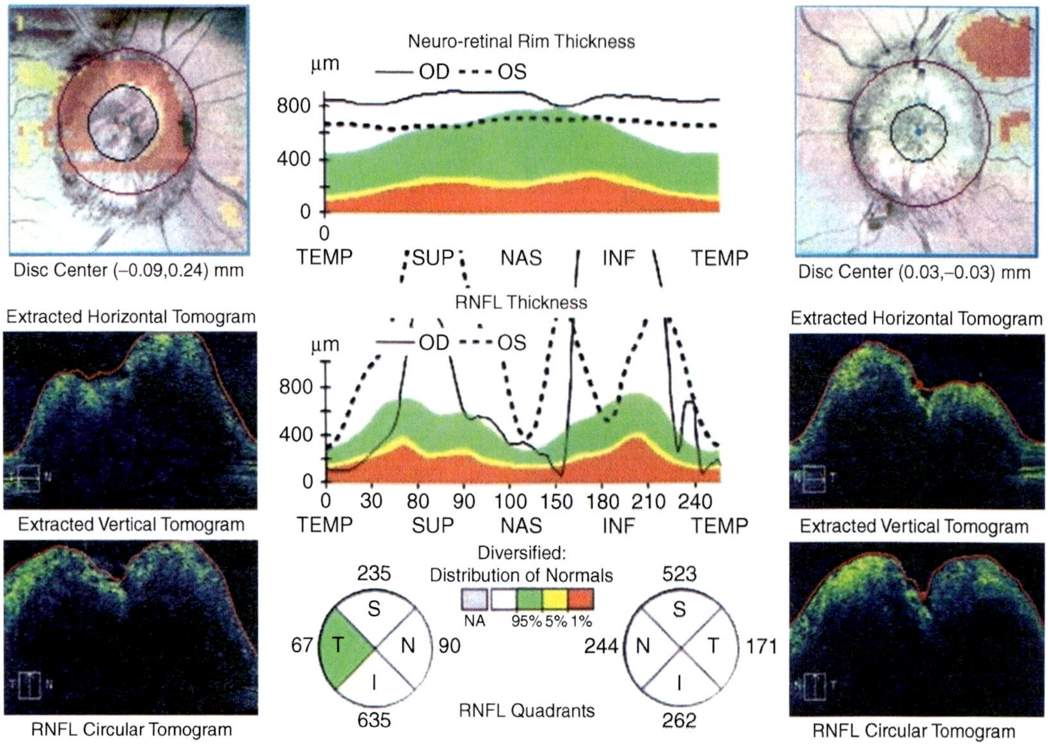

Fig. 52.5 OCT RNFL thickness analysis printouts. The peripapillary RNFL thickness increased significantly in both eyes

along which the optic nerve fiber runs from the temporal side of the retina. However, the above explanations are hardly proven clinically. According to the case report of symmetric binasal visual field defects, the causes include the following [1–4]: (a) arachnoiditis at the optic chiasm; (b) meningioma originating from the lesser wing of the sphenoid bone; (c) spinal tuberculous optic atrophy; (d) multiple sclerosis; (e) glaucoma; and (f) internal carotid aneurysm (which pushes the optic chiasm to the other side). Salinas Garcia et al. reported eight patients with incomplete binasal hemianopsia, and the causes included ischemic optic neuropathy, optic disc drusen, glaucoma, and achromatic retinitis pigmentosa. In addition to other diseases, the two cases described in this section both have empty sella, so the following discussion will focus on empty sella or empty sella syndrome (ESS).

ESS is a series of clinical symptoms caused by empty sella, such as headache, hypertension, cerebrospinal fluid rhinorrhea, endocrine hormone disorders, benign intracranial hypertension, and visual impairment. Headache is usually considered to be associated with increased intracranial pressure, while the endocrine disorders are associated with damage to the pituitary, which may result from atrophy of the pituitary caused by entrance of the arachnoid into the pituitary fossa along the pressure gradient under the intracranial pressure. After pituitary injury, manifestations of hyperpituitarism may occur, such as acromegaly, amenorrhea, and hyperprolactinemia. There are also clinical symptoms of anterior pituitary hypofunction [5, 6].

An empty sella that occurs following pituitary radiation or pituitary surgery is classified as secondary ESS. These patients present with symptoms such as sella hollowness, vision loss, and visual field defects. Even growth regression was seen in rare cases. The authors once saw a female patient, who underwent a surgery at 8 years old to remove the tumor mass of "pituitary macroadenoma." She had been not administered with a

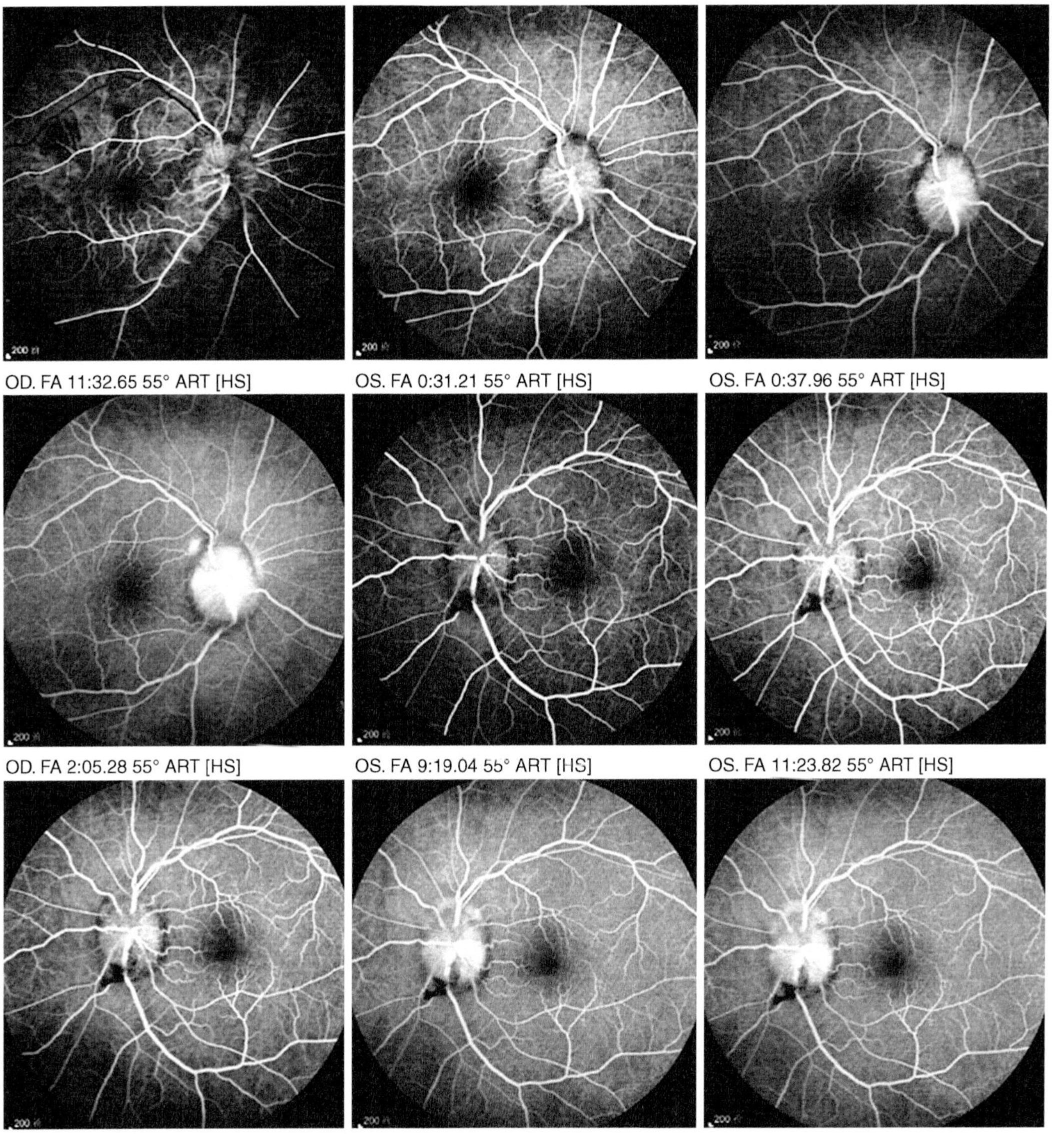

Fig. 52.6 FFA images. Diffuse telangiectasis on the surface of the edematous optic disc in both eyes and flaky hemorrhage blocking the fluorescence in the inferior optic disc of the left eye could be seen. Minimal dye leakage was seen over time. Late-phase angiography showed hyperfluorescent staining of the disc associated with blurring margins

postoperative hormone replacement therapy, so growth retardation was seen. After the age of 13, she became shorter and shorter, which was accompanied by alopecia, facial edema, and decline in language skills and intelligence. At 17 years old, she was only 88 cm in height and 16.5 kg in weight, with thin hair and a pale edema puffy face. She could only count from 1 to 100 and could not speak a complete sentence at that time. Her intelligence was similar to that of a 3-year-old normal child. After 17 years old, she received levothyroxine, prednisone, and other medications. Later on, she experienced physical and intellectual growth again.

Empty sella can be a primary or secondary condition. Primary empty sella is most commonly caused by congenital sellar diaphragm defects, whereas secondary empty sella is often

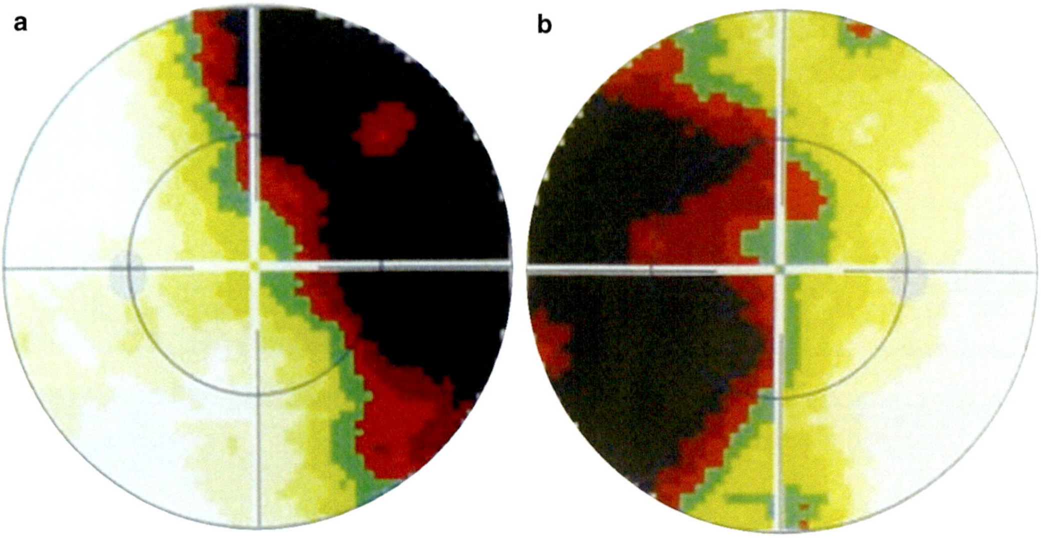

Fig. 52.7 The grayscale maps of Octopus perimeter visual field analysis. The 30-2 test showed nasal visual field defects in both eyes. Panel a, left eye; Panel b, right eye

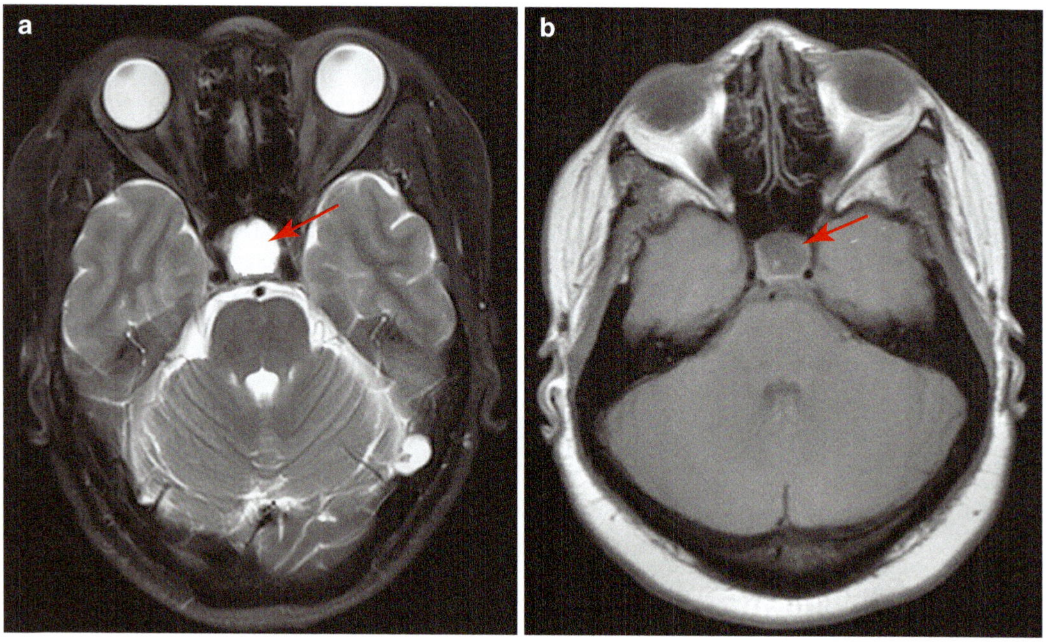

Fig. 52.8 Orbital MRI images. The optic nerve signals were normal without signs of compression in both eyes. Long T1 and long T2 signals suggested that the sella was filled with cerebrospinal fluid (red arrow), consistent with the clinical manifestations of empty sella. Panel a: T2-weighted fat suppression image; Panel b: T1-weighted image

associated with pituitary atrophy following the treatment of pituitary adenoma or spontaneous pituitary atrophy, both of which cause relative enlargement of the sella. In addition, absolute enlargement of the sella is caused by bone destruction and absorption in the sellar region. Figure 52.9 shows the underlying pathogenesis of empty sella.

Studies have demonstrated that 38% of patients with empty sella syndrome have a vari-

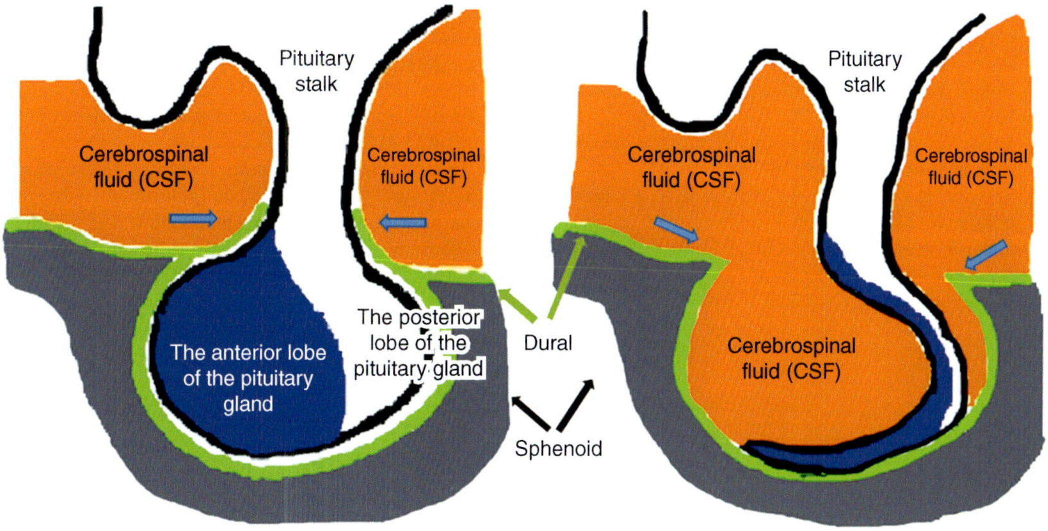

Fig. 52.9 Schematic diagram of the pathogenesis of empty sella. Weakened sellar diaphragm (blue arrow in A) or pituitary atrophy let the cerebrospinal fluid (blue arrow in B) flow into the pituitary fossa

ety of concomitant eye damage, including decreased visual acuity, visual field defects, optic disc edema, and optic nerve atrophy [6–8]. Visual field changes can manifest as unilateral temporal hemianopsia, bitemporal hemianopsia, and binasal hemianopsia. The visual field changes in empty sella syndrome are related to the location of arachnoid hernia in the pituitary fossa and the anatomical relationship between the optic chiasm and the pituitary gland. The position of the optic chiasm above the sella is divided into three types: prefixed type, postfixed type, and normal type. Therefore, the cerebrospinal fluid compresses the optic chiasm from different directions, resulting in different visual field defects.

Different from that of the visual field defects arising from direct compression of the optic chiasm by a tumor (such as pituitary adenoma), the possible mechanisms of binasal hemianopsia produced by empty sella include the following [6]: (a) the optic chiasm is pushed toward the intrasellar side; (b) the anterior part of the third ventricle herniates into the sella, causing changes in the position and shape of the optic nerve (such as tortuosity); and (c) the optic chiasm incarceration. Binasal hemianopsia may be symmetrical or irregular, and the patients often have other head abnormalities which may not be related to the ocular diseases (such as empty sella). Therefore, routine cranial MRI examinations should be done.

Active intervention for the eye disorders should be undertaken in patients with binasal hemianopsia. No treatment is indicated for patients with mild symptoms of empty sella. Medical interventions which can alleviate symptoms and hormone replacement therapy should be undertaken if symptoms of empty sella become severe. In cases of severe visual impairment and visual field changes, severe headaches, cerebrospinal rhinorrhea, and intracranial hypertension accompanied with signs of gyrus compression and even separation of cranial sutures, surgical treatment should be considered. The operation scheme depends on the condition of the patient. If the optic chiasm or the intracranial segment of the optic nerve was elongated or distorted, artificial diaphragm implantation may be helpful.

References

1. Cushing H, Walker CB. Distortions of the visual fields in cases of brain tumor (third paper): binasal hemianopsia. Arch Ophthalmol. 1912;41:559–98.

2. Ashwin PT, Quinlan M. Interpreting binasal hemianopia: the importance of ocular examination. Eur J Intern Med. 2006;17(2):144–5.
3. Pringle E, Bingham J, Graham E. Progressive binasal hemianopia. Lancet. 2004;363(9421):1606.
4. Salinas-Garcia RF, Smith JL. Binasal hemianopia. Surg Neurol. 1978;10(3):187–94.
5. Shinder R, Wolansky L, Turbin RE. Congenital homonymous hemianopia and cortical migration abnormalities in a young adult. J Pediatr Ophthalmol Strabismus. 2009;46(1):38–41.
6. Wang H, Li S, Wang N, et al. Ocular characteristics of empty Sella syndrome. J Ophthalmol. 2012;21(5):309–12.
7. Bryan BT, Pomeranz HD, Smith KH. Complete binasal hemianopia. Proc (Bayl Univ Med Cent). 2014;27(4):356–8.
8. Yamabayashi S, Yamamoto T, Sasaki T, Tsukahara S. A case of 'low tension glaucoma' with primary empty sella. Br J Ophthalmol. 1988;72(11):852–5.

Part VI

Lesions in Posterior Visual Pathway

53 Characteristic Visual Field Defects of Patients with Occipital Lobe Infarction: Homonymous Hemianopia and Macular Sparing

Xiaobin Xie, Ning Fan, and Ningli Wang

Occipital lobe lesions are usually caused by trauma or infarction. The most characteristic visual field defect is symmetrical homonymous hemianopia, which is usually accompanied by macular sparing. This section will discuss the possible pathological mechanism of macular sparing in two cases.

53.1 Case 1

53.1.1 Case Presentation

A 70-year-old female patient had a complaint that her visual field of the left eye had narrowed for 1 month, affecting her daily life, including walking. No spotted vision or floaters, visual distortion, red eye, sore eye, or other accompanying discomforts were present. She had no dizziness or headache, either. The patient had suffered from hypertension for years controlled with medication. Half a month before, she had been diagnosed with cerebral infarction in another hospital. History of systemic diseases, other ocular diseases, trauma, or familial diseases was denied.

The uncorrected visual acuity (UCVA) was 20/25 OU, and the best corrected visual acuity (BCVA) was 20/20 OU with refractive correction (−2.00DS). The intraocular pressure (IOP) was normal OU. Slit-lamp examination of her anterior segments was unremarkable, with sensitive direct light reflex of each pupil, except for an increased density of the lens in both eyes. Fundus examination revealed that the optic disc was pink with clear margin and a cup-to-disc (C/D) ratio of 0.3, and the macula and peripheral retina were normal in both eyes (Fig. 53.1).

Standardized automated perimetry demonstrated left homonymous hemianopia with macular sparing (Fig. 53.2).

Optical coherence tomography (OCT) scan showed the thickness of retinal nerve fiber layers (RNFL) was within normal limits in both eyes (Fig. 53.3).

The latency and amplitude values of P100 in the pattern visual evoked potential (P-VEP) were within normal limits in both eyes (Fig. 53.4).

Computed tomography (CT) in axial view of the head from another hospital revealed a hypodense patch-like lesion in the right occipital lobe (Fig. 53.5).

X. Xie
Eye Hospital of China Academy of Chinese Medical Sciences, Beijing, China

N. Fan
Shenzhen Eye Hospital, Shenzhen University, Shenzhen, China

N. Wang (✉)
Department of Ophthalmology, Beijing Tongren Hospital, Capital Medical University, Beijing, China

N. Wang et al. (eds.), *Optic Disorders and Visual Field*, Advances in Visual Science and Eye Diseases 2, https://doi.org/10.1007/978-981-13-2502-1_53

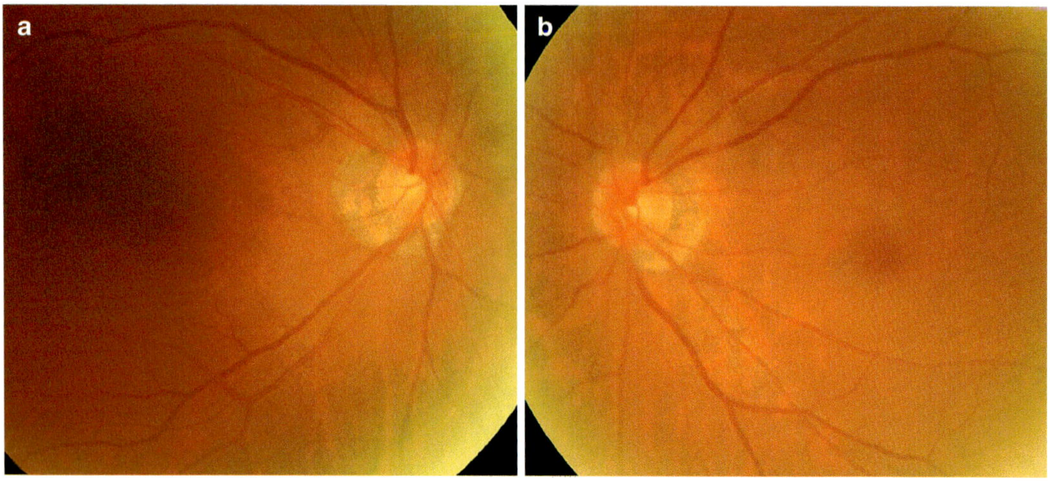

Fig. 53.1 Fundus photographs. In both eyes, the optic disc was pink with clear margin and a C/D ratio of 0.3. No abnormalities were found in the macula and retina in either eye (Note: the image quality was slightly affected by small pupil size and increased lens density). Panel a: right eye. Panel b: left eye

Magnetic resonance imaging (MRI) in axial view of the head performed with diffusion weighted imaging (DWI) from another hospital showed a flaky hyperintense signal in the right occipital lobe, suggesting infarction (Fig. 53.6).

53.1.2 Case Analysis

Visual field of the patient's left eye was noted narrowed. No significant abnormality was found in the fundus of either eye. RNFL thickness was within normal limits. Standardized automated perimetry found homonymous hemianopia accompanied by macular sparing. The light reflexes of both pupils are normal. According to these findings, it was considered to be diseases in posterior visual pathway. Given the history of right occipital lobe infarction half a month before, the change in the visual field was caused by the occipital lobe infarction.

53.1.3 Final Diagnosis

The final diagnosis was right occipital lobe infarction.

53.1.4 Case Review

In this case, the time from disease onset was relatively short, and the visual fields showed typical homonymous hemianopia with macular sparing in both eyes, which is a specific manifestation of damages in the visual radiation and visual cortex. The homonymous hemianopia is caused by the contralateral damages in the optic radiation or primary visual cortex. The borderline in the visual fields between the impaired part and the intact one was not straight, and the whole function or vision of the macula, i.e., the central vision, was preserved. Its mechanism is still not clear.

a

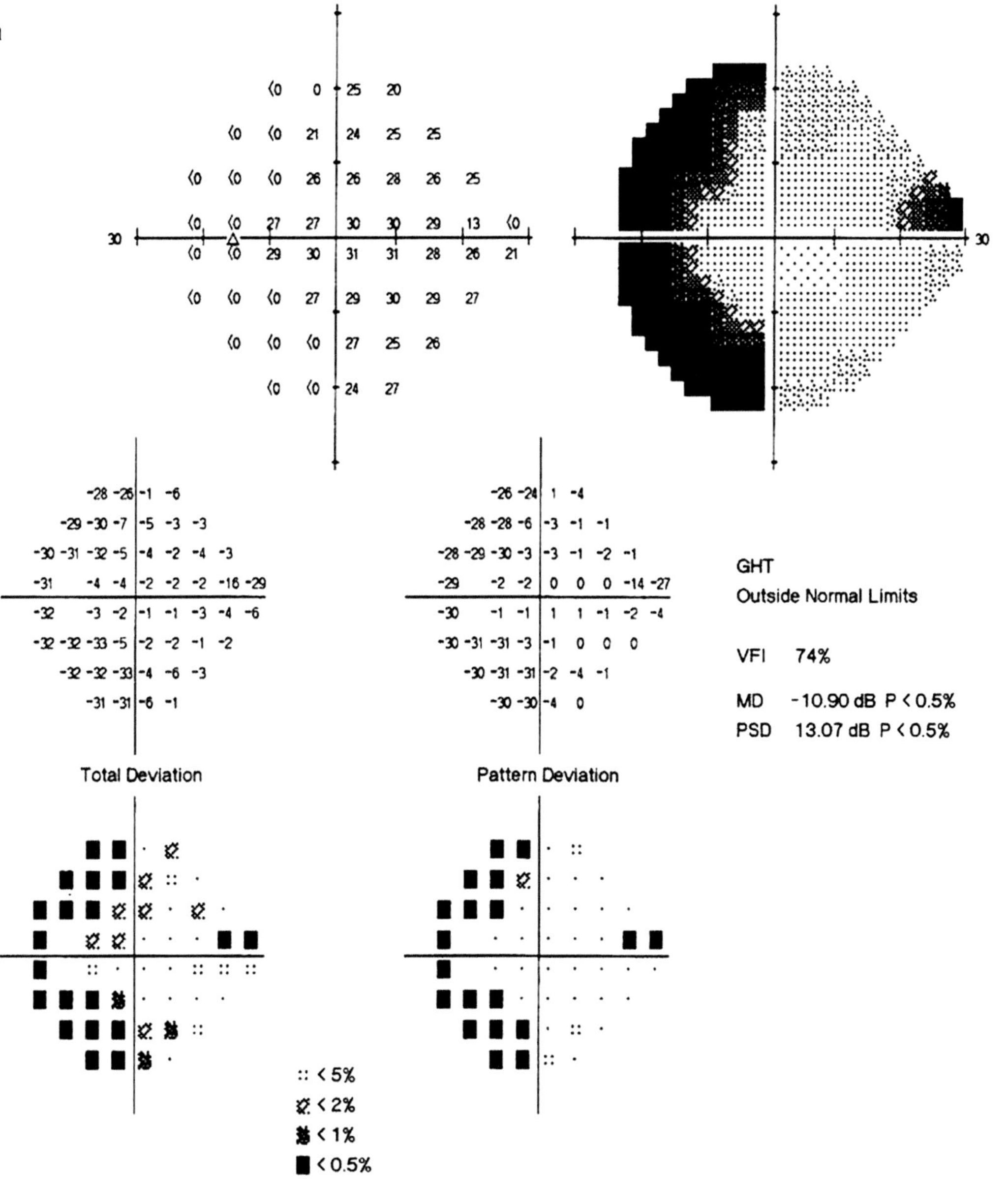

Fig. 53.2 Humphrey visual field analysis printouts. 24-2 test demonstrated left homonymous hemianopia with macular sparing. Panel a: left eye. Panel b: right eye

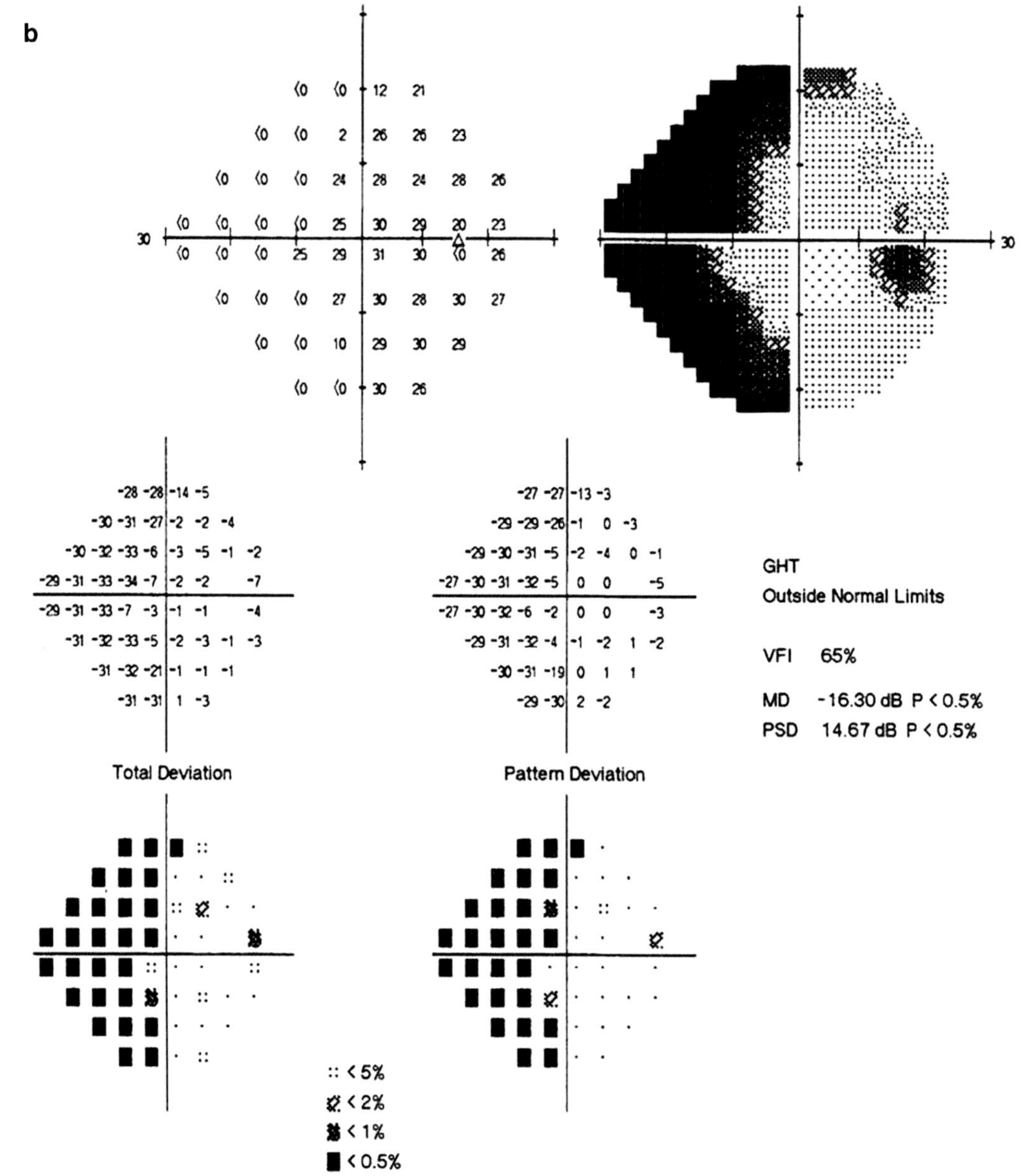

Fig. 53.2 (continued)

53.2 Case 2

53.2.1 Case Presentation

A 56-year-old female patient complained of blurred vision in both eyes for 1 week without any other discomforts such as floaters, visual distortion, red eyes, or sore eyes. There were no signs of dizziness or headache. The patient had suffered from hypertension for many years and denied any history of other systemic, ocular, or familial diseases and trauma.

The UCVA was 20/33 OU and the BCVA was 20/20 OU with refractive correction

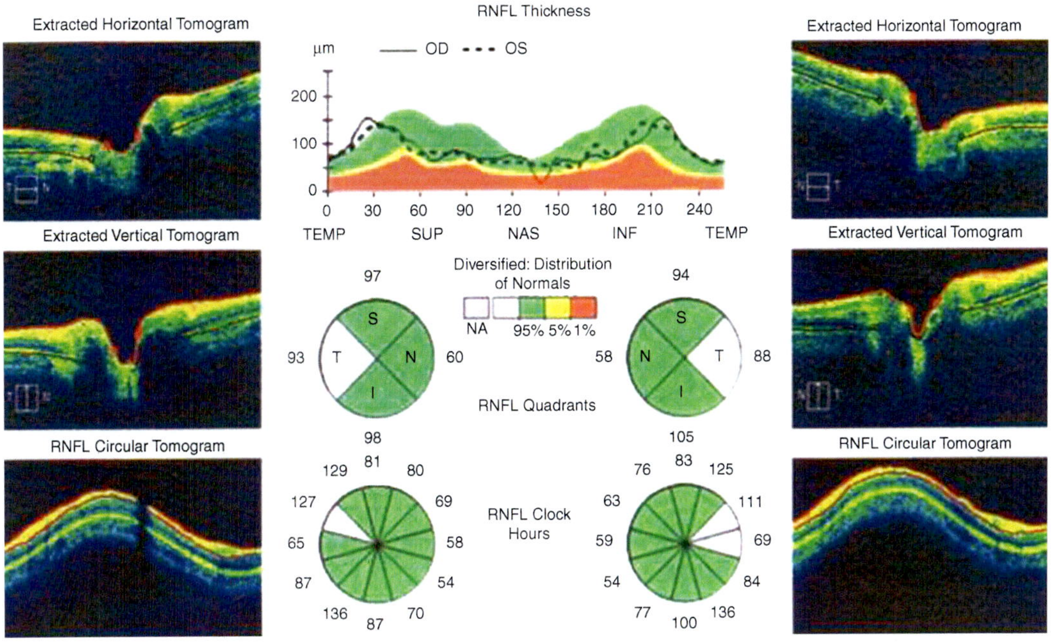

Fig. 53.3 RNFL thickness analysis printout in OCT. RNFL thickness was within normal limits in both eyes

Pattern-VEP

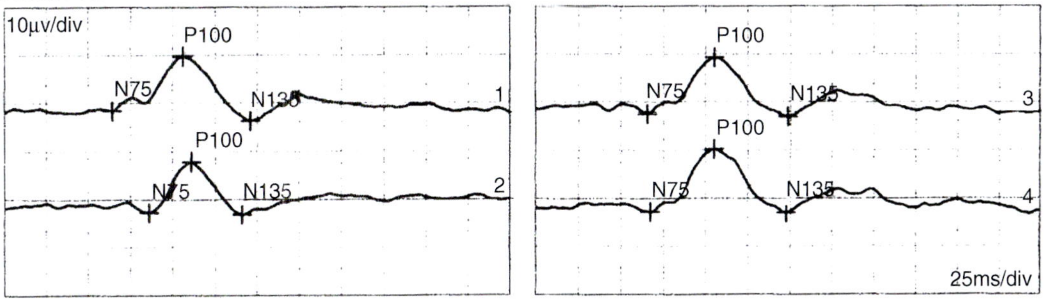

Channel	N75 [ms]	P100 [ms]	N135 [ms]	N75-P100	P100-N135
1 R-1 1,0	65	106	146	11.4µv	13.4µv
3 L-1 1,0	66	106	149	11.9µv	12.5µv
2 R-1 0,15	86	112	141	10.4µv	10.9µv
4 L-1 0,15	68	106	148	13.1µv	13.3µv
Normals	-	90-120-90-120	-	-	-

Channel	Stimulus	Ampl., Range, Filter
1 R-1 1,0	MON Patt. Rev. CB, 1?Full Field, Ctr:97% 1.5Hz, Avg:72	1, +/-100µv 1-50Hz
2 R-1 0,15	MON Patt. Rev. CB, 0?5' Full Field, Ctr:97% 1.5Hz, Avg:75	1, +/-100µv 1-50Hz
3 L-1 1,0	MON Patt. Rev. CB, 1?Full Field, Ctr:97% 1.5Hz, Avg:74	1, +/-100µv 1-50Hz
4 L-1 0,15	MON Patt. Rev. CB, 0?5' Full Field, Ctr:97% 1.5Hz, Avg:72	1, +/-100µv 1-50Hz

Fig. 53.4 P-VEP examination printout. The waveform, latency, and amplitude values of the P100 waves were normal in both eyes

(−1.50DS). IOP was normal OU. Slit-lamp examination of her anterior segments was unremarkable, with sensitive direct light reflexes of both pupils. Fundus examination revealed that the optic disc was pink with clear margin and the retinal arteries became thinner in both eyes (Fig. 53.7).

Standardized automated perimetry demonstrated right homonymous hemianopia in both eyes (Fig. 53.8).

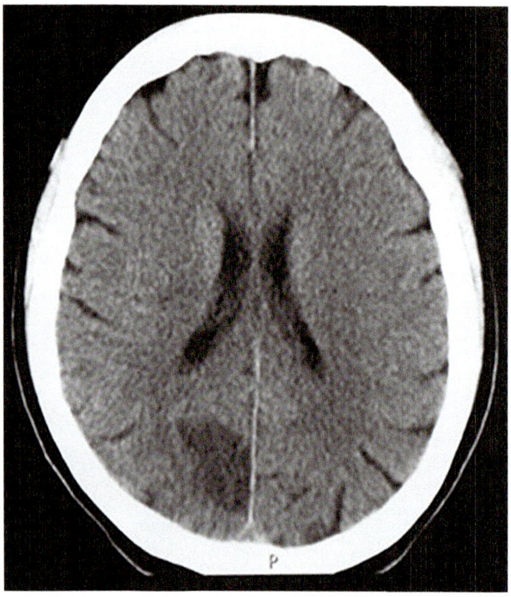

Fig. 53.5 Head CT image in axial view. A hypodense patch-like lesion was found in the right occipital lobe

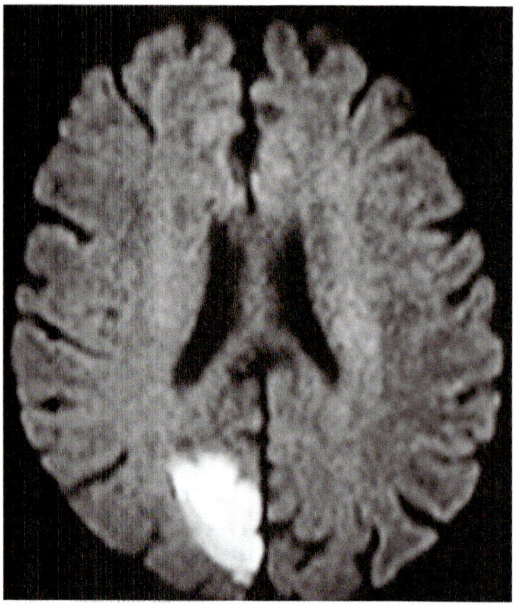

Fig. 53.6 Head MRI image in axial view. Right occipital lobe infarction was observed

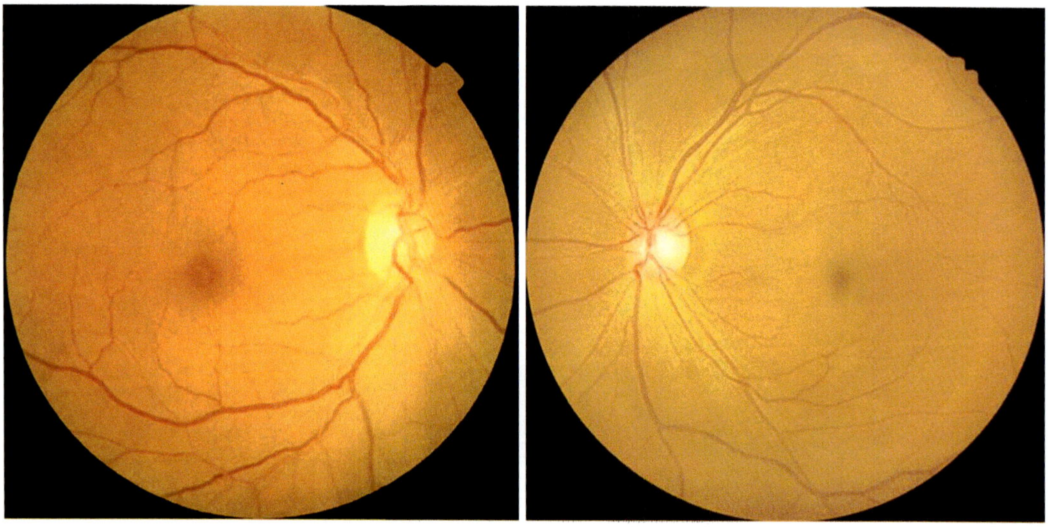

Fig. 53.7 Fundus photographs. The optic disc was pink with clear margin and the retinal arteries became thinner in both eyes

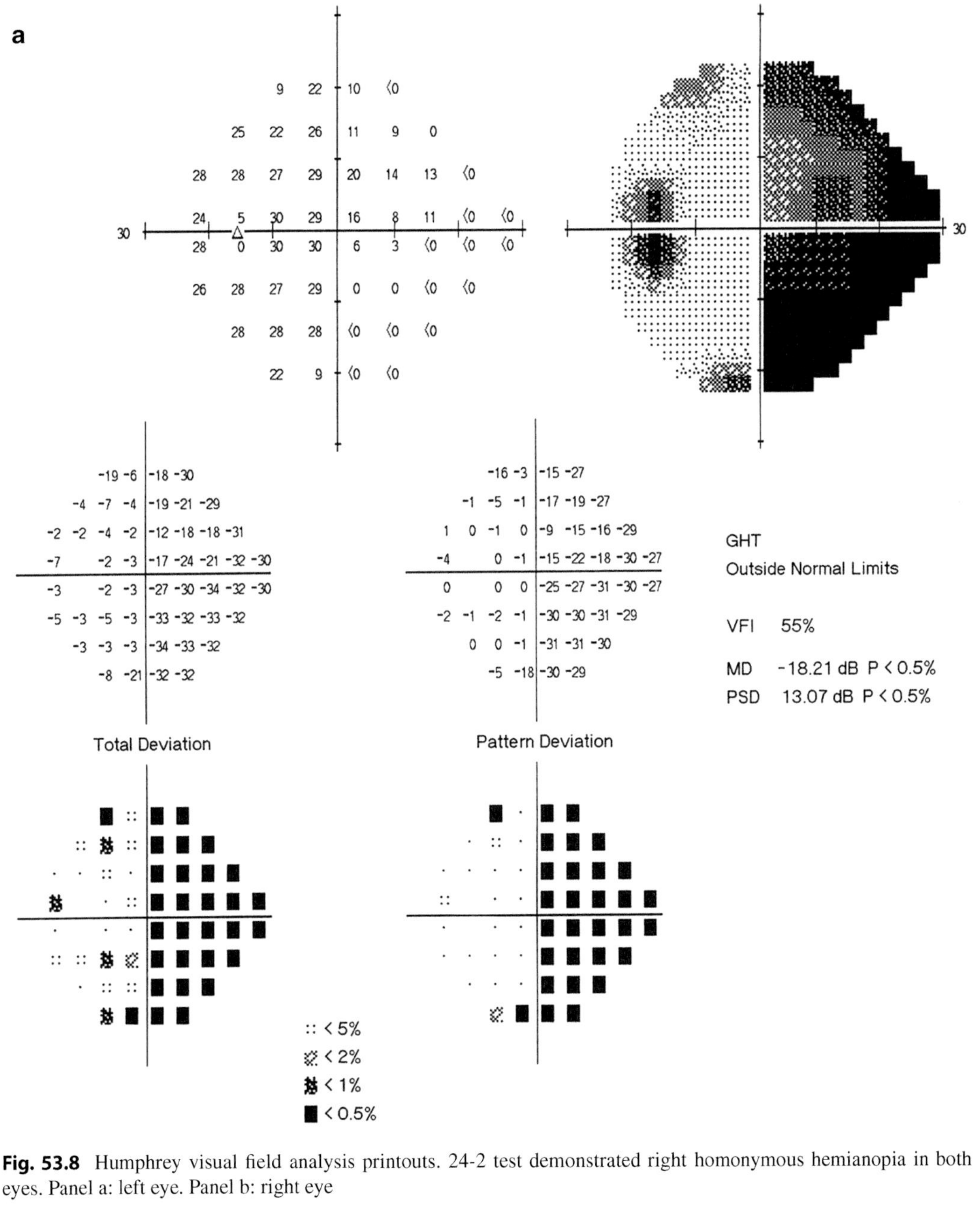

Fig. 53.8 Humphrey visual field analysis printouts. 24-2 test demonstrated right homonymous hemianopia in both eyes. Panel a: left eye. Panel b: right eye

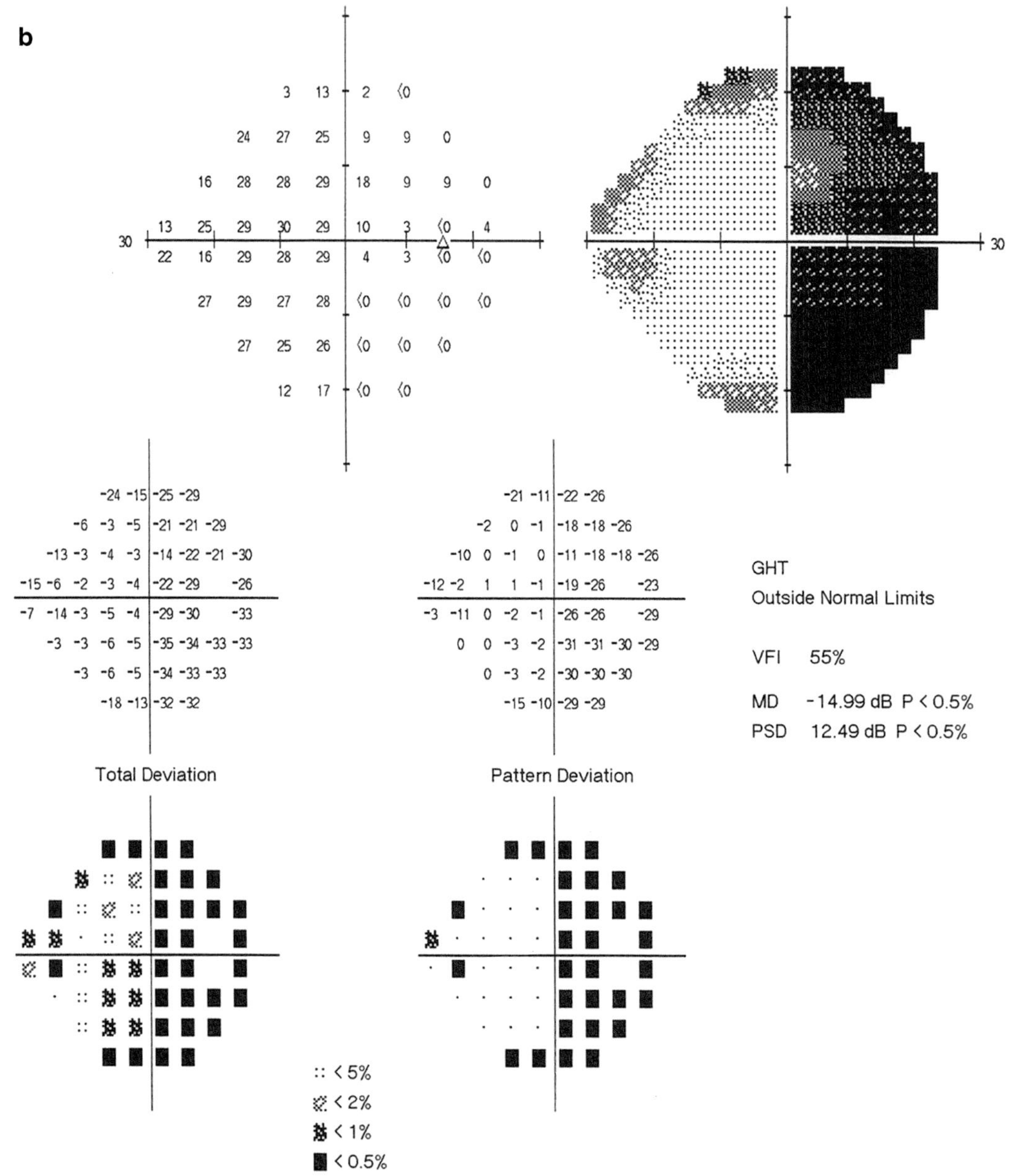

Fig. 53.8 (continued)

Head MRI in axial view showed a large infarction lesion in the left parieto-occipital lobe (Fig. 53.9).

53.2.2 Final Diagnosis

The final diagnosis was left occipital lobe infarction.

53.3 Discussion

Both patients were elderly women complaining of narrowed visual field and blurred vision. However, routine examinations on the anterior and posterior segments as well as the pupils showed no abnormalities in either eye. RNFL thickness in OCT and the P100 wave in P-VEP also showed normal

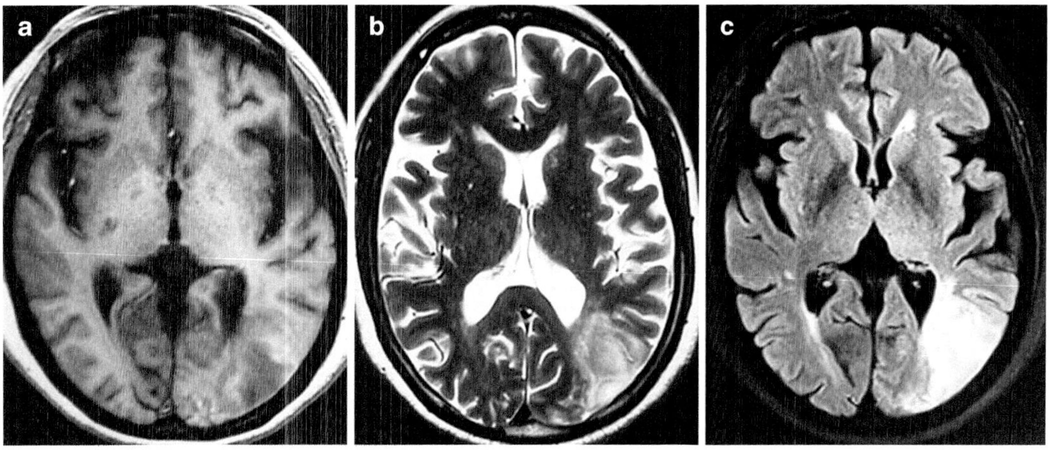

Fig. 53.9 Head MRI images in axial view. Extensive wedge-shaped abnormal signals were seen in the left parieto-occipital lobe. Panel a: slightly hypointense signal was shown on T1-weighted image (T1WI). Panel b: slightly hyperintense signal was shown on T2WI. Panel c: marked hyperintense signal was shown on the fluid-attenuated inversion-recovery image (FLAIR)

results. Therefore, the standardized automated perimetry was particularly important. Especially when patients show no other sensory or motor dysfunctions except for the only clinical manifestation of unilateral blurred vision, clinicians tend to focus on the ocular examination, so that misdiagnosis or missed diagnosis occurs. Because of the difficulty to perceive nasal visual field defects and the presence of normal nasal visual field with defected temporal visual field in the contralateral eye, the complaints are mainly narrowed visual field and blurred vision in the contralateral eye. For the patients with homonymous hemianopia accompanied by macular sparing and adequate central vision, the ophthalmologists need to consider the possibility of occipital lobe lesions.

In addition, it should be noted that although there are obvious occipital lobe damages even involving both sides, the patients still think they are capable of seeing and deny visual field defects. This condition is considered as Anton's syndrome [1].

Cerebrovascular disease is a common cause of occipital lobe damages, and ischemia may lead to infarction. Occipital lobe infarction often affects elderly patients. The most common reasons of occipital lobe infarction include arterial stenosis or occlusion caused by the sclerosis of the posterior cerebral arteries and their branches. In some cases, occipital lobe infarction may be caused by bleeding. The posterior cerebral arteries are the terminal branches of the basilar artery, which send out central branches and cortical branches. The cortical branches are further divided into the calcarine artery and the parieto-occipital artery, which mainly supply the occipital lobe except for the lateral parts of some occipital lobe and the inferior and inferolateral edge of the temporal lobe except for the temporal pole. In addition to the posterior cerebral artery, other arteries also participate in the blood supplying to the occipital lobe in most people, such as the posterior temporal artery, the parieto-occipital artery, and sometimes the middle cerebral artery.

Due to the special structure of the striate cortex of the occipital lobe, its damage only affects the visual field, i.e., almost identical visual field defects in both eyes without any other neurological dysfunctions or damages in the anterior optic pathway will result; for example, there is no pale optic disc or relative afferent pupillary defect (RAPD), and the central visual acuity is often not affected.

Unilateral occipital lobe infarction will cause contralateral homonymous hemianopia, but the morphology of visual field defects varies with the location and size of infarction. For example, if the lesion impairs the entire striated cortex on one side, the visual field may demonstrate complete homonymous hemianopia on the opposite side; if the lesion is located at the cuneus or gyrus lingualis on one side, the visual field may demonstrate quadrantanopia on the opposite side. Please find the details in other chapters. Both of the patients described above were elderly women suffering from cerebral infarction. Their visual fields manifested as homonymous hemianopia contralateral to the lesion, and the defects in the two eyes were identical, but only one patient showed macular sparing, which is worth exploration.

Macular sparing manifests as preservation of the central vision and the pupillary light reflex. The mechanism of macular sparing is still not clear at present. Presumably, the possible mechanisms include [2, 3]:

(a) Dual projections of the macula: in the visual radiation, the fibers from the macula cross at the splenium, so the macular fibers from one side terminate in both the ipsilateral and contralateral visual centers; the corpus callosum is the main transverse tract of fibers that connects the two cerebral hemispheres. It is the main component of the centrum ovale, and its splenium connects the two occipital lobes. In other words, the central visual field is perceived by the visual cortex on both sides.
(b) Wide distribution of macular fibers: macular fibers are quite scattered before they terminate. They are widely located and terminate in the entire visual cortex. Usually, it is difficult for a single lesion to completely destroy the whole macular projecting fibers.
(c) Dual blood supplies: the macular fibers finally terminate in the occipital cortex, which are supplied by the branches originated from the posterior cerebral arteries and middle cerebral arteries with their anastomoses. When the lesion only blocks the blood circulation of one artery, the macular function is not impaired. If the lesion destroys the vascular territory of the macular projecting fibers, there is no macular sparing, and vice versa.

All of above are just speculation. The protection mechanism of human central visual field during the biological evolution may be far more complicated than what we have known.

In addition, it is noteworthy that these patients usually show inconsistencies between visual field injuries and occipital damages. For example, some obvious unilateral occipital infarctions can be seen, but visual fields only show contralateral homonymous hemianopia involving a very small central area, as shown in Sect. 53.2 of this chapter.

Based on the above analyses, it is speculated that a part of the striated cortex on one side was damaged in Case 1, and hence the visual field defects were accompanied by macular sparing; however, the area of cerebral infarction in Case 2 was larger, so the absence of macular sparing is considered to be related to the impairment of the entire striated cortex, including the occipital pole.

References

1. Tong Y, Wei S, You S. Basis and clinical Progress of visual pathway diseases. Beijing: People's Medical Publishing House; 2010.
2. Brysbaert M. The importance of interhemispheric transfer for foveal vision: a factor that has been overlooked in theories of visual word recognition and object perception. Brain Lang. 2004;88(3):259–67.
3. Chokron S, Perez C, Peyrin C. Behavioral consequences and cortical reorganization in homonymous hemianopia. Front Syst Neurosci. 2016;28(10):57.

A Case of Wallenberg Syndrome with Unilateral Occipital Lobe Infarction

54

Xiaobin Xie, Ning Fan, and Ningli Wang

A young healthy woman suddenly experienced sore eyes, headache, and unstable gait. It was finally identified that these symptoms were caused by multiple cerebral infarction due to detached tumor emboli from the mitral valve. After surgery and 2 years of rehabilitation, the patient gradually returned to normal life and work. However, the patient could not produce tears in the right eye during crying. Although the visual acuities were 20/20 in both eyes, she always complained of blurred vision. What is the reason behind it?

54.1 Case

54.1.1 Case Presentation

A 29-year-old female patient complained of alacrima during crying in the right eye and blurred vision in both eyes for 2 years. The patient had experienced sudden sore eye pain, headache, and unstable gait 2 years before. She had been treated in several hospitals in China. Via echocardiography (ECG) and head MRI, she was finally diagnosed with multiple cerebral infarctions caused by detached tumor emboli from the mitral valve. Then, the patient received the surgery of valve replacement and was pathologically diagnosed with "papillary fibroelastoma in the mitral valve." After more than 2 years of rehabilitation since then, the patient gradually recovered but still suffered from alacrima in the right eye during crying and blurred vision with a central visual acuity of 20/20. Her sensation of pain and temperature on the left side of the body below the neck disappeared, but the sensation of touch was normal. She could normally sweat and her ability of physical exercise was not affected. She had mild dyskinesia and ataxia on the right side of the body without sensation disturbance.

The uncorrected visual acuity (UCVA) was 20/20 OU. The intraocular pressure (IOP) was normal OU. Slit-lamp examination of her anterior segments and fundus examination were unremarkable with normal pupil, disc, macula, and retinal vessels in both eyes.

Standardized automated perimetry demonstrated right inferior homonymous quadrantanopia within the central 10° in both eyes (Fig. 54.1).

X. Xie
Eye Hospital of China Academy of Chinese Medical Sciences, Beijing, China

N. Fan
Shenzhen Eye Hospital, Shenzhen University, Shenzhen, China

N. Wang (✉)
Department of Ophthalmology, Beijing Tongren Hospital, Capital Medical University, Beijing, China

N. Wang et al. (eds.), *Optic Disorders and Visual Field*, Advances in Visual Science and Eye Diseases 2, https://doi.org/10.1007/978-981-13-2502-1_54

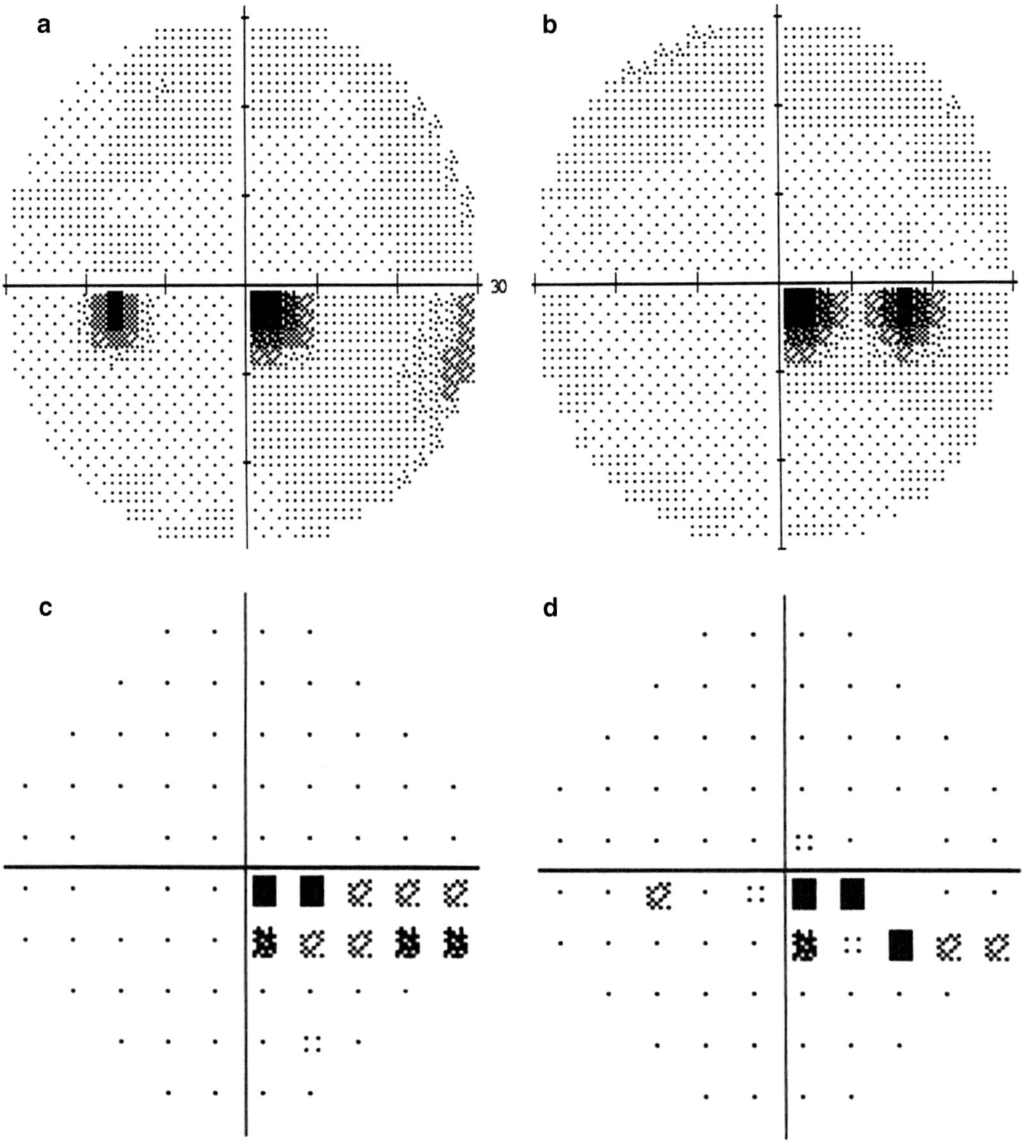

Fig. 54.1 Humphrey grayscale maps and pattern deviation probability plots. 30-2 test demonstrated right inferior homonymous quadrantanopic central scotomas. Panel a: grayscale map of the left eye. Panel b: grayscale map of the right eye. Panel c: pattern deviation probability plot of the left eye. Panel d: pattern deviation probability plot of the right eye

Computed tomography (CT) in axial view of the head exhibited a hypodense lesion in the left occipital lobe, lesions of cerebral infarction, and no compression on the ventricles (Fig. 54.2).

Magnetic resonance imaging (MRI) in axial view of the head showed a right posterior lesion in the inferior part of the pons, hypointense on T1-weighted image (T1WI) with no enhancement and hyperintense on T2WI. This indicated that the lesion was cerebral infarction involving the right superior salivary nuclei, right lateral spinothalamic tract, and posterior spinocerebellar tract (Fig. 54.3).

54.1.2 Case Analysis

Papillary fibroelastoma (PFE) is a less common but the third frequent benign primary cardiac tumor following myxoma and lipoma with a proportion of 8% [1]. This tumor may occur at any age and affects men and women alike. PFE often occurs on the surface of the valves, mostly in the aortic valve, mitral valve, and tricuspid valve. The clinical symptoms depend on the location, size, and growth rate of the tumor as well as the trend of embolization. Most patients are asymptomatic before the onset of embolization, which is the most serious complication of PFE. Coronary artery embolism, cerebral embolism, and pulmonary embolism have all been reported [2–4].

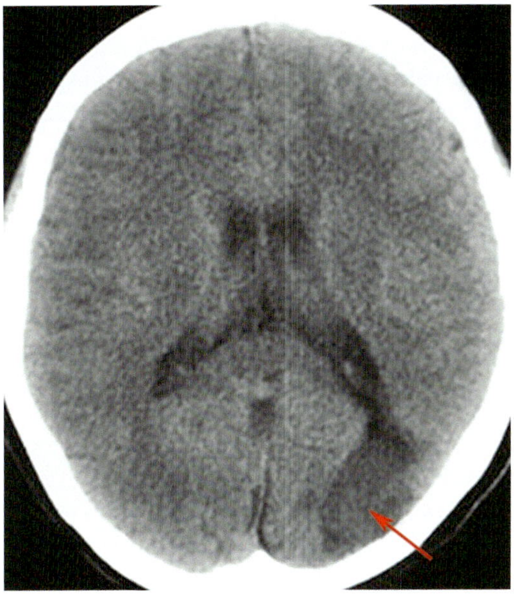

Fig. 54.2 Head CT image in axial view. A patch-like hypodense lesion was seen in the left occipital lobe (red arrow)

54.1.3 Final Diagnosis

The final diagnosis was Wallenberg syndrome, left occipital infarction, and mitral valve PFE.

54.1.4 Case Review

Wallenberg syndrome, also known as dorsolateral medullary syndrome or dorsolateral medullary infarction, is a syndrome located in the nuclei and conductive bundles in the dorsolateral medulla caused by posterior inferior cerebellar artery embolism. Depending on the involved regions, the following manifestations can be observed:

(a) Damage to the vestibular nuclei: dizziness, nausea, vomiting, and nystagmus
(b) Damage to the superior salivary nuclei: alacrimia of the affected eye
(c) Damages to the nucleus ambiguous, glossopharyngeal nerve, and vagus nerve: paralyses of muscles in the velum and pharyngolarynx

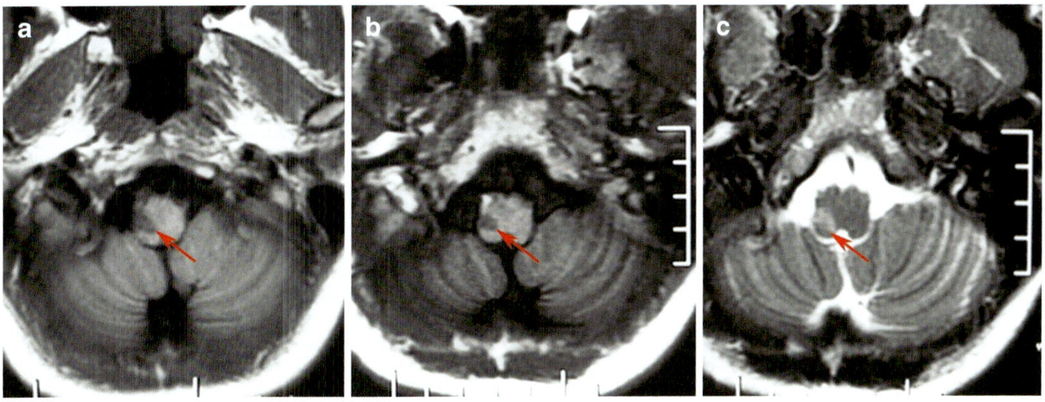

Fig. 54.3 Head MRI images. a right posterior lesion was noticed in the inferior part of the pons (red arrow). Panel a: hypointense on T1WI. Panel b: no enhancement on T1WI. Panel c: hyperintense on T2WI

at the affected side, which manifest as dysphagia, dysarthria, ipsilateral soft palate drooping, and disappearance of pharyngeal reflex

(d) Damage to the corpora restiformia: ataxia at the affected side

(e) Damage to the descending sympathetic fibers: Horner's syndrome

(f) Damages to the spinal trigeminal tract and its nucleus: alternate hemianesthesia, i.e., loss of sensations in temperature and pain on the affected face and reduction or loss of sensations in temperature and pain on the contralateral side of the body, suggesting damages to the lateral spinothalamic tract

MRI showed that the medullary infarction involved the right lateral spinothalamic tract and the posterior spinocerebellar tract. On one hand, the lateral spinothalamic tract is originated from the second neurons of the spine cord for sensations of pain and temperature, crosses via the anterior commissure, and runs upward along the lateral cord to the reticular structure and the thalamic ventral posterolateral nucleus. Therefore, the patient experienced a loss of sensation in temperature and pain on the skin at the left side of the body. On the other hand, the posterior spinocerebellar tract does not cross and travels upward along the lateral cord to the vermis of the cerebellum, providing the fine coordination for the posture and limb muscle movement at the subconscious level. So the patient had dyskinesia and ataxia on the right side of the body. When the patient had suffered acute dorsolateral medullary infarction 2 years before, there were other typical symptoms of Wallenberg syndrome, some of which were alleviated or disappeared after treatment.

54.2 Discussion

The visual center is located in the visual cortex on both sides of the calcarine sulcus on the medial surface of the occipital lobe. The visual cortex is called as Brodmann area 17, also known as the striate cortex or the first visual area. There is an exact anatomical relationship between the visual cortex and the retina: The visual information from the left halves of visual fields in both eyes is projected onto the right visual cortex, and vice versa; the visual information from the superior halves of visual fields in both eyes is projected onto the inferior visual cortex, and vice versa; most of the visual information from the central visual field is projected onto the posterior visual cortex, while the visual information from the peripheral visual field is projected onto the anterior visual cortex [5]. The central 10° of the visual field corresponds to at least 50–60% of the posterior visual cortex, and the central 30° of the visual field corresponds to 80% of the posterior visual cortex. The visual cortex corresponding to the centermost visual field is comparable to the visual cortex corresponding to the 50° of peripheral visual field. The magnifying effect of the visual cortex reflects the theory of biological evolution, and the central visual field is more important for the survival of living organisms.

Almost all of the visual field defects caused by occipital lobe lesions are characteristic homonymous hemianopia. The more posterior the location of the lesions, the greater the size of visual field defects. The left occipital lobe of this patient showed an infarction lesion, and her visual field defects were manifested as right inferior homonymous quadrantanopia in the central 10°. Therefore, the location of the occipital lesion was further determined to be the superior half of the left posterior visual cortex. Due to central visual field defects in both eyes, she still felt blurred vision, although her visual acuity was 20/20 in both eyes.

This case tells us that we should also pay attention to the changes in visual function when we are treating systemic diseases. Perimetry of this patient only showed small-scale homonymous hemianopia, while the imaging studies suggested a large unilateral lesion of occipital lobe infarction, although its pathogenesis is not yet fully understood. The previous section has mentioned that macular fibers are quite scattered before they terminate. They are widely located and terminate in the entire visual center. Therefore, it is difficult for a single lesion to completely destroy the region of its distribution. Therefore, in the perimetry printouts, even a relatively small and slight defect involving the central area is considered to be a significant visual field damage, because the area of lesion represented by the defect is not small at all, especially the damage to the posterior visual pathway.

The lacrimal glands are controlled by the parasympathetic fibers of the facial nerve and the sympathetic nerve fibers from the superior cervical ganglion. Emotional tearing is caused by the secretion of the lacrimal glands activated by the signal that reaches the facial nerve through the central bypass. The superior salivatory nucleus is located in the inferior part of the pons and sends out general visceral motor fibers, a part of the parasympathetic preganglionic fibers, into the major petrous nerve of the facial nerve. After neurotransmission in the pterygopalatine ganglion, the postganglionic fibers are distributed throughout the lacrimal glands, thus controlling the tear secretion of them. MRI of this patient indicated the right posterior cerebral infarction in the inferior part of the pons, which involved the right superior salivary nucleus and caused the lack of tears when the patient was crying.

Finally, it is worth mentioning that we have followed this patient for many years and hence witnessed her miraculous recovery. Although greatly injured by the disease, she maintained a healthy and optimistic attitude and undauntedly fought the disease. Starting from practicing sit-ups and walking, she is able to do strenuous exercises, such as surfing now. This is one of the most inspirational examples we have seen during long-term follow-ups, which fully demonstrates that a healthy mentality is so important for recovery from diseases.

References

1. Val-Bernal JF, Mayorga M, Garijo MF, et al. Cardiac papillary fibroelastoma: retrospective clinicopathologic study of 17 tumors with resection at a single institution and literature review. Pathol Res Pract. 2013;209(4):208–14.
2. Law KB, Phillips KRB, Cusimano RJ, et al. Multifocal "tapete" papillary fibroelastoma. J Clin Pathol. 2009;62(12):1066–70.
3. Khair T, Mazidi P, Laos LF. Cardiac papillary fibroelastoma: case report and review of the literature. Int J Cardiol. 2010;139(1):102–4.
4. Jha NK, Khouri M, Murphy DM, et al. Papillary fibro elastoma of the aortic valve—a case report and literature review. J Cardiothorac Surg. 2010;5:84.
5. Miller NR. Walsh & Hoyt's clinical neuro-ophthalmology (translated by Zhang Xiaojun, Wei Wenbin). Beijing: Science Press; 2009.

55 A Case of Spontaneously Improved Homonymous Hemianopia

Xiaobin Xie, Ning Fan, and Ningli Wang

Homogeneous hemianopia is a characteristic change of the visual field in postchiasmatic visual pathway diseases, usually caused by vascular lesion, tumor, infection and trauma, etc. In general, the brain damage is considered to be irreversible. However, the following is a case of visual field damage that improved spontaneously. The mechanism for such spontaneous improvement will be analyzed.

55.1 Case

55.1.1 Case Presentation

A 36-year-old male patient complained of a shadow in vision in both eyes for 1 week, especially obvious on the temporal side of the right eye after fatiguing work, without any accompanying discomfort, such as red eye or sore eye, blurred vision, pain upon eye movement, double vision, dizziness, headache, nausea, vomiting, or tinnitus. He denied the history of trauma, other ocular diseases, and systemic or familial diseases.

The uncorrected visual acuity (UCVA) was 20/20 OU. The intraocular pressure (IOP) was normal OU. Slit-lamp examination of his anterior segments and fundus examination were unremarkable in both eyes, with normal pupil, optic disc, retinal blood vessels, and macula (Fig. 55.1).

Standardized automated perimetry demonstrated right homonymous hemianopia with macular sparing in both eyes (Fig. 55.2).

Optical coherence tomography (OCT) scan showed normal retinal nerve fiber layer (RNFL) thickness in both eyes (Fig. 55.3) and no abnormalities in the macular fovea of either eye (Fig. 55.4).

The pattern visual evoked potential (P-VEP) showed that the latencies and amplitudes of the P100 wave were normal in both eyes (Fig. 55.5).

Magnetic resonance imaging (MRI) of head revealed no abnormalities, i.e., no occipital lobe lesions were found.

The computed tomography angiography (CTA) of the head and neck showed no abnormalities.

Routine blood tests produced normal results.

Because no cause of the visual field defects was identified, the patient was suggested to return for follow-up visits regularly. During the follow-ups, we noticed the following changes in the visual field:

X. Xie
Eye Hospital of China Academy of Chinese Medical Sciences, Beijing, China

N. Fan
Shenzhen Eye Hospital, Shenzhen University, Shenzhen, China

N. Wang (✉)
Department of Ophthalmology, Beijing Tongren Hospital, Capital Medical University, Beijing, China

N. Wang et al. (eds.), *Optic Disorders and Visual Field*, Advances in Visual Science and Eye Diseases 2, https://doi.org/10.1007/978-981-13-2502-1_55

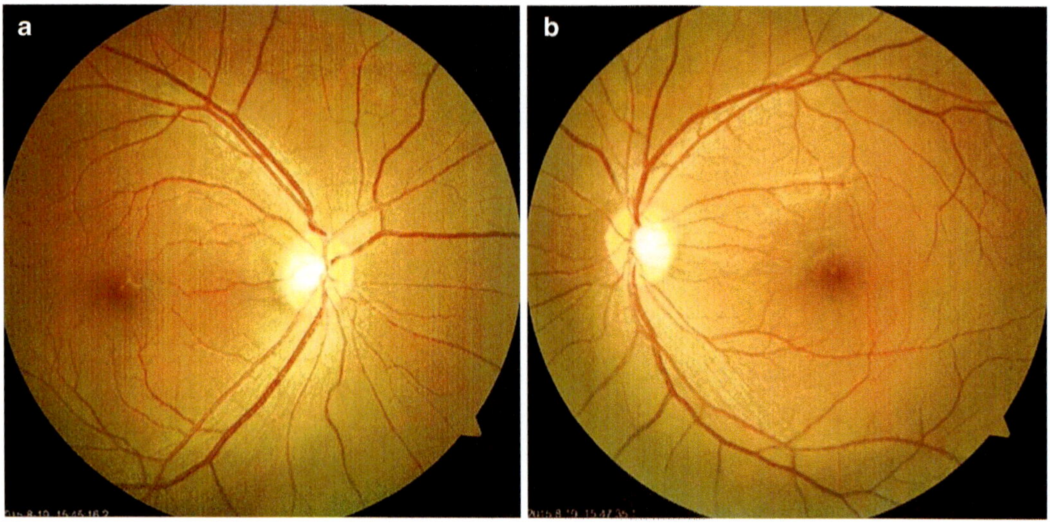

Fig. 55.1 Fundus photographs. In both eyes, the optic disc was pink with clear margin, the courses of blood vessels were normal, and the fovea reflex was noticed in both eyes. Panel a: right eye. Panel b: left eye

At the first month of follow-up, obvious reduction in the size of the visual field defect and residual right superior quadrantanopia was seen in both eyes (Fig. 55.6).

At the third month of follow-up, further reduction in the size of right superior quadrantanopia was noticed in both eyes (Fig. 55.7).

At the sixth month of follow-up, the size of right superior quadrantanopia diminished gradually in both eyes (Fig. 55.8).

At the ninth month of follow-up, the right superior quadrantanopia in the left eye improved, while the condition in the right eye was roughly the same as previously seen (Fig. 55.9).

55.1.2 Case Analysis

The visual field defects of both eyes showed such symmetrical spontaneous improvement, and visual field defects were always symmetrical in location, while the head MRI did not show lesions in the optic tracts, optic radiations, or occipital lobes. Further examinations were needed to exclude vascular lesions.

Magnetic resonance venography (MRV) of the head revealed that the left transverse sinus was relatively thin near torcular herophili, while the conditions of the superior and inferior sagittal sinuses, the two transverse sinuses, and sigmoid sinuses were good (Fig. 55.10).

Therefore, we speculated that venous edema was triggered in the corresponding tissues of the left occipital lobe due to the stenosis in the left transverse sinus and the consequent obstruction of the venous drainage from the left occipital lobe into the transverse sinus, thus causing the corresponding visual field defects. With the establishment of collateral circulation, venous drainage was improved and the visual field defects gradually ameliorated.

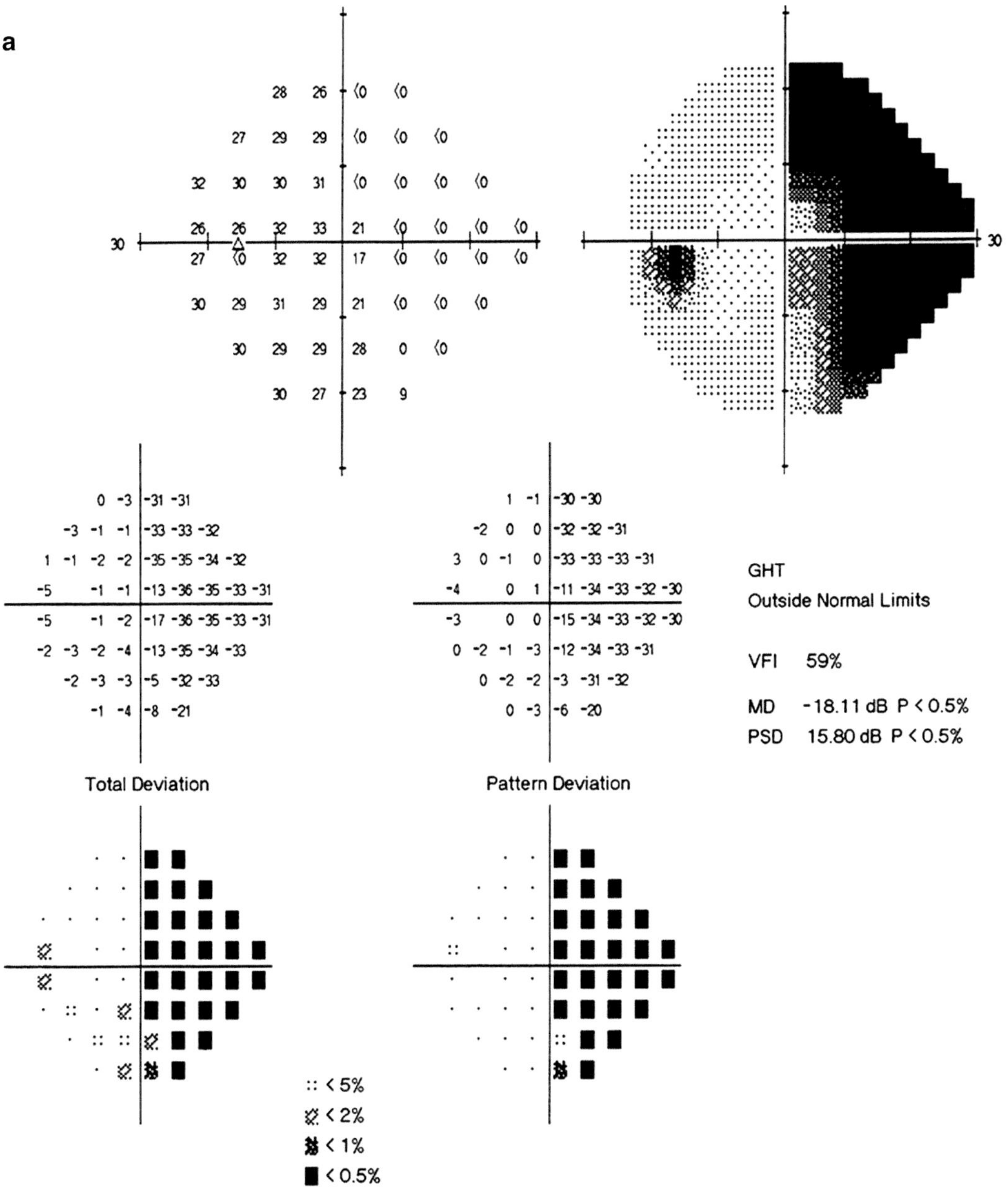

Fig. 55.2 Humphrey visual field analysis printouts (1 week after onset). 24-2 test demonstrated right homonymous hemianopia with macular sparing in both eyes. Panel a: left eye. Panel b: right eye

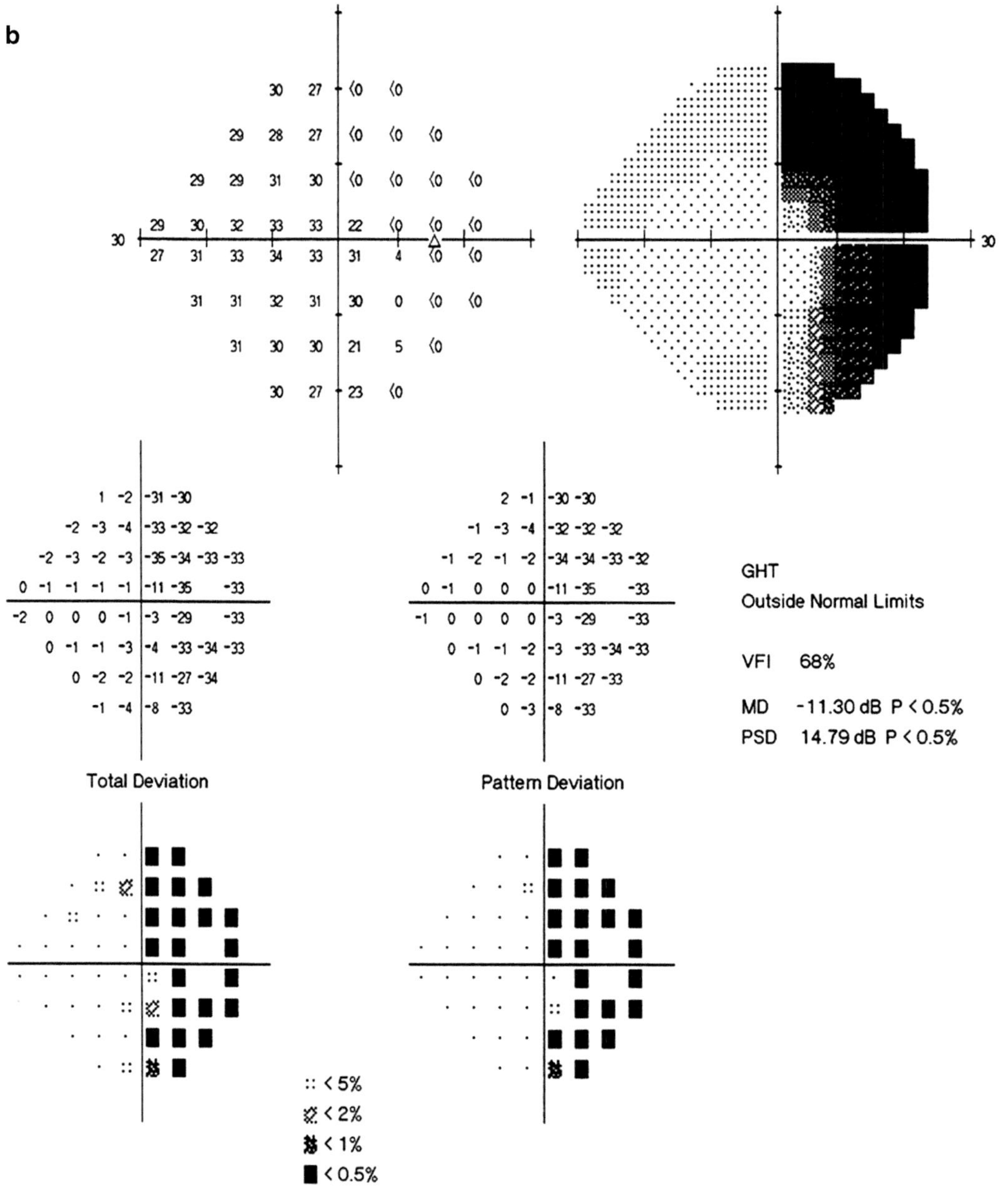

Fig. 55.2 (continued)

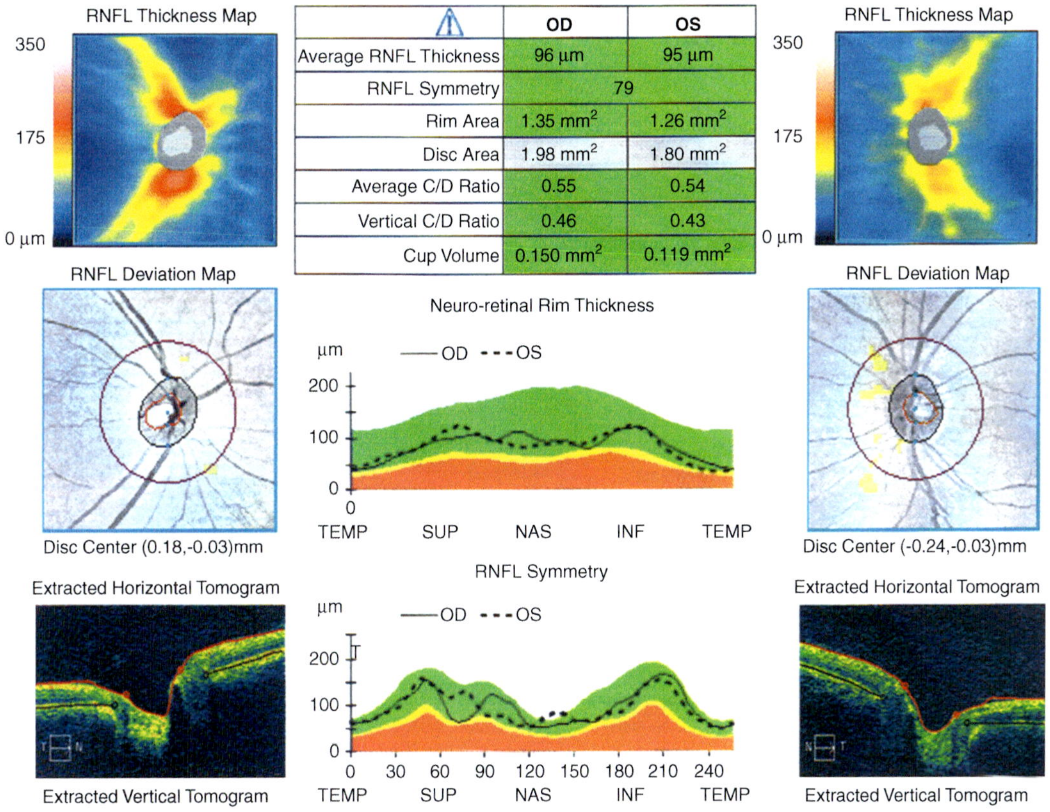

Fig. 55.3 RNFL thickness analysis printout in OCT. The peripapillary RNFL thickness was normal in both eyes

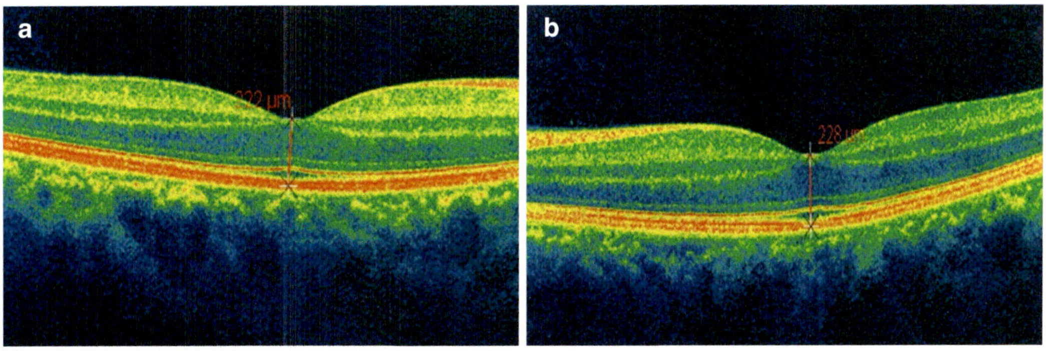

Fig. 55.4 Macula analysis printouts in OCT. The images showed normal macula in both eyes. Panel a: right eye. Panel b: left eye

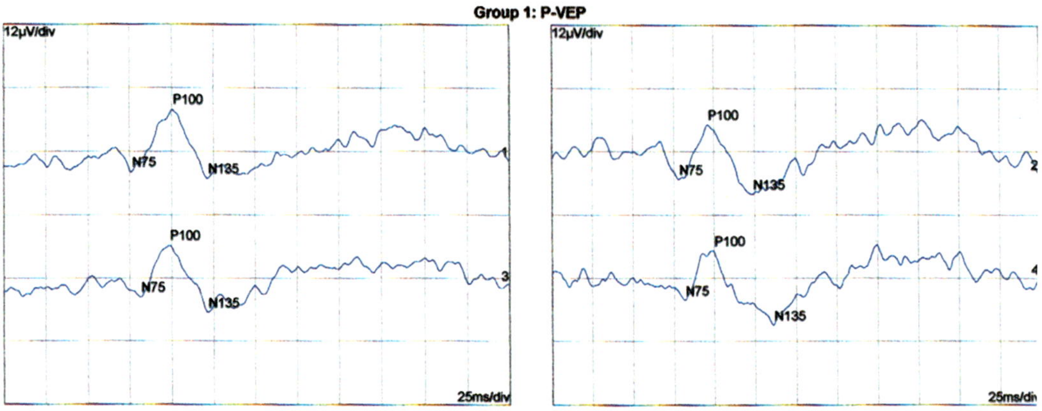

Diagnostic data:

Channel	N75 [ms]	P100 [ms]	N135 [ms]	N75-P100	P100-N135
1 right P-VEP	76	100	121	12.4µV	13.6µV
2 right P-VEP	78	96	124	10.9µV	13.8µV
3 left P-VEP	81	98	121	10.3µV	13.4µV
4 left P-VEP	81	100	136	9.87µV	14.9µV

Test parameter:

Channel	Stimulus	Ampl., Range, Filter
1 right P-VEP	Patt. Rev. CB, 1° Full Field, Ctr:97% 1.5Hz, Avg:100	1, +/-100µV 1-100Hz
2 right P-VEP	Patt. Rev. CB, 0°31' Full Field, Ctr:97% 1.5Hz, Avg:100	1, +/-100µV 1-100Hz
3 left P-VEP	Patt. Rev. CB, 1° Full Field, Ctr:97% 1.5Hz, Avg:100	1, +/-100µV 1-100Hz
4 left P-VEP	Patt. Rev. CB, 0°31' Full Field, Ctr:97% 1.5Hz, Avg:100	1, +/-100µV 1-100Hz

Fig. 55.5 P-VEP examination printout. The waveform, amplitude, and latency values of P100 were normal in both eyes

55.1.3 Final Diagnosis

The final diagnosis was left transverse sinus stenosis and possible left occipital lobe lesions.

55.1.4 Case Review

In this case, the head MRV showed conspicuous stenosis of the left transverse sinus, which was considered to be due to congenital dysplasia. When the patient was in fatigue or psychological stress, the induced hypercoagulability of the blood caused local occlusion of venous drainage in the non-dominant transverse sinus, thus resulting in venous edema of corresponding brain tissue and special bilateral visual field defects; according to the characteristics of such visual field defects, it was speculated that the damaged brain tissue was in the left occipital lobe, especially in the lingual gyrus. Due to the presence and compensation from collateral circulation, vein drainage disturbance was gradually alleviated, and the temporary edema of the brain tissue was also ameliorated, thus causing the "gradual spontaneous improvement" of the visual field defects. Vein drainage disturbance occurred in the non-dominant

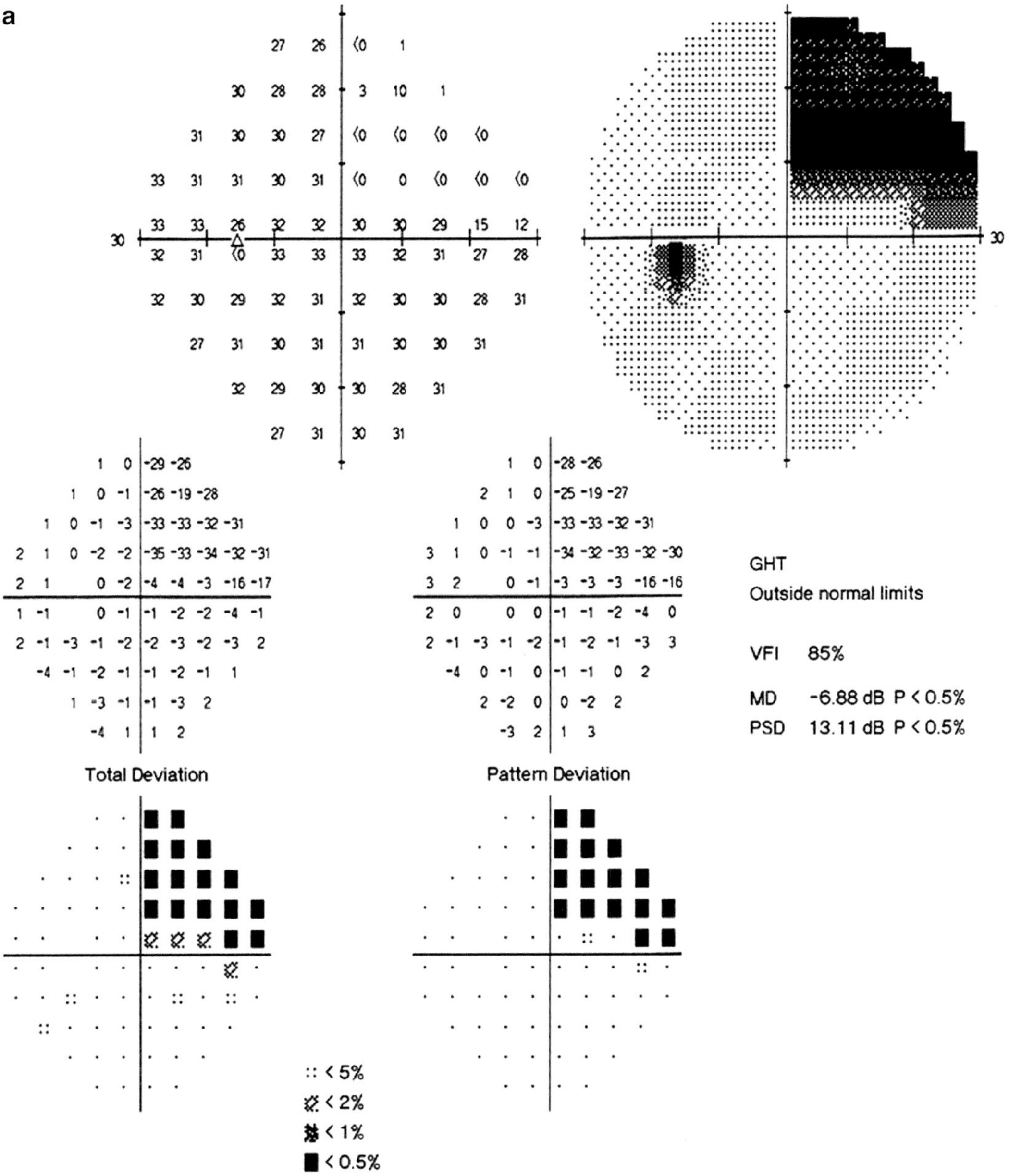

Fig. 55.6 Humphrey visual field analysis printouts (1 month after onset). 30-2 test demonstrated right superior quadrantanopia in both eyes. Panel a: left eye. Panel b: right eye

b

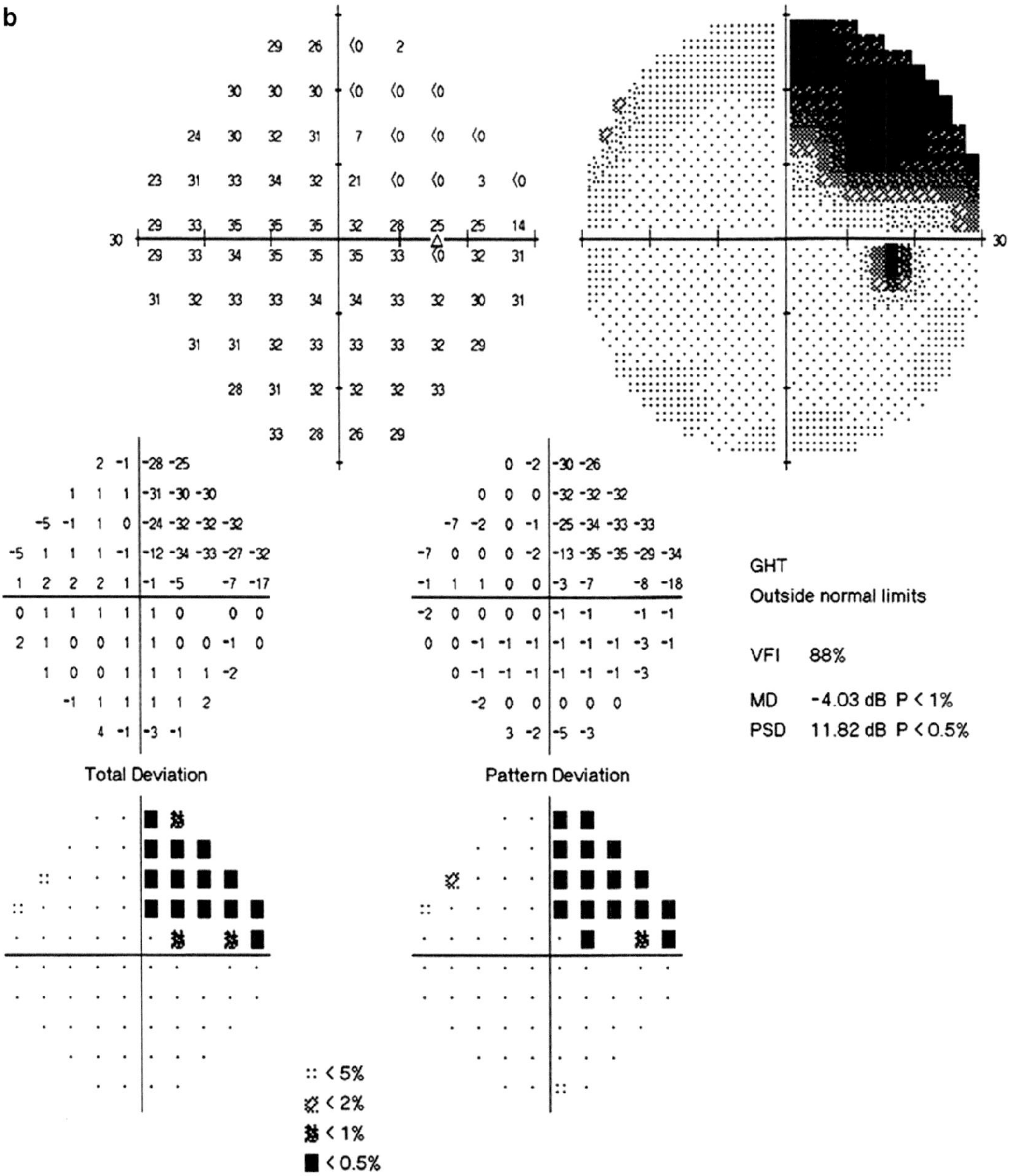

Fig. 55.6 (continued)

a

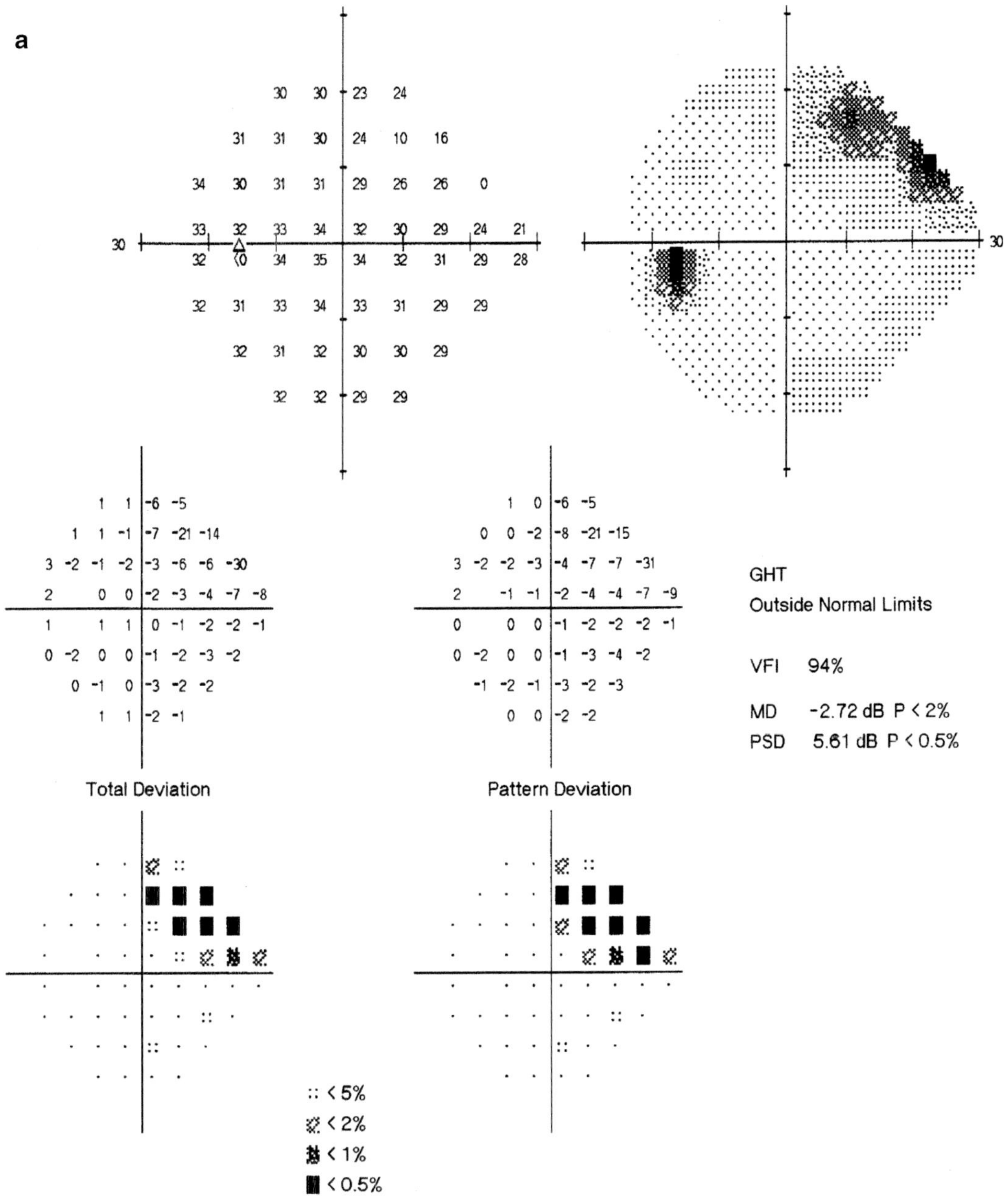

Fig. 55.7 Humphrey visual field analysis printouts (3 months after onset). 24-2 test demonstrated that the size of right superior quadrantanopia decreased in both eyes. Panel a: left eye. Panel b: right eye

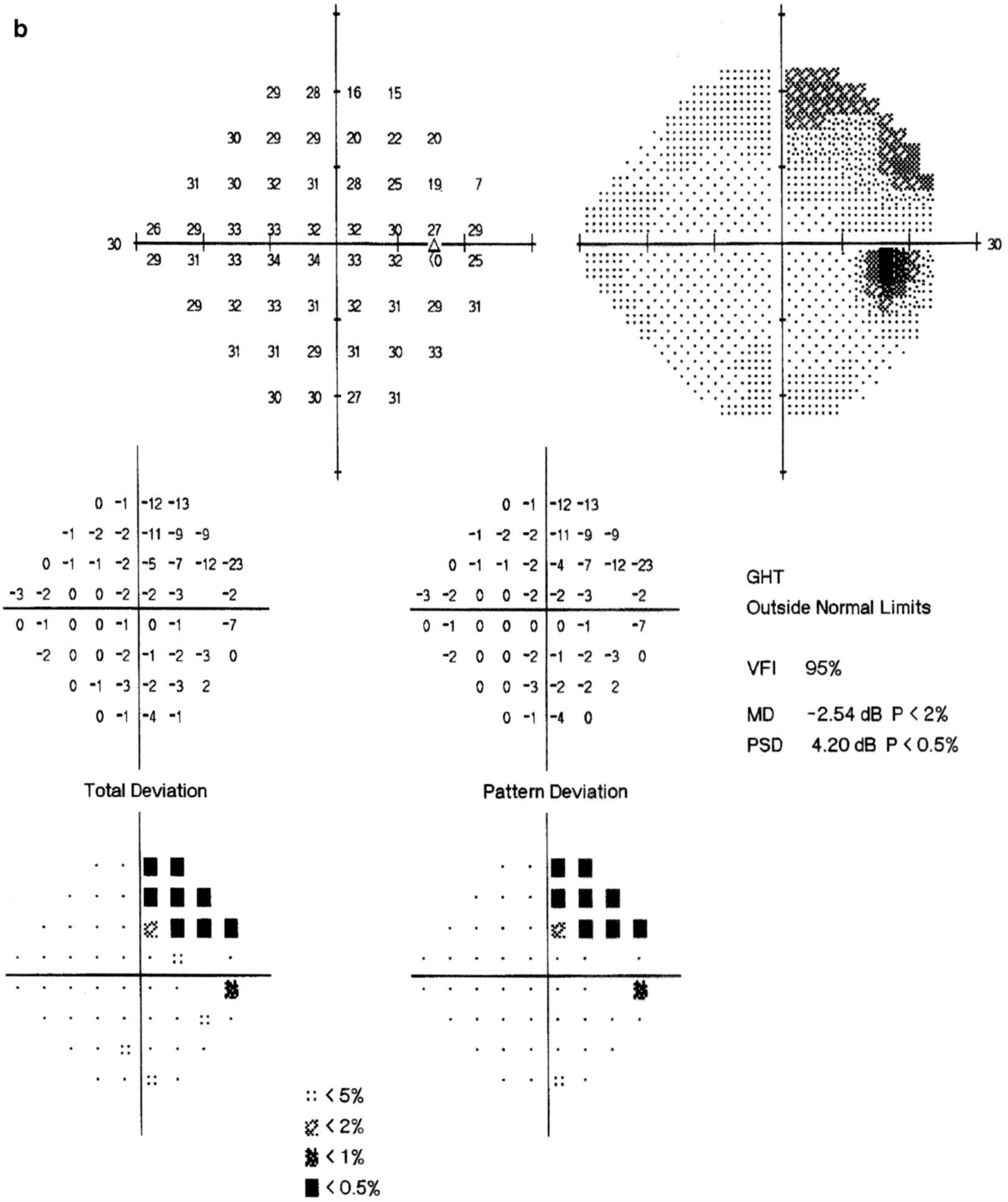

Fig. 55.7 (continued)

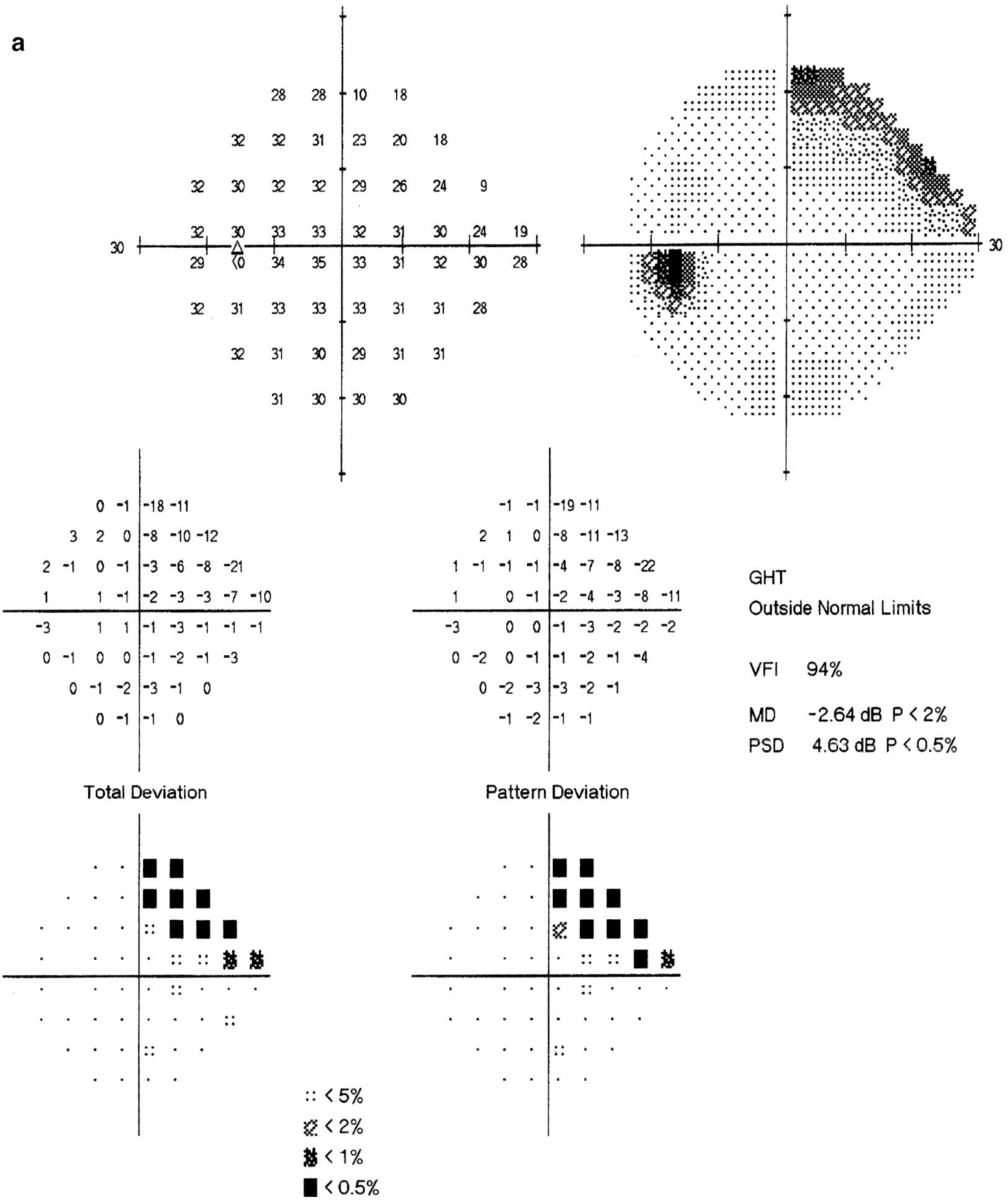

Fig. 55.8 Humphrey visual field analysis printouts (6 months after onset). 24-2 test demonstrated that the size of right superior quadrantanopia diminished gradually in both eyes. Panel a: left eye. Panel b: right eye

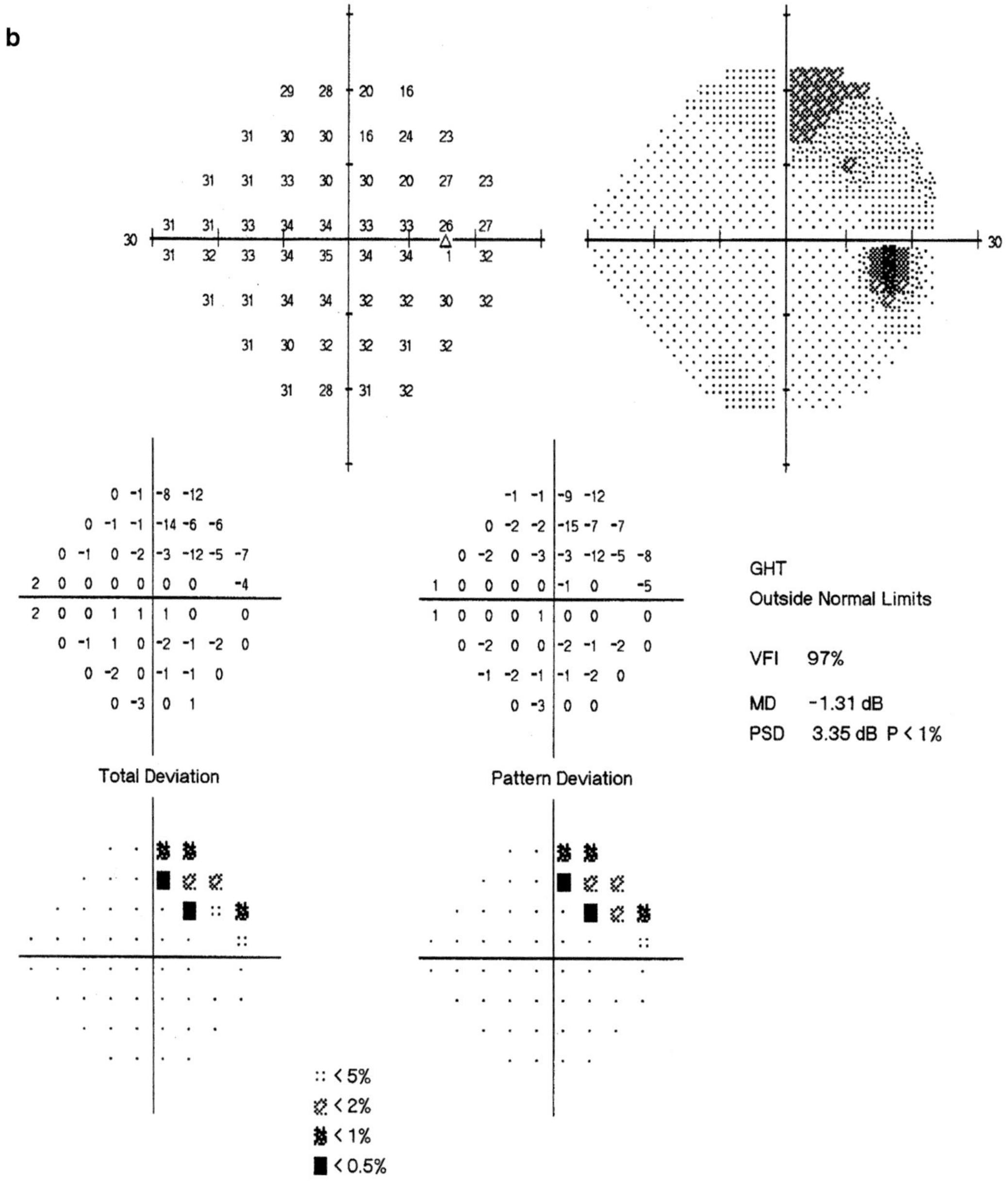

Fig. 55.8 (continued)

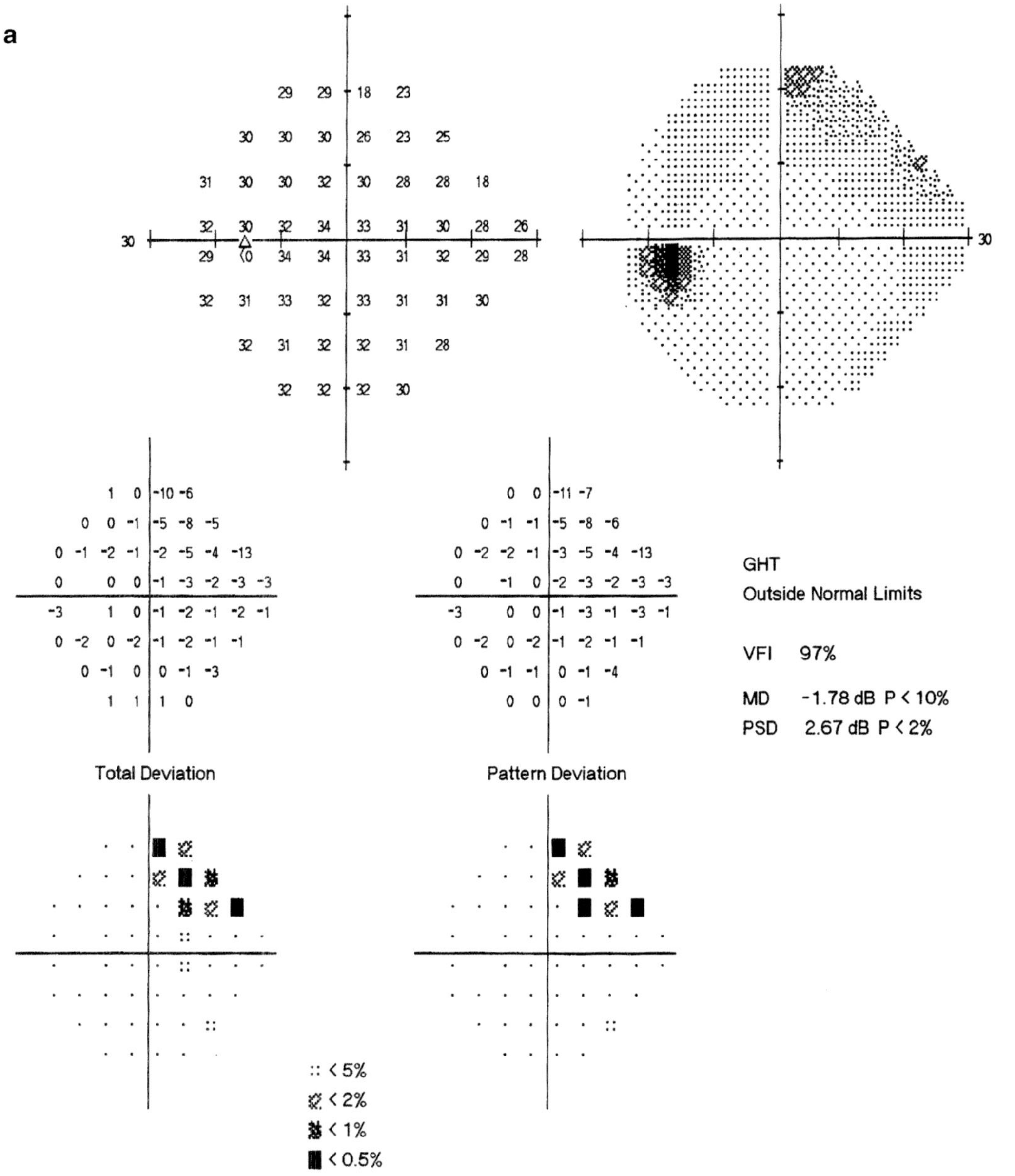

Fig. 55.9 Humphrey visual field analysis printouts (9 months after onset). 24-2 test demonstrated that the right superior quadrantanopia in the left eye improved, while the condition in the right eye was roughly the same as that observed 3 months before. Panel a: left eye. Panel b: right eye

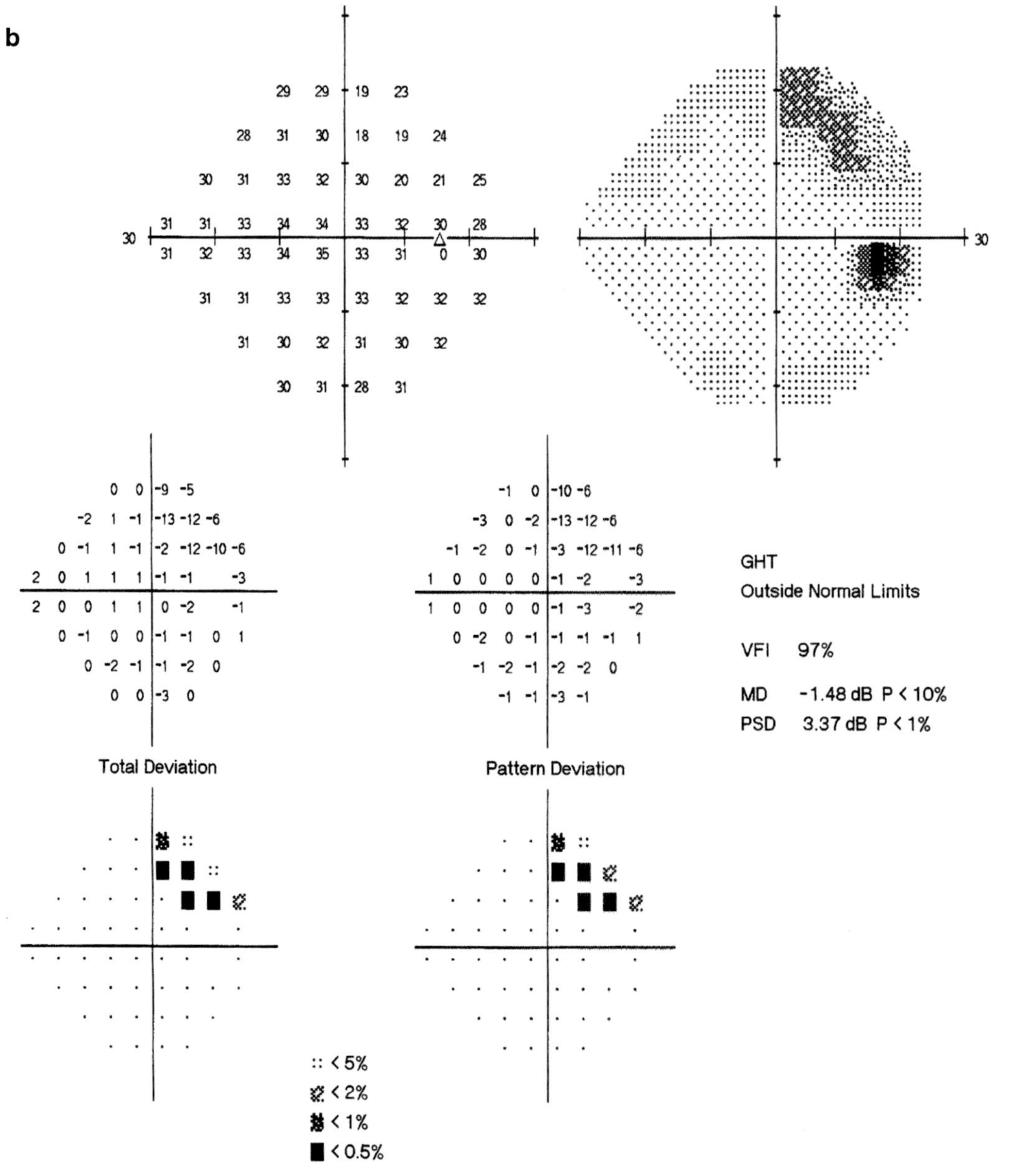

Fig. 55.9 (continued)

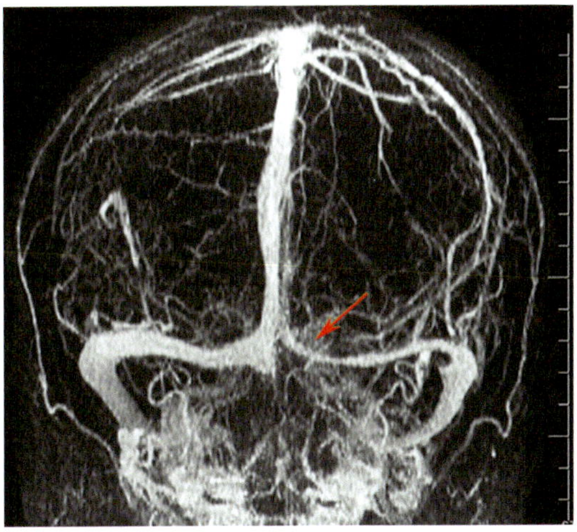

Fig. 55.10 Head MRV image in coronal view. The left transverse sinus was relatively thin near the torcular herophili (red arrow), while the conditions of the superior and inferior sagittal sinuses, the two transverse sinuses, and sigmoid sinuses were good

transverse sinus, so the symptoms from the lesions in the dominant transverse sinus did not appear.

55.2 Discussion

Homonymous hemianopia caused by lesions of cerebral venous sinuses has not been reported yet.

There are a large number of veins in the head and face. The venous blood is drained into the internal jugular vein through venous sinuses and finally into the right atrium. Cerebral sinuses, also known as dural sinuses, are cavities between the duras or between the dura and the internal lamina of the skull. They include the transverse sinuses, sigmoid sinuses, superior and inferior sagittal sinuses, and straight sinuses [1].

The physiological functions of the transverse sinuses include the following: (a) drainage of the cerebral venous blood to the right atrium and (b) regulation of the intracranial pressure. The subendothelial layer of the transverse sinuses has smooth muscle cells. Therefore, the intracranial volume can be regulated through the contraction and relaxation of the smooth muscle as well as the siphon effect created by the intracranial veins. Drainage via the dominant transverse sinus is seen in some normal individuals, whose right transverse sinus is bigger than the left one in the development. However, because of the existence of collateral circulation, it does not affect the intracranial venous drainage [2].

There are many reasons for transverse sinuses stenosis, including congenital dysplasia, trauma, arachnoiditis, cancer, etc. [3]. When stenosis occurs in the dominant transverse sinus, its common complications include venous stasis, cerebral edema, elevated intracranial pressure, sinus thrombosis, and in severe cases, cerebral infarction or hemorrhage, which may produce some common symptoms, such as refractory headache, vomiting, pulsatile tinnitus, optic disc edema, visual impairment and abducens paralysis, etc.

In this case, although the presence of right hemianopia and its spontaneous improvement may be explained by the stenosis of the left transverse sinus, the detailed mechanism still needs to be explored. We have consulted with neurosurgeons and administered patients with oral aspirin treatment, and the changes in the visual field will be monitored through follow-up observation.

References

1. Park HK, Bae HG, Choi SK, et al. Morphological study of sinus flow in the confluence of sinuses. Clin Anat. 2008;21(4):294–300.
2. Li B, Liang Y, Cao X, et al. Discussion on the imaging anatomy characteristics of cerebral sinus stenosis and its clinical diagnosis and treatment. Natl Med J China. 2015;95(43):3505–8.
3. Sultan AE, Hassan T. Infantile dural arteriovenous fistula of the transverse sinus presenting with ocular symptoms, case reports and review of literature. J Korean Neurosurg Soc. 2016;59(3):296–301.

56 Schizencephaly and Homonymous Hemianopia

Xiaobin Xie, Ning Fan, and Ningli Wang

Schizencephaly is a congenital craniocerebral deformity caused by neuronal migration disorders, possibly involving the frontal, frontoparietal, parieto-occipital, and temporal lobes. There will be characteristic visual field changes when the temporal or parietal lobe is involved.

56.1 Case

56.1.1 Case Presentation

A 28-year-old male patient had suffered poor vision in the left eye since childhood. He had not experienced red eye or sore eyes, visual distortion, fixed shadow, or other discomforts and had not received any diagnosis and treatment. The patient had never worn glasses. He began to have recurrent convulsion of the limbs and unconsciousness from the age of 12. The symptoms were improved after antiepileptic therapy, but the patient did not take medications regularly. There is no history of trauma or other diseases, including familial diseases.

The uncorrected visual acuity (UCVA) was 20/33 OD and 20/400 OS. The best corrected visual acuity (BCVA) was 20/40 OD with refractive correction (−3.00DS) and 20/125 OS with refractive correction (−9.00DS−1.25DC*25). The intraocular pressure (IOP) was normal OU. Slit-lamp examination of his anterior segments in both eyes was unremarkable, with sensitive direct and indirect light reflexes of both pupils. In fundus examination, the optic disc was pale in color and the cup-to-disc ratio (C/D) was 0.8 in both eyes, and a giant atrophy area was seen temporal to the optic disc in the left eye (Fig. 56.1). There were no other abnormalities.

Standardized automated perimetry demonstrated left homonymous hemianopia in both eyes. The defect in the left eye extended across the vertical midline (Fig. 56.2).

The pattern visual evoked potential (P-VEP) revealed that the latency of the P100 wave was prolonged.

Magnetic resonance imaging (MRI) in axial view of the head showed schizencephaly in the right temporal lobe in a shape of open lip accompanied by ectopic gray matter (Fig. 56.3).

X. Xie
Eye Hospital of China Academy of Chinese Medical Sciences, Beijing, China

N. Fan
Shenzhen Eye Hospital, Shenzhen University, Shenzhen, China

N. Wang (✉)
Department of Ophthalmology, Beijing Tongren Hospital, Capital Medical University, Beijing, China

N. Wang et al. (eds.), *Optic Disorders and Visual Field*, Advances in Visual Science and Eye Diseases 2, https://doi.org/10.1007/978-981-13-2502-1_56

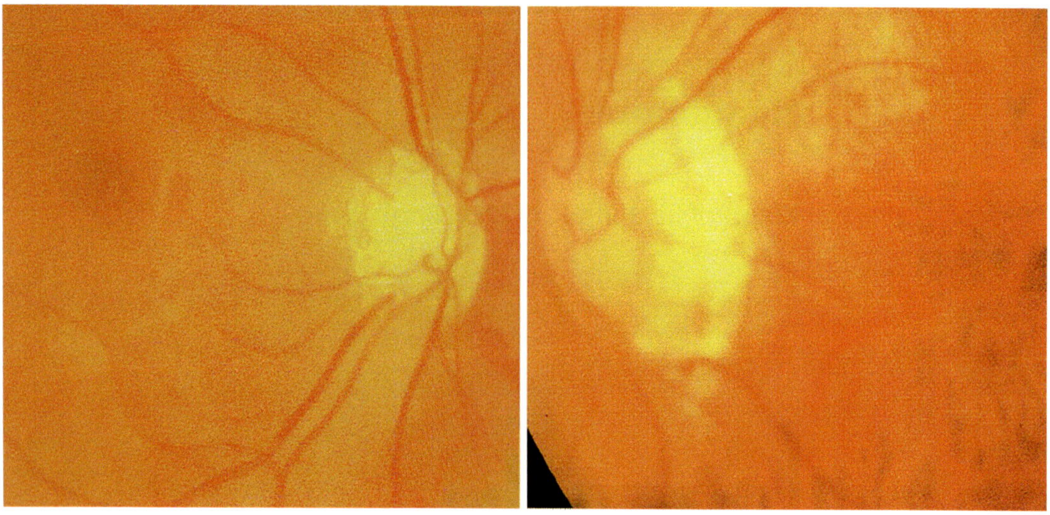

Fig. 56.1 Fundus photographs. The optic disc was pale in color with a C/D ratio of 0.8 in both eyes. A giant atrophy area was seen temporal to the left optic disc

Furthermore, there was an absence of septum pellucidum, right hippocampus atrophy and sclerosis, and a few lesions of demyelination in white matter in head MRI (Fig. 56.4).

56.1.2 Final Diagnosis

The final diagnosis was right schizencephaly.

56.1.3 Case Review

The lesions of posterior visual pathway often lead to characteristic visual field defects. The occurrence of schizencephaly often leads to the rupture of the nerve fibers in the posterior visual pathway and then the characteristic visual field defects. Depending on the involved region of the optic tract, there may be different changes in the visual fields in the two eyes. For example, schizencephaly involving the entire optic radiation at the posterior limb of internal capsule induces homonymous hemianopia, schizencephaly involving the temporal lobe at the inferior part of the optic radiation induces homonymous superior quadrantanopia, and schizencephaly involving the parietal lobe at the superior part of the optic radiation induces homonymous inferior quadrantanopia. The patient's head MRI showed schizencephaly of the right temporal lobe in a shape of open lip with ectopic gray matter, and perimetry presented typical left homonymous hemianopia due to the rupture of nerve fibers in the optic radiation caused by schizencephaly.

56.2 Discussion

Schizencephaly, first reported by Yakovlev and Wadsworth in 1946, refers to a fissure lined with gray matter involving the full thickness of one or both cerebral hemisphere(s). Gray matter at the edge of the fissure is abnormal and composed of multiple cerebellar gyri. It may be accompanied by ectopic gray matter and is a congenital neuronal migration dysplasia [1]. Forty-four percent of them were found in the frontal lobe, 30% in the frontoparietal lobe, 19% in the parieto-occipital lobe, 7% in the temporal lobes alone, and 35% were bilateral. The etiology of this disease has not yet been completely elucidated, and it is presumably induced by the damage to the embryonic stroma in the seventh week of pregnancy. It is known that the neurons in the cerebral cortex come from the neural tube epithelium of the ventricular wall during the embryonic period. If the neurons are disturbed during migration or the germinal stroma layers cannot develop normally, the neuronal migration will be blocked or stopped prematurely. The involved cortex often shows thickening and disorders of neuronal arrangement, i.e., abnormal accumulation of neurons whose migration stops, thus leading to schizencephaly and loss of cells that can normally migrate to the cortex [2]. Its typical cases often manifest epileptic seizures, while other neurological symptoms vary with the

a

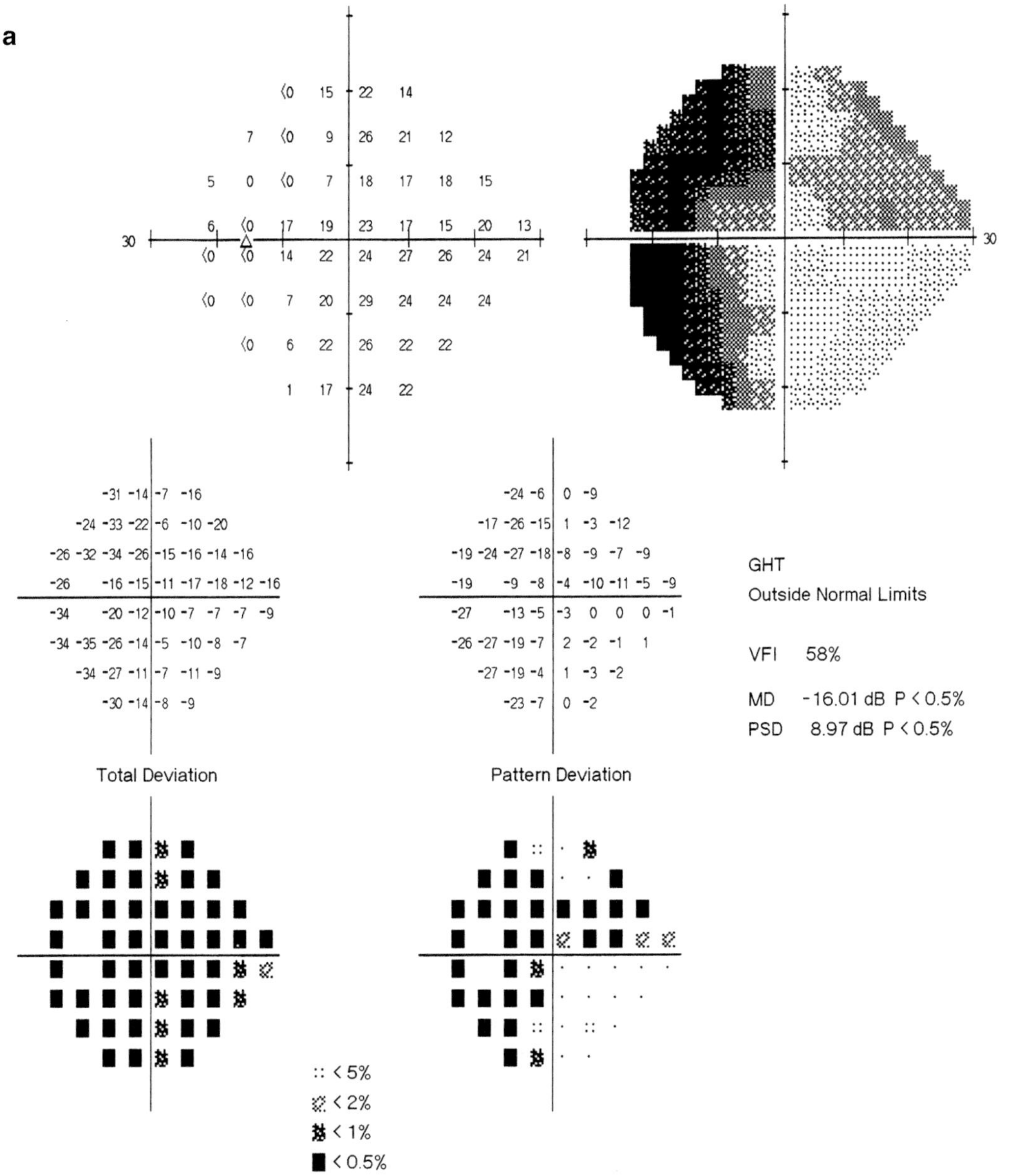

Fig. 56.2 Humphrey visual field analysis printouts. 24-2 test demonstrated left homonymous hemianopia in both eyes, with the defect in the left eye extending across the vertical midline. Panel a: left eye. Panel b: right eye

b

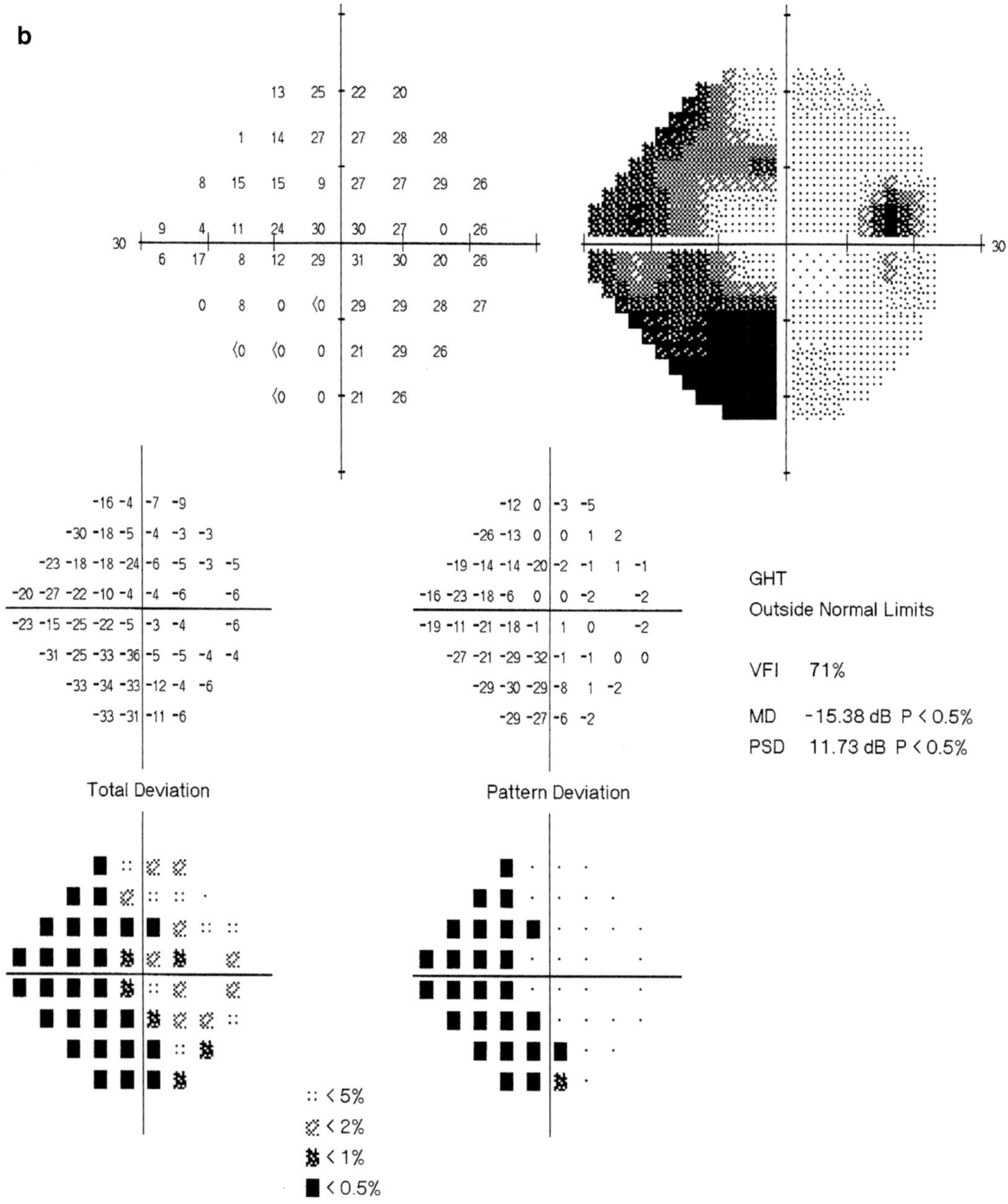

Fig. 56.2 (continued)

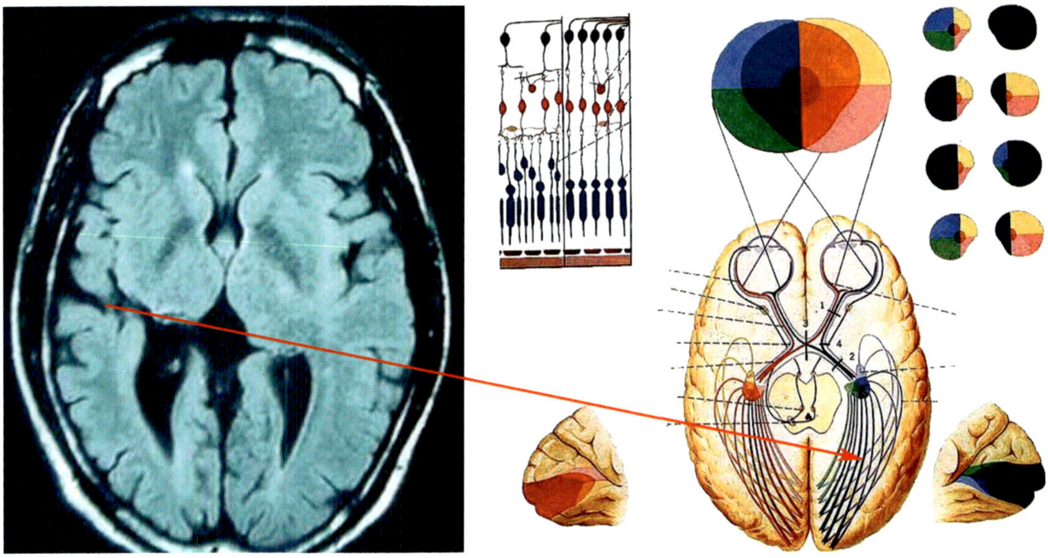

Fig. 56.3 Head MRI image in axial view and lesion localization. Schizencephaly with ectopic gray matter in a shape of open lip was found in the right temporal lobe

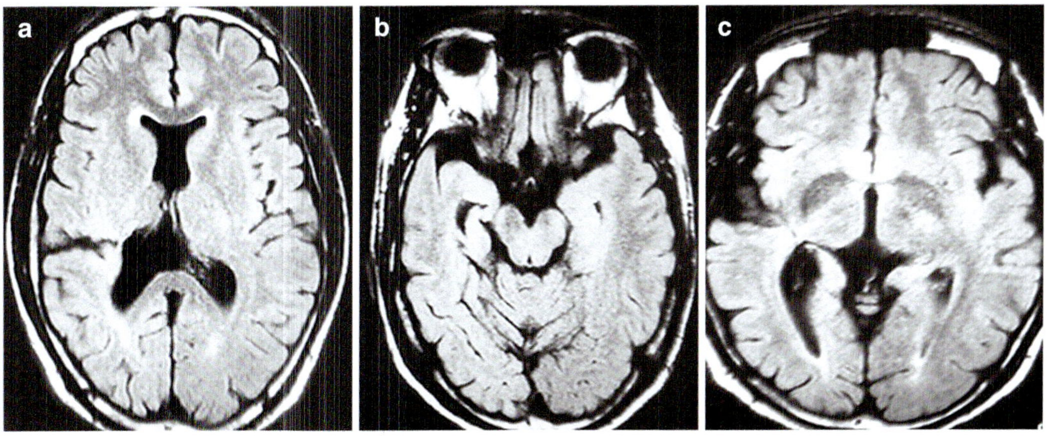

Fig. 56.4 Head MRI images in axial view. Panel a: absence of septum pellucidum. Panel b: right hippocampus atrophy and sclerosis. Panel c: a few lesions of demyelination in white matter

disease condition and the severity of the rupture in the defected brain tissue.

The epilepsy in this case disappeared after the patient entered adulthood. The lesions mainly involved the visual pathway, and the patient's schizencephaly was presumably mild. The optic disc dysplasia of the patient may be related to it.

References

1. Wang H. Modern neurophthalmology. Beijing: People's Medical Publishing House; 2005.
2. Granata T, Freri E, Caccia C, et al. Schizencephaly: clinical spectrum, epilepsy, and pathogenesis. J Child Neurol. 2005;20(4):313–8.

A Case of False Foster-Kennedy Syndrome

57

Xiaobin Xie, Ning Fan, and Ningli Wang

The etiology of Foster-Kennedy syndrome, also known as Kennedy's syndrome or basilar frontal lobe syndrome, involves space-occupying lesions at the basilar part of the frontal lobe, such as abscess, hemangioma, meningioma of the sphenoid ridge, carotid atherosclerosis, arachnoiditis, and brain trauma. In typical Foster-Kennedy syndrome cases, unilateral tumor in the anterior cranial fossa compresses the ipsilateral optic nerve, resulting in ipsilateral optic atrophy, and meanwhile space-occupying lesions induce intracranial hypertension, leading to contralateral optic disc edema. The patient in the case below suffered from Foster-Kennedy syndrome with optic disc edema in one eye and a pale optic disc in the other. What is the mechanism behind this condition?

X. Xie
Eye Hospital of China Academy of Chinese Medical Sciences, Beijing, China

N. Fan
Shenzhen Eye Hospital, Shenzhen University, Shenzhen, China

N. Wang (✉)
Department of Ophthalmology, Beijing Tongren Hospital, Capital Medical University, Beijing, China

57.1 Case

57.1.1 Case Presentation

A 46-year-old male patient complained of decreased vision in his left eye for more than 1 year.

He had developed decreased vision in his left eye without any trigger 1 year before, without any discomforts such as red eye, sore eye, and visual distortion and had received no diagnosis or treatment. The history of trauma, other ocular diseases, and systemic or familial diseases was denied.

The uncorrected visual acuity (UCVA) was 20/66 OD and 20/400 OS, and the best corrected visual acuity (BCVA) was 0.9 OD with refractive correction (+4.00DS) and 20/50 OS with refractive correction (+4.50DS). The intraocular pressure (IOP) measured by standard Goldmann applanation tonometry was 17 mmHg OD, 15 mmHg OS. Slit-lamp examination of his anterior segments was normal in both eyes except for the slow direct light reflex in the left pupil with a diameter of 4 mm. Fundus examination showed that the right optic disc was pink with unclear raised margin and edema, while the left optic disc was pale in color with clear margin, and star-like exudate was seen in the left macula (Fig. 57.1).

Standardized automated perimetry demonstrated residual central tubular visual field in the

N. Wang et al. (eds.), *Optic Disorders and Visual Field*, Advances in Visual Science and Eye Diseases 2, https://doi.org/10.1007/978-981-13-2502-1_57

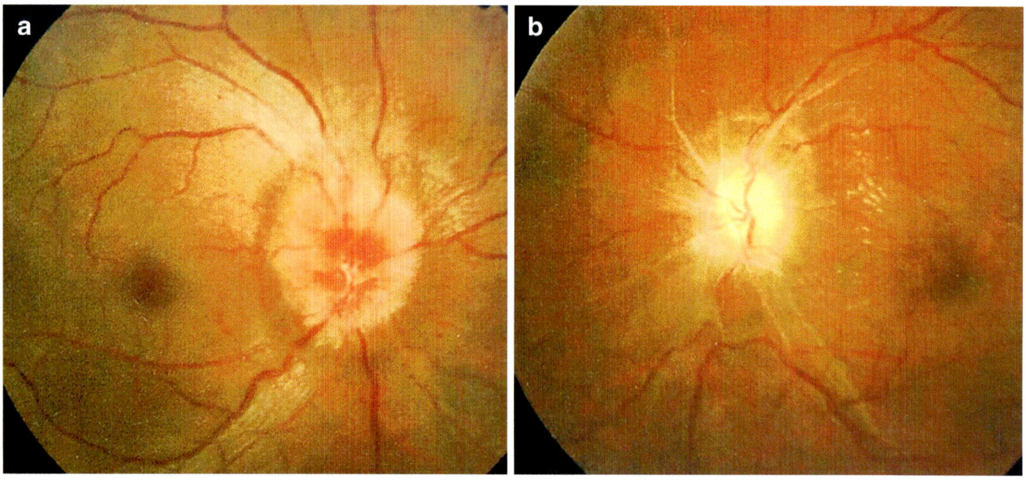

Fig. 57.1 Fundus photographs. Panel a: right eye, the optic disc was pink with unclear raised margin and showed edema. Panel b: left eye, the optic disc was pale in color with clear margin, and star-like exudate was seen in the macula

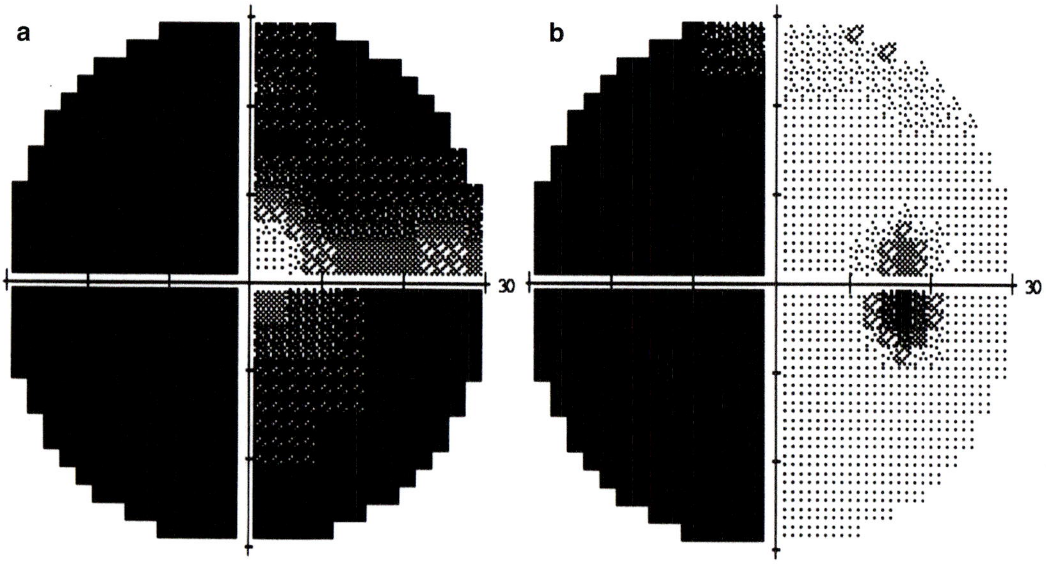

Fig. 57.2 Grayscale maps in Humphrey visual field. Panel a: residual central tubular visual field in the left eye. Panel b: nasal hemianopia in the right eye

left eye and nasal hemianopia in the right eye (Fig. 57.2).

Magnetic resonance imaging (MRI) in axial view of the head showed an irregular massive space-occupying lesion (7.7 cm × 7.1 cm × 6.2 cm) above the right tentorium with quite a lot of blood vessels in it. The right temporal lobe, insula, and midbrain were compressed. Based on these findings, huge right tentorial meningioma was suspected, which might compress the right optic radiation and lead to the above visual field defects (Fig. 57.3).

57.1.2 Case Analysis

According to the patient's visual field, the possibility of space-occupying lesions was pretty high.

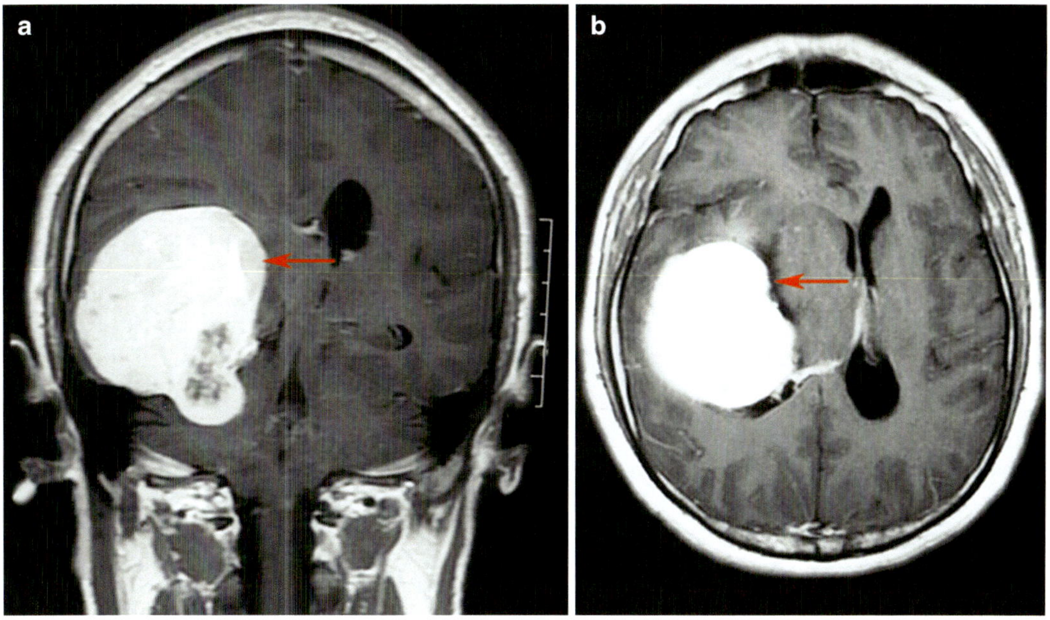

Fig. 57.3 Head MRI images. There was an irregular massive space-occupying lesion above the right tentorium with quite a lot of blood vessels in it (7.7 cm × 7.1 cm × 6.2 cm) (arrow), which compressed the right temporal lobe, insula, and midbrain. Panel a: coronal view. Panel b: axial view

MRI images showed an irregular massive space-occupying lesion on the right tentorium with quite a lot of blood vessels in it. The right temporal lobe, insula, and midbrain were compressed. Our preliminary consideration was that the meningioma on the right tentorium compressed the optic radiation and leaded to visual field defects.

The tumor was located in the right middle cranial fossa and involved the right optic radiation. So the visual field should exhibit left hemianopia, but this patient also showed nasal hemianopia in the left eye additionally, which was obviously related to the pale optic disc and optic atrophy in the left eye.

The patient mainly complained of decreased vision in the left eye. It was suspected that the left eye suffered from the previous optic nerve disease leading to optic atrophy according to the manifestations in the left fundus. In addition, the extent of the nasal visual field defect was inconsistent with that of the temporal one (the left eye part of the homonymous hemianopia) in the left eye. The former was less severe.

Therefore, there was optic disc edema in the right eye because of the intracranial hypertension resulting from the giant space-occupying lesion in the right middle cranial fossa, whereas there was no optic disc edema in the left eye due to the previous optic atrophy. The fundus manifestations of both eyes were similar to those in Foster-Kennedy syndrome. However, their pathological mechanisms are completely different.

If the patient did not have any intracranial tumor, his visual fields might present themselves as follows (Fig. 57.4).

57.1.3 Final Diagnosis

The final diagnosis was right tentorial meningioma, left optic atrophy, and right optic disc edema.

57.2 Discussion

In a typical case of Foster-Kennedy syndrome, unilateral tumor in the anterior cranial fossa compresses the ipsilateral optic nerves, resulting in ipsilateral optic atrophy, and meanwhile intracra-

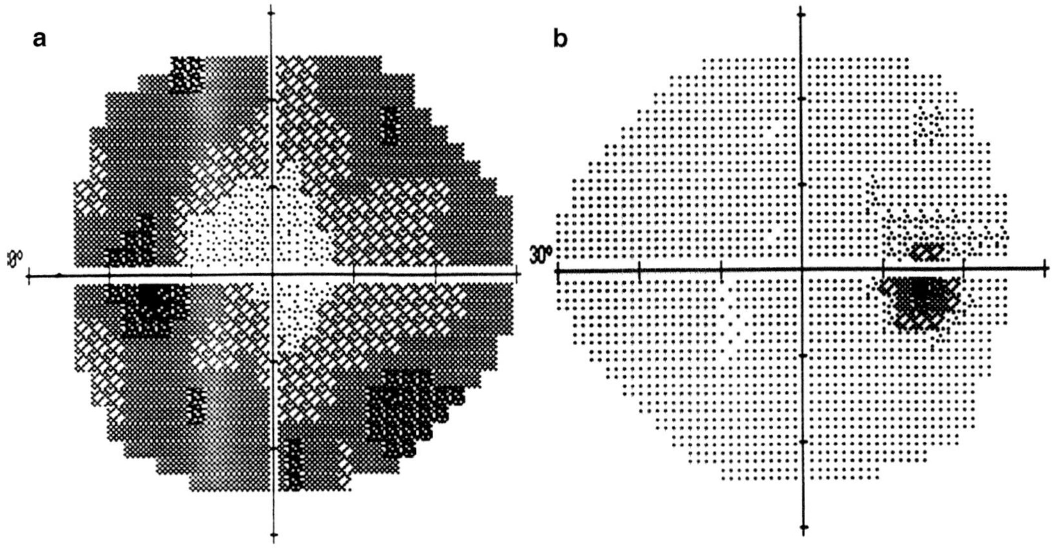

Fig. 57.4 Hypothetical grayscale maps of the visual fields. The possible manifestations of the visual fields if the patient had no intracranial tumor. Panel a: left eye. Panel b: right eye

nial hypertension induced by the huge tumor leads to contralateral optic disc edema [1]. In the present case of "Foster-Kennedy syndrome," the optic disc edema in one eye and the optic atrophy in the other were caused by a huge space-occupying lesion in the middle cranial fossa that compressed the optic radiation and induced homonymous hemianopia and intracranial hypertension. The left optic disc did not show edema due to the presence of optic atrophy, while the right disc showed edema due to intracranial hypertension.

When a patient shows homonymous hemianopia accompanied by total blindness in one eye, the possible ocular diseases and intracranial lesions should be carefully analyzed, and the relationship between them should be explored [2].

References

1. Acebes X, Arruga J, Acebes JJ, et al. Intracranial meningiomatosis causing Foster Kennedy syndrome by unilateral optic nerve compression and blockage of the superior sagittal sinus. J Neuroophthalmol. 2009;29(2):140–2.
2. Bansal S, Dabbs T, Long V. Pseudo-Foster Kennedy syndrome due to unilateral optic nerve hypoplasia: a case report. J Med Case Rep. 2008;2(1):1–2.

Retrograde Transneuronal Injury: From the Posterior Optic Pathway to Retinal Ganglion Cells

58

Xiaobin Xie, Ning Fan, and Ningli Wang

Retrograde transneuronal injury refers to damage from superior neurons to their inferior neurons across synapse retrogradely in the course of the nerve conduction pathway. Common pathological changes are those lesions in the lateral geniculate body (LGB), mainly including the vascular lesions, tumor, infections, and trauma on the occipital or temporal lobes, which may lead to damage to the retinal ganglion cells (RGCs) and their axons (nerve fibers). In this section, we will describe two cases and tentatively explore the mechanism.

58.1 Case 1

58.1.1 Case Presentation

A 32-year-old female patient complained of blurred vision in both eyes for 6 months after the temporal lobe meningioma excision. She had neither accompanying symptoms including visual distortion, red eye, and sore eye nor discomforts such as headache, nausea, and vomiting. Three months before, the patient had been found with left hemianopia in both eyes during the visual field test. She had been given neurotrophic drugs for improving microcirculation. The history of trauma, other ocular diseases, and systemic diseases was denied.

The uncorrected visual acuity (UCVA) was 20/20 OU. The intraocular pressure (IOP) was normal OU. Slit-lamp examination of her anterior segments was unremarkable in both eyes, with sensitive direct light reflexes of both pupils. Fundus examination revealed that the optic disc was pale in color with clear margin in both eyes, and many vascular branches were distributed above the right optic disc, while macula fovea reflection was present in both eyes (Fig. 58.1).

Standardized automated perimetry demonstrated left homonymous hemianopia that partially extended across the vertical midlines, more severe in the left eye (3 months after the onset, Fig. 58.2).

Optical coherence tomography (OCT) scan of the ganglion cell layer (GCL) thickness at the macula showed that, bounded by a vertical midline through the macular fovea, GCL thickness of the temporal retina at the right macula and GCL thickness of the nasal retina at the left macula decreased significantly (Fig. 58.3).

X. Xie
Eye Hospital of China Academy of Chinese Medical Sciences, Beijing, China

N. Fan
Shenzhen Eye Hospital, Shenzhen University, Shenzhen, China

N. Wang (✉)
Department of Ophthalmology, Beijing Tongren Hospital, Capital Medical University, Beijing, China

N. Wang et al. (eds.), *Optic Disorders and Visual Field*, Advances in Visual Science and Eye Diseases 2, https://doi.org/10.1007/978-981-13-2502-1_58

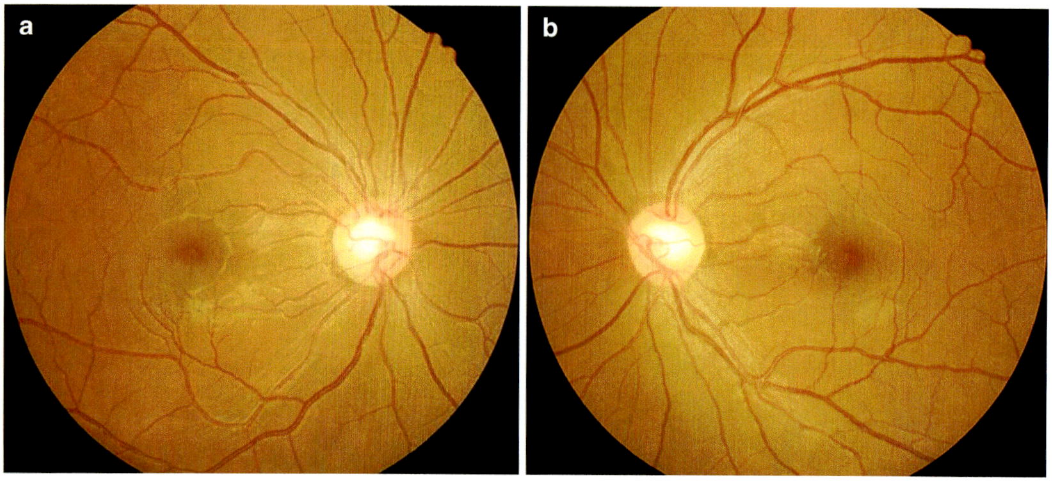

Fig. 58.1 Fundus photographs. The optic disc was pale in color with clear margins, and foveal reflection was present in both eyes. Many vascular branches were seen above the optic disc in the right eye. Panel a: right eye. Panel b: left eye

OCT scan of the macula thickness showed that, with a vertical midline through the macular fovea as the boundary, the GCL thickness decreased significantly at its temporal side in the right eye and at its nasal side in the left eye (Fig. 58.4).

Pattern visual evoked potential (P-VEP) showed decreased amplitudes of P100 with normal latency in both eyes (Fig. 58.5).

Magnetic resonance imaging (MRI) in axial view of the head revealed multiple patch-like hypointense signals on T1-weighed image (T1WI) and hyperintense T2WI in the right temporal lobe, basal ganglion, and thalamus, suggesting multiple softening lesions (Fig. 58.6).

58.1.2 Final Diagnosis

The final diagnosis was postoperative complications of temporal lobe meningioma resection.

58.1.3 Case Review

The visual field damages of the patient in this case are left homonymous hemianopia, mainly due to the damage on the right LGB and the visual pathway behind it caused by the meningioma in the right temporal lobe, basal ganglia, and thalamus. In addition to left hemianopia, the bilateral visual field damages partially crossed over the vertical midline. The reason may be the damage on the anterior visual pathway from transient intracranial hypertension or ischemia during the preoperative or perioperative period. It is noteworthy that, with a vertical midline through the fovea as the boundary, the RGCs and the thickness of macula decreased significantly on the nasal side in the right eye and temporal side in the left eye. Especially in the layer of RGCs, such manifestations were more prominent. In this case, there were no abnormalities in either eye in the past, and the visual field defects and retinal changes both occurred secondary to the meningioma. Therefore, we speculated that retrograde transneuronal injury was the theoretical basis for the damage to the RGCs in both his eyes.

In the visual pathway, nerve fibers originated from RGCs converge and form optic nerves, which perform neurotransmissions in the LGB. The fibers from the LGB form the optic radiation and project to the visual center of the occipital lobe. In this case, the damage on the LGB and the visual pathway behind it crossed synapses retrogradely and run backward to cause damage to its inferior neurons, RGCs. Clinically, we have also observed optic nerve damages, mainly manifested as thinning of peripapillary retinal nerve fiber layers. However, the distribution of the thinning regions was more complicated. The anatomical correspondence between such changes and the lesion locations of the posterior visual pathway were not as consistent as that observed between the distribution of the thinning of the GCL and the lesion locations. Therefore, no in-depth analysis of the optic nerve damage is made here.

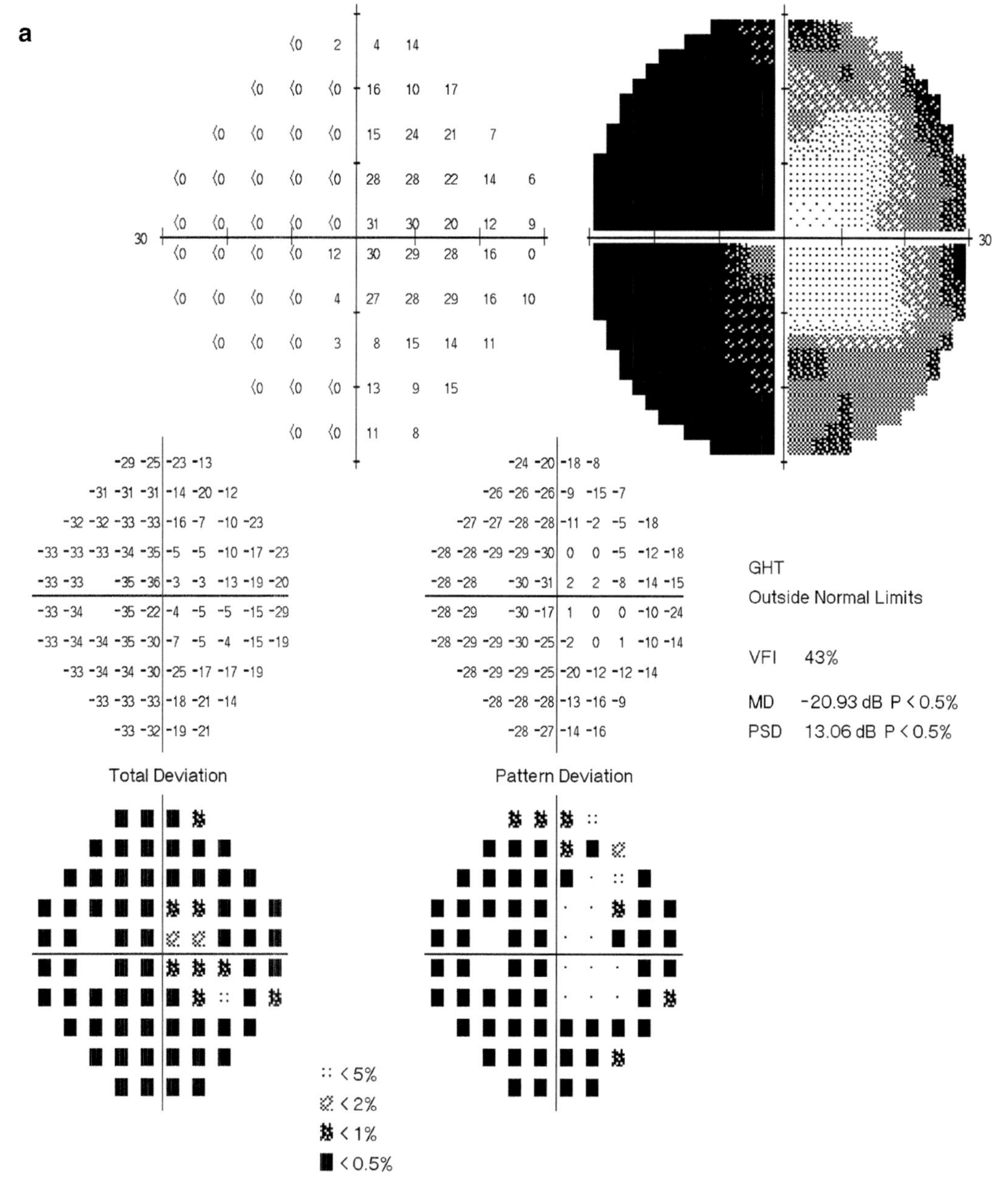

Fig. 58.2 Humphrey visual field analysis printouts. 30-2 test demonstrated left homonymous hemianopia that partially extended across the vertical midline in both eyes, more severe in the left eye. Panel a: left eye. Panel b: right eye

b

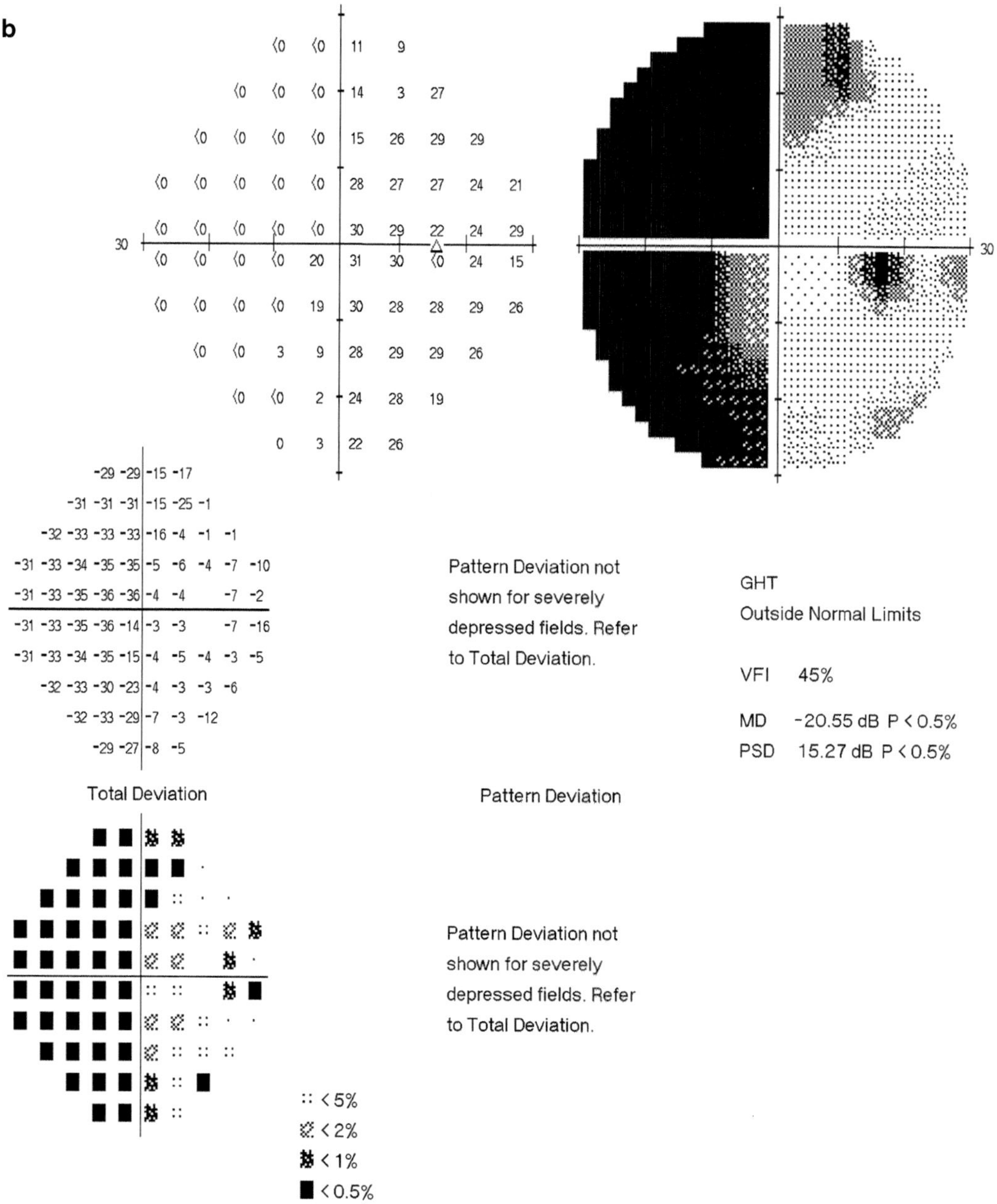

Fig. 58.2 (continued)

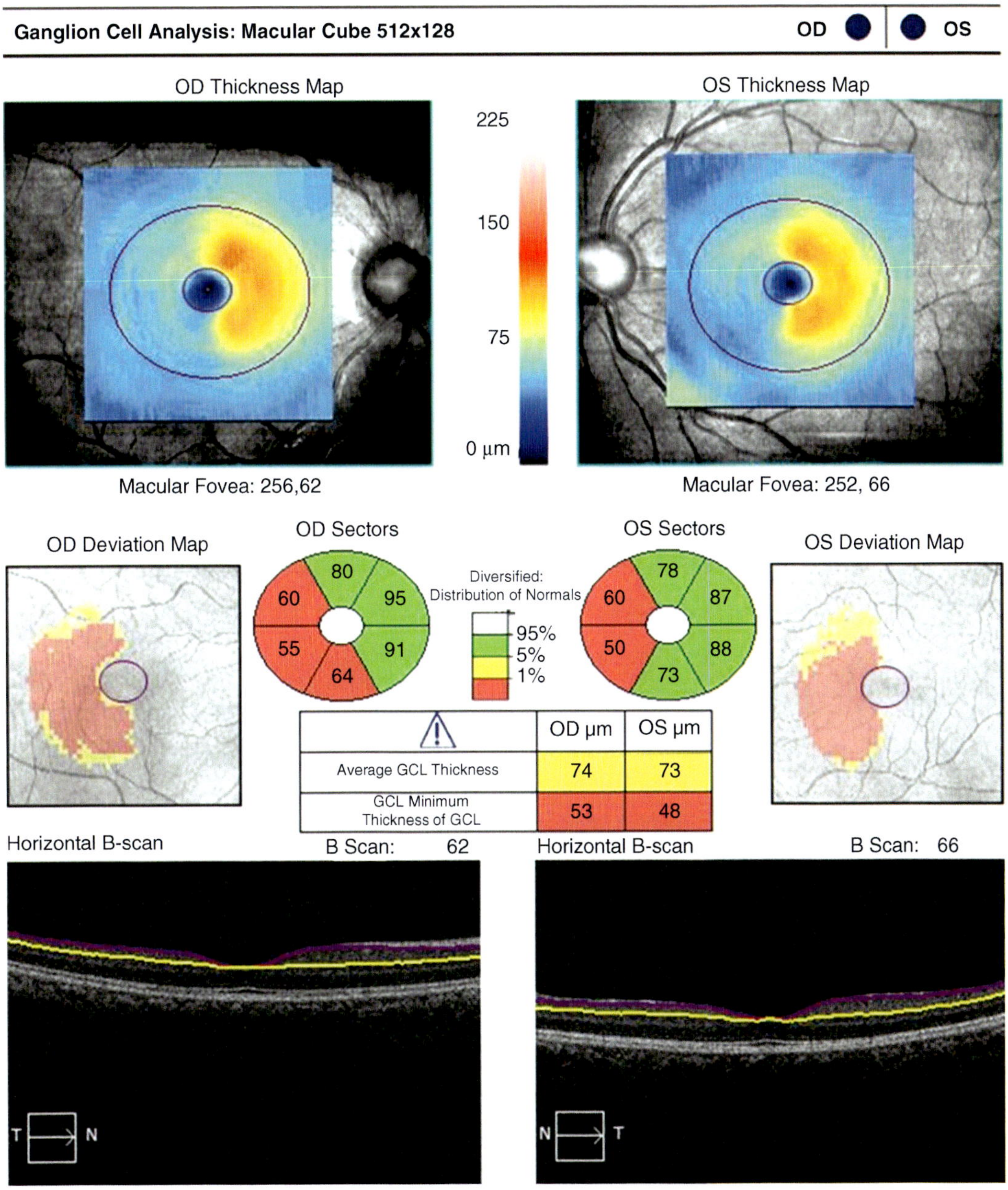

Fig. 58.3 GCL thickness analysis printout in OCT. With a vertical midline through the macular fovea as the boundary, the GCL thickness decreased significantly at its temporal side in the right eye and at its nasal side in the left eye

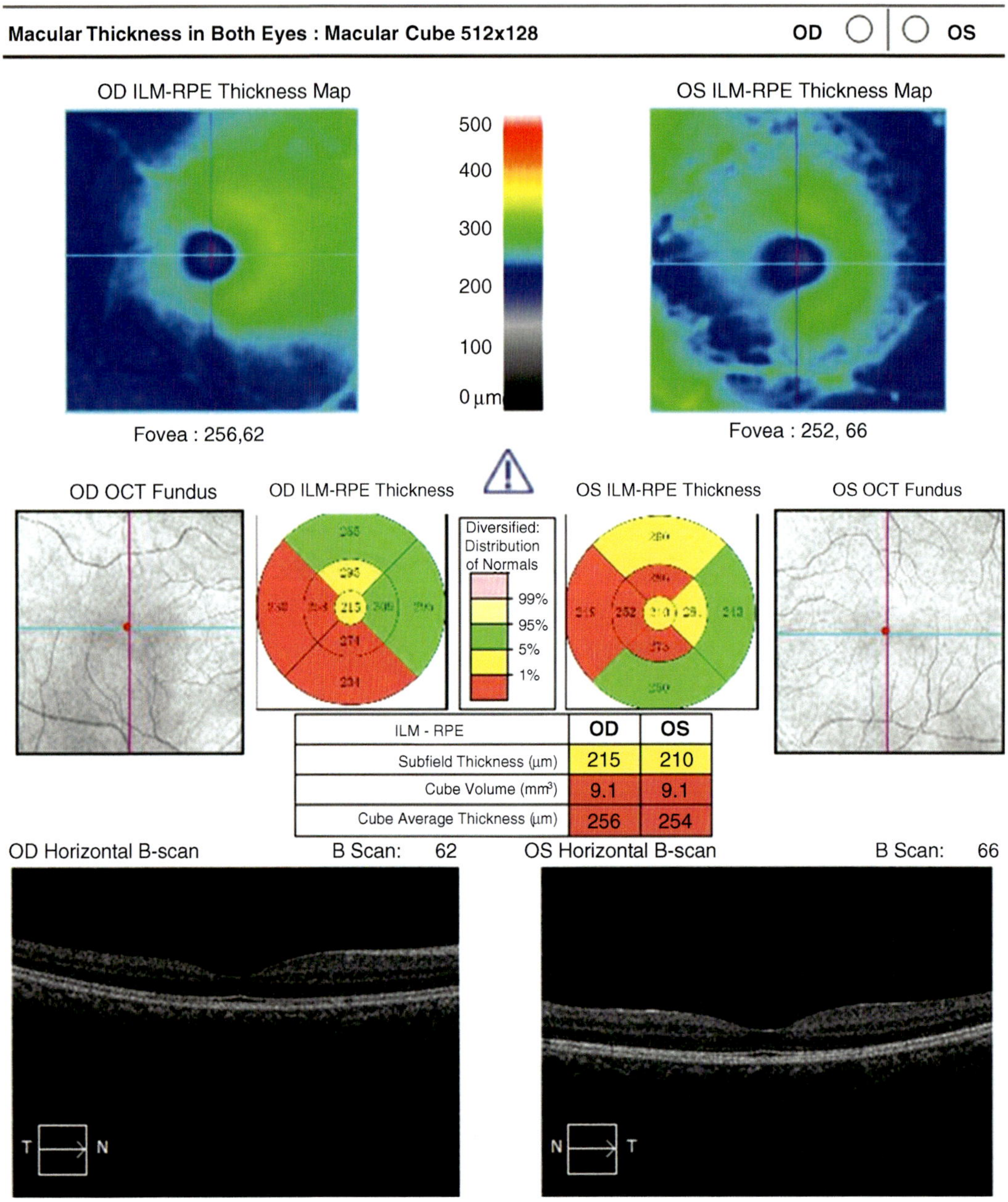

Fig. 58.4 Macula thickness analysis printout in OCT. With a vertical midline through the macula fovea as the boundary, the GCL thickness decreased significantly at its temporal side in the right eye and at its nasal side in the left eye

58.2 Case 2

58.2.1 Case Presentation

A 47-year-old male patient had suffered from a shadow over half of the visual field in both eyes for 1 year. He had felt blurred vision during driving 1 year before. There had been no accompanying ocular symptoms such as visual distortion, red eye, or sore eye and no systemic discomforts such as dizziness, headache, nausea, vomiting, and tinnitus. The patient had visited a local hospital and was treated with drugs, but the details were not clear. However, his visual acuities in

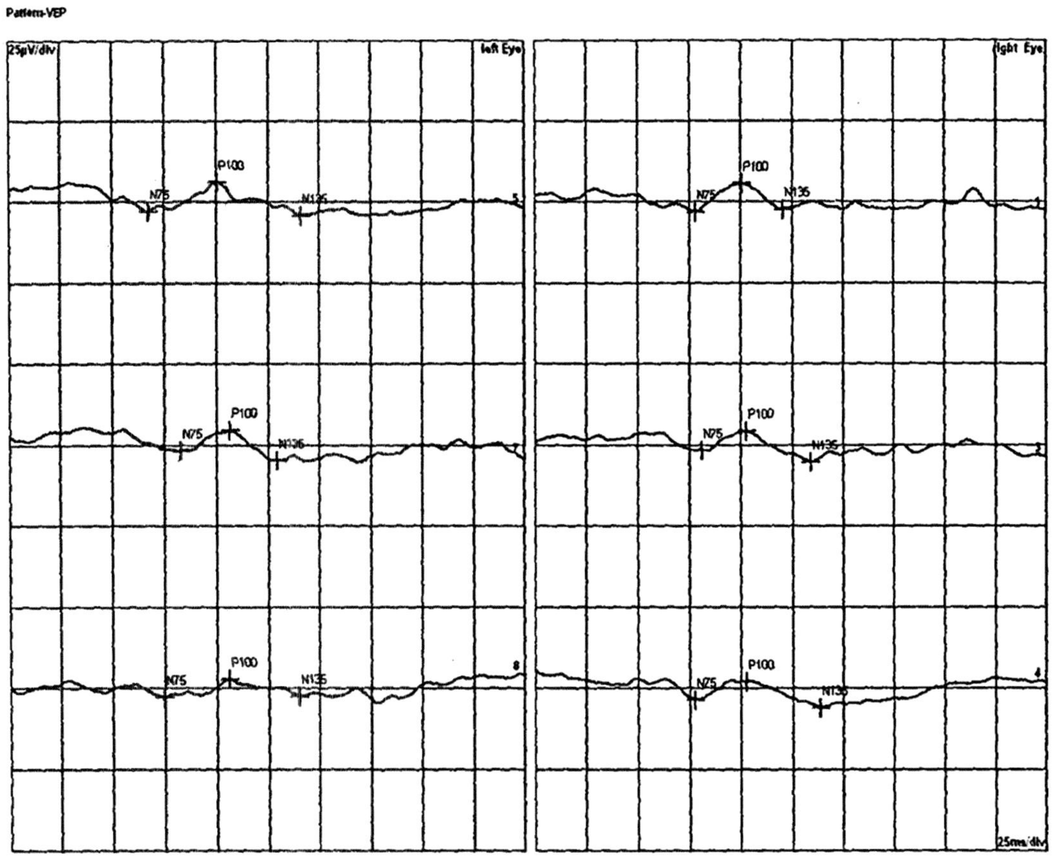

Fig. 58.5 P-VEP examination printout. The latency values of P100 were normal but their amplitudes decreased in both eyes

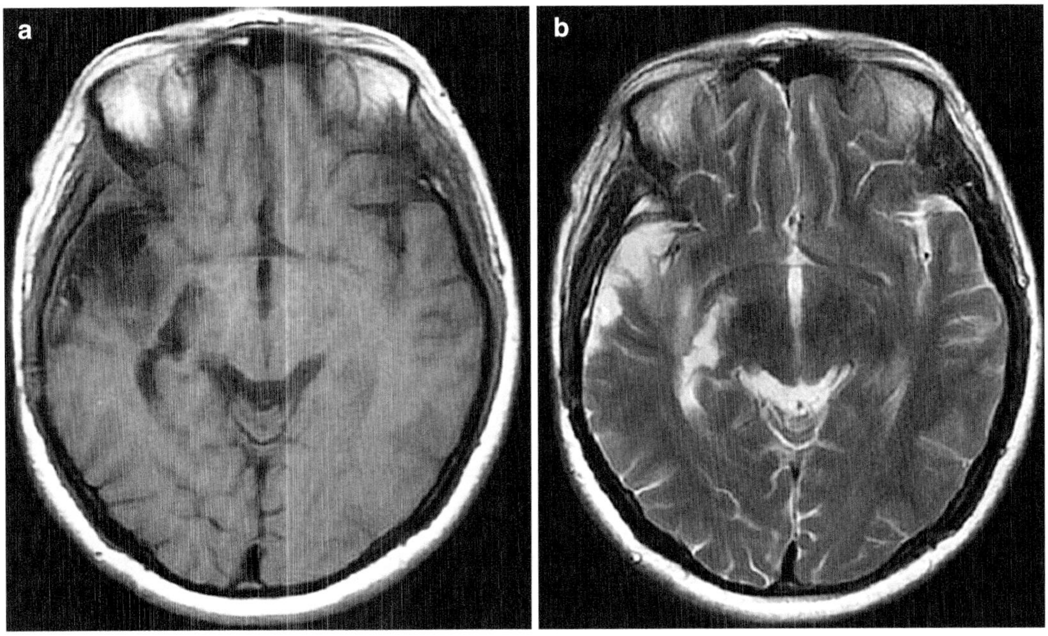

Fig. 58.6 Head MRI on axial images. Panel a: Hypointense signal on T1WI in the right temporal lobe. Panel b: Hyperintense signal on T2WI in the right temporal lobe

both eyes decreased progressively accompanied by left limb weakness. Visual field test showed left homonymous hemianopia. The brain MRI image showed infarction in the right occipital lobe, temporal lobe, and thalamus. Then the patient was diagnosed with cerebral infarction and was treated with drugs for improving circulation and neurotrophy. After that, the symptoms of left limb weakness improved, but the shadow in visual fields of both eyes had no significant relief. The patient had suffered from hyperlipidemia and fatty liver for 5 years and denied the history of trauma, other ocular diseases, or familial diseases.

The uncorrected visual acuity (UCVA) was 20/25 OD and 20/50 OS, and the best corrected visual acuity (BCVA) was 1.0 OU. The intraocular pressure (IOP) was normal OU. Slit-lamp examination of his anterior segments in both eyes was unremarkable, except for slightly increased density of both lenses. Fundus examination revealed pink optic disc with clear margin and normal retinal vessels in both eyes (Fig. 58.7).

Standardized automated perimetry demonstrated left homonymous hemianopia in both eyes (Fig. 58.8).

OCT scan of GCL thickness at the macula showed that the color representing the thickness of RGCs temporal to the right macula and nasal to the left macula significantly faded (arrow) in the pseudo-color thickness maps, suggesting local GCL thickness is decreasing. The measurements of sector thickness showed that the GCL thickness in the temporal sector of the right macula and the GCL thickness in the nasal sector of the left macula became thinner than those of the contralateral sectors (Fig. 58.9).

Pseudo-color images in OCT scan of macular thickness showed no significant changes in either eye, but the topographic maps showed that the macular thickness in the temporal region of the right macula and in the nasal region of the left macula were slightly smaller than those in the corresponding contralateral regions (Fig. 58.10).

P-VEP revealed the amplitude values of the P100 wave decreased with normal latencies in both eyes (Fig. 58.11).

Head MRI demonstrated an extensive softening lesion involving the right occipital lobe, temporal lobe, and thalamus (Fig. 58.12).

58.2.2 Final Diagnosis

The final diagnosis was infarction in the right occipital lobe, temporal lobe, and thalamus.

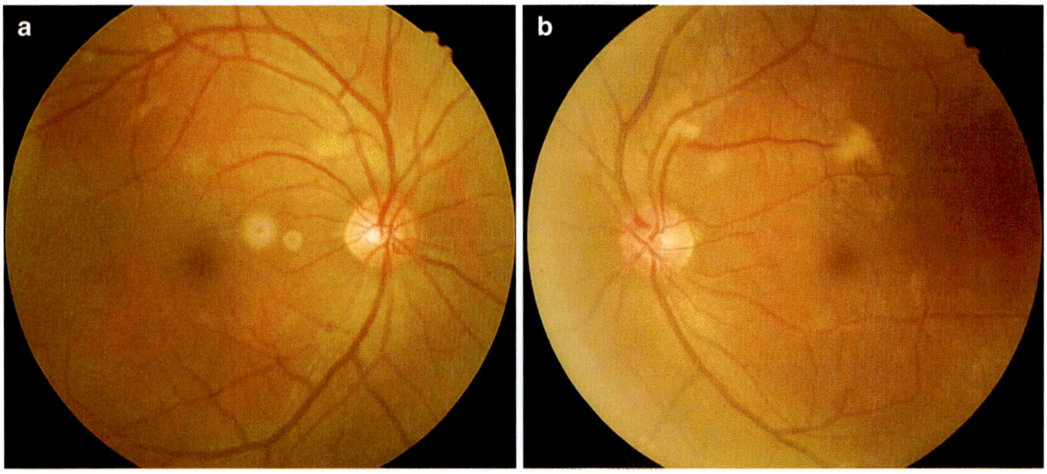

Fig. 58.7 Fundus photographs. The optic disc was pink in color with clear margin, and the macula was normal in both eyes. Panel a: right eye. Panel b: left eye (Note: the image quality was affected by camera lens contamination)

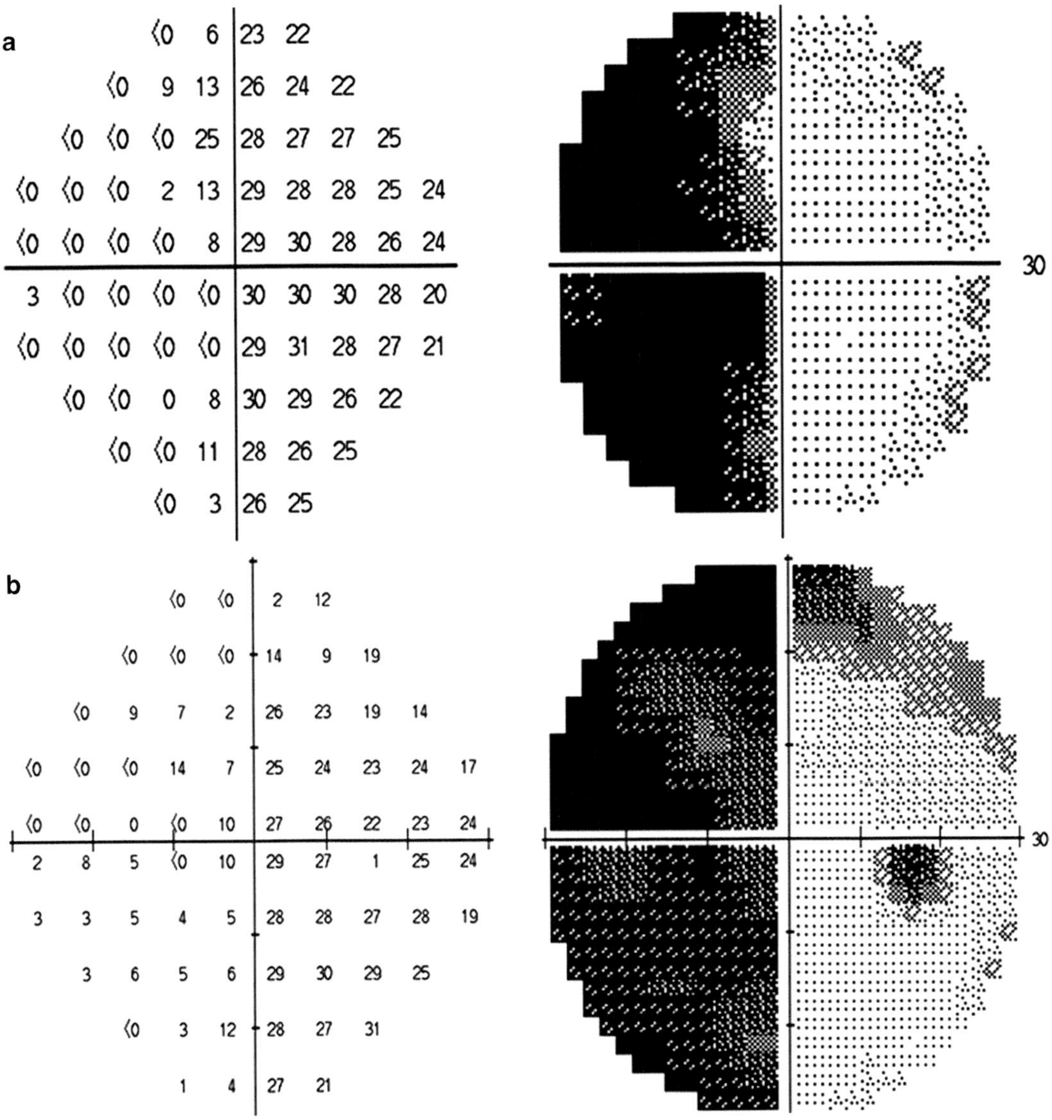

Fig. 58.8 Humphrey visual field analysis printouts. 30-2 test demonstrated left homonymous hemianopia (12 months after onset). Panel a: left eye. Panel b: right eye

58.2.3 Case Review

The visual field of this patient was also manifested as left hemianopia, which was mainly due to the damage on the visual pathway behind the LGB and the occipital center, which was caused by the infarction involving the right occipital lobe, basal ganglia, and thalamus. OCT results showed that, with a vertical midline through the fovea as the boundary, GCL thickness decreased significantly on its temporal side in the right eye and its nasal side in the left eye, as compared with those on the contralateral sides. In this case, there were no abnormalities in either eye in the past, and visual field defects and GCL thickness changes both occurred secondary to cerebral infarction. Therefore, we speculated that the loss of RGCs in both eyes was due to the damage retrograding from the occipital lobe or the posterior visual pathway behind the LGB to the retina after the cerebral infarction, i.e., retrograding across one level of neurons or two levels of neurons, respectively.

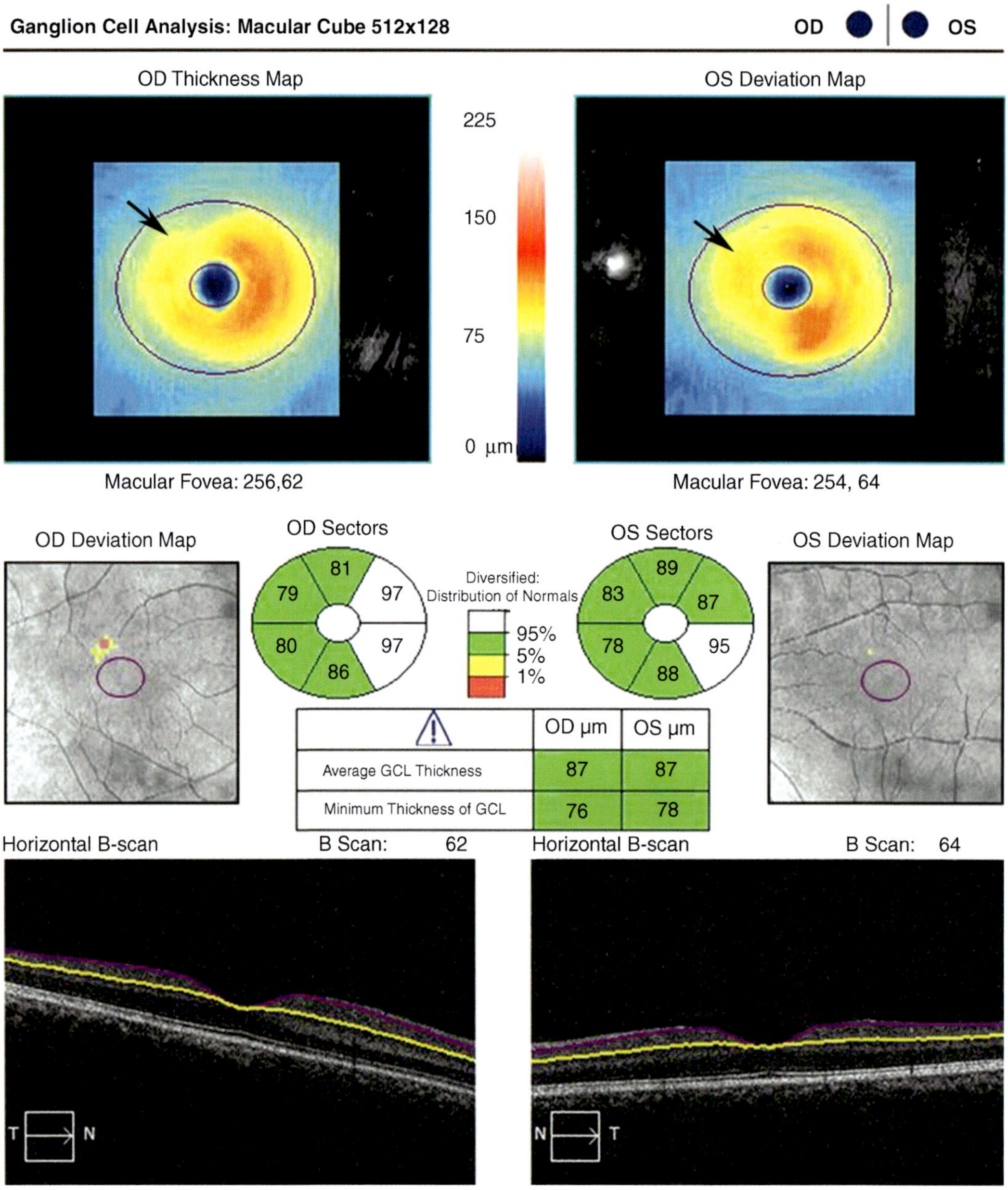

Fig. 58.9 GCL thickness analysis printout in OCT. The color representing the region temporal to the right macula and the region nasal to the left macula (arrow) significantly faded, suggesting that decreased GCL thickness is there; the GCL in the temporal sector of the right macula and in the nasal sector of the left macula became thinner than those of the contralateral sectors

Compared with case 1, the loss of RGCs in case 2 occurred later and less severely. The reason may be that the lesion of case 1 was located more anteriorly in the visual pathway and more severe, which lead to the damage on RGCs from retrograding across one level of neurons. In case 2, the lesion was located closer to the posterior visual pathway, and the damage on RGCs resulted from retrograding across two levels of neurons; furthermore, there might be collateral synapse

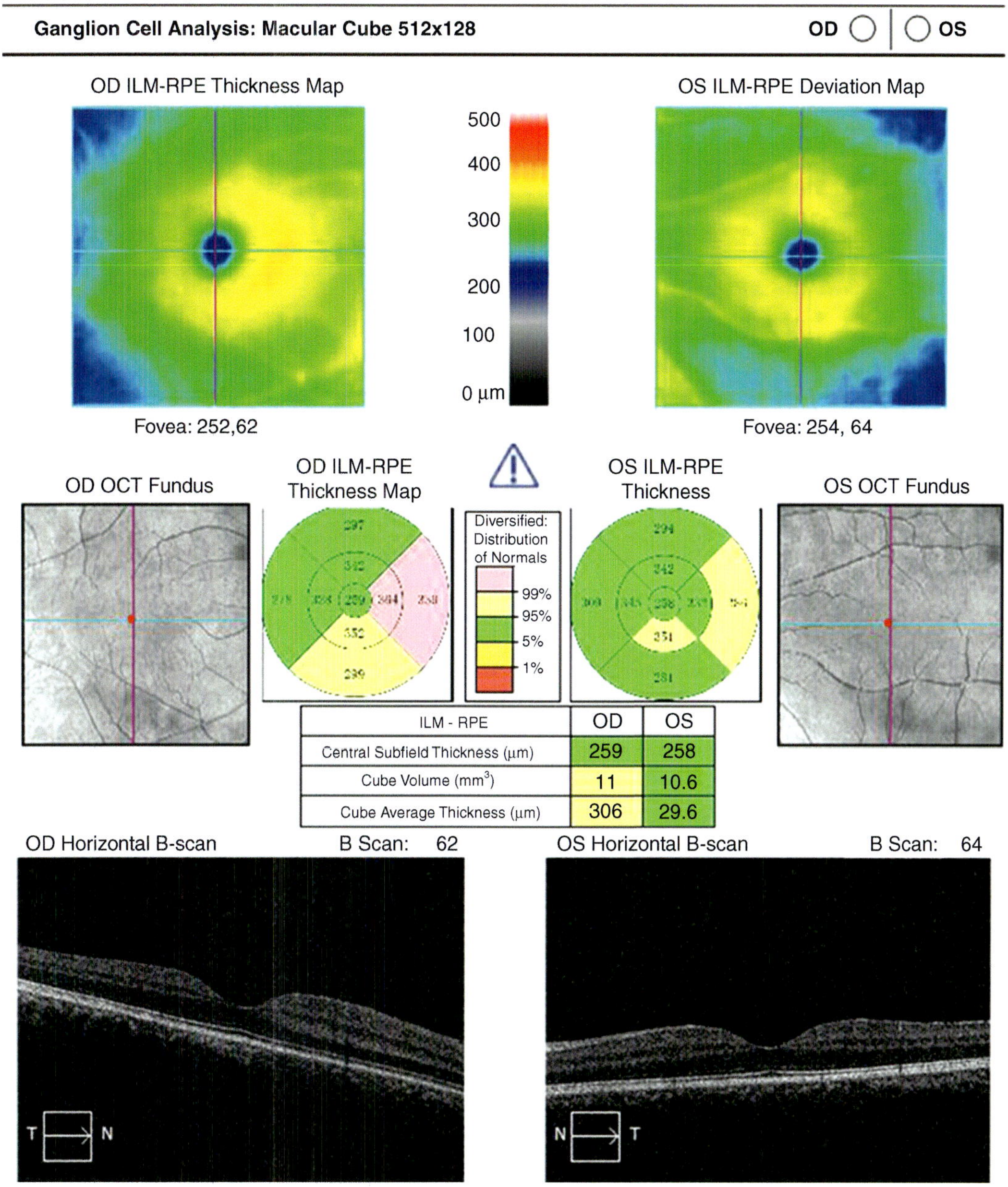

Fig. 58.10 Macular thickness analysis printout in OCT. Pseudo-color images in OCT scan of macular thickness showed no significant changes in either eye, but the topographic maps showed that the macular thickness in the temporal region of the right macula and in the nasal region of the left macula were slightly smaller than those in the corresponding contralateral regions (thickness value in green areas is smaller than that in the faint yellow and pink areas)

connections, so the damage to RGCs was less severe. In addition, in OCT printout, it can be seen that RGCs in case 2 showed a significant loss, but the change in retinal thickness was still not obvious. Therefore, the observation of GCL thickness is more sensitive than that of macular thickness for the detection of a retrograde transneuronal injury.

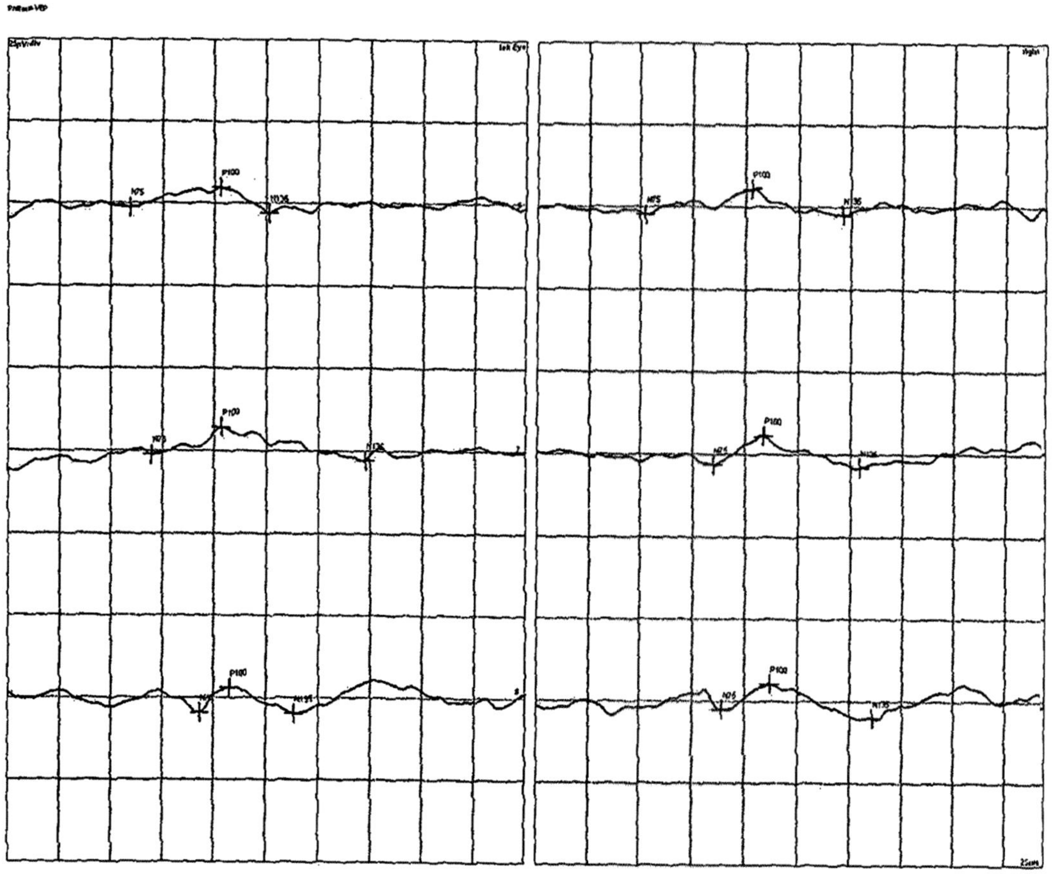

Fig. 58.11 P-VEP examination printout. P-VEP revealed the amplitude values of the P100 wave decreased with normal latencies in both eyes

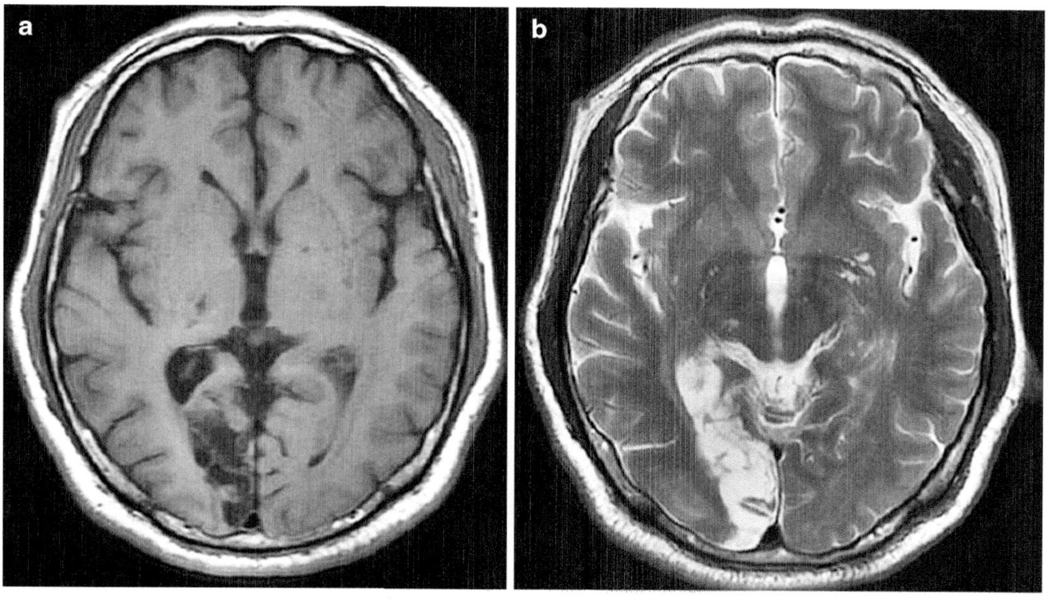

Fig. 58.12 Head MRI axial images. Panel a: hypointense signal in the occipital lobe on T1WI. Panel b: hyperintense signal in the occipital lobe on T2WI

58.3 Discussion

Transneuronal injury refers to the damage from a level of neurons to its upper or lower level of neurons via crossing the synapses along the nerve conduction pathway. Such injury is also known as transsynaptic degeneration. In other words, the loss of extraneous projecting nerve fibers will lead to neurons' atrophy and death. There are two types of transneuronal injuries. If the optic nerve is damaged in one eye, the neurons in the LGB will undergo atrophy and then disappear, which is called ascending transneuronal degeneration. Otherwise, the degeneration and apoptosis of RGCs occurring after the onset of occipital lobe lesions are called retrograde or descending transneuronal damage. The ones discussed in this section belong to the latter.

Clinically, visual field damages of homonymous hemianopia are caused by the damage to the visual pathway behind the optic chiasm especially the posterior visual pathway behind LGB. The retrograde transneuronal damage on the optic nerve from the lesions in the occipital visual center or the posterior visual pathway behind the LGB has already been confirmed by autopsy and animal studies but is still in controversy in clinical practice. Therefore, this theory had not been confirmed until the introduction of OCT, which can be used to objectively and dynamically observe the change in the thickness of the retinal nerve fiber layers [1]. At the same time, it also suggests that the synapses not only transmit visual signals via neurotransmitters but also help superior neurons to exert neurotrophic and supportive effects on inferior neurons.

The first common reason of the damages on the posterior visual pathway behind the LGB is vascular lesions in the temporal lobe and the occipital lobe, such as cerebral hemorrhage and infarction. A common clinical manifestation is a sudden occurrence of contralateral homonymous hemianopia, often accompanied by the symptoms of limbs ipsilateral to the lesion. The second reason is space-occupying lesions, such as meningioma, neuroglioma, hemangioma, and acoustic neuroma in the temporal or occipital lobes. These lesions also clinically manifest homonymous hemianopia with chronic onset and gradual severity, often accompanied by the intracranial hypertension manifestations such as headache. In addition, traumatic injury to the temporal or occipital lobe is more easily diagnosed as there is usually a definite history of trauma. Homonymous hemianopia is also a characteristic visual field change of them.

We also found that the loss of RGCs and their fibers was not always detectable in patients with homonymous hemianopia, which is also one of the main reasons why this theory is controversial. This may be related to the patient's age of disease onset, the severity of intracranial lesions, the lesion location in the visual pathway, and the time from disease onset. Studies have shown that the loss of RGCs and their fibers caused by occipital lobe damage can be detected as early as 3.6 months after onset, and the most significant loss is within 2 years after onset, and the loss will continue in the progression of disease, with the loss rate of peripapillary RNFL being about 9.08 μm reduction in thickness every 10 years [2].

There are also some authors who do not believe in retrograde transneuronal injury. They believe that even there is such a phenomenon, RGCs damage is secondary to the damage on the white matter of the visual pathway or due to the influence of the blood supply in the visual pathway, including the LGB. However, animal experiments confirmed that, after the cortex receiving the macular projecting in the occipital lobe was removed, RGCs in macula experienced significant loss or degeneration [3]. Obviously, the removal of partial occipital cortex will not affect the LGB or the posterior visual pathway; therefore, only the theory of retrograde transneuronal damage can explain the loss of RGCs under this condition.

The visualization of the optic nerve and the high resolution of OCT not only enable the confirmation of the existence of retrograde transneuronal damage but also provide a platform for further studies [1]. However, due to the great individual differences in the optic nerves and retina, retrograde transneuronal damages are greatly influenced by gender, age, ocular axis, refractive status, and optic disc dysplasia. With regard to the study of retrograde transneuronal damages using OCT, longitudinal studies with large sample sizes and control groups are more convincing.

In addition, it is also worth investigating whether the visual field changes caused by retrograde transneuronal damages will aggravate the visual field damages caused by the original disease and how to judge the retrograde transneuronal damage by perimetry.

References

1. Jindahra P, Petrie A, Plant GT. Retrograde trans-synaptic retinal ganglion cell loss identified by optical coherence tomography. Brain. 2009;132(Pt 3):628–34.
2. Jindahra P, Petrie A, Plant GT. The time course of retrograde trans-synaptic degeneration following occipital lobe damage in humans. Brain. 2012;135(Pt 2):534–41.
3. Johnson H, Cowey A. Transneuronal retrograde degeneration of retinal ganglion cells following restricted lesions of striate cortex in the monkey. Exp Brain Res. 2000;132(2):269–75.

59 Visual Field Changes and Prognosis of Hysteria

Xiaobin Xie, Ning Fan, and Ningli Wang

Hysterical visual function damage can manifest itself in a wide range of forms, such as double vision, visual field constriction, anomalopia, cyclospasm, etc. Its visual field manifestations are generally bilateral changes. Before the diagnosis of hysteria is established, it is very important to exclude organic diseases to avoid misdiagnosis.

59.1 Case

59.1.1 Case Presentation

A 46-year-old female patient complained of blurred vision in both eyes for half a year, which was more serious at night.

The patient had felt blurred vision 1 year before and the symptoms aggravated gradually over time, especially at night. The patient had visited the local hospital 10 days before. Her visual field test showed "tubular visual field in both eyes," and thus the patient was suspected of "retinitis pigmentosa" and was referred to a higher-level hospital for treatment. History of trauma, ocular and systemic diseases, or familial diseases was denied.

The uncorrected visual acuity (UCVA) was 20/100 OU, and the best corrected visual acuity (BCVA) was 20/20 OU. The intraocular pressure (IOP) measured by standard Goldmann applanation tonometry was 18 mmHg OD, 16 mmHg OS. Slit-lamp examination of her anterior segments and dilated fundus examination were both unremarkable in both eyes (Fig. 59.1).

Standardized automated perimetry demonstrated concentric constriction, and only a central tubular visual field was left in both eyes (Fig. 59.2).

Fluorescence fundus angiography (FFA) showed no obvious abnormalities in either eye (Fig. 59.3).

Pattern visual evoked potential (P-VEP) revealed that the waveform, latency, and amplitude values of P100 wave were within normal limits in both eyes (Fig. 59.4).

59.1.2 Case Analysis

The clinical features of this case are as follows: (a) subjective impaired vision and poor night

X. Xie
Eye Hospital of China Academy of Chinese Medical Sciences, Beijing, China

N. Fan
Shenzhen Eye Hospital, Shenzhen University, Shenzhen, China

N. Wang (✉)
Department of Ophthalmology, Beijing Tongren Hospital, Capital Medical University, Beijing, China

N. Wang et al. (eds.), *Optic Disorders and Visual Field*, Advances in Visual Science and Eye Diseases 2, https://doi.org/10.1007/978-981-13-2502-1_59

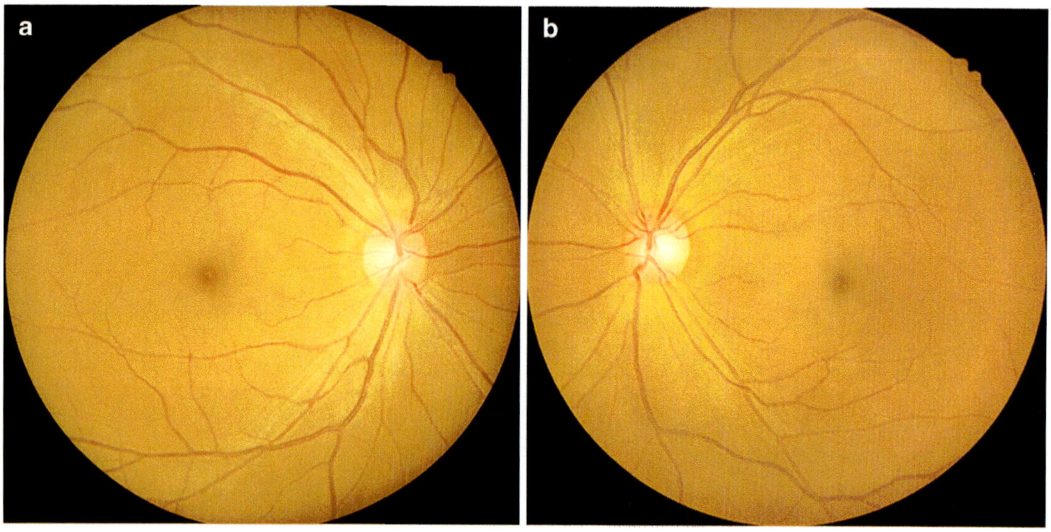

Fig. 59.1 Fundus photographs. The optic discs were pink with clear margin, and foveal reflections were present in both eyes. Panel a: right eye. Panel b: left eye

vision was present in both eyes, but BCVA was 20/20 OU; (b) only a central tubular visual field was left in both eyes; (c) there were no abnormalities in the examination of the anterior and posterior segments; and (d) pupillary light reflex, P-VEP, and FFA were all normal.

The tubular visual fields in both eyes of the patient could not be explained, especially when the visual field test reliability indicators were within the normal limits and the objective ocular examination showed no abnormalities. During the communication with the patient, we found that the patient was anxious. She was particularly worried about the diagnosis of "retinitis pigmentosa." So we suspected the existence of functional visual field changes was caused by mental factors. We gave her some enlightening and soothing words and advised her to receive treatment at Beijing Tongren Hospital with an easy mind. After the anxiety was relieved, the patient became obviously relaxed in expression. She underwent the retest of visual fields after that, and further optical coherence tomography (OCT) and flash electroretinogram (F-ERG) examinations ruled out organic diseases.

Humphrey visual field assessment with 24-2 test during recheck exhibited a normal central visual field in both eyes (Fig. 59.5).

The morphology of the macular fovea in both eyes was normal in OCT examination (Fig. 59.6).

F-ERG examination revealed normal responses in both eyes (Fig. 59.7).

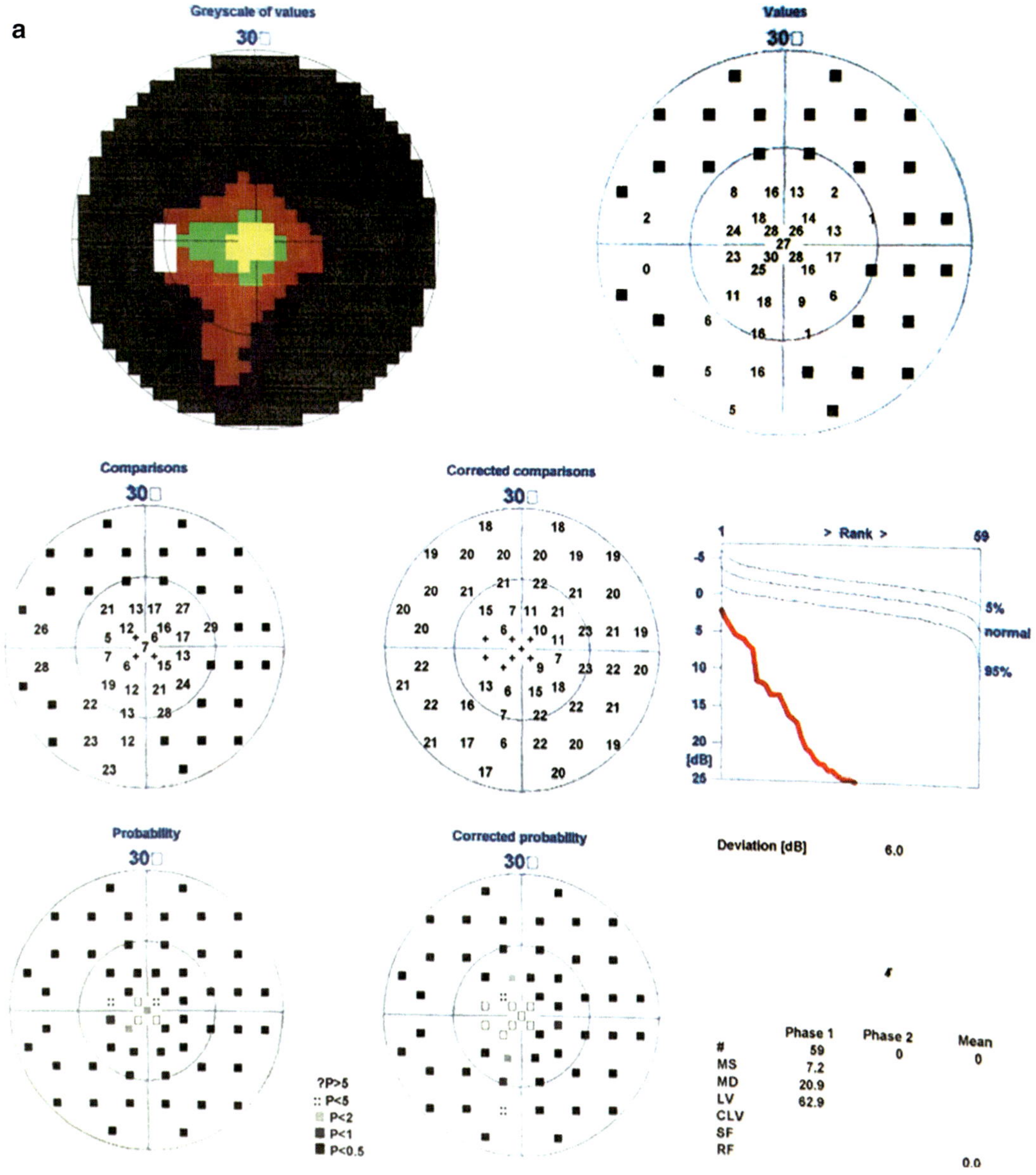

Fig. 59.2 Octopus visual field analysis printouts. There was a tubular visual field in both eyes. Panel a: left eye. Panel b: right eye

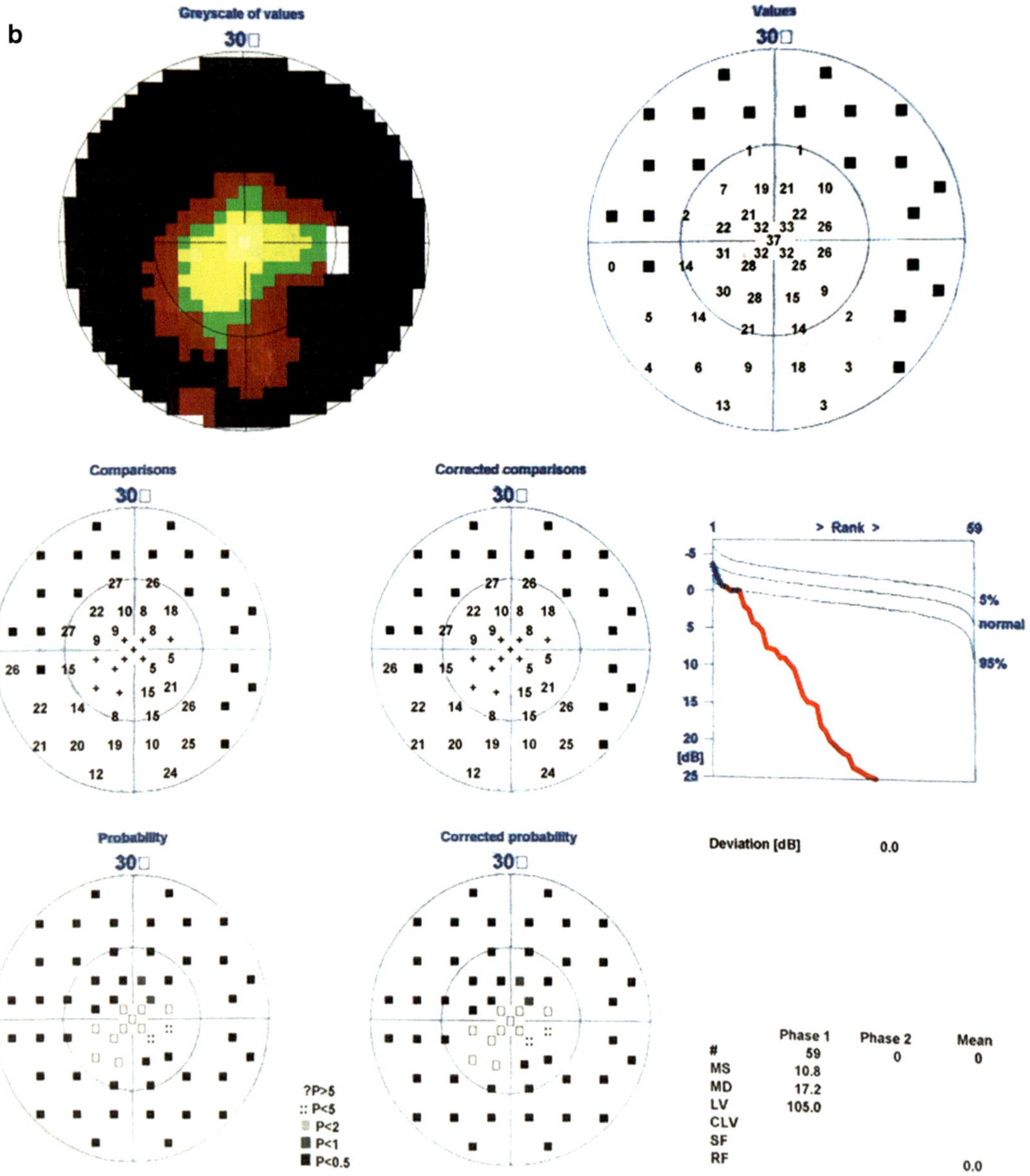

Fig. 59.2 (continued)

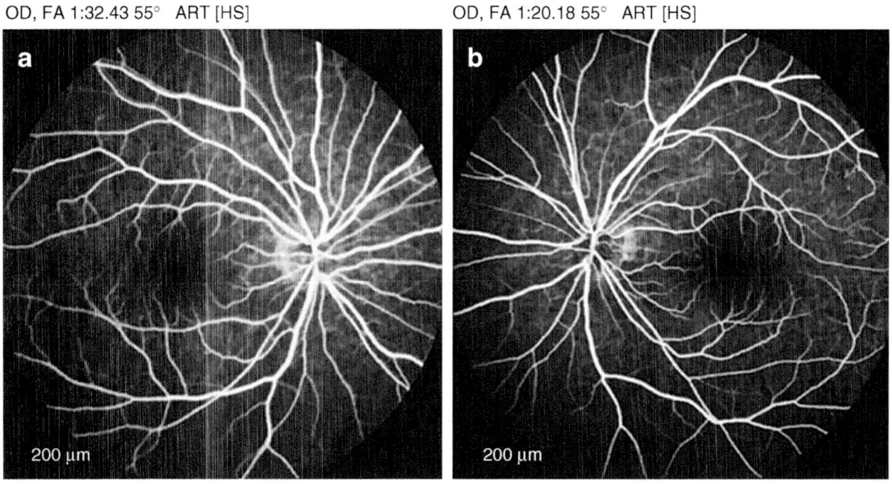

Fig. 59.3 FFA images. No abnormalities were seen in the imaging process in either eye. Panel a: right eye. Panel b: left eye

1_Pattern-VEP 1,0 deg (M)

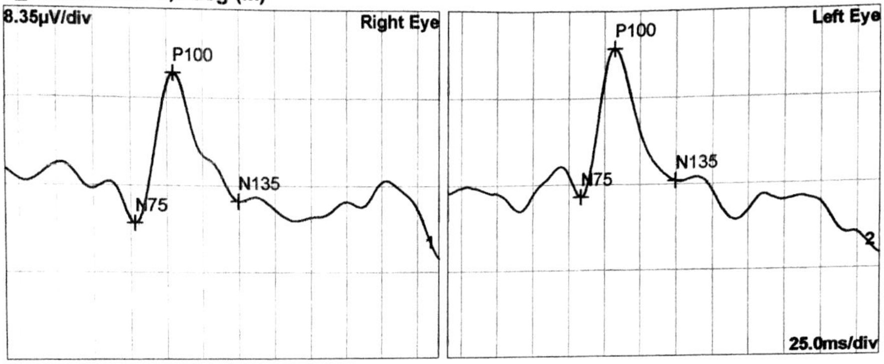

Normals	-	96-109	-	7.70μV-16.7μV	
Channel	N75 [ms]	P100 [ms]	N135 [ms]	N75-P100	P100-N135
1 R-1 1,0 deg	78.7	105.1	150.3	14.3μV	12.2μV
2 L-1 1,0 deg	84.0	108.0	150.3	14.3μV	12.8μV

2_Pattern-VEP 15 min (M)

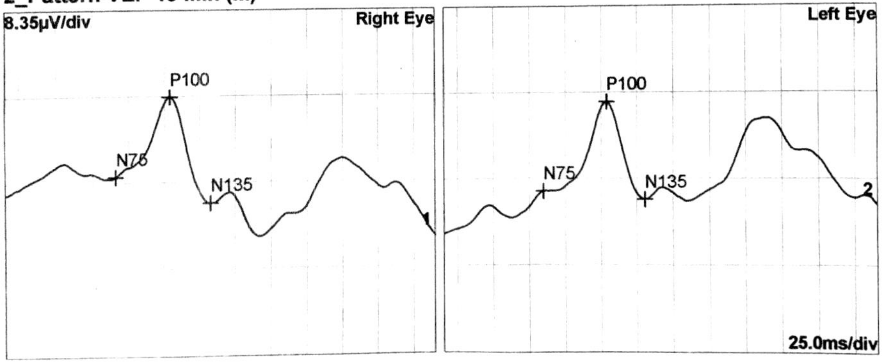

Normals	-	96-109	-	7.70μV-16.7μV	
Channel	N75 [ms]	P100 [ms]	N135 [ms]	N75-P100	P100-N135
1 R-1 15 min	66.9	104.5	133.9	7.72μV	10.2μV
2 L-1 15 min	60.5	104.5	131.5	8.67μV	9.49μV

Fig. 59.4 P-VEP examination printouts. The waveform, latency, and amplitude values of P100 were normal in both eyes

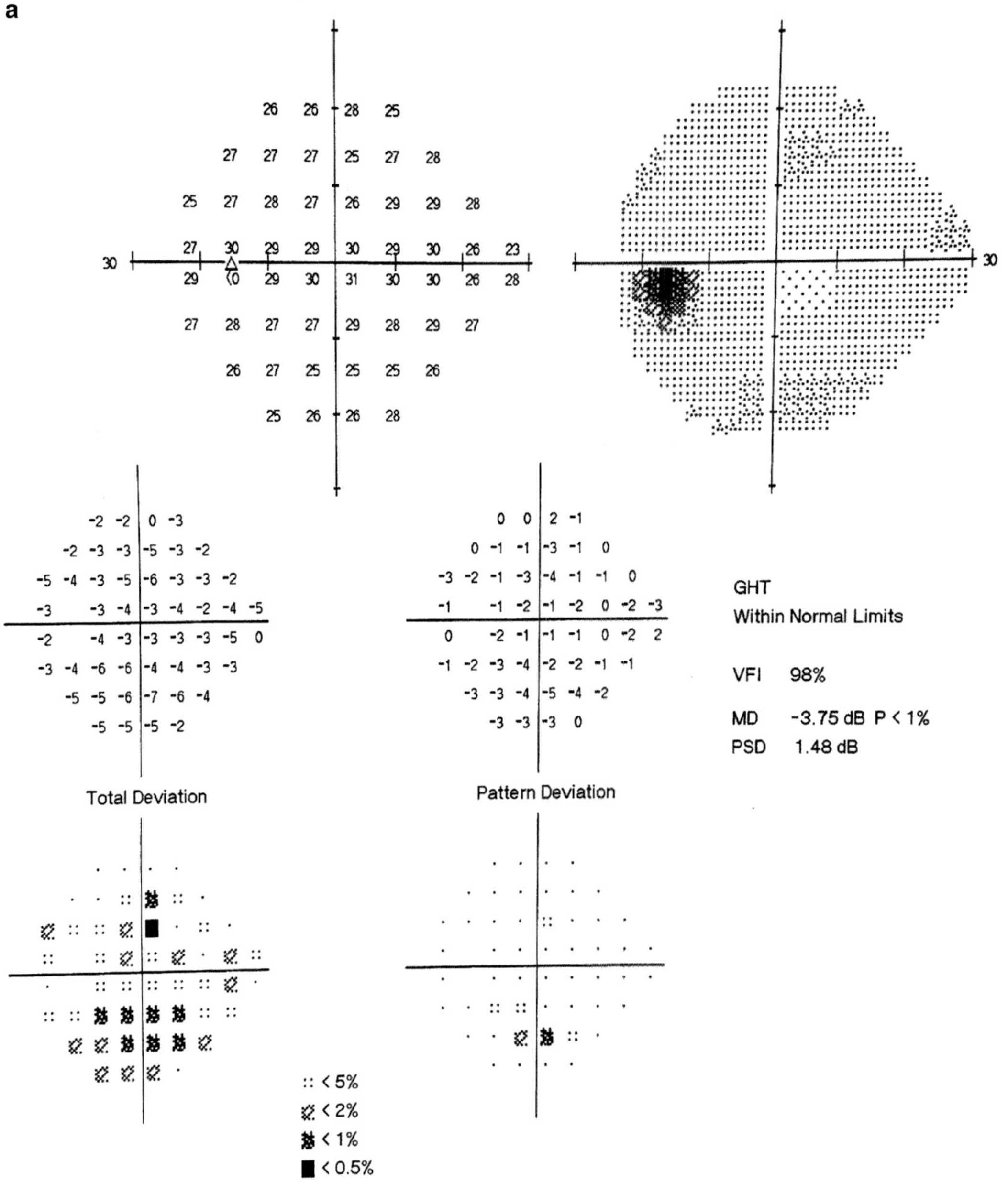

Fig. 59.5 Humphrey visual field reassessment printouts. Recheck of the visual field with 24-2 test showed no abnormalities in either eye. Panel a: left eye. Panel b: right eye

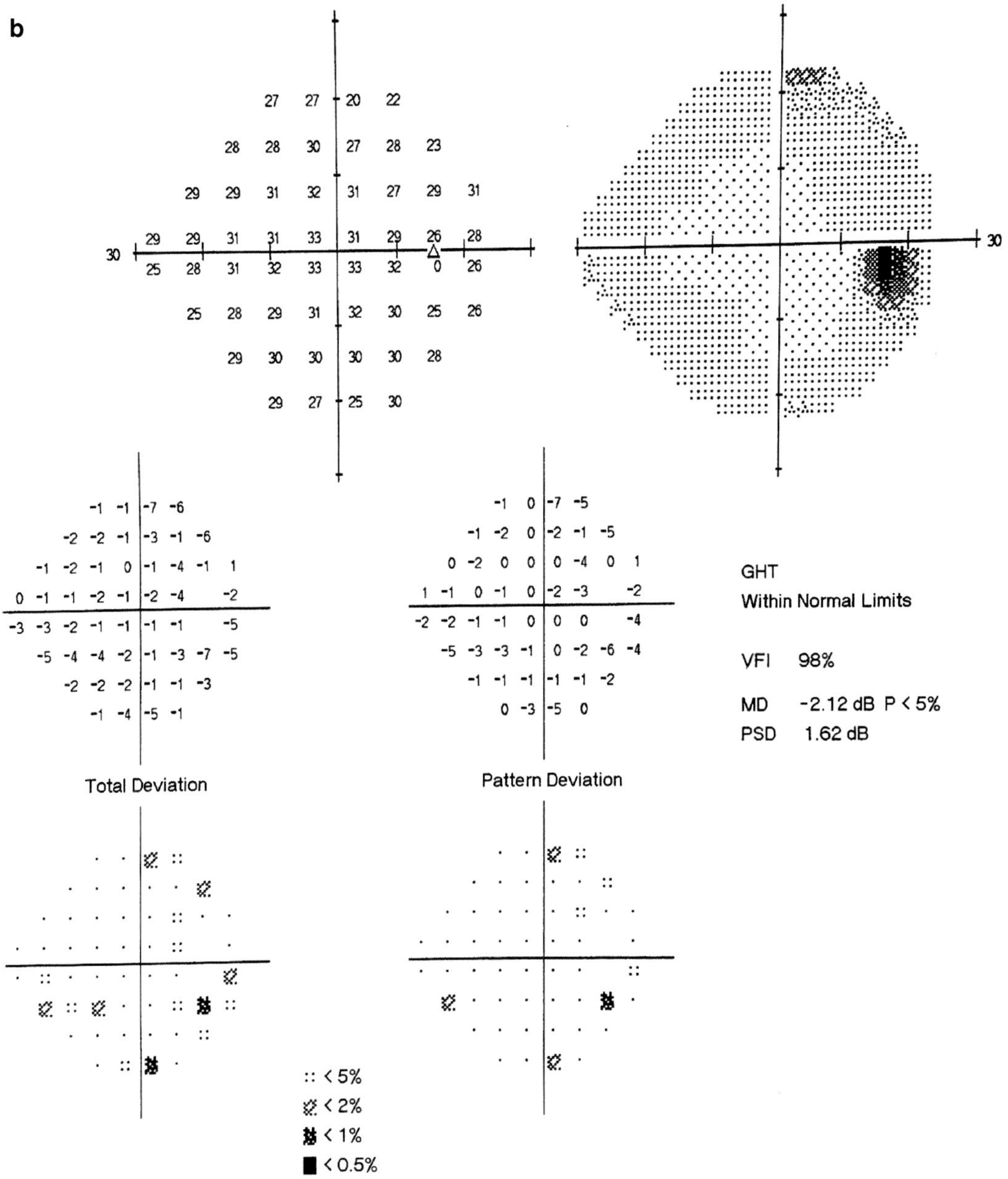

Fig. 59.5 (continued)

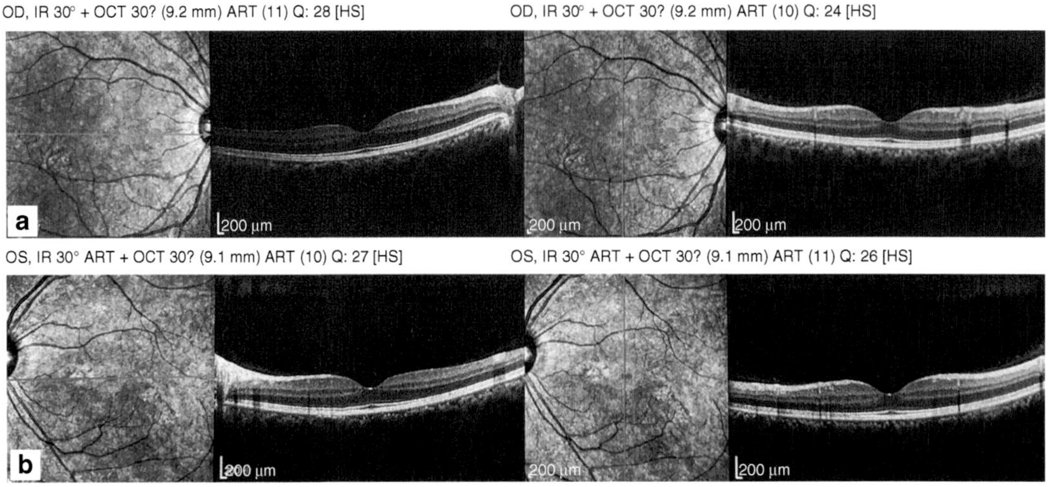

Fig. 59.6 Macula scan images in OCT. No abnormalities were seen at the macula in either eye. Panel a: right eye. Panel b: left eye

59.1.3 Final Diagnosis

The final diagnosis was hysteria.

59.2 Discussion

The patient in this case showed concentric constriction and tubular visual field in both eyes, while the final diagnosis was hysteria. Because the patient had no organic lesions and there were no specific visual field changes, it is so easy to make misdiagnosis or missed diagnosis.

Hysteria belongs to dissociative conversion disorders, which impairs the abilities of conscious selection and control, and the degree of impairment can vary from day to day or even from hour to hour [1].

Hysteria patients often manifest amblyopia, blindness, tubular visual field, visual field constriction, or monocular diplopia. Other possible symptoms include photophobia, foreign body sensation, pain in the eyeball or orbit, anomalopia, ocular motility disorders, nystagmus, blepharospasm, cyclospasm, or cycloplegia, etc. [2]. It often happens suddenly but can also suddenly disappear during treatment. It is mainly caused by a strong mental stimulation and local inhibition in the projection area of the visual cortex. Such inhibition is not homogenous or complete. Although the patients may complain of vision loss and cannot see large objects in front of them, they can surprisingly accomplish adequate physical activities and can even read books or newspapers, etc. The visual evoked potentials of them are often normal. Under the effects of psychological suggestion, the symptoms can be aggravated, alleviated, or disappear. The main treatment for such disease is psychological treatment.

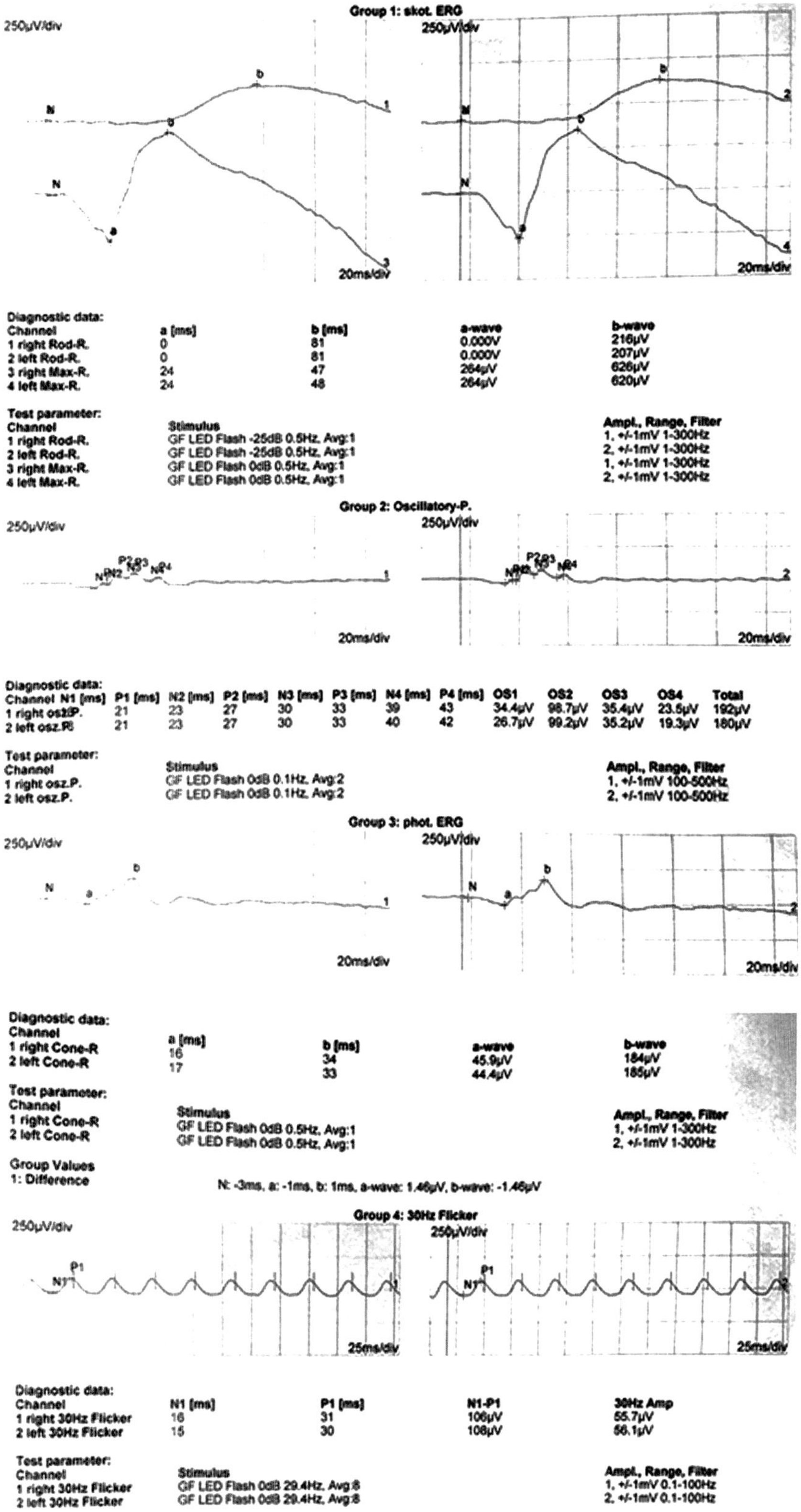

Fig. 59.7 F-ERG analysis printouts. No abnormalities were seen in each response during F-ERG examination in either eye

References

1. Hao W, Yu X. Psychiatry. 7th ed. Beijing: People's Health Press; 2013.
2. Zhao K. Ophthalmology. 7th ed. Beijing: People's Medical Publishing House; 2008.

Part VII

Ocular-cranial Pressure Gradient-Related Disorders

The Manifestation of the Optic Nerve Head Under Simultaneous Intraocular Pressure and Intracranial Pressure Elevation

60

Xiaobin Xie and Ningli Wang

From the anatomical and biomechanical standpoints, the optic nerve fibers travel through two different fluid pressure cavities, the intraocular pressure space and the retrobulbar cerebrospinal pressure space. The lamina cribrosa forms the border between the higher-pressure intraocular space and the lower-pressure retrobulbar and cerebrospinal fluid space and hence is susceptible to pressure-induced mechanical damage. The pressure gradient that occurs across the lamina cribrosa (intraocular pressure–intracranial pressure) is called as "translaminar pressure gradient" in ophthalmology [1, 2, 4–6, 7]. From the perspective of integrative medicine, it is also referred to as the "ocular-cranial pressure gradient" [8]. The variation of the ocular-cranial pressure gradient plays a pathophysiologic role in optic nerve head damage [1–4, 9]. When the optic nerve is experiencing elevated intraocular pressure and cerebrospinal fluid pressure, and the two pressures eventually stabilize at a new equilibrium, how will the optic nerve head respond to this new environment?

X. Xie
Eye Hospital of China Academy of Chinese Medical Sciences, Beijing, China

N. Wang (✉)
Department of Ophthalmology, Beijing Tongren Hospital, Capital Medical University, Beijing, China

60.1 Case

60.1.1 Case Presentation

A 51-year-old female patient presented with bilateral progressive vision loss, accompanied by headache of greater than 1 year's duration. She denied previous ocular and systemic diseases, trauma, or a family history of related disease. A complete review of systems was negative.

On ophthalmological examination, her uncorrected visual acuity (UCVA) was 20/200 OD and 20/100 OS, and her best-corrected visual acuity (BCVA) was 20/63 OD and 20/25 OS. Intraocular pressure (IOP) was measured as 11 mmHg OD and 38 mmHg OS. Slit-lamp examination showed a shallow central anterior chamber depth, a peripheral anterior chamber depth that was 1/3 of the corneal thickness, and mild cataracts in both eyes. Fundus examination in the right eye revealed optic disc edema and elevation, as well as a blurred disc margin for 360° in the right eye with the presence of tortuous retinal vessels and retinal folds at the posterior pole. In the left eye, the optic disc was not elevated, but its nasal margin was blurred and included the presence of a narrowed inferior disc rim and retinal nerve fiber layer (RNFL) defect at the corresponding site; retinal mild edema, retinal folds, and tortuous blood vessels were also observed at the posterior pole (Fig. 60.1). Gonioscopy revealed bilaterally

N. Wang et al. (eds.), *Optic Disorders and Visual Field*, Advances in Visual Science and Eye Diseases 2, https://doi.org/10.1007/978-981-13-2502-1_60

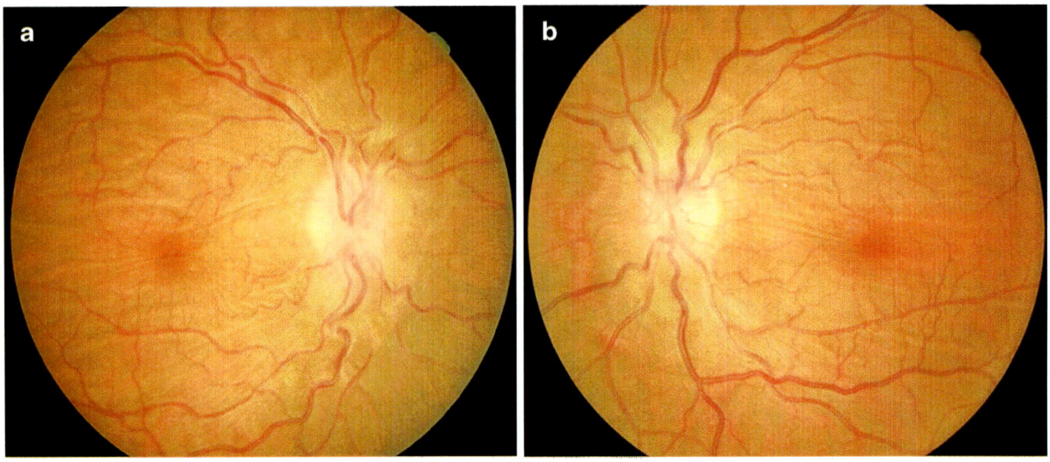

Fig. 60.1 Fundus photographs. Panel a: In the patient's right eye, the optic disc was swollen, the disc margin was blurred, the retinal blood vessels were tortuous, and the retina was edematous and folded at the posterior pole. Panel b: In the patient's left eye, the optic disc was not elevated, but nasal margin of the optic disc was blurred. The optic disc rim was narrowed and had retinal nerve fiber layer defects. Retinal vessels were tortuous, and the retina was slightly folded at the posterior pole

narrow angles: N1~N2 in the right eye and N2~N3 with the presence of the peripheral anterior synechia in the superior quadrant of the left eye.

Standardized automated perimetry demonstrated an enlarged blind spot with a central scotoma in both eyes (Fig. 60.2).

60.1.2 Case Analysis

Even though this patient's IOP in the left eye had reached 38 mmHg, this eye's visual acuity was notably better than that of the right eye (20/25 vs. 20/63), and the visual field examination was unremarkable except for an enlarged blind spot; her IOP in the right eye, however, was not nearly so high, but this eye's visual field and visual acuity impairment were worse. Why was the visual field less damaged in the left eye compared to the right eye, despite a substantially higher intraocular pressure? Why did the right eye have an abnormal visual field and vision, despite a normal intraocular pressure? Given the fundus manifestations of tortuous retinal veins, retinal folds, and the blurring of the optic disc boundary, the following initial diagnoses could be considered: (a) glaucoma in the left eye; (b) optic disc edema in both eyes; (c) Vogt-Koyanagi-Harada (VKH) disease in both eyes.

Given the medical history and symptoms of the patient, the diagnosis of VKH disease should be ruled out. The patient presented with progressively decreased vision accompanied by headache; VKH is unlikely given the absence of these symptoms and signs: eye pain, eye redness, photophobia, sharp decline in visual acuity, and obvious signs of uveitis.

The patient was transferred to the neurology department for lumbar puncture: her cerebrospinal fluid pressure was measured as 280 mmH_2O (21 mmHg), which is much higher than the normal value of 80~180 mmH_2O (6~13 mmHg). The cerebrospinal fluid composition was normal.

Thus, it can be seen that bilateral optic disc edema in this patient was caused by increased intracranial pressure. This asks the question: why are the appearances of the optic discs inconsistent in this patient? How does one diagnose and treat this patient?

The patient's IOP was 11 mmHg OD and 38 mmHg OS, while her intracranial pressure (ICP) was 21 mmHg. By analyzing the relationship between the IOP and intracranial pressure, we found that her ocular-cranial pressure gradient was −10 mmHg in the right eye and 17 mmHg in the left eye. The normal range of ocular-cranial pressure gradient is 4–8 mmHg. Therefore, the patient's right eye showed optic disc edema, venous tortuosity, and retinal folds due to the higher retrolaminar cerebrospinal fluid pressure (retrograde translaminar pressure gradient). Although the left eye showed venous tortuosity and retinal folds, also under the influence of increased orbital cerebrospinal fluid pressure, there was no manifestation of optic disc edema because of the presence of elevated IOP (positive ocular-cranial pressure gradient). The elevated IOP did, however, induced optic nerve damage (disc rim narrowing, retinal nerve fiber layer defect).

It follows that the patient should be treated for the intracranial hypertension and intraocular hypertension in the left eye. She first underwent Nd:YAG laser peripheral iridotomy in both eyes. After the Nd:YAG laser therapy, ophthalmic

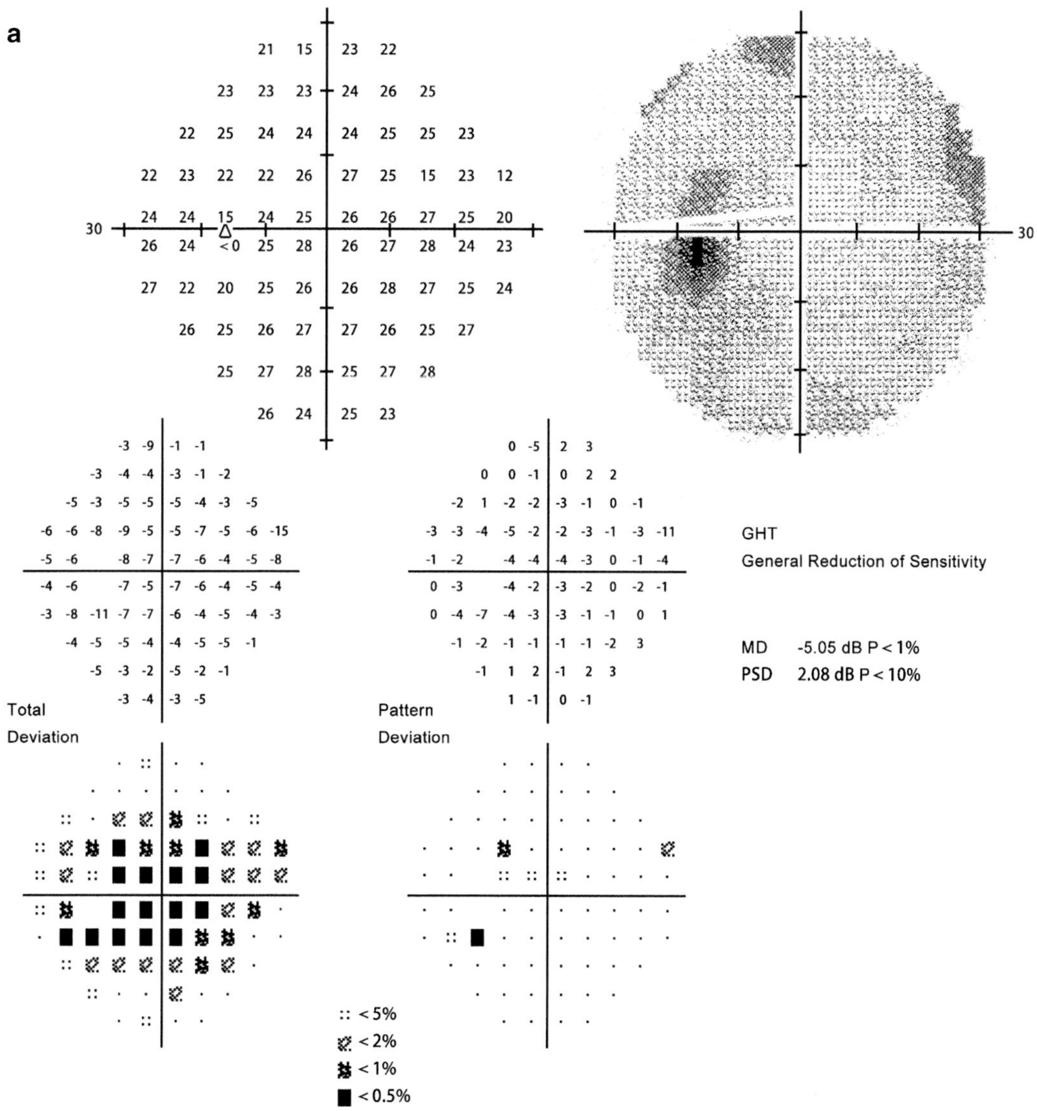

Fig. 60.2 Humphrey visual field analysis printout. Enlarged physiological blind spots in both eyes, accompanied by central scotoma, were shown via 30-2 test. Panel a: Left eye. Panel b: Right eye

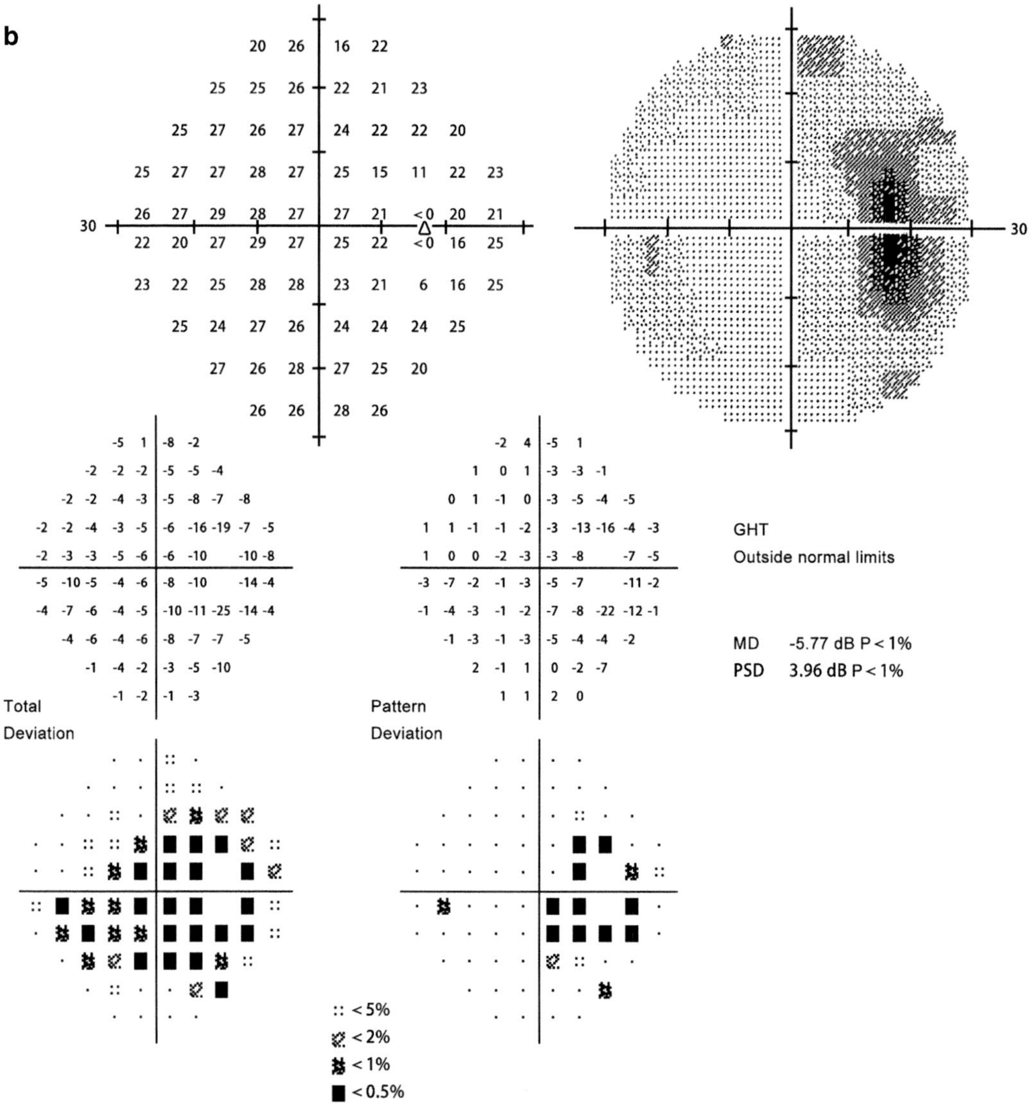

Fig. 60.2 (continued)

ultrasound biomicroscope (UBM) showed the angle between the iris, and the surface of trabecular meshwork became wide, and significant deepening was revealed in the peripheral anterior chamber of the left eye, and a normal ciliary body was seen in both eyes. Her IOP was 8.8 mmHg OD and 20.2 mmHg OS. Subsequently, she underwent cerebrospinal fluid lumbo-peritoneal shunt surgery, and her ICP was reduced to 120 mmH_2O (8.8 mmHg).

She was followed-up with after the surgery. One year after lumbo-peritoneal shunt surgery, the optic disc edema in the right eye was obviously relieved, as expected. It is noteworthy that, in the left eye, even though the IOP and ICP were basically under control, fundus photograph showed an enlarged cup/disc ratio, optic disc rim thinning and retinal nerve fiber layer defect in the superior and inferior quadrants (Figs. 60.3 and 60.4).

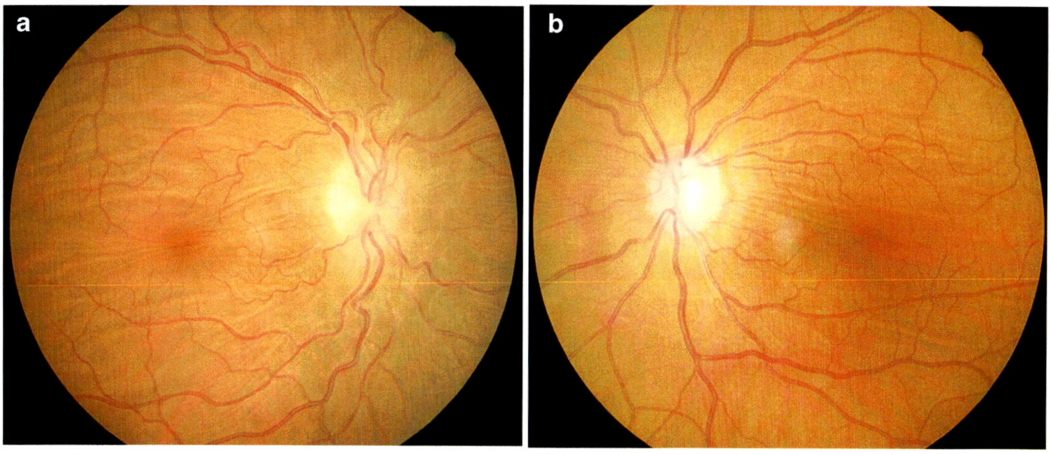

Fig. 60.3 Fundus photographs (1 year after lumbo-peritoneal shunt surgery). Panel a: The optic disc edema in the right eye was obviously relieved. Panel b: The left eye showed the superior and inferior rim narrowing and corresponding retinal nerve fiber layer defects

Comparing the fundus photographs obtained before and after the bilateral Nd:YAG laser therapy and lumbo-peritoneal shunt surgery, we could distinctly see the changes in the fundus. After the lumbo-peritoneal shunt surgery, the retinal venous tortuosity in both eyes was clearly relieved. In the right eye, the optic disc edema was reduced, and the disc became pale. An enlarged cup/disc ratio, thinner optic disc rim, and retinal nerve fiber layer defects in the superior and inferior segments were observed in the left eye (Fig. 60.4).

60.1.3 Final Diagnosis

The final diagnosis was primary chronic angle-closure glaucoma in the left eye, accompanied by intracranial hypertension (causes to be investigated).

60.2 Discussion

Glaucoma is a disease which often manifests with IOP elevation and posterior displacement of the lamina cribrosa. Conversely, intracranial hypertension syndrome often manifests as lamina cribrosa protrusion and optic disc edema. Both diseases lead to optic nerve damage. From the biomechanical point of view, the pressure factors in the translaminar pressure gradient, which is also referred to as the ocular-cranial pressure gradient, act in opposite directions in these two diseases, thus resulting in dramatically different clinical manifestations. In this case, the patient suffered from intracranial hypertension syndrome in both eyes and angle-closure glaucoma in only the left eye. Her right eye showed typical signs of optic disc edema which did not appear in the left eye due to the fact that, to a certain extent, the intraocular hypertension was counterbalanced by the intracranial hypertension. However, after we corrected her high intraocular pressure and high intracranial pressure, her glaucomatous optic nerve damage in the left eye was witnessed due to the decreased intracranial pressure.

In this case, we have recognized that the lamina cribrosa is subject to both IOP from the anterior direction and retrolaminar pressure from the posterior direction of the optic nerve head; in healthy individuals these pressures reach a normal equilibrium (or a normal translaminar pressure gradient). Any abnormal increase of the pressure in either direction will cause an increase in the intraocular-intracranial pressure gradient in either the positive or negative direction, which then causes changes in the optic disc structure and can damage the optic

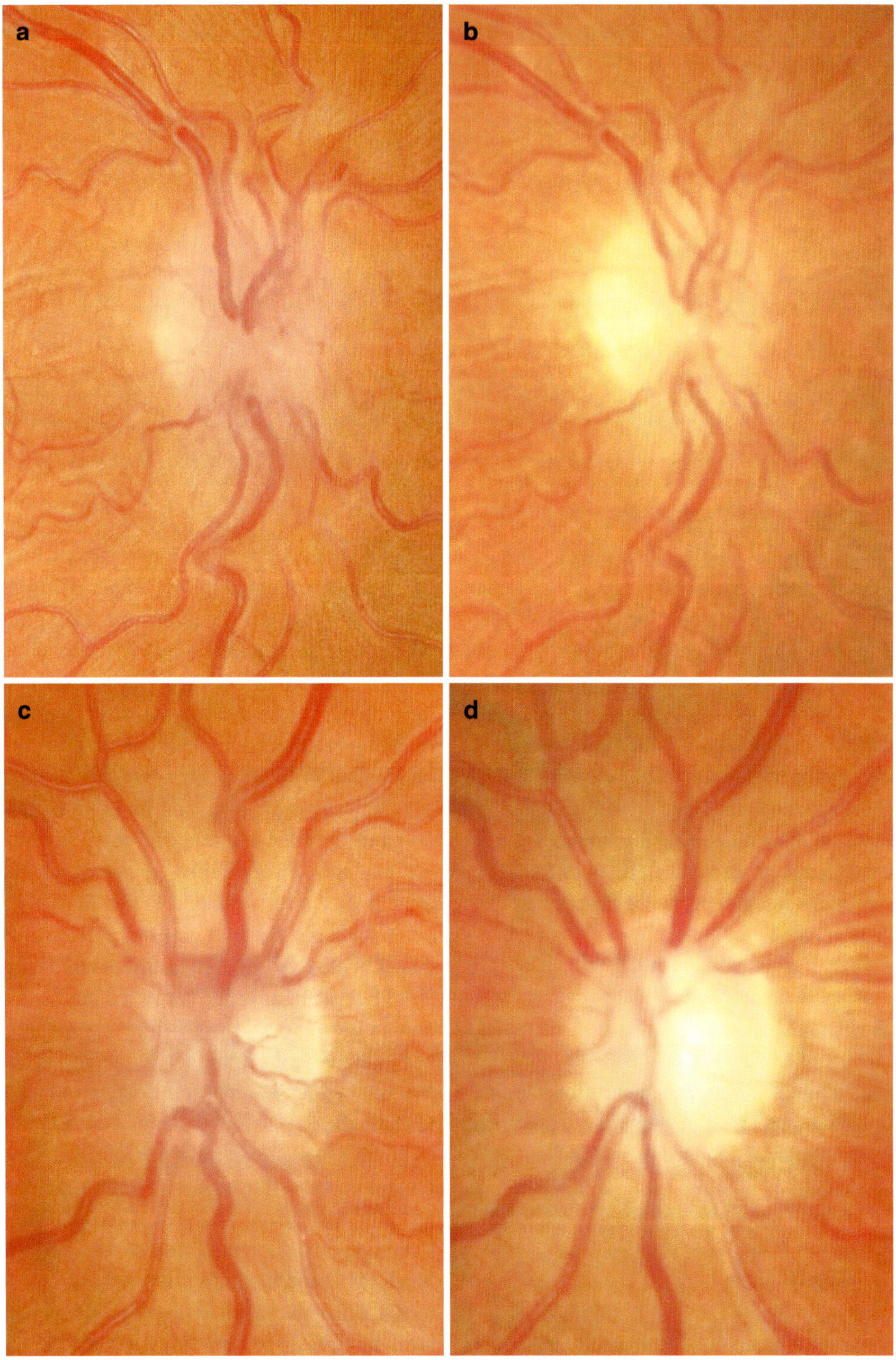

Fig. 60.4 Fundus photographs (1 year after lumbo-peritoneal shunt surgery). Panel a: Before lumbo-peritoneal shunt surgery, the optic disc was swollen, and retinal veins were tortuous in the right eye. Panel b: After lumbo-peritoneal surgery, the retinal vein tortuosity was obviously relieved, and the optic disc edema was reduced, and the disc became pale in the right eye. Panel c: Before lumbo-peritoneal shunt surgery, the optic disc was swollen, and retinal veins were tortuous in the left eye. Panel d: After lumbo-peritoneal surgery, the retinal venous tortuosity was notably relieved, while optic disc rim thinning and retinal nerve fiber layer defects that appeared in the superior and inferior quadrants were found in the left eye

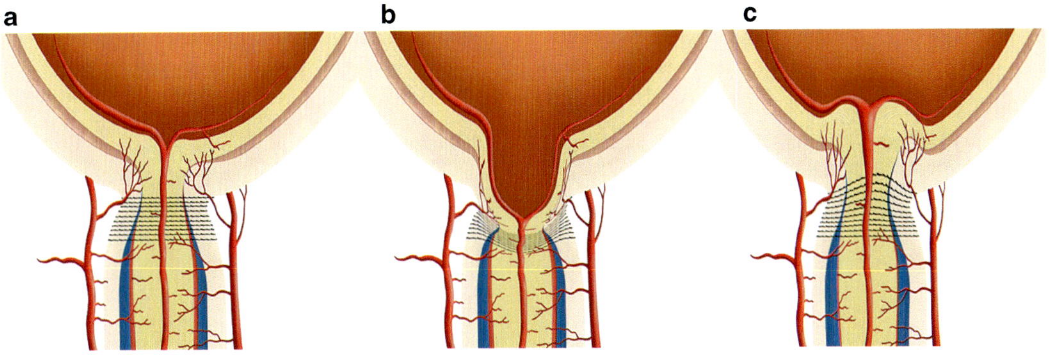

Fig. 60.5 Schematic diagrams to demonstrate the ocular-cranial pressure gradient-related damage. Panel a: Normal ocular-cranial pressure gradient. Panel b: IOP is higher than ICP, and the ocular-cranial pressure gradient increases anterogradely, causing posterior displacement of the lamina cribrosa. Panel c: ICP is higher than IOP, and the ocular-cranial pressure gradient increases retrogradely, causing anterior displacement of the lamina cribrosa and optic disc swelling

nerve (Fig. 60.5) [4–6]. Therefore, when we encounter patients with intraocular hypertension without optic disc damage, we should examine whether they also have intracranial hypertension. On the contrary, when we encounter patients with normal IOP but glaucomatous optic disc damage, we should determine whether they have intracranial hypotension. Specifically, intracranial hypotension should be ruled out for patients with normal tension glaucoma. Patients with normal tension glaucoma and people with relatively low ICP often share similar population characteristics, such as an especially slim, weak, and tall body, so careful examination is warranted.

For patients with intracranial hypertension syndrome, their IOPs should also be considered. The continuous reduction of ICP may increase the ocular-cranial pressure gradient, thus leading to glaucomatous optic nerve damage.

In this case, the confusion originated from the counterintuitive visual field changes in both eyes. Specifically, the eye with a higher intraocular pressure showed less visual field loss instead. The translaminar pressure gradient, also known as the ocular-cranial pressure gradient, progressed throughout the evolution and prognosis of the disease, prompting us to extend our effort from the pre-laminar to the post-laminar area and to similarly extend our focus from glaucoma to the cranium to consider a whole integrated disease, thus helping us to understand glaucoma from the perspective of holistic integrative medicine [8].

In the clinical settings, this situation is somehow similar to that of patients suffering from "intraocular hypertension" with increased intracranial pressure, which results in an unchanged ocular-cranial pressure gradient across the lamina cribrosa, thus alleviating the potential optic nerve damage caused by high intraocular pressure. Of course, this is just one possible explanation.

References

1. Ren R, Jonas JB, Tian G, et al. Cerebrospinal fluid pressure in glaucoma: a prospective study. Ophthalmology. 2010;117:259–66.
2. Ren R, Wang N, Zhang X, et al. Trans-lamina cribrosa pressure difference correlated with neuroretinal rim area in glaucoma. Graefes Arch Clin Exp Ophthalmol. 2011;249(7):1057–63.
3. Wang N, Xie X, Yang D, et al. Orbital cerebrospinal fluid space in glaucoma: the Beijing intracranial and intraocular pressure (iCOP) study. Ophthalmology. 2012;119(10):2065–73.
4. Wang N, Yang DY, Jonas JB. Low cerebrospinal fluid pressure in the pathogenesis of primary open-angle glaucoma: epiphenomenon or causal relationship? The Beijing Intracranial and Intraocular Pressure (iCOP) Study. J Glaucoma. 2013;22(7):S11–2.
5. Jonas JB, Yang D, Wang N. Intracranial pressure and glaucoma. J Glaucoma. 2013;22(5 Suppl):S13–4.

6. Zhang Z, Wang X, Jonas JB, et al. Valsalva manoeuver, intraocular pressure, cerebrospinal fluid pressure, optic disc topography: Beijing intracranial and intraocular pressure study. Acta Ophthalmol. 2014;92(6):e475–80.
7. Jonas JB, Wang NL, Yang DY, et al. Facts and myths of cerebrospinal fluid pressure for the physiology of the eye. Prog Retin Eye Res. 2015;46:67–83.
8. Wang N. Holistic integrative ophthalmology. Beijing: People's Medical Publishing House; 2014.
9. Yang D, Fu J, Hou R, et al. Optic neuropathy induced by experimentally reduced cerebrospinal fluid pressure in monkeys. Invest Ophthalmol Vis Sci. 2014;55(5):3067–73.

"Push Me, Pull You"

61

Xiaobin Xie and Ningli Wang

In the case described in the previous section, we analyzed the relationship between the ocular-cranial pressure gradient and morphological changes in the optic disc. We noted that under a dynamic balance between high intraocular and high intracranial pressure, glaucomatous cupping of the optic disc may be postponed or not occur. However, when the eye is instead subject to low intraocular pressure and high intracranial pressure, what changes does this bring to the optic disc?

61.1 Case

61.1.1 Case Presentation

An 80-year-old female patient presented with progressively decreased vision in her left eye that had been affecting her for the entire past year. She underwent trabeculectomy 1 year ago for primary open-angle glaucoma (POAG), and optic disc edema in her left eye was found by chance after operation. Over the past year, she had chronically and progressively decreased vision in her left eye, accompanied by a progressive narrowing of the visual field. By tracing her family history, we found that her father had glaucoma. In her past medical history, she had undergone binocular cataract phacoemulsification combined with intraocular lens implantation.

On ophthalmological examination, UCVA was observed to be 20/20 OD and 20/100 OS. Vision correction was ineffective in her left eye. Intraocular pressure was measured as 16 mmHg OD and 5 mmHg OS. An elevated and well-formed filtering bleb was found in both eyes. The cornea was transparent, and the anterior chamber was clear with a normal depth. The iridotomy was unobstructed. The pupillary light reflex was positive. The intraocular lenses were in place. Fundus examination showed that, in the right eye, the cup-to-disc (C/D) ratio was 0.95, and the optic disc had a clear boundary, with a notch at its inferior margin; in the left eye, the optic disc was remarkably swollen and pale in color, with disappearance of the retinal nerve fiber layer reflections (Fig. 61.1).

Threshold perimetry demonstrated a superior arcuate scotoma in the right eye and an annular visual field defect in the left eye (Fig. 61.2).

X. Xie
Eye Hospital of China Academy of Chinese Medical Sciences, Beijing, China

N. Wang (✉)
Department of Ophthalmology, Beijing Tongren Hospital, Capital Medical University, Beijing, China

N. Wang et al. (eds.), *Optic Disorders and Visual Field*, Advances in Visual Science and Eye Diseases 2, https://doi.org/10.1007/978-981-13-2502-1_61

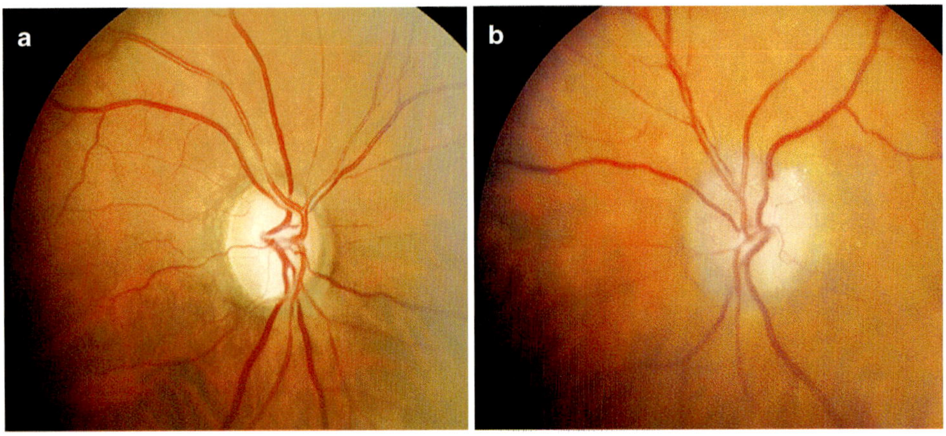

Fig. 61.1 Fundus photographs. Panel a: In the right eye, the cup-to-disc ratio was 0.95, and the optic disc had a clear boundary with a notch at its inferior margin. Panel b: In the left eye, the optic disc was remarkably swollen and pale in color with disappearance of the retinal nerve fiber layer reflections

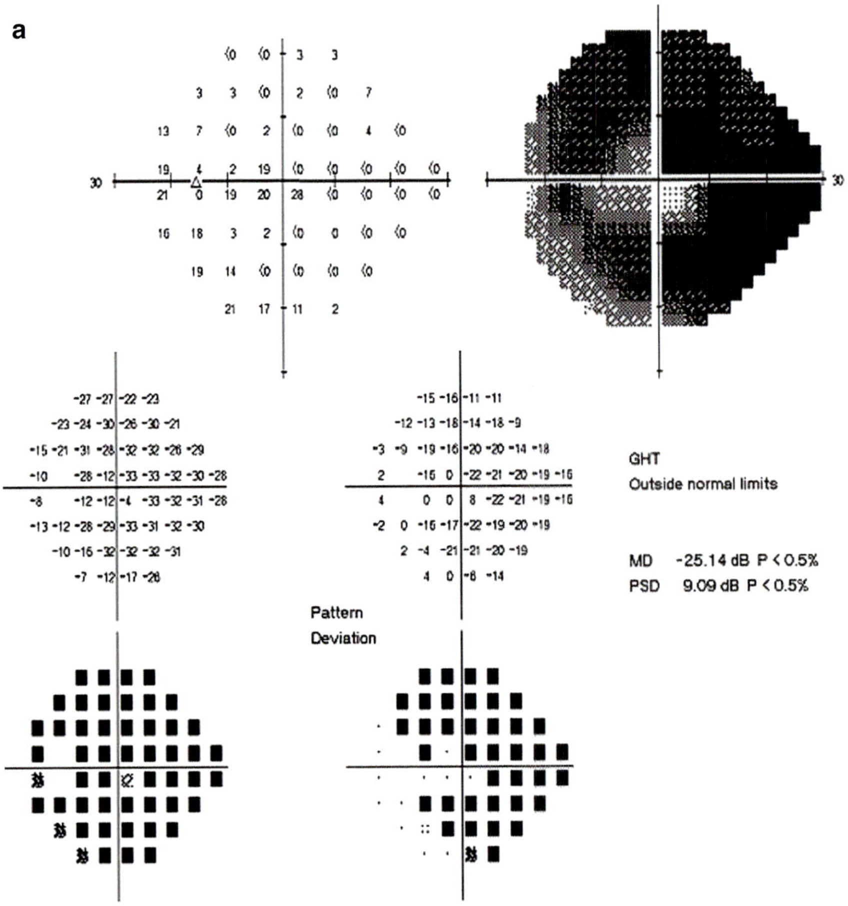

Fig. 61.2 Humphrey visual field analysis printouts. Panel a: The 24-2 test showed an annular visual field defect in the left eye. Panel b: A superior arcuate scotoma in the right eye

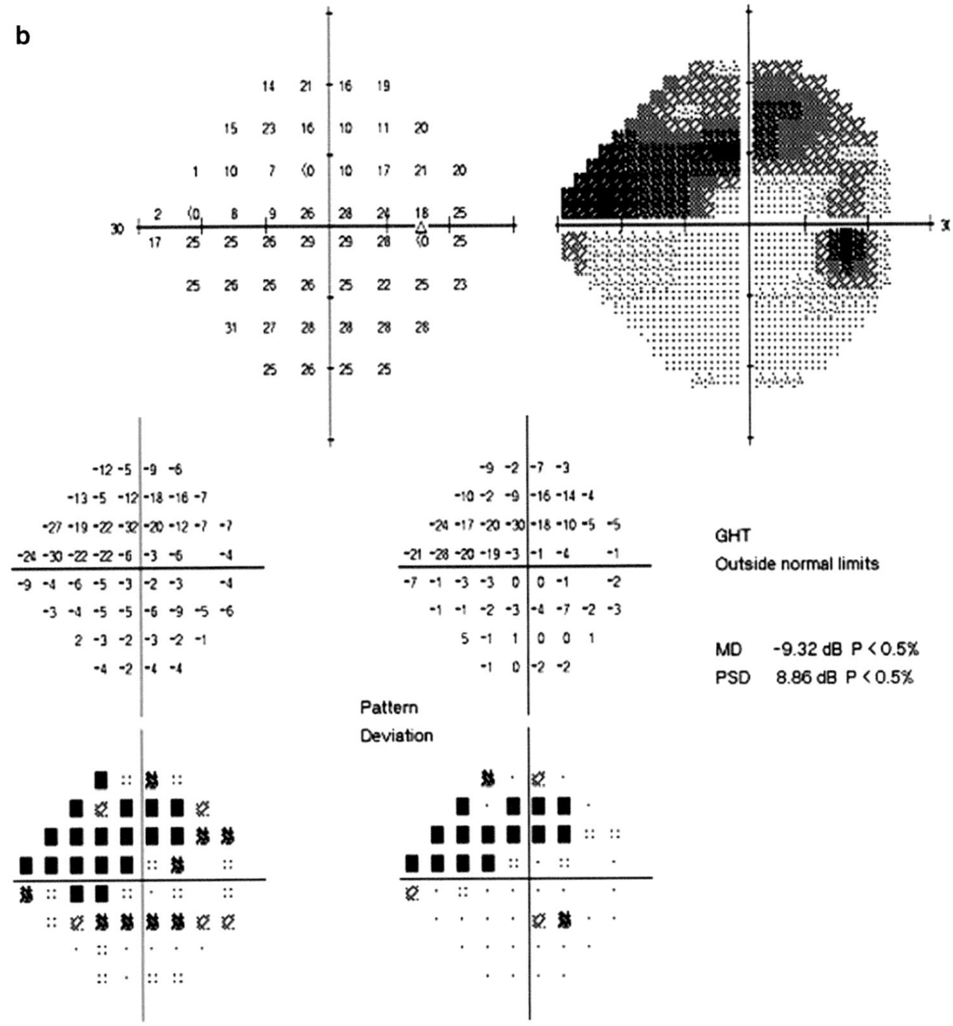

Fig. 61.2 (continued)

61.1.2 Case Analysis

This elderly female patient was clearly diagnosed with glaucoma in both eyes. In the right eye, fundus examination displayed typical glaucomatous optic disc damage, and visual field examination showed a corresponding arcuate scotoma. In the left eye, fundus examination revealed the optic disc was swollen and pale in color, and visual field examination indicated a tubular visual field. As optic disc edema is not characteristic of glaucoma, the possibility of other coexisting diseases besides glaucoma in her left eye should be taken into consideration, including inflammation and ischemia arising from the intracranial lesions or the optic nerve itself. The patient was an elderly woman with no previous systemic inflammatory and immune diseases. No specific symptoms were found associated with optic neuropathy, such as pain upon eye movement or abnormalities in pupillary light reflex. While the ophthalmology department continued excluding other etiologies for the disease, the patient was directed to take further tests to facilitate a differential diagnosis, including

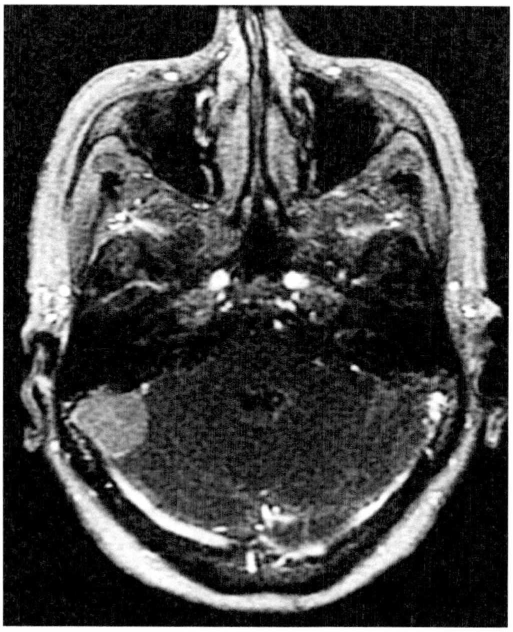

Fig. 61.3 Cranial MRI. A 2.2 cm × 2.0 cm mass in the right cerebellopontine angle

an intracranial magnetic resonance imaging (MRI) examination, cerebrospinal fluid pressure measurement, and blood and cerebrospinal fluid tests.

Cranial MRI revealed that there was a 2.2 cm × 2.0 cm mass in the right cerebellopontine angle, which was highly suspected to be as meningioma (Fig. 61.3).

Lumbar puncture showed an opening pressure of 240 mmH_2O (17.6 mmHg), notably higher than the normal pressure values for this test (which range from 6 to 13 mmHg). The routine cerebrospinal fluid test was unremarkable.

The results of the hematological examination showed that erythrocyte sedimentation rate (ESR) was 34 mm/h; serum protein electrophoresis (SPEP), antinuclear antibody (ANA), rapid plasma reagin (RPR), and lysozyme were unremarkable, and angiotensin-converting enzyme (ACE) was slightly increased.

61.1.3 Final Diagnosis

The final diagnosis was POAG in both eyes, right meningioma, intracranial hypertension, and optic disc edema in the left eye.

61.2 Discussion

The lamina cribrosa region of the optic nerve head is considered as the primary site of pressure-induced optic retinopathy in glaucomatous optic disc cupping [1]. From an anatomical perspective, the lamina cribrosa is the pressure barrier between the intraocular space and the retrolaminar space, which is filled with the cerebrospinal fluid. Within the eye, the intraocular pressure generates a posteriorly directed force on the prelaminar tissue, whereas within the retrolaminar subarachnoid space, the lamina cribrosa bears the pressure of the cerebrospinal fluid, which generates an anterior force on the lamina cribrosa. The difference between the intraocular pressure anteriorly and the cerebrospinal fluid pressure posteriorly forms an "ocular-cranial pressure difference" [2] . With an elevation of intraocular pressure, the ocular-cranial pressure difference increases, potentially leading to posterior bowing of the lamina cribrosa, which can ultimately result in optic nerve damage [3–6]. However, if either the intracranial pressure increased or the intraocular pressure decreased, the ocular-cranial pressure gradient would amplify in the negative direction, resulting in anterior optic disc cupping and optic disc edema [7–9].

After bilateral filtration surgery, the patient developed unilateral optic disc edema in the left eye. Optic disc swelling was principally caused by increased intracranial pressure induced by intracranial tumors. However, with the same intracranial pressure acting on both eyes, why was optic disc edema not detected in the right eye? Perhaps the different ocular-cranial pressure gradient in the two eyes could explain. Her intraocular pressure was 16 mmHg OD and 5 mmHg OS, while the cerebrospinal fluid pressure was 17.6 mmHg. Thus, the ocular-cranial pressure difference was −1.6 mmHg OD and −12.6 mmHg OS, respectively. Clearly, the left optic nerve head bore a greater negative ocular-cranial pressure difference, which then resulted in resulting in optic disc swelling.

From a visual field point of view, these following conditions should be taken into account. Assuming that the preoperative glaucomatous optic nerve damages in both eyes of this patient were nearly equal, that is to say the C/D ratio in both eyes was approximately 0.95, then the visual field loss in the left eye should be at least similar to, if not heavier than, that in the right eye, since there was a remarkably lower postoperative intraocular pressure in the left eye. In fact, the visual field defect in the left eye was significantly worse. It is reasonable for us to speculate then that, in addition to glaucoma, the visual impairment in the left eye may be related to further optic nerve damage rising from intracranial hypertension, worsening her condition. For this reason, in this type of patient, it is significantly beneficial to reduce intracranial pressure.

In fact, this case can be considered to be an "ocular-cranial pressure difference-related diseases" [2]. Results from serial, prospective, observational studies conducted by Beijing Intracranial and Intraocular Pressure Study Group in patients with high-pressure glaucoma, normal-pressure glaucoma, and ocular hypertension in Beijing Tongren Hospital support the notion of a potential role of elevated ocular-cranial pressure gradient (i.e., the so-called translaminar pressure gradient) in the pathogenesis of POAG [3]. A lower cerebrospinal fluid pressure could result in an increased ocular-cranial pressure gradient and be associated with glaucomatous optic neuropathy in normal-pressure glaucoma. Conversely, a higher cerebrospinal fluid pressure in ocular hypertensive subjects could counterbalance against an increased intraocular pressure such that the ocular-cranial pressure gradient would be in the normal range, which might delay or prevent the occurrence of glaucomatous optic nerve damage [7–9].

References

1. Meiyu L. Storz ophthalmology manual. Beijing: People's Medical Publishing House; 2000.
2. Ningli W. Holistic integrative ophthalmology. Beijing: People's Medical Publishing House; 2014.
3. Ren R, Wang N, Zhang X, et al. Trans-lamina cribrosa pressure difference correlated with neuroretinal rim area in glaucoma. Graefes Arch Clin Exp Ophthalmol. 2011;249(7):1057–63.
4. Yang D, Fu J, Hou R, et al. Optic neuropathy induced by experimentally reduced cerebrospinal fluid pressure in monkeys. Invest Ophthalmol Vis Sci. 2014;55(5):3067–73.
5. Jonas JB, Wang NL, Yang DY, et al. Facts and myths of cerebrospinal fluid pressure for the physiology of the eye. Prog Retin Eye Res. 2015;46:67–83.
6. Wang N, Xie X, Yang D, et al. Orbital cerebrospinal fluid space in glaucoma: The Beijing intracranial and intraocular pressure (iCOP) study. Ophthalmology. 2012;119(10):2065–73.
7. Ren R, Zhang X, Wang N, et al. Cerebrospinal fluid pressure in ocular hypertension. Acta Ophthalmol. 2015;89(2):e142–8.
8. Jonas JB, Wang N, Wang YX, et al. Ocular hypertension: general characteristics and estimated cerebrospinal fluid pressure. The Beijing Eye Study 2011. Plos One. 2014;9(7):e100533.
9. Xie X, Chen W, Li Z, et al. Noninvasive evaluation of cerebrospinal fluid pressure in ocular hypertension: a preliminary study. Acta Ophthalmol. 2018;96(5):e570–6.

62 A Case Report: Intracranial Hypertension-Caused Visual Dysfunction

Xiaobin Xie and Ningli Wang

What diagnosis and treatment methods can ophthalmologists provide to support neurologists in the treatment of a patient with highly suspected, but unconfirmed through physical examination, elevated intracranial pressure-induced severe optic neuropathy? What is the patient's clinical outcome in these circumstances?

62.1 Case

62.1.1 Case Presentation

A 25-year-old female patient complained of progressively decreased vision in both eyes for 1 month but which had aggravated over the past 2 weeks. One month ago, she had developed blurred vision in both of her eyes, accompanied by a mild headache. No other discomforts, such as dizziness, nausea, or vomiting, were reported. Her visual acuity was 20/16 OD and 20/25 OS on ocular examination in a local hospital. Intracranial hypertension syndrome was highly suspected according to the local neurologist. However, considering her physical condition which included "obesity that rendered the length of a lumbar puncture needle insufficient," measurement of intracranial pressure was impossible by routine lumbar puncture. So, a definitive diagnosis remained elusive. Two weeks ago, her visual acuity worsened to 20/100 OD and 20/200 OS. Consequently, she was transferred to Beijing Tongren Hospital for further treatment and diagnosis. No medical history of trauma, other ocular diseases, systemic diseases, or familial diseases was found.

On physical examination, her height was 172 cm and her weight was 124 kg. Her blood pressure was measured as 110/70 mmHg. Her waist circumference and hip circumference were 120 and 128 cm, respectively. She had concentric obesity with adequate muscle strength. No abnormalities were found on neurological examination.

On ophthalmological examination, the UCVA was hand motion in both eyes, which showed no improvement with correction. Intraocular pressure was measured as 16 mmHg OD and 18 mmHg OS by an applanation tonometer. No abnormality was found in the anterior segment of both eyes. Fundus examination indicated elevation and edema of the optic discs, tortuous and dilated retinal veins, and presence of the foveal reflex in both eyes (Fig. 62.1).

Total blindness in both eyes was demonstrated by perimetry (Fig. 62.2).

X. Xie
Eye Hospital of China Academy of Chinese Medical Sciences, Beijing, China

N. Wang (✉)
Department of Ophthalmology, Beijing Tongren Hospital, Capital Medical University, Beijing, China

N. Wang et al. (eds.), *Optic Disorders and Visual Field*, Advances in Visual Science and Eye Diseases 2, https://doi.org/10.1007/978-981-13-2502-1_62

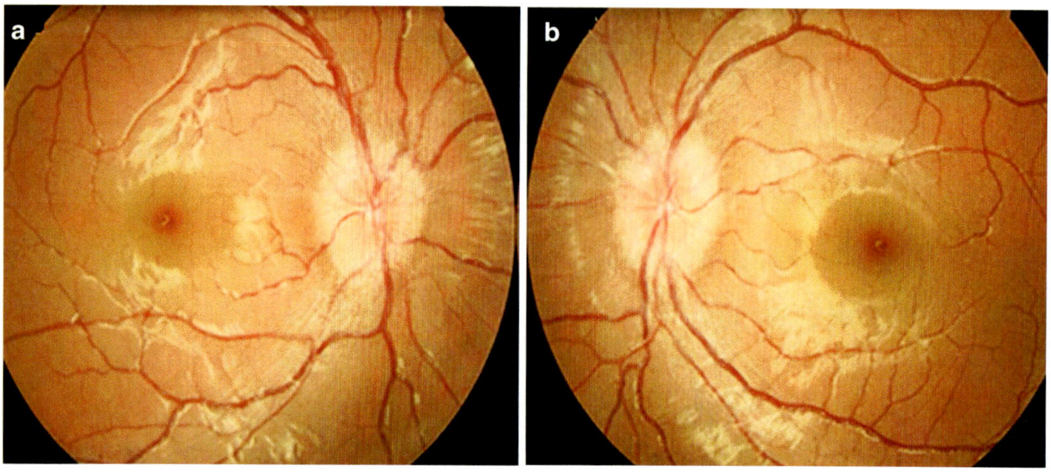

Fig. 62.1 Fundus photographs. Elevation and edema of the optic disc with tortuous and dilated retinal veins in both eyes. Panel a: Right eye. Panel b: Left eye

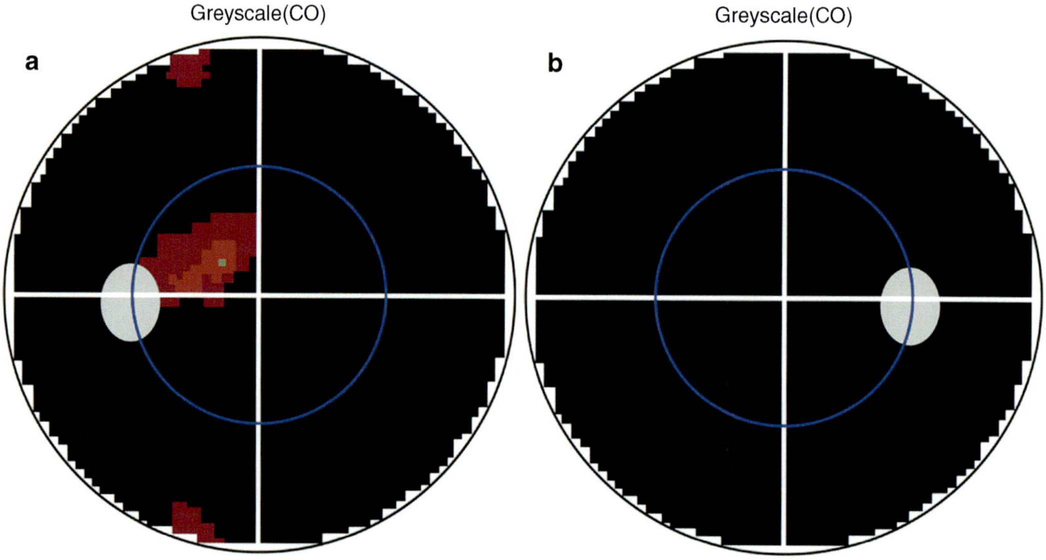

Fig. 62.2 The Octopus grayscale images of visual field. Total blindness in both eyes. Panel a: Left eye. Panel b: Right eye

62.1.2 Case Analysis

This patient was a young obese woman with progressive vision loss and optic disc edema in both eyes. An initial diagnosis of bilateral optic disc swelling secondary to intracranial hypertension was made, but which needed to be differentiated from bilateral optic papillitis. Brain MRI and magnetic resonance venography (MRV) ruled out the possibility of intracranial hypertension secondary to brain arteriovenous malformations and mass lesions of the brain. Was the condition idiopathic intracranial hypertension? Further lumbar puncture was warranted to measure the pressure and composition of the cerebrospinal fluid.

However, spinal needle insertion failed, due in part to the contributions of obesity and hypertrophy of the subcutaneous fat layer. In the process of making a lumbar puncture, it was determined that the lumbar puncture needle was not long enough to be inserted into her lumbar cistern, and it was thus unable to access the cerebrospinal fluid, both in the neurology department at the previous hospital and the neurosurgery department at Beijing Tongren Hospital.

Although her clinical manifestations closely resembled idiopathic intracranial hypertension, given that there was no knowledge of the actual value of her intracranial pressure by routine diagnostic lumbar puncture, the patient and her family developed a suspicious attitude toward the neurosurgeons' recommendations of medications for the treatment of raised intracranial pressure and cerebrospinal fluid shunt surgery. At the same time, the neurosurgeons risked iatrogenic injury if they imprudently performed surgery on this patient. Since the intracranial pressure could not be measured by lumbar puncture, it was very difficult for neurologists to perform further diagnosis and treatment. Meanwhile, the patient's visual acuity continued to deteriorate.

What can ophthalmologists do confronting such a situation?

One possibility is that ophthalmologists could directly measure the cerebrospinal fluid pressure of retrobulbar subarachnoid space around the optic nerve using a piercing needle. However, the process is as invasive and, in fact, even more aggressive than a lumbar puncture. Thus, it is not widely applied in clinical practice.

In an observational study conducted by the Beijing Intracranial and Intraocular Pressure (iCOP) Study Group [1], Xie and colleagues showed that the width of the cerebrospinal fluid space width surrounding the optic nerve, measured using 3.0 T MRI, correlated well with lumbar cerebrospinal fluid pressure in 72 patients with various neurological conditions (intracranial hypotension, meningitis, multiple sclerosis, and so forth). A simple and rapid T2-weighted fat-suppressed sequence was used to noninvasively measure the width of the cerebrospinal fluid space surrounding the optic nerve (Fig. 62.3). Using a stepwise multivariate linear regression analysis, Xie and colleagues have developed a relatively simple formula to predict intracranial pressure noninvasively, based on three independent variables: the cerebrospinal fluid width surrounding the optic nerve, body mass index, and blood pressure to predict intracranial pressure noninvasively.

$$\text{non-invasive ICP} = 16.95 \times \text{SASW9} + 0.39 \times \text{BMI} + 0.14\text{MAP} - 20.90[1]$$

Noninvasive ICP refers to noninvasive calculation of intracranial pressure, SASW9 refers to orbital subarachnoid space width at 9 mm behind the globe, BMI refers to body mass index, and MAP refers to the mean arterial pressure.

In this patient's case, could intracranial pressure be noninvasively estimated by using MRI-based measurements of the width of the orbital subarachnoid space?

After measuring the width of the orbital subarachnoid space, we substituted the measured value into the formula and calculated the intracranial pressure as 266 mm H_2O (19.6 mmHg), which is above the normal range for intracranial pressure. Reference values for the MRI-based measurement of the width of the subarachnoid space, which were used to assess the intracranial pressure, are shown in Table 62.1 (The patient's measured values are expressed in bold).

62.1.3 Final Diagnosis

The final diagnosis was idiopathic intracranial hypertension and optic disc edema in both eyes.

After the diagnosis of idiopathic intracranial hypertension was established, the patient and her family consented to undergo the cerebrospinal fluid lumbo-peritoneal shunt surgery. During the surgery, the cerebrospinal fluid pressure was measured to be 280 mm H_2O (20.6 mmHg), only 1 mmHg higher than the MRI-based noninvasive intracranial pressure assessment.

Three days after the cerebrospinal fluid lumbo-peritoneal shunt surgery, her visual acuity in both eyes recovered to finger counting at 1 m. We estimated cerebrospinal fluid pressure noninvasively by using MRI once more, obtaining a pressure of 191.1 mm H_2O (14.5 mmHg), which was coinciding with the set point of the cerebrospinal fluid shunt valve.

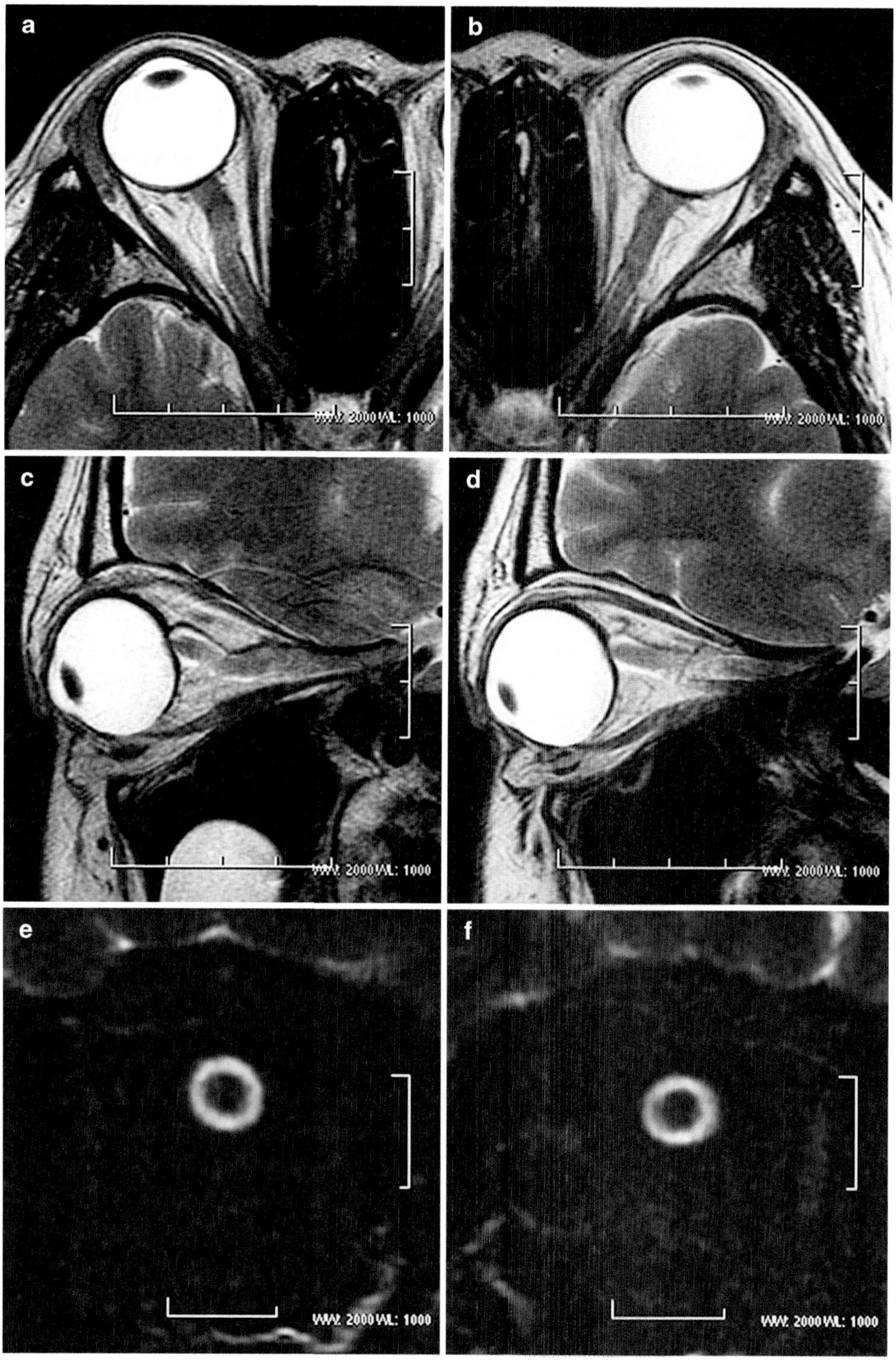

Fig. 62.3 3.0 T MRI scan of the retrobulbar optic nerve/sheath complex. Panel a: Transversal section in the right eye. Panel b: Transversal section in the left eye. Panel c: Oblique sagittal section in the right eye. Panel d: Oblique sagittal section in the left eye. Panel e: Oblique MRI of the retrobulbar optic nerve sheath complex in the right eye. Panel f: Oblique MRI of the retrobulbar optic nerve sheath complex in the left eye

Table 62.1 Reference values for the MRI-based measurement of the orbital subarachnoid space width that were used to assess the intracranial pressure

	Very High	High	Moderately Increased	Medium	Moderately Decreased	Low	Very Low
OSASW 3 mm	>1.85	1.85–1.46	**1.46–1.07**	1.07–0.83	0.83–0.77	0.77–0.51	<0.51
OSASW 9 mm	>1.38	**1.38–0.92**	0.92–0.76	0.76–0.64	0.64–0.62	0.62–0.46	<0.46
OSASW 15 mm	>1.23	1.23–0.79	0.79–0.73	**0.73–0.63**	0.63–0.47	0.47–0.39	<0.39
ICP mm H_2O	>355	**355–225**	225–195	195–160	160–140	140–100	<100
ICP mmHg	>26.1	**26.1–16.5**	16.5–14.3	14.3–11.8	11.8–10.3	10.3–7.4	<7.4

OSASW orbital subarachnoid space width, *ICP* intracranial pressure

Following 3 months of a gradual decrease in the set pressure of the cerebrospinal fluid shunt valve, her visual acuity was restored to 20/20, and her visual field was significantly improved.

62.2 Discussion

In general, idiopathic intracranial hypertension is rarely associated with significant visual impairment [2]. In this case, however, the patient had optic disc edema and significant visual impairment concurrently. Her visual acuity in both eyes dropped acutely. For this young and obese female patient, the presumed and unsurprising cause of bilateral optic disc edema was intracranial hypertension. However, due to her obesity, she failed to undergo a lumbar puncture for the measurement of intracranial pressure. Under these conditions, the ophthalmologists used their anatomical and biomechanical analysis of the optic nerve and cerebrospinal fluid, as well as findings from previous studies, to help neurosurgeons obtain reliable clinical evidence, accurately estimate the patient's intracranial pressure, and ultimately cure the patient.

Conventionally, ophthalmologists measure the cerebrospinal fluid pressure by puncturing the retrobulbar orbital subarachnoid space. However, like lumbar puncture, this method has its own limitations and disadvantages as it is an invasive (but even more challenging) examination. Therefore, it should not be extensively employed in clinical practice. Through cooperating with radiologists and neurologists, the authors developed a noninvasive method, based on MRI-assisted orbital subarachnoid space width measurements with adjustment for body mass index and mean arterial blood pressure, to indirectly estimate cerebrospinal fluid pressure in the orbital subarachnoid space. The estimated cerebrospinal fluid pressure was approximately equal to the pressure value acquired by lumbar puncture, with no significant difference found between the pressure values obtained by each method [1]. This new method shows good reproducibility and can be used not only for estimating cerebrospinal fluid pressure but also for evaluating the translaminar pressure difference in various ocular diseases.

This case, along with the other two cases described in the previous two sections, warrant serious consideration. For a long time, the optic neuropathy caused by abnormal intraocular pressure and the optic neuropathy caused by abnormal intracranial pressure have been diagnosed and treated, respectively, in two separate areas, the ophthalmology and the neurology, respectively [2, 4], between which there is a substantial gap. Each subspecialist focuses on only the diagnosis and treatment of diseases in the scope of their expertise, often neglecting interdisciplinary integration and collaboration. Thus, it is difficult for each to consider the unfamiliar perspectives of a different discipline in the diagnosis and treatment of disease. Neglecting the role of the ocular-cranial pressure gradient in optic neuropathy is a clear example of the limitations of a narrower focus, especially for patients with problems involving both intraocular and intracranial pressure. Their diseases cannot be completely resolved by addressing only a single clinical problem from a single disciplinary perspective. This is one reason why difficulties in the diagnosis and treatment of ocular-cranial pressure gradient-related diseases still persist widely [3].

In summary, a much more sensible choice to conquer ocular-cranial pressure gradient-related diseases could be adopting the concept of integrative medicine in the diagnosis, management, and further investigation of such diseases. We have sufficient reason to believe that this concept can also bring about a deeper understanding, or even a complete re-interpretation, of the relationship between ocular disease and other systemic diseases [4].

In this light, we consider integrative medicine and integrative ophthalmology are considered to be powerful means for improving both our clinical proficiency and the level of our scientific research level [4].

References

1. Xie X, Zhang X, Fu J, et al. Beijing iCOP Study Group. Noninvasive intracranial pressure estimation by orbital subarachnoid space measurement: the Beijing Intracranial and Intraocular Pressure (iCOP) study. Crit Care. 2013;17(4):R162.
2. Savino PJ, Danesh-Meyer HV. Neuro-ophthalmology: color atlas and synopsis of clinical ophthalmology—Wills Eye Institute Translated by Dai Yi, Jin Xiaohong, Kong Xiangmei et al. Shanghai: Shanghai Scientific and Technical Publisher; 2005.
3. Wang NL, Yang D, Jonas JB. Low cerebrospinal fluid pressure in the pathogenesis of primary open-angle glaucoma: epiphenomenon or causal relationship? The Beijing Intracranial and Intraocular Pressure (iCOP) Study. J Glaucoma. 2013;22(5 Suppl):S11–2.
4. Wang N. Holistic integrative ophthalmology. Beijing: People's Medical Publishing House; 2014.